# Drug
# Resistance
# in
# Oncology

# BASIC AND CLINICAL ONCOLOGY

*Editor*

**Bruce D. Cheson, M.D.**

*National Cancer Institute*
*National Institutes of Health*
*Bethesda, Maryland*

**ADDITIONAL VOLUMES IN PREPARATION**

# Drug Resistance in Oncology

### edited by

## Samuel D. Bernal
*UCLA San Fernando Valley Program*
*Sepulveda Veterans Administration Medical Center*
*Sepulveda, California*

MARCEL DEKKER, INC.    NEW YORK · BASEL · HONG KONG

**Library of Congress Cataloging-in-Publication Data**

Drug resistance in oncology / edited by Samuel D. Bernal.
    p.  cm. — (Basic and clinical oncology ; 13)
    Includes bibliographical references and index.
    ISBN 0-8247-9295-5 (hardcover : alk. paper)
    1. Drug resistance in cancer cells. I. Bernal, Samuel D. II. Series.
    [DNLM: 1. Antineoplastic Agents—therapeutic use. 2. Drug Resistance, Neoplasm.
3. Neoplasms—drug therapy. W1 BA813W v.13 1997 / QZ 267 D79382 1997]
RC271.C5D77753  1997
616.99'4061—dc21
for Library of Congress

                                             97-22375
                                              CIP

The publisher offers discounts on this book when ordered in bulk quantities. For more information, write to Special Sales/Professional Marketing at the address below.

This book is printed on acid-free paper.

MARCEL DEKKER, INC.
270 Madison Avenue, New York, New York 10016
*http://www.dekker.com*

Current printing (last digit):
10  9  8  7  6  5  4  3  2  1

**PRINTED IN THE UNITED STATES OF AMERICA**

*To my mother, Loreto D. Bernal, and in memory of my father, Teofilo Z. Bernal. To my children, Elise, Ariel, and Laure.*

*In appreciation of Fred Elizalde and family for their encouragement and support of cancer research.*

*In memory of Manuel Soriano, who struggled with multiple cancers that developed drug resistance. Special thanks to Gerry and Marite de Luzuriaga for their encouragement of cancer research.*

# Series Introduction

The current volume, *Drug Resistance in Oncology*, is the tenth in the Basic and Clinical Oncology series. Many of the advances in oncology have resulted from close interaction between the basic scientist and the clinical researcher. The current volume illustrates the success of this relationship as demonstrated by new insights into clinical drug resistance and means of circumventing this potential obstacle to effective cancer treatment.

As editor of the series, my goal is to recruit volume editors who not only have established reputations based on their outstanding contributions to oncology, but who also have an appreciation for the dynamic interface between the laboratory and the clinic. To date, the series has consisted of monographs on topics that are of a high level of current interest. *Drug Resistance in Oncology* certainly fits into this category and is a most important addition to the series.

Volumes in progress focus on chronic myelogenous leukemia, an updated volume on chronic lymphocytic leukemia, and the current use of paclitaxel. I anticipate that these books will provide a valuable contribution to the oncology literature.

*Bruce D. Cheson*

# Preface

This book brings together work by laboratory scientists and clinicians on mechanisms of resistance of specific cancers to various chemotherapeutic drugs. The idea for this book came after the publication of *Lung Cancer Differentiation*, edited by S. Bernal and P. Hesketh (Marcel Dekker, Inc., 1992). In that volume, several chapters were devoted to the relationship between the differentiation phenotypes and response to chemotherapy. This relationship is explored further in this volume, and emphasizes the mechanisms of drug resistance in different histological types of cancer. In addition, strategies for overcoming drug resistance in various tumor types are presented.

Chapters 1–3 address drug resistance in small cell and non–small cell lung cancer. Chapter 4 reviews selective targeting of chemotherapeutic drugs to tumors using liposomes, especially those incorporating differentiation/adhesion proteins. Chapters 5–7 discuss breast cancer resistance to hormone and cytotoxic agents. Strategies for overcoming drug resistance are described for ovarian cancer (Chap. 8) and colon cancer (Chap. 9). The clinical relevance of P-glycoprotein in hematological malignancies and the prediction of drug resistance in acute leukemia are presented in Chapters 10 and 11.

Strategies for overcoming resistance are discussed for various drugs, including estramustine, a drug used in the treatment of prostate cancer (Chap. 12), anthracyclines (Chap. 13), and platinum compounds (Chap. 14). The efficacy of radiation therapy for treatment of chemotherapy-resistant tumors is described in Chapter 15. Finally, the use of preclinical in vivo models for developing clinically relevant approaches for overcoming drug resistance is presented in Chapter 16.

This book offers a comprehensive view of drug resistance by bringing together the work of clinical and basic laboratory investigators who are leading authorities in their fields. Clinical insights into the problem of drug resistance will be useful not only for physicians involved in the management of specific cancers but also for scientists developing practical applications of basic laboratory investigations. An update on the cell and molecular biology of drug resistance will be useful for basic scientists and also for clinicians involved in research protocols for improving response rates to anticancer drugs.

I am grateful to Graham Garratt and the staff of Marcel Dekker, Inc., for their patience, support, and encouragement. I also wish to thank my secretary, Bonnie R. Hunnicutt, for her assistance in correspondence with the various authors and to my mother Loreto Bernal and my children Elise, Ariel, and Laure, for their understanding when I could not spend some vacation times with them.

*Samuel D. Bernal*

# Contents

# Contributors

**Philip J. Bergman, D.V.M.**  Department of Cell Biology, The University of Texas M.D. Anderson Cancer Center, Houston, Texas

**Samuel D. Bernal, M.D., Ph.D.**  UCLA San Fernando Valley Program, Sepulveda Veterans Administration Medical Center, Sepulveda, California

**Gloria Bernas, Ph.D.**  UCLA San Fernando Valley Program, Sepulveda Veterans Administration Medical Center, Sepulveda, California, and University of Santo Tomas, Manila, Philippines

**Bonne Biesma, M.D., Ph.D.**  Department of Pulmonology, Free University Hospital, Amsterdam, The Netherlands

**Daniel J. Booser, M.D., F.R.C.P.C.**  Department of Breast Medical Oncology, The University of Texas M.D. Anderson Cancer Center, Houston, Texas

**Daniel R. Ciocca, M.D., Ph.D.**  Laboratory of Reproduction and Lactation, Regional Center for Scientific and Technological Research (CRICYT), Mendoza, Argentina

**Susan P. C. Cole, Ph.D.**  Cancer Research Laboratories, Queen's University, Kingston, Ontario, Canada

**Michael W. DeGregorio, Pharm.D.**  Department of Internal Medicine, Division of Hematology/Oncology, University of California, Davis, California

**Romulo de Villa, M.D., Ph.D.**  UCLA San Fernando Valley Program, Sepulveda Veterans Administration Medical Center, Sepulveda, California, and Far Eastern University, Manila, Philippines

**E. G. E. de Vries, M.D., Ph.D.**  University Hospital Groningen, Groningen, The Netherlands

**Karen R. Gravitt, M.S.**  Department of Cell Biology, The University of Texas M.D. Anderson Cancer Center, Houston, Texas

**Krishna P. Gupta, Ph.D.**   Department of Cell Biology, The University of Texas M.D. Anderson Cancer Center, Houston, Texas

**Constantin G. Ioannides, Ph.D.**   Department of Cell Biology, The University of Texas M.D. Anderson Cancer Center, Houston, Texas

**Rolf Larsson, M.D., Ph.D.**   Department of Clinical Pharmacology, Uppsala University Hospital, Uppsala, Sweden

**Per E. Lønning, M.D., Ph.D.**   Department of Oncology, Haukeland University Hospital, Bergen, Norway

**Gerrit Los, Ph.D.**   University of California, San Diego, Cancer Center, La Jolla, California

**Patrick Miller, M.D.**   Department of Radiation Oncology, University of Arizona Health Sciences Center, Tucson, Arizona

**Shelagh E. L. Mirski, Ph.D.**   Cancer Research Laboratories, Queen's University, Kingston, Ontario, Canada

**Michael Nejad, B.S.**   Department of Molecular and Cellular Biology, University of Arizona Health Sciences Center, Tucson, Arizona

**Catherine A. O'Brian, Ph.D.**   Department of Cell Biology, The University of Texas M.D. Anderson Cancer Center, Houston, Texas

**Jeroen Oldenburg, M.D.**   Division of Experimental Therapy, The Netherlands Cancer Institute, Amsterdam, The Netherlands

**Petra C. Pasman, M.D.**   Department of Internal Medicine, University Hospital Maastricht, Maastricht, The Netherlands

**Pieter E. Postmus, M.D., Ph.D.**   Department of Pulmonology, Free University Hospital, Amsterdam, The Netherlands

**Harry C. Schouten, M.D., Ph.D.**   Department of Internal Medicine, University Hospital Maastricht, Maastricht, The Netherlands

**David S. Shimm, M.D.**   Department of Radiation Oncology, University of Arizona Health Sciences Center, Tucson, Arizona

**Egbert F. Smit, M.D., Ph.D.**   Department of Pulmonology, University Hospital Groningen, Groningen, The Netherlands

**Lin Soe, M.B., B.S., M.P.H.**   Department of Internal Medicine, Division of Hematology/Oncology, University of California, Davis, California

**Lisa A. Speicher, Ph.D.**   Department of Oncology, Wyeth-Ayerst Research, Philadelphia, Pennsylvania

**Beverly A. Teicher, Ph.D.**   Departments of Medicine and Radiation Oncology, Dana Farber Cancer Institute, Harvard Medical School, Boston, Massachusetts

**Kenneth D. Tew, Ph.D., D.Sc.**   Department of Pharmacology, Fox Chase Cancer Center, Philadelphia, Pennsylvania

**A. G. J. van der Zee, M.D., Ph.D.**   University Hospital Groningen, Groningen, The Netherlands

**Laura M. Vargas Roig, M.D., Ph.D.**   Laboratory of Reproduction and Lactation, Regional Center for Scientific and Technological Research (CRICYT), Mendoza, Argentina

**G. J. Veldhuis, M.D.**   University Hospital Groningen, Groningen, The Netherlands,

**Nancy E. Ward, M.S.**   Department of Cell Biology, The University of Texas M.D. Anderson Cancer Center, Houston, Texas

**David W. Wilbur, M.D., Ph.D.**   Oncology Section, Department of Medicine, Loma Linda University School of Medicine and J. L. Pettis Memorial Veterans Medical Center, Loma Linda, California

**P. H. B. Willemse, M.D., Ph.D.**   Department of Medical Oncology, University Hospital Groningen, Groningen, The Netherlands

**Yuk-Chor Wong, Ph.D.**   UCLA San Fernando Valley Program, Sepulveda Veterans Administration Medical Center, Sepulveda, California

# 1

## Chemotherapy Resistance in Small Cell Lung Cancer: Consequences for the Clinician and Future Prospects

**Bonne Biesma and Pieter E. Postmus**
*Free University Hospital, Amsterdam, The Netherlands*

**Egbert F. Smit**
*University Hospital Groningen, Groningen, The Netherlands*

### INTRODUCTION

Lung cancer is the leading cause of cancer death in men and its incidence is rising worldwide. In the United States, lung cancer–related mortality exceeds that of breast cancer in women (1,2). A clear relationship between cigarette smoking and lung cancer incidence and mortality has been demonstrated (3). There are four major histological subtypes of lung cancer: adenocarcinoma, large cell carcinoma, squamous cell carcinoma, and small cell carcinoma. Around 1970, it became apparent that different treatment modalities were necessary for the different types of tumor. Squamous cell carcinoma, adenocarcinoma, and large cell carcinoma are generally referred to as non–small cell lung cancer (NSCLC). Although chemotherapy is increasingly being used in clinical trials in NSCLC, the only treatment modality offering real chances for long-term survival is surgery. In contrast, small cell lung cancer (SCLC), accounting for approximately 20% of the lung carcinomas, is more sensitive to both radiotherapy and chemotherapy than NSCLC both in patients and in tumor model systems (1,2,4). In SCLC—unlike NSCLC—surgery offers a solution in only a small minority of patients (5). Subsequently, chemotherapy has become the cornerstone of treatment for this disease. In the late 1960s, the first randomized placebo-controlled trial with cyclophosphamide demonstrated improvement of survival in patients with SCLC (6). Several cytotoxic drugs have demonstrated efficacy, some of which (for instance, methotrexate and CCNU) have been replaced by more active drugs. It is generally accepted that combination chemotherapy should be used for the treatment of SCLC, because by this approach it is expected that the development of tumor cell resistance will be prevented or delayed. These combinations contain two or, in most cases, three active drugs. The most frequently used induction regimens are cyclophosphamide-doxorubicin-vincristine (CAV), cyclophosphamide-doxorubicin-etoposide (CDE), and cisplatin-etoposide (PE).

During the past two decades, clinical research has resulted in the design of chemotherapeutic regimens that produce an initial overall response rate of 80–90% to combination chemotherapy. Complete response (CR) rates vary from 15–30% for extensive disease (ED); CR rates higher than 50% have been reported for limited disease (LD). Unfortunately, relapse occurs in the vast majority of patients, resulting in a fatal outcome for most. Long-term disease-free survival is achieved in approximately 10% of patients with LD and in less than 1% of patients with ED. Median survival has reached 14 months and 7 months in patients with LD and ED, respectively.

Although finding drugs active against SCLC has obviously been the main goal in many trials, one other important question that has been raised concerned the duration of treatment (7–10). Until the early 1980s, chemotherapy for SCLC was given continuously for 1 to 2 years, a period often coinciding with the duration of the patient's life. In a large (687 patients) multicenter randomized trial, nonprogressing patients were randomized, after induction chemotherapy consisting of five CDE courses, either to receive a further seven cycles of the same chemotherapy or to follow-up and treatment at progression (7). Although the patients randomized to the maintenance chemotherapy arm had a significantly longer progression-free survival time, no difference in overall survival between the two arms was observed. Results from other studies have been mixed. Some studies favored maintenance chemotherapy over no further chemotherapy (11,12); other studies demonstrated no beneficial effect of maintenance chemotherapy on survival compared to treatment at relapse (8,13). From the data of the randomized trials, it was recommended that, "After selection of those patients considered to be fit enough to receive induction chemotherapy, they should be treated with 4–6 courses of an adequately dosed and proved effective combination chemotherapy regime. At progression or relapse, they should be treated with the same or another adequately dosed and proved combination chemotherapy regime" (14).

The very high relapse rates and the very modest survival rates can be explained by the existence of chemotherapy-resistant cell clones at the beginning of treatment or the emergence of such drug-resistant clones during treatment. In vitro data support this assumption (15–17). As a result, chemotherapeutic drugs and regimens demonstrate significantly less activity in previously treated patients compared with previously untreated patients.

This chapter focuses on clinical drug resistance to standard and second-line chemotherapy in SCLC and on approaches to circumvent this drug resistance, keeping in mind the basic mechanisms responsible for multidrug resistance.

## ALTERNATING CHEMOTHERAPY

A simple mathematical model of the probability of the development of resistant cell clones within a tumor has been proposed by Goldie and Coldman (18). In this model, it is assumed that tumors grow exponentially and that each course of chemotherapy results in log cell kill. The outcomes of two treatment strategies, alternation of two non–cross-resistant chemotherapy regimens and sequential administration of these regimens, were evaluated by computer simulation. Given the assumption that there was symmetry between the two regimens (i.e., the same log cell kill and same rate of mutation leading to cells resistant to the combination used), the cure rate of alternating chemotherapy was superior to sequential chemotherapy. Although it is impossible to prove whether these two assumptions concerning the tumor are correct, previous clinical experience with hematological malignancies (19) made it worthwhile to test the Goldie-Coldman hypothesis in SCLC.

Essentially, two conditions have to be fulfilled before the Goldie-Coldman hypothesis can be tested clinically to its full merit:

1. The two combination chemotherapy regimens have to be equipotent with regard to tumor cell kill—i.e., to have comparable response rates.
2. There should be non-cross-resistance between the two regimens.

The latter assumption implies a reasonable response rate to chemotherapy regimen B in relapsing patients after initial treatment with regimen A and vice versa (20).

The Goldie-Coldman hypothesis predicts that optimal results would be obtained if all active chemotherapeutic agents would be used simultaneously early in the treatment of the malignant disease. However, cumulative toxicity of the different drugs, primarily myelosuppression, prevents the clinical application of such schemes. Theoretically, rapid alternation of non-cross-resistant chemotherapeutic regimens would be the second-best alternative.

Alternating chemotherapy for SCLC has been evaluated in clinical trials since 1979 (21). In a review by Elliott et al. in 1984, all controlled trials performed at that time had failed to show any consistent benefit for patients treated with alternating regimens (22). In their conclusion, it was suggested that the time at which alternate cycles of treatment were introduced might be of critical importance. A study in which alternating chemotherapy was preceded by an initial period of induction chemotherapy showed no improvement in response duration (23). These results were in contrast with data from the Finsen group demonstrating a prolonged duration of remission after alternating chemotherapy (24). Furthermore, in future trials, confounding variables such as radiotherapy should be eliminated.

Since then, several large controlled trials have focused on alternating chemotherapy. These trials have varied extensively with regard to both the regimens tested and the patients (LD, ED, or both groups) included. Very few, if any, have met the above-mentioned criteria concerning the conditions of the two potentially non-cross-resistant regimens. In some studies, the chemotherapeutic regimen in the control arm differed from the regimens used in the alternating arm completely (25) or just in detail (26). Another factor complicating the interpretation of the results, primarily response duration and survival, was the use of maintenance chemotherapy in some studies (8). Radiotherapy of the primary tumor was used only in patients with LD and, in addition, in some studies only after completion of chemotherapy (25,27) or only in responding patients (27).

In the first large randomized trial, Evans et al. (28) treated 289 patients with ED with CAV or CAV alternating with cisplatin and etoposide (PE). Patients receiving alternating chemotherapy demonstrated significantly better response rates, progression-free survival, and overall survival compared with patients treated with CAV. However, if patients with locoregional disease were excluded from the analysis—and sex and performance score were taken into account—overall survival was no longer statistically significant, but time to progression still was. In two large randomized trials (29, 30), CAV and PE were compared with alteration of these regimens (CAV/PE). Both studies differed in the dosages and the time scheduling of the drugs. In addition, the Japanese study included LD and ED patients (288 evaluable patients), whereas the patients in the SCSG study (437 eligible patients) all had ED. In the latter study, no significant differences in treatment outcome for CAV, PE, and CAV/PE could be demonstrated. Overall response rates were 51%, 61%, and 59%, and CR rates were 7%, 10%, and 7%, respectively. Median survival was 8.3, 8.6, and 8.1 months, respectively, with a (statistically nonsignificant) trend toward a longer median time to progression in the alternating arm. Of major importance in this study are the response rates in patients who received crossover second-line chemotherapy at time of progression after initial CAV or PE treatment. One hundred patients were evaluable for response to crossover chemotherapy. Of 28 patients initially responding to PE, only 4 (14%) responded to CAV; only one of 13 PE nonresponders (8%) achieved a response. Of the 32 responders to first-line CAV, nine (28%) responded to second-line PE, whereas four of 27 (15%) nonresponders did. Certainly, the lack of responses to CAV after first-line PE treatment suggests that there is no true non-cross-resistance between the two regimens. In the study by Fukuoka et al., response rates for PE (78%) and CAV/PE (76%) were significantly higher than for CAV (55%), albeit that the CR rates were similar for the three groups (29). Nine of 39 patients (23%) not responding to the initial CAV regimen responded to second-line PE, but only one of 13 patients (8%) responded to second-line CAV after failing to respond to PE. Both observations are in clear conflict with the conditions to be fulfilled for a test of the Goldie-Coldman hypothesis. The combination CAV/PE has been the combination most widely used in alternating studies so far. Although some studies have demonstrated similar efficacy for the CAV and PE regimen (30,31), other studies appear to demonstrate that the two regimens are not equipotent (27,29). Furthermore, other data support the assumption that CAV and PE are not true non-cross-resistant chemotherapeutic regimens (32).

Wolf et al. (33) compared alternating chemotherapy (ifosfamide/etoposide [IE] and CAV) with response-oriented chemotherapy (IE) for a maximum of six cycles in a multicenter randomized trial with 321 patients (LD and ED). In the response-oriented arm, patients were treated with IE to a maximal response and subsequently were switched to CAV. Patients with stable disease (SD), also after only one cycle, were also given CAV in the next cycle. In the alternating treatment arm, patients were shifted to second-line treatment only if progression occurred. Patients with LD received chest radiotherapy following chemotherapy. Overall response rates were 77% and 70% for the alternating and response-oriented arm, respectively. The CR rate was 26% in both arms. Median survival times were 9.7 and 10.7 months, and 2-year survival rates were 11% and 9% for the alternating and response-oriented groups, respectively. The study did not demonstrate advantages for alternating chemotherapy over the response-oriented treatment. Although the above-described studies suggest that no relevant clinical benefit can be expected from the use of alternating chemotherapy regimens instead of standard regimens, the most important conclusion that can be drawn is that the studies have been performed without testing in advance the possible non-cross-resistance of the regimens in properly designed phase II trials. This has led to resource- and time-consuming phase III studies. Recently, data have become available from a phase II study of the EORTC Lung Cancer Cooperative Group testing the possible non-cross-resistance of the CDE regimen and ifosfamide-mesna-carboplatin (IMP) (34). In a previous study, it was shown that these two regimens were almost equipotent (35). Sixty-eight patients previously treated with CDE, IMP, or vincristine and carboplatin (VP), who had documented tumor progression within 3 months after the last chemotherapy, were entered in the study. Twenty-five patients clinically resistant to

CDE were treated with vincristine plus IMP (VIMP). This resulted in 1 CR and 14 PR; overall response rate, 60%. Patients clinically resistant to VP (n=22) or IMP (n=21) were treated with CDE, resulting in 6 CR and 16 PR, with an overall response rate of 51%. Median survival was 24 weeks for patients responding to CDE and 21 weeks for patients responding to VIMP. These data are slightly better than those for nonresponders to second-line chemotherapy, with a median survival of 11 and 12 weeks after CDE and VIMP, respectively. In order to evaluate whether this degree of non-cross-resistance is sufficient to enhance survival rates in comparison with the standard CDE regimen, the EORTC Lung Cancer Cooperative Group has performed a randomized trial comparing CDE with alternating CDE and VIMP in 148 patients with ED (36). The best overall response rates for the CDE and CDE/VIMP groups were 69% and 70%, respectively. The median duration of response was 7 months and 6.8 months, and the median survival time was 7.6 months and 8.7 months, respectively. These differences were not statistically significant. Furthermore, hematological toxicity (WHO grade III–IV) was encountered more frequently in the alternating arm. This study demonstrates that CDE and VIMP are not truly non-cross-resistant regimens. Of interest, in the previous phase II study, nearly all patients responding to VIMP had responded to CDE induction chemotherapy, which again suggests no complete non-cross-resistance between the two regimens.

It has been 15 years since Goldie and Coldman published their mathematical model, and so far all attempts to test their hypothesis in the clinic have failed because of the lack of regimens with a high degree of non-cross-resistance. This may be partially related to the fact that in the past decade only a limited number of new drugs have demonstrated efficacy in SCLC. Other important factors are a still incomplete knowledge of the mechanisms that cause drug resistance and of the mechanisms of cross-resistance. After identification of such non-cross-resistant regimens, it will require large randomized studies to demonstrate possible enhanced survival rates after alternating chemotherapy, given the expected differences according to the Goldie-Coldman hypothesis.

## CHEMOTHERAPY DOSE INTENSIFICATION

For many tumors, there appears to be a clear relationship between the chemotherapy dose administered and the tumor response (37,38). The explanation for this might be the prevention or delay of development of tumor cell resistance. In a small randomized study testing dose intensification for SCLC, an increase in the response rate was found with increasing cyclophosphamide, methotrexate, and CCNU doses (39). Several approaches with regard to dose intensification are possible, some of which have been in use for quite some time; others were developed more recently. Next, these different approaches are discussed separately.

### High-Dose Induction Chemotherapy

High-dose chemotherapy followed by autologous bone marrow transplantation (ABMT) as initial treatment in patients with SCLC was first tested in 1982 (40). Souhami et al. administered cyclophosphamide (160–200 mg/kg), followed by ABMT, to 16 patients and achieved an overall response rate of 87% (7 CR and 7 PR). Since then, several small trials have been conducted, mainly in patients with good performance status. Although initial response rates were at least similar to those after standard-dose chemotherapy, there was no improvement in survival after high-dose chemotherapy and ABMT (40–44). High-dose chemotherapy followed by ABMT in patients with recurrent or refractory SCLC also demonstrated promising response rates; however, responses were of short duration (45).

Although these results appear to discourage further attempts at dose intensification in SCLC, the character of the intensive treatment regimens used was very high-dose pulse therapy. This approach was associated with considerable toxicity and could only be applied in a limited number of institutes in small studies involving patients with good performance status. As a consequence, one was never able to demonstrate small differences in long-term survival rates, and the assumption that dose-intensification might be worthwhile should not be rejected on the basis of these data alone.

## Late-Intensification Therapy

Norton and Simon have developed a mathematical model based on the assumption that tumors have a Gompertzian growth pattern (46). Based on this model, late chemotherapy dose intensification might result in eradication of residual disease in patients responding to induction treatment. Humblet et al. conducted a randomized phase III trial in selected SCLC patients that included ABMT after late intensification (47). The CR rate increased from 39% to 79% after high-dose chemotherapy. Furthermore, high-dose chemotherapy led to a significant increase in relapse-free survival: 28 weeks versus 10 weeks in the standard treatment group. However, the study failed to show significant improvement in the prognosis of the late intensification group, as the median survival was 68 weeks for the intensified group and 65 weeks for the standard-treatment group. In eight ED patients treated with late-intensive chemotherapy combined with radiotherapy and followed by ABMT, the median survival time was less than 1 year, with no 2-year survivors (48). In a Southwest Oncology Group study, 58 previously untreated LD patients received induction chemoradiotherapy and consolidation chemotherapy (49). Twenty-one patients received high-dose cyclophosphamide (150 mg/kg) as late intensification without ABMT. Of these 21 patients, five relapsed and died, four succumbed to treatment-related toxicity, and three died of other causes but were in CR at that time. At the time of evaluation, the remaining nine patients were in CR with a median survival of 27 months. For the complete group, this treatment strategy did not result in an increase in survival compared with standard treatment.

## Increased Dose of Standard Chemotherapy

In the above-mentioned trials, dose intensification was achieved by administering a single high-dose chemotherapy course. Dose intensification, however, can also be achieved by increasing the doses of the drugs in the standard regimens or by reducing the time intervals between consecutive standard-dose chemotherapy courses. It is conceivable that these methods may lead to enhanced toxicity, especially myelotoxicity, resulting in an increase in episodes of febrile neutropenia and bleeding complications caused by thrombocytopenia. Furthermore, progressive myelotoxicity is a feature of many of the standard regimens, resulting in chemotherapy dose reduction or postponement of the next chemotherapy course because of insufficient bone marrow recovery.

As a result, the achieved relative dose intensity is less than anticipated, even after standard-dose regimens.

Randomized studies comparing different doses of chemotherapy in regimens are scarce. In an early randomized study, a higher dose of cyclophosphamide correlated with improved response rates and median survival rates (39). In two large trials, the assumed beneficial effect of increased doses of cyclophosphamide and doxorubicin in the CAV regimen was studied (50,51). Although the CR rate improved in one of the studies (50), both studies failed to demonstrate an increase in survival in the high-dose group. Ihde et al. performed a prospective randomized trial of previously untreated ED patients comparing high-dose and standard-dose PE (52). Ninety patients were randomized for the study (44 patients receiving high-dose treatment); another 25 patients were excluded from randomization and were assigned to standard treatment. High-dose PE (cisplatin 27 mg/m$^2$ and etoposide 80 mg/m$^2$ both days 1–5 q 3 weeks) was administered only during cycles 1 and 2, followed by standard-dose PE (cisplatin 80 mg/m$^2$ day 1 and etoposide 80 mg/m$^2$ days 1–3 q 3 weeks). Complete responders received PE in cycles 5 through 8; other patients received second-line treatment. At the cost of significantly increased myelotoxicity, a 68% higher dose and a 46% higher dose-rate intensity was achieved in the high-dose group. Despite this dose intensification, there was no increase in CR rate and median survival duration in the high-dose group (23% and 10.7 months, respectively) compared with the standard-dose group (22% and 11.4 months, respectively). In contrast, a recent prospective randomized study of 105 patients with LD demonstrated improved disease-free survival and overall survival after initial higher doses of cyclophosphamide and cisplatin (53). In this French trial, patients were randomized to one cycle of high-dose chemotherapy (doxorubicin 40 mg/m$^2$ day 1, etoposide 75 mg/m$^2$ days 1–3, cisplatin 100 mg/m$^2$ day 2, cyclophosphamide 300 mg/m$^2$ days 2–5) or lower dose chemotherapy (cisplatin 80 mg/m$^2$, cyclophosphamide 225 mg/m$^2$, similar doses of etoposide and doxorubicin) during cycle 1. Subsequent cycles were identical for both groups. Six cycles of chemotherapy were given, alternating with three cycles of radiotherapy. The high-dose chemotherapy group demonstrated a superior 2-year survival rate (45% vs. 26%, $P=.02$) and 2-year disease-free survival rate (28% vs. 8%, $P=.02$). There was no significant difference in CR rate at 6 months (67% vs. 54%). Patients in the high-dose group experienced WHO grade IV neutropenia more frequently after the first cycle, but no differences were observed during the following cycles. The authors did not mention any myelotoxicity-related complications. At this stage, it remains unclear why the French study demonstrated enhanced survival after just one cycle of higher dose chemotherapy, which seems in contrast with the results of the majority of the randomized studies.

## Increased Dose Intensity by Interval Reduction

Multiple studies have investigated the efficacy of frequent administration of chemotherapy. These studies include cyclic alternating chemotherapy, a subject discussed earlier in this chapter. Murray et al. designed the CODE regimen (cisplatin, vincristine, doxorubicin, etoposide) to reduce myelotoxicity, which enabled weekly administration of chemotherapy (54). Supportive drugs included prednisone, cimetidine, trimethoprim-sulfamethoxazole, and ketoconazole. Forty-eight patients, all with ED and good performance score, were included in the study. The dose intensity compared to the original CAV/PE schedule was increased by reducing the intervals between treatment rather than increasing the doses of the different drugs: 9–12 weeks vs. 18 weeks. After chemotherapy, the overall response rate was 94%, including 40% CR. After thoracic irradiation, the CR rate improved to 56%. With a median follow-up period of 2.5 years, the median time to progression and the median survival time were 43 and 61 weeks, respectively. The authors recommended 9 weeks of therapy rather than 12 weeks, a treatment schedule resulting in an approximately twofold dose intensification. Miles et al. treated LD patients (n=45) and ED patients with good prognostic factors (n=25) with almost the same drugs, except ifosfamide was substituted for cyclophosphamide (55). The overall response rate was 91%, with a 50% CR. Response rates for LD and ED patients were similar. Median survival was 58 weeks for the LD group and 42 weeks for the ED group (overall, 54 weeks). Recently, data from a large randomized phase III study comparing multiple-drug weekly chemotherapy with standard (CDE) chemotherapy became available (56). Two-hundred twenty-five patients were randomized to receive six courses of a multiple-drug combination (doxorubicin 25 mg/m$^2$, etoposide 120 mg/m$^2$, cyclophosphamide 500 mg/m$^2$, all on day 1; cisplatin 60 mg/m$^2$, vindesine 3 mg/m$^2$, both on day 8; vincristine 2 mg and methotrexate 100 mg/m$^2$ on day 15) or CDE. Overall objective response rates were 69% and 62% for the multidrug and CDE group, respectively (NS). In addition, there was no significant difference in median survival duration and 2-year survival between the multidrug group (49 weeks and 8.5%, respectively) and the CDE group (43 weeks and 7.9%, respectively). However, for the LD patients there was a significant increase in the overall response rate in favor of the multiple-drug schedule. Patients receiving CDE experienced more frequent hematological toxicity, WHO grade III–IV. Because of increased treatment delays, the total relative dose intensity was significantly higher in the CDE arm. In contrast to the previously described nonrandomized trials, this randomized trial failed to demonstrate improved efficacy and survival after multidrug treatment. Another randomized trial, including 311 good performance status patients (195 LD, 116 ED), also failed to demonstrate improved response and survival rates in the intensified treatment arm (57). Standard treatment consisted of PE alternating 3-weekly with cyclophosphamide, doxorubicin, and vincristine. Intensified chemotherapy comprised PE alternating weekly with ifosfamide and doxorubicin. The overall response rates for the 3-weekly and weekly treatment groups were 78% (CR 33%) and 81% (CR 30%), respectively. Median survival time was 44 and 46 weeks. Neutropenia was the most frequently encountered dose-limiting toxicity in the weekly treated group.

### Increased Dose Intensity by Hematopoietic Growth Factor Support

In several of the studies described above, the desired chemotherapy dose intensification or relative dose intensity was not achieved because of dose-limiting myelotoxicity. The introduction of recombinant human hematopoietic colony-stimulating factors (rhCSFs) has provided a tool to reduce chemotherapy-induced myelosuppression (58–61). The first phase I/II trial with rhG-CSF (granulocyte CSF) was performed in patients with SCLC (62). Two large multicenter randomized placebo-controlled trials in chemotherapy-naive patients with SCLC demonstrated that administration of rhG-CSF (230 $\mu$g/m$^2$/day subcutaneously) for up to 14 days after chemotherapy reduced both the incidence of severe neutropenia and the incidence of febrile neutropenia (63,64).

**Table 1** Chemotherapy Dose Intensification with rhG-CSF

| Method | Intensification | Ref. |
|---|---|---|
| Less dose reduction | Yes | 65 |
| Interval reduction | Yes | 66 |
| Chemotherapy dose increased | Yes | 67 |
| Interval reduction | Yes | 68 |
| Less dose reduction | No | 69 |

Since it became apparent that rhCSFs could reduce chemotherapy-related neutropenia, several investigators have attempted chemotherapy dose intensification with the aid of rhCSFs. In Table 1, some studies with rhG-CSF are summarized. An increased dose intensity was achieved by either less chemotherapy dose reduction or by shortening the interval between courses. However, certainly not in all studies did the application of rhG-CSF lead to an increased dose intensity (66,69). Despite an increase in dose intensity in patients treated with rhG-CSF (5 $\mu$g/kg/day) after each of six cycles of the VICE (vincristine, ifosfamide, carboplatin, and etoposide) regimen compared with a control group, the overall response rate in that study did not differ significantly (94.1% in the rhG-CSF group and 93.5% in the control group) (68). CR rates were 55.9% and 58.1%, respectively. Although the rhG-CSF group had more chemotherapy-related deaths (six vs. one), this group demonstrated a better 2-year survival rate (32% vs. 15%). The median survival time for the rhG-CSF group and the control group was 69 and 65 weeks, respectively (NS). In this study, patients received prophylactic cranial irradiation after cycle 1 and thoracic irradiation after cycle 3.

RhGM-CSF (rh granulocyte-macrophage CSF) has also demonstrated efficacy in reducing chemotherapy-induced neutropenia in patients with SCLC (70,71). In Table 2, some trials using rhGM-CSF to increase chemotherapy dose intensity are summarized. In a study conducted by Paccagnella et al., with the addition of rhGM-CSF (10 $\mu$g/kg/day sc), the relative dose intensity was significantly increased by 29% for cisplatin and etoposide and by 63% for epirubicin compared with the control group (74). The overall response rate was 95% (40% CR) in the rhGM-CSF groups and 72% (24% CR) in the control group. Median response duration for the rhGM-CSF groups and the control group was 10.8 months and 8.8 months, respectively.

RhG-CSF and rhGM-CSF predominantly reduce the duration of chemotherapy-induced neutropenia. In comparison, rhIL-3 (interleukin-3) has proved to be a more

**Table 2** Chemotherapy Dose Intensification with rhGM-CSF

| Method | Intensification | Ref. |
|---|---|---|
| Interval reduction | Yes | 72 |
| Interval reduction | Yes | 73 |
| Chemotherapy dose increased | Yes | 74 |
| Chemotherapy dose increased | No | 75 |

potent stimulator of megakaryopoiesis in vitro (76,77). Clinical studies with rhIL-3 administered to patients with advanced malignancies, myelodysplastic syndromes, aplastic anemia, or bone marrow failure demonstrated its multilineage stimulation of hematopoiesis in vivo (78–81). Therefore, rhIL-3 could be a potent CSF for the reduction of chemotherapy-induced neutropenia and thrombocytopenia. In a phase I/II trial, Postmus et al. administered rhIL-3 subcutaneously for 14 days after the second course of second-line chemotherapy to 19 patients with a relapse of SCLC (82). At rhIL-3 doses of 8 and 16 $\mu$g/kg/day, patients treated with VIMP demonstrated a significantly hastened neutrophil recovery. At 8 $\mu$g/kg/day rhIL-3, the platelet counts also were increased. Headache was the dose-limiting toxicity. In a placebo-controlled randomized Belgian study, 28 patients with newly diagnosed SCLC were treated with carboplatin, etoposide, and epirubicin (83). RhIL-3 (0.25 to 10 $\mu$g/kg/day) was administered during 7 days following the second cycle of chemotherapy. At 7.5 and 10 $\mu$g/kg/day rhIL-3, patients demonstrated a significantly faster platelet recovery. There was also a trend toward a faster neutrophil recovery, albeit not statistically significant. Chemotherapy postponement due to myelotoxicity was less frequent at the higher ($\geq$ 2.5 $\mu$g/kg/day) rhIL-3 dose steps. Compared with an age-matched historical control group treated with identical chemotherapy, patients who received the addition of rhIL-3 did not show improved disease-free survival and overall survival rates. However, given the phase I character of the study and the limited number of patients included, this was not the primary aim of the study. Dose-limiting toxicity was not encountered up to 10 $\mu$g/kg/day rhIL-3.

Finally, rh erythropoietin (rhEpo), administered three times weekly at doses of 150 and 300 IU/kg, delayed the onset of anemia and reduced the red blood cell transfusion requirements in patients with SCLC treated with the VICE regimen (84). However, in attempts to intensify chemotherapy, it appears to be of greater importance to reduce neutropenia and thrombocytopenia, rather than anemia.

## SECOND-LINE CHEMOTHERAPY

As stated earlier, until less than two decades ago, patients with SCLC were usually treated continuously with chemotherapy for the greater part of their remaining life. As a result, patients were seldom treated with a second-line chemotherapy regimen. Furthermore, if such patients were treated with second-line chemotherapy at time of relapse or progression, these patients could be considered to have true refractory disease and, as a result, response rates were very disappointing. More recently, new ideas about the duration of induction chemotherapy in SCLC (7,14) have led to the development of induction chemotherapy regimens consisting of four to six courses. Given the very high relapse rates, this necessitated developing second-line regimens. Several studies have given us much more insight into the role of clinical resistance and the efficacy of second-line treatment.

Second-line treatment became more attractive and effective, as the patients were usually off treatment for some time, allowing time for recovery from side effects. In addition, the lower cumulative dose of chemotherapy saves a much larger bone marrow reserve capacity and causes less chemotherapy-induced tumor cell resistance; this is probably dependent on the length of the therapy-free interval. In pretreated patients, a distinction should be made between relapsing and refractory patients: in the former group the tumor still may be sensitive to chemotherapy, whereas the latter group should be considered truly chemoresistant. Unfortunately, most studies with second-line chemotherapy do not differentiate between the two groups, thus hampering both the interpretation and comparison of the results.

Three types of chemotherapy regimens are used in relapsing or refractory patients:

1. Re-treatment with the same chemotherapy regimen as initially administered.
2. Regimens thought to be at least partially non-cross-resistant with the induction regimen.
3. New drugs usually tested in phase II trials.

### Re-Treatment with Induction Chemotherapy

Distinguishing refractory patients from relapsing patients is of critical importance if reinduction treatment is considered. In 1983, Batist et al. reported a response to reinduction chemotherapy in 4 of 6 patients with an initial response duration of more than 27 months (85). Postmus et al. treated 37 patients, initially responding to CDE, at relapse again with this schedule (86). In 62% of the patients, a second response was obtained. Patients obtaining a CR after first-line treatment responded significantly better to second-line treatment compared to patients with a PR after induction chemotherapy. In addition, re-treatment was significantly more effective in patients with an initial response duration over 34 weeks in comparison with patients relapsing earlier. Giaccone et al. treated 13 patients, initially responsive to induction chemotherapy, at relapse with the same chemotherapy regimen (87). Patients had been off treatment for a median of 30 weeks. Overall response rate was 50%. The median survival from start of second-line chemotherapy was 26 weeks, and 94 weeks from start of any therapy. In a Belgian study, six patients with an initial CR duration of more than 1 year demonstrated responses to re-treatment at relapse (2 CR, 4 PR), with a response duration ranging from 6 to over 15 months (88). Further evidence of a relation between the initial response duration and the response duration to second-line treatment can be derived from data of Vincent et al., who observed a 67% PR in 15 patients previously responding to various chemotherapy regimens (89). The median response duration to second-line treatment was related to the response duration to first-line treatment: if the primary response has lasted more than 8 months, a second response duration longer than 2 months was more likely to occur.

These data stress the vital importance of the elapsed time between the last course of the induction regimen and the moment of relapse with regard to the strategy in second-line chemotherapy. In patients treated with teniposide (VM-26) as second-line treatment after initial treatment with mostly CDE, it was demonstrated that both the effectiveness of the prior chemotherapy and the time interval between both chemotherapy regimens affected the patient response (90). Of the patients responding to induction chemotherapy, 42% responded also to VM-26. In contrast, in the group of the nonresponders to the initial regimen, no responses to VM-26 were observed. Furthermore, only 12% of the patients whose last chemotherapy course had been administered in the past 2.6 months responded to VM-26. In patients with a treatment-free interval of more than 2.6 months, the response rate was 53%.

Andersen et al. reviewed the literature on second-line chemotherapy for the period 1979–1989 (91). At that time, a total of 35 reports, all phase II trials, had been published. The authors differentiated between three groups according to treatment:

Reinduction with the initial chemotherapy regimen
Cisplatin and/or etoposide with or without other agents
Other drugs believed to be non-cross-resistant

Information from the different studies was often incomplete with regard to duration of response after induction chemotherapy and the drug-free interval. However, with the information available, the three groups appeared to be balanced with regard to age, sex, performance score, and tumor stage. The overall response rates after reinduction with the initial regimen (64%) and after cisplatin and etoposide (45%) were superior to response rates obtained with other supposedly non-cross-resistant regimens (< 20%). The overall response rate for second-line regimens was 30%, with 5% of the patients obtaining a CR. As the duration of response was reported in roughly only one quarter of the studies, data on that subject were inconclusive. It was concluded that truly non-cross-resistant regimens or drugs had yet to be identified (although the PE combination demonstrated definite activity). Furthermore, the favorable response rates in trials using reinduction chemotherapy might be related to selected patients, given the fact that these patients all responded during primary treatment. Also, this last group of patients had a drug-free interval before second-line chemotherapy was administered. From these data, it was derived that patients achieving a response on first-line chemotherapy had a response rate of over 50% when re-treated with the induction regimen at relapse.

Nowadays, it is recognized that patients relapsing within 3 months after the last induction chemotherapy course should be considered truly resistant to the drugs applied during the initial treatment and, therefore, second-line schedules should consist of other non-cross-resistant drugs. Patients relapsing at a later stage may benefit from re-treatment with the initial chemotherapy scheme, although the duration of response still is limited.

## Second-Line Treatment with Drugs Supposedly Non-Cross-Resistant to the Induction Regimen

As stated earlier, a major problem with developing non-cross-resistant chemotherapy regimens is the uncertainty about the definition of such a regimen. The assumption that a second-line "non-cross-resistant" scheme should demonstrate reasonable activity in relapsing patients is confounded by the observation that second-line response rates appear to be related to both the primary response duration and the effectiveness of the induction chemotherapy (90).

Among the second-line schedules that have been studied, the PE combination is one of the most active, with an overall response rate of approximately 50% (92–94). In 1979 Sierocki et al. first described a PR in four of six heavily pretreated patients with SCLC (95). In the 1980s, response rates in larger phase II trials varied from 12% (96) to 55% (94). The median survival time varied from 12 to 35 weeks, the latter in LD patients (94). In the majority of the patients, first-line treatment consisted of CAV. Again, results were negatively affected by a short off-treatment period or progression during first-line treatment (96). As described earlier, with the VIMP regimen, a response rate of 60% in patients clinically resistant to CDE was achieved, albeit that the number of patients in the study was limited (34). However, median survival in responding patients was a mere 21 weeks. A disappointing feature in virtually all the second-line studies is that responses almost never were complete and that the response was of short duration. This is in line with the assumption that completely non-cross-resistant regimens are needed to eradicate the remaining resistant cell clones.

## New Drugs

As mentioned earlier, until the early 1980s, patients with SCLC were treated with chemotherapy for the larger part of their remaining life. New chemotherapeutic drugs were tested only in relapsing or refractory patients who had been heavily pretreated. As could be expected, the response rates of such new drugs were very disappointing. Since new prognostic factors with regard to second-line response rates (treatment-free interval, response rates to induction therapy) have been recently stipulated, it is acknowledged that the antitumor activity of some of these drugs was underestimated. For example, such was the case with teniposide (VM-26). In a phase II trial, 33 previously untreated elderly patients were treated with VM-26 (97). VM-26 yielded a response rate of 90.9%, including 30% CR. The median duration of survival was nearly 9 months. Although a similar response rate was not met in other previously untreated patients (90), results were superior to those in previously treated patients with response rates of less than 25% (98–100).

VP-16 also demonstrated feeble activity if administered to pretreated patients (101–103), but in untreated patients overall response rates up to 89% were achieved if VP-16 was administered as a single agent (104,105). Of notice is the importance of etoposide scheduling, as a 5-day schedule has demonstrated superior activity over a 1-day schedule in patients with ED, with overall response rates of 89% and 10%, respectively (105). In the latter study, the median response duration was 4.5 months for the patients treated with the 5-day schedule.

Carboplatin, a second-generation platinum analogue, demonstrated a high degree of activity in previously untreated patients with ED. In a study conducted at the Royal Marsden Hospital, an overall response rate of 60% was observed (10% CR); response rates of 24% and 11% were achieved in relapsing patients and refractory patients, respectively (106). The median duration of survival was 8 months for previously untreated patients and 4.5 months if all patients are included. Other studies have confirmed the promising activity of carboplatin in untreated patients with ED (107,108). In patients with recurrent or progressive brain metastases, carboplatin yielded an overall response rate of 40%, with a median response duration of 8 weeks (109). Almost all patients had been previously treated with teniposide.

Two other drugs that demonstrated promising activity in SCLC in the 1980s were ifosfamide, an isomer of cyclophosphamide (110), and epirubicin, the 4′ epimer of doxorubicin. Blackstein et al. administered epirubicin (100 or 200 mg/m$^2$ IV every 3 weeks) to 40 previously untreated patients (111). Twenty patients (50%) achieved an objective response, while three patients had CR. Median duration of response was 212 days. Patients failing to respond to epirubicin were given the opportunity to be treated with cisplatin and VP-16. This increased the response rate to 62.5%, with a median survival of 8.3 months. In an EORTC study of previously untreated elderly or unfit patients, a response rate of 57% after epirubicin (110 mg/m$^2$) was observed, with a median survival time for the whole group of 6.61 months (112). Other studies have demonstrated promising activity, with response rates of 33–57% (113–115). Rosenthal et al. (116) treated 20 patients with recurrent or refractory SCLC with epirubicin (85 mg/m$^2$ IV every 3 weeks). The overall response rate in this study was 21% (2 CR and 2 PR in 19 evaluable patients). The median survival time of all patients from the moment of commencement of epirubicin treatment was 9 weeks. Three of the 14 responders to induction chemotherapy responded to epirubicin; such was the case in only one of the six who failed to respond to first-line treatment. Furthermore, median time from cessation of first-line treatment until the start of epirubicin administration was 35 and 14 weeks for the responders and nonresponders to epirubicin, respectively.

More recently, CPT-11, a water-soluble derivative of camptothecin and inhibitor of topoisomerase I, demonstrated remarkable activity in patients with refractory or recurrent SCLC (117). Sixteen patients were treated with CPT-11 (100 mg/m$^2$ IV) on a weekly basis. All patients were initially treated with a cisplatin-based regimen. The median time off treatment was 7.3 months. Among 15 evaluable patients, seven (47%) patients responded (all PR), with a median response duration of 58 days. The major toxicities encountered were myelosuppression (mainly neutropenia), diarrhea, and pulmonary toxicity. Given this response rate, the authors suggest at least a partial non-cross-resistance between cisplatin and CPT-11. However, results may have been favored by the relatively long elapsed period between initial and second-line treatment.

Another semisynthetic camptothecin analogue and inhibitor of topoisomerase I, topotecan, is currently also under clinical investigation. In a multicenter phase II study, the EORTC assessed the activity and toxicity of topotecan in pretreated SCLC patients (118). Topotecan was administered intravenously at a dose of 1.5 mg/m$^2$ during 5 consecutive days, every 3 weeks. Treatment was discontinued if disease progression or unacceptable toxicity was encountered. Two groups of patients were studied: "sensitive" patients responding to induction chemotherapy but relapsing after more than 3 months, and "refractory" patients not responding to primary treatment or relapsing within 3 months. In 45 sensitive patients 5 CR and 13 PR were observed (overall response rate 38%). In 49 resistant patients, 1 CR and 3 PR were achieved. Grade III–IV neutropenia was encountered in 78% of the courses. Grade III–IV thrombocytopenia and anemia was observed in 54% and 29% of the patients, respectively. Dose reduction was necessary in 10% of the courses, while postponement of the next cycle was required in 18% of the courses.

Finally, Taxol (paclitaxel) is under study in SCLC patients. Paclitaxel is the active constituent of the bark of the Pacific yew, *Taxus brevifolia*. The mechanism of action has been elucidated and is based on a unique disruptive effect on the dynamic equilibrium between tubulin heterodimers and microtubules (119). In vivo, paclitaxel has demonstrated promising response rates in platinum-resistant ovarian cancer (120), breast cancer (121), and NSCLC (122). In a phase II study, 36 previously untreated patients with ED received four courses of paclitaxel 250 mg/m$^2$ IV over 24 h every 3 weeks (123). A PR was achieved in 34% of the patients; no CRs were observed. Nineteen percent of the patients had SD. Induction (paclitaxel) and salvage therapy (PE) resulted in a response in 53% of the patients. The dose-limiting toxicity was leukopenia, grade IV, in 56% of the patients.

Despite promising results, administration of investigational drugs in previously untreated patients has been subject to debate (124,125). Two of the major concerns raised were a decrease in overall survival and a poor response rate to standard chemotherapy if the initially administered investigational drug proved to be ineffective (126, 127). If an investigational drug is ineffective, it is likely that the tumor mass during the period of administration and evaluation increases. Subsequently, so will the number of resistant tumor cells. As a consequence, selected patients groups with certain prognostic factors (elderly patients, patients with very extensive disease) were selected for trials with new drugs (104,106). In the study published by Blackstein et al., patients with ED not responding to epirubicin were treated with PE (111). Results were comparable with survival times after first-line CAV in a large randomized trial (28). In a randomized trial, Ettinger et al. (128) administered either CAV or a phase II drug (menogaril) to previously untreated patients with ED (n=86). Nonresponders received PE as salvage treatment. Treatment of responders varied. The overall response after CAV was significantly better than that after menogaril (42% vs. 5%, $P$=.0001). The estimated median survival was 45 and 37 weeks for CAV and menogaril, respectively ($P$=.28). The 1-year survival rates were 27.9% and 24.4% for CAV and menogaril, respectively. Because of the wide confidence intervals, the authors were unable to demonstrate whether the evaluation of a new drug in this selected patient group had adverse effects on survival. However, the data suggested that their study design did not negatively affect the overall survival of ED patients initially treated with an investigational phase II drug, despite the poor response rate. It was concluded that it was safe to conduct such a trial, provided that the following inclusion criteria were met: good performance score, absence of vena cava superior syndrome, and no liver involvement or other illnesses that would not allow salvage chemotherapy if needed.

From these data, several conclusions may be derived:

The use of investigational drugs in previously untreated patients should be limited to selected patients with ED, provided that a standard non-cross-resistant regimen is administered at time of progression.

In previously treated patients, the use of an investigational drug may be considered if the majority of the patients included in the study have responded to first-line chemotherapy and if the elapsed time between initial treatment and the use of an investigational drug is at least 3 months.

If one wants to test the potential non-cross-resistance to the previously given drugs, the new drugs should be given to patients with so-called resistant tumors within 3 months after the last chemotherapy course or at any time of progression during first-line chemotherapy.

## MULTIDRUG RESISTANCE (MDR) MODULATORS

With the advent of new tissue culture techniques, experimental techniques, and growth factors at the beginning of the 1980s, it became possible to establish lung cancer cell lines. In the past 15 years numerous mechanisms of resistance have been identified in (small cell) lung cancer cell lines. Unfortunately, the translation of such knowledge gathered in the laboratory has not yet led to improvement in the outcome of patients with resistant SCLC. Still, chemotherapy for relapsing or therapy-resistant SCLC is administered on a trial-and-error basis.

The development of rapid methods for in vitro drug sensitivity testing renewed interest in pretreatment chemosensitivity testing of patients with lung cancer. When fresh tumor cells are subjected to drug sensitivity testing in vitro, a major problem is assurance of enough viable tumor cells (129). A way to circumvent these problems is to establish cell lines before in vitro drug sensitivity testing. Gazdar et al. (130) found a nonsignificant difference between the response rate of relapsing SCLC patients with ED after cisplatin and etoposide therapy receiving an in vitro best regimen (n=16, RR 25%) or vincristine, doxorubicin, and cyclophosphamide (VAC) on an empirical basis (n=43, response rate 7%). Survival data for both subsets of patients after secondary therapy were not provided. Other investigators found significant differences in tumor chemosensitivity between pretreated patients in contrast to untreated SCLC patients, but in vitro/in vivo correlations were not provided (131–133). Apart from practical problems—one being the requirement for close cooperation between oncologists and research laboratory personnel—a disadvantage of this approach is that during the establishment of cell lines, selection of tumor cell populations may occur. Consequently, results of drug sensitivity testing may not apply to all tumor cell clones present in vivo, and associations with clinical response based on these results are apt to be poor (134). In conclusion, second-line therapy based on drug sensitivity testing in vitro, although theoretically attractive, has not found widespread acceptance.

A way to cope with some of these problems may be to investigate specific properties of tumor cells thought to be associated with drug resistance rather than looking at cell kill in vitro. The best-studied mechanism of resistance is P-glycoprotein (Pgp) mediated multidrug resistance. Pgp, a 180-kd membrane-bound glycoprotein, acts as an energy-dependent drug efflux pump. Overexpression or amplification of the *MDR*-1 gene leads to resistance of several structurally unrelated cytotoxic drugs in vitro by reducing intracellular levels of these drugs. Competition for the substrate of Pgp with noncytotoxic compounds such as calcium antagonists, antiestrogens, and cyclosporin has led to successful reversal of drug resistance both in vitro and in vivo. It is still not known whether the MDR phenotype is of clinical importance in drug-resistant SCLC. Depending on the method of detection of P-glycoprotein expression (e.g., mRNA levels and the use of various monoclonal antibodies), the reported incidence of MDR in clinical samples varies. However, this mechanism of resistance is likely to play a minor role in SCLC. Two studies have investigated modulation of Pgp-mediated multidrug resistance in SCLC. Milroy et al. randomized 226 untreated SCLC patients to four cycles of CAV chemotherapy with or without orally administered verapamil (480 mg daily × 5), an agent known to reverse MDR in vitro (135). Apart from more severe alopecia, no differences in toxicity were observed. Noteworthy, there was no difference in cardiac and hematological toxicity although lower white blood cell counts were found after the first course in the experimental arm, leading to chemotherapy dose reductions that were significant. Response rates and survival were equal in both study groups. Serum levels of verapamil found in 18 of 111 patients were well below those known to reverse MDR in vitro, which was, according to the authors, the major reason for lack of treatment effect in the verapamil arm. Figueredo and coworkers included 58 consecutive untreated SCLC patients with ED in a phase I/II study of verapamil and tamoxifen in addition to standard-dose AVE (doxorubicin, vincristine, and etoposide) (136). The dose of verapamil and tamoxifen could be escalated to 480 mg daily times 4 and 100 mg daily times 4, respectively. From the data presented, it is not clear why the phase I part of the study was finished at this dose level. No toxicity of the resistance modifiers was observed. Response rates and survival compared favorably to historical controls but remained in the usually reported range: 58% total response rate and median survival of 46 weeks. Pharmacokinetic data for neither resistance modifier were reported. It is important to note that in both studies no data on the Pgp status of the SCLC patients were provided. The absence of a positive effect from the addition of resistance modifiers to the chemotherapy used may therefore be the result of the absence of Pgp-positive tumors. At present, no studies are reported that randomize exclusively SCLC patients with enhanced Pgp expression in their tumors. Such a study is mandatory to assess the value, if any, of MDR1 modulation in SCLC.

Atypical drug resistance is mediated by topoisomerase IIa. This essential enzyme is the intracellular target for one of the most active single agents in SCLC—etoposide and its congener teniposide. Topoisomerase II reduces supercoiling of DNA induced by transcription and replication processes by the formation of transient double-strand DNA breaks. Topoisomerase II inhibitors stabilize these breaks, leading to cell death by an as yet unknown mechanism. In vitro resistance to topoisomerase inhibitors is caused by a decrease of cellular topoisomerase II content or mutations of the gene encoding for this protein. Currently, there are no data available on whether this phenomenon occurs in SCLC in vivo. The understanding of the mechanism of action of topoisomerase II inhibitors has led to a more rational use of these compounds in the clinic.

The translation of other resistance mechanisms found in vitro in lung cancer cell lines to clinical research has not yet taken place. Because it is likely that apart from MDR1 and topoisomerase II mediated resistance, a variety of other mechanisms— among others, increased DNA repair mechanisms, increased detoxifying capacity, and failure of tumor cells to undergo apoptotic death—simultaneously are activated, this area remains important for future clinical studies.

## CONCLUSIONS AND FUTURE PROSPECTS

On first sight, it may appear that little has changed in past decades concerning the clinical outcome in patients with SCLC. Although response rates after first-line chemotherapy are promising, this cannot be said about the overall survival rates. However, the results of the clinical trials and in vitro studies have provided us with more detailed information on the treatment of SCLC. Several attempts to cope with resistance that is already present or developing have been performed.

With regard to alternating chemotherapy regimens, it is still premature to reject the Goldie-Coldman hypothesis, as true non-cross-resistant regimens have yet to be developed. With an increasing knowledge of the basic mechanisms of drug resistance and the introduction of several new drugs in the treatment of SCLC, it seems not unreasonable to expect the development of such non-cross-resistant regimens in the not too far distant future. However, large randomized trials will be needed to demonstrate improved response rates compared to standard multidrug treatment. As a consequence, the Goldie-Coldman hypothesis needs testing in carefully designed phase II trials prior to such number- and time-consuming phase III studies.

Until now, there has been little evidence that resistance can be overcome by increased doses of chemotherapy in SCLC. However, it should be noted that studies of high-dose pulse chemotherapy, sometimes followed by ABMT, have been conducted with very few patients. Given the expected limited improvement in survival rates after intensified chemotherapy treatment, studies need large numbers of patients to demonstrate such an effect. Therefore, we first must try to demonstrate a dose-response relationship in SCLC by increasing the standard dose of chemotherapy, with the aid of rhCSFs if necessary. If such attempts fail, then studies with high-dose chemotherapy—followed by bone marrow reinfusion or the reinfusion of peripheral stem cells—seem to no avail.

Concerning second-line treatment, certainly one of the most important features is the recognition of two types of patients: relapsing and refractory. Patients relapsing more than 3 months after first-line treatment are considered candidates for re-treatment with the induction chemotherapy regimen. In contrast, patients relapsing within 3 months after induction chemotherapy, and those patients with progressive disease during initial treatment, nowadays are considered refractory patients and preferably should be treated with non-cross-resistant chemotherapeutic drugs.

On the application of new drugs in SCLC, several new insights have arisen. In previously treated patients who initially responded to first-line chemotherapy and who have been off treatment for more than 3 months, new chemotherapeutic drugs may demonstrate considerable activity. Furthermore, it has become clear that chemotherapeutic drugs demonstrating less than 20% overall response rates in previously treated patients may show considerable activity in chemotherapy-naive patients; therefore, such drugs should not be excluded from further investigational trials.

In previously untreated patients, it remains uncertain whether the use of an investigational drug, which may have poor response rates, will negatively effect the clinical outcome in patients due to development of resistance to standard drugs. Recently, some data suggested that this will not be the case. Until firm evidence is provided, the use of new investigational drugs as first-line treatment should be limited to selected patients with ED, provided that standard chemotherapy is given at any time of progression.

Finally, increasing knowledge of the basic mechanisms of drug resistance may provide us with new drugs that significantly enhance the survival time of patients with SCLC. Given the marginally increased survival time over the past 10 to 20 years, it appears logical to believe that such new drugs are really necessary to improve the clinical outcome of patients with SCLC significantly.

## REFERENCES

1. Ginsberg RJ, Kris MG, Armstrong JG. Cancer of the lung, non-small cell lung cancer. In: DeVita Jr VT, Hellman S, Rosenberg SA, eds. Cancer: Principles & Practice of Oncology. 4th ed. Philadelphia: Lippincott, 1993:673–722.
2. Ihde DC, Pass HI, Glatstein EJ. Cancer of the lung, small cell lung cancer. In: DeVita Jr VT, Hellman S, Rosenberg SA, eds. Cancer: Principles & Practice of Oncology. 4th ed. Philadelphia: Lippincott, 1993:723–758.
3. Wynder EL, Hoffmann D. Smoking and lung cancer: scientific challenges and opportunities. Cancer Res 1994; 54:5284–5295.
4. Gazdar AF, Giaccone G. The relevance of xenografts and in vitro drug sensitivity testing in human small cell lung cancer. Cancer Ther Contr 1991; 2:3–11.
5. Smit EF, Groen HJM, Timens W, de Boer WJ, Postmus PE. Surgical resection for small cell carcinoma of the lung: a retrospective study. Thorax 1994; 49:20–22.
6. Green RA, Humphrey E, Close H, Patno ME. Alkylating agents in bronchogenic carcinoma. Am J Med 1969; 46:516–525.

7. Giaccone G, Dalesio O, McVie GJ, et al. Maintenance chemotherapy in small-cell lung cancer: long-term results of a randomized trial. J Clin Oncol 1993; 11:1230–1240.

8. Ettinger DS, Finkelstein DM, Abeloff MD, Ruckdeschel JC, Aisner SC, Eggleston JC. A randomized comparison of standard chemotherapy versus alternating chemotherapy and maintenance versus no maintenance therapy for extensive-stage small-cell lung cancer: a phase III study of the Eastern Cooperative Oncology Group. J Clin Oncol 1990; 8:230–240.

9. Spiro SG, Souhami RL, Geddes DM, et al. Duration of chemotherapy in small cell lung cancer: a Cancer Research Campaign trial. Br J Cancer 1989; 59:578–583.

10. Bleehen NM, Fayers PM, Girling DJ, et al. Controlled trial of twelve versus six courses of chemotherapy in the treatment of small-cell lung cancer. Br J Cancer 1989; 59:584–590.

11. Maurer LH, Tulloh M, Weiss RB, et al. A randomized combined modality trial in small cell carcinoma of the lung. Comparison of combination chemotherapy-radiation therapy versus cyclophosphamide-radiation therapy effects of maintenance chemotherapy and prophylactic whole brain irradiation. Cancer 1980; 45:30–39.

12. Cullen M, Morgan D, Gregory W, et al. Maintenance chemotherapy for anaplastic small cell carcinima of the bronchus: a randomised, controlled trial. Cancer Chemother Pharmacol 1986; 17:157–160.

13. Lebeau B, Chastang Cl, Allard P, et al. Six vs twelve cycles for complete responders to chemotherapy in small cell lung cancer: definitive results of a randomized clinical trial. Eur Respir J 1992; 5:286–290.

14. Splinter TAW. Chemotherapy of SCLC: duration of treatment. Lung Cancer 1989; 5:186–195.

15. Berendsen HH, de Leij L, de Vries EGE, et al. Characterization of three small cell lung cancer cell lines established from one patient during longitudinal follow-up. Cancer Res 1988; 48:6891–6899.

16. de Vries EGE, Meijer C, Timmer-Bosscha H, et al. Resistance mechanisms in three human small cell lung cancer cell lines established from one patient during clinical follow-up. Cancer Res 1989; 47:4175–4178.

17. Berendsen HH, de Leij L, Postmus PE, et al. Small cell lung cancer. Tumor cell phenotype detected by monoclonal antibodies and response to chemotherapy. Chest 1987; 91 (suppl): 11–12.

18. Goldie JH, Coldman AJ, Gudauskas GA. Rationale for the use of alternating non-cross-resistant chemotherapy. Cancer Treat Rep 1982; 66:439–449.

19. Santoro A, Bonadonna G, Bonfante V, Valagussa P. Alternating drug combinations in the treatment of advanced Hodgkin's disease. N Engl J Med 1982; 306:770–775.

20. Viallet J, Ihde DC. Systemic therapy for small-cell lung cancer: old themes replayed, new ones awaited. J Clin Oncol 1989; 8:985–987.

21. Cohen MH, Ihde DC, Bunn PA, et al. Cyclic alternating combination chemotherapy for small cell bronchogenic carcinoma. Cancer Treat Rep 1979; 63:163–170.

22. Elliott JA, Osterlind K, Hansen HH. Cyclic alternating "non-cross resistant" chemotherapy in the management of small cell anaplastic carcinoma of the lung. Cancer Treat Rev 1984; 11:103–113.

23. Aisner J, Whitacre M, Van Echo DA, Wiernik PH. Combination chemotherapy for small cell carcinoma of the lung: continuous versus alternating non-cross-resistant combinations. Cancer Treat Rep 1982; 66:221–230.

24. Osterlind K, Sörensen S, Hansen HH, et al. Continuous versus alternating combination chemotherapy for advanced small cell carcinoma of the lung. Cancer Res 1983; 43:6085–6089.

25. Havemann K, Wolf M, Holle R, et al. Alternating versus sequential chemotherapy in small cell lung cancer. Cancer 1987; 59:1072–1082.

26. Goodman GE, Crowley JJ, Blasko JC, et al. Treatment of limited small-cell lung cancer with etoposide and cisplatin alternating with vincristine, doxorubicin, and cyclophosphamide ver-

sus concurrent etoposide, vincristine, doxorubicin, and cyclophosphamide and chest radiotherapy: a Southwest Oncology Group study. J Clin Oncol 1990; 8:39–47.

27.  Feld R, Evans WK, Coy P, et al. Canadian multicenter randomized trial comparing sequential and alternating administration of two non-cross-resistant chemotherapy combinations
in patients with limited small-cell carcinoma of the lung. J Clin Oncol 1987; 5:1401–1409.

28.  Evans WK, Feld R, Murray N, et al. Superiority of alternating non-cross-resistant chemotherapy in extensive small cell lung cancer. A multicenter, randomized clinical trial by the
National Cancer Institute of Canada. Ann Intern Med 1987; 107:451–458.

29.  Fukuoka M, Furuse K, Saijo N, et al. Randomized trial of cyclophosphamide, doxorubicin,
and vincristine versus cisplatin and etoposide versus alternation of these regimens in small-
cell lung cancer. J Natl Cancer Inst 1991; 83:855–861.

30.  Roth BJ, Johnson DH, Einhorn LH, et al. Randomized study of cyclophosphamide, doxorubicin, and vincristine versus etoposide and cisplatin versus alternation of these two regimens
in extensive small-cell lung cancer: a phase III trial of the Southeastern cancer study group.
J Clin Oncol 1992; 10:282–291.

31.  Evans WK, Shepherd FA, Feld R, et al. VP-16 and cisplatin as first-line therapy for small-cell
lung cancer. J Clin Oncol 1985; 3:1471–1479.

32.  Shepherd FA, Evans WK, MacCormick R, Feld R, Yau JC. Cyclophosphamide, doxorubicin, and vincristine in etoposide- and cisplatin-resistant small cell lung cancer. Cancer
Treat Rep 1987; 71:941–944.

33.  Wolf M, Pritsch M, Drings P, et al. Cyclic-alternating versus response-oriented chemotherapy in small-cell lung cancer: a German multicenter randomized trial of 321 patients. J Clin
Oncol 1991; 9:614–624.

34.  Postmus PE, Smit EF, Kirkpatrick A, Splinter TAW. Testing the possible non-cross resistance
of two equipotent combination chemotherapy regimens against small-cell lung cancer: a phase
II study of the EORTC lung cancer cooperative group. Eur J Cancer 1993; 29A:204–207.

35.  Postmus PE, Splinter TAW, Palmen FMLHG, et al. Comparison of two carboplatin-con-
taining regimens with standard chemotherapy for small cell lung cancer in a randomised
phase II study. Eur J Cancer 1992; 28:96–100.

36.  Scagliotti GV, Postmus PE, Splinter TAW, et al. EORTC phase III trial of standard versus
alternating chemotherapy in extensive disease small cell lung cancer. Proc Am Soc Clin
Oncol 1995; 14:384.

37.  DeVita VT. Dose-response is alive and well. J Clin Oncol 1986; 4:1157–1159.

38.  Frei III E, Canellos GP. Dose: a critical factor in cancer chemotherapy. Am J Med 1980;
69:585–594.

39.  Cohen MH, Creavenn PJ, Fossieck BE, et al. Intensive chemotherapy of small cell bronchogenic carcinoma. Cancer Treat Rep 1977; 61:349–354.

40.  Souhami RL, Harper PG, Linch D, et al. High-dose cyclophosphamide with autologous
marrow transplantation as initial treatment of small cell carcinoma of the bronchus. Cancer
Chemother Pharmacol 1982; 8:31–34.

41.  Farha P, Spitzer G, Valdivieso M, et al. High-dose chemotherapy and autologous bone
marrow transplantation for the treatment of small cell lung carcinoma. Cancer 1983; 52:
1351–1359.

42.  Johnson DH, DeLeo MJ, Hande KR, Wolff SN, Hainsworth JD, Greco FA. High-dose
induction chemotherapy with cyclophosphamide, etoposide, and cisplatin for extensive-
stage small-cell lung cancer. J Clin Oncol 1987; 5:703–709.

43.  O'Donnell MR, Ruckdeschel JC, Baxter D, McKneally MF, Caradonna R, Horton J. Intensive induction chemotherapy for small cell anaplastic carcinoma of the lung. Cancer Treat
Rep 1985; 69:571–575.

44.  Littlewood TJ, Bentley DP, Smith AP. High-dose etoposide with autologous bone marrow
transplantation as initial treatment of small cell lung cancer—a negative report. Eur J Respir
Dis 1986; 68:370–374.

45. Postmus PE, Mulder NH, De Vries-Hospers HG, et al. High-dose cyclophosphamide and high-dose VP16-213 for recurrent or refractory small cell lung cancer. A phase II study. Eur J Cancer Clin Oncol 1985; 21:1467–1470.
46. Norton L, Simon R. Tumor size, sensitivity to therapy, and design of treatment schedules. Cancer Treat Rep 1977; 61:1307–1317.
47. Humblet Y, Symann M, Bosly A, et al. Late intensification chemotherapy with autologous bone marrow transplantation in selected small-cell carcinoma of the lung: a randomized study. J Clin Oncol 1987; 5:1864–1873.
48. Ihde DC, Deisseroth AB, Lichter AS, et al. Late intensive combined modality therapy followed by autologous bone marrow infusion in extensive-stage small-cell lung cancer. J Clin Oncol 1986; 4:1443–1454.
49. Goodman GE, Crowley J, Livingston RB, Rivkin SE, Albain K, McCulloh JH. Treatment of limited small-cell lung cancer with concurrent etoposide/cisplatin and radiotherapy followed by intensification with high-dose cyclophosphamide: a Southwest Oncology Group study. J Clin Oncol 1991; 9:453–457.
50. Johnson DH, Einhorn LH, Birch R, et al. A randomized comparison of high-dose versus conventional-dose cyclophosphamide, doxorubicin, and vincristine for extensive-stage small-cell lung cancer: a phase III trial of the Southeastern Cancer Study Group. J Clin Oncol 1987; 5:1731–1738.
51. Figueredo AT, Hryniuk WM, Strautmanis I, Frank G, Rendell S. Co-trimoxazole prophylaxis during high-dose chemotherapy of small-cell lung cancer. J Clin Oncol 1985; 3:54–64.
52. Ihde DC, Mulshine JL, Kramer BS, et al. Prospective randomized comparison of high-dose and standard-dose etoposide and cisplatin chemotherapy in patients with extensive-stage small-cell lung cancer. J Clin Oncol 1994; 12:2022–2034.
53. Arriagada R, Le Chevalier T, Pignon J-P, et al. Initial chemotherapeutic doses and survival in patients with limited small-cell lung cancer. N Engl J Med 1993; 329:1848–1852.
54. Murray N, Shah A, Osoba D, et al. Intensive weekly chemotherapy for the treatment of extensive-stage small cell lung cancer. J Clin Oncol 1991; 9:1632–1638.
55. Miles DW, Earl HM, Souhami RL, et al. Intensive weekly chemotherapy for good-prognosis patients with small-cell lung cancer. J Clin Oncol 1991; 9:280–285.
56. Sculier JP, Paesmans M, Bureau G, et al. Multiple-drug weekly chemotherapy versus standard combination regimen in small-cell lung cancer: a phase III randomized study conducted by the European lung cancer working party. J Clin Oncol 1993; 11:1858–1865.
57. Miles DW, Souhami RL, Spiro SG, et al. A randomised trial comparing "standard" 3 weekly with weekly chemotherapy in patients with small cell lung cancer. Proc Am Soc Clin Oncol 1992; 11:289.
58. Gabrilove JL, Jakubowski A, Scher H, et al. Effect of granulocyte colony-stimulating factor on neutropenia and associated morbidity due to chemotherapy for transitional-cell carcinoma of the urothelium. N Engl J Med 1988; 318:1414–1422.
59. Antman KS, Griffin JD, Elias A, et al. Effect of recombinant human granulocyte-macrophage colony-stimulating factor on chemotherapy-induced myelosuppression. N Engl J Med 1988; 319:593–598.
60. Brandt SJ, Peters WP, Atwater SK, et al. Effect of recombinant human granulocyte-macrophage colony-stimulating factor on hematopoietic reconstitution after high-dose chemotherapy and autologous bone marrow transplantation. N Engl J Med 1988; 318:869–876.
61. Biesma B, Willemse PHB, Mulder NH, et al. Effects of interleukin-3 after chemotherapy for advanced ovarian cancer. Blood 1992; 80:1141–1148.
62. Bronchud MH, Scarffe JH, Thatcher N, et al. Phase I/II study of recombinant human granulocyte colony-stimulating factor in patients receiving intensive chemotherapy for small cell lung cancer. Br J Cancer 1987; 56:809–813.

63. Crawford J, Ozer H, Stoller R, et al. Reduction by granulocyte colony-stimulating factor of fever and neutropenia induced by chemotherapy in patients with small-cell lung cancer. N Engl J Med 1991; 325:164–170.

64. Trillet-Lenoir V, Green J, Manegold C, Von Pawel J, Gatzemeier U, Lebeau B, et al. Recombinant granulocyte colony stimulating factor reduces the infectious complications of cytotoxic chemotherapy. Eur J Cancer 1992; 29A:319–324.

65. Gatzemeyer U, European Lung Cancer Study Group. Recombinant G-CSF with combination chemotherapy in small cell lung cancer: results of a double blind, placebo controlled, randomised trial. Lung Cancer 1991; 7(suppl):131.

66. Kudoh S, Fukuoka M, Negoro S, et al. Weekly dose-intensive chemotherapy in patients with small cell lung cancer. Am J Clin Oncol 1992; 15:29–34.

67. Eguchi K, Etou H, Miyachi S, et al. A study of dose escalation of teniposide (VM-26) plus cisplatin (CDDP) with recombinant human granulocyte colony-stimulating factor (rhG-CSF) in patients with advanced small cell lung cancer. Eur J Cancer 1994; 30A:188–194.

68. Woll PJ,. Hodgetts J, Lomax L, Bildet F, Cour-Chabernaud V, Thatcher N. Can cytotoxic dose-intensity be increased by using granulocyte colony-stimulating factor? A randomized controlled trial of lenograstim in small-cell lung cancer. J Clin Oncol 1995; 13:652–659.

69. Miles DW, Fogarty O, Ash CM, et al. Received dose-intensity: a randomized trial of weekly chemotherapy with and without granulocyte colony-stimulating factor in small-cell lung cancer. J Clin Oncol 1994; 12:77–82.

70. Hamm J, Schiller JH, Cuffie C, et al. Dose-ranging study of recombinant human granulocyte-macrophage colony-stimulating factor in small-cell lung carcinoma. J Clin Oncol 1994; 12:2667–2676.

71. Gurney H, Anderson H, Radford J, et al. Infection risk in patients with small cell lung cancer receiving intensive chemotherapy and recombinant human granulocyte-macrophage colony-stimulating factor. Eur J Cancer 1992; 28:105–112.

72. Ardizzoni A, Sertoli MR, Corcione A, et al. Accelerated chemotherapy with or without GM-CSF for small cell lung cancer: a non-randomised pilot study. Eur J Cancer 1990; 26: 937–941.

73. Ardizzoni A, Venturini M, Crinò L, et al. High dose-intensity chemotherapy, with accelerated cyclophosphamide-doxorubicin-etoposide and granulocyte-macrophage colony stimulating factor, in the treatment of small cell lung cancer. Eur J Cancer 1993; 29A:687–692.

74. Paccagnella A, Favaretto A, Riccardi A, et al. Granulocyte-macrophage colony-stimulating factor increases dose intensity of chemotherapy in small cell lung cancer. Cancer 1993; 72: 697–706.

75. Shepherd FA, Goss PE. Phase I trial of granulocyte-macrophage colony-stimulating factor with high-dose cisplatin and etoposide for treatment of small-cell lung cancer: a study of the national Cancer Institute of Canada clinical trials group. J Natl Cancer Inst 1992; 84:59–60.

76. Bruno E, Briddell R, Hoffman R. Effect of recombinant and purified hematopoietic growth factors on human megakaryocyte colony formation. Exp Hematol 1988; 70:371–377.

77. Lu L, Briddell RA, Graham CD, Brandt JE, Bruno E, Hoffman R. Effect of recombinant and purified human haematopoietic growth factors on in vitro colony formation by enriched populations of human megakaryocyte progenitor cells. Br J Haematol 1988; 70:149–156.

78. Ganser A, Lindemann A, Seipelt G, et al. Effects of recombinant human interleukin-3 in patients with normal hematopoiesis and in patients with bone marrow failure. Blood 1990; 76:666–676.

79. Ganser A, Seipelt G, Lindemann A, et al. Effects of recombinant human interleukin-3 in patients with myelodysplastic syndromes. Blood 1990; 76:455–462.

80. Ganser A, Lindemann A, Seipelt G, et al. Effects of recombinant human interleukin-3 in aplastic anemia. Blood 1990; 76:1287–1292.

81. Kurzrock R, Talpaz M, Estrov Z, Rosenblum MG, Gutterman JU. Phase I study of recombinant human interleukin-3 in patients with bone marrow failure. J Clin Oncol 1991; 9:1241–1250.

82. Postmus PE, Gietema JA, Damsma O, et al. Effects of recombinant human interleukin-3 in patients with relapsed small-cell lung cancer treated with chemotherapy: a dose-finding study. J Clin Oncol 1992; 10:1131–1140.

83. D'Hondt V, Weynants P, Humblet Y, et al. Dose-dependent interleukin-3 stimulation of thrombopoiesis and neutropoiesis in patients with small-cell lung carcinoma before and following chemotherapy: a placebo-controlled randomized phase Ib study. J Clin Oncol 1993; 11:2063–2071.

84. de Campos E, Radford J, Steward W, et al. Clinical and in vitro effects of recombinant human erythropoietin in patients receiving intensive chemotherapy for small-cell lung cancer. J Clin Oncol 1995; 13:1623–1631.

85. Batist G, Ihde DC, Zabell A, et al. Small-cell carcinoma of lung: reinduction therapy after late relapse. Ann Intern Med 1983; 98:472–474.

86. Postmus PE, Berendsen HH, van Zandwijk N, Splinter TAW, Burghouts ThM, Bakker W. Retreatment with the induction regimen in small cell lung cancer relapsing after an initial response to short term chemotherapy. Eur J Cancer Clin Oncol 1987; 23:1409–1411.

87. Giaccone G, Ferrati P, Donadio M, Testore F, Calciati A. Reinduction chemotherapy in small cell lung cancer. Eur J Cancer Clin Oncol 1987; 23:1697–1699.

88. Collard Ph, Weynants P, Francis Ch, Rodenstein DO. Treatment of relapse of small cell lung cancer in selected patients with the initial combination chemotherapy carboplatin, etoposide, and epirubicin. Thorax 1992; 47:369–371.

89. Vincent M, Evans B, Smith I. First-line chemotherapy rechallenge after relapse in small cell lung cancer. Cancer Chemother Pharmacol 1988; 21:45–48.

90. Giaccone G, Donadio M, Bonardi G, Testore F, Calciati A. Teniposide in the treatment of small-cell lung cancer: the influence of prior chemotherapy. J Clin Oncol 1988; 6:1264–1270.

91. Andersen M, Kristjansen PEG, Hansen HH. Second-line chemotherapy in small cell lung cancer. Cancer Treat Rev 1990; 17:427–436.

92. Lopez JA, Mann J, Grapski RT, et al. Etoposide and cisplatin salvage chemotherapy for small cell lung cancer. Cancer Treat Rep 1985; 69:369–371.

93. Porter III LL, Johnson DH, Hainsworth JD, Hande KR, Greco FA. Cisplatin and etoposide combination chemotherapy for refractory small cell carcinoma of the lung. Cancer Treat Rep 1985; 69:479–481.

94. Evans WK, Osoba D, Feld R, Shepherd FA, Bazos MJ, DeBoer G, Etoposide (VP-16) and cisplatin: an effective treatment for relapse in small-cell lung cancer. J Clin Oncol 1985; 3: 65–71.

95. Sierocki JS, Hilaris BS, Hopfan S, et al. Cis-Dichlorodiammineplatinum(II) and VP-16-213: an active induction regimen for small cell carcinoma of the lung. Cancer Treat Rep 1979; 63:1593–1597.

96. Batist G, Carney DN, Cowan KH, et al. Etoposide (VP-16) and cisplatin in previously treated small-cell lung cancer: clinical trial and in vitro correlates. J Clin Oncol 1986; 4:982–986.

97. Bork E, Hansen M, Dombernowsky P, Hansen SW, Pedersen AG, Hansen HH. Teniposide (VM-26), an overlooked highly active agent in small-cell lung cancer. Results of a phase II trial in untreated patients. J Clin Oncol 1986; 4:524–527.

98. Woods RL, Fox RM, Tattersall MHN. Treatment of small cell bronchogenic carcinoma with VM-26. Cancer Treat Rep 1979; 63:2011–2013.

99. Creech RH, Tritchler D, Ettinger DS, et al. Phase II study of PALA, amsacrine, teniposide, and zinostatin in small cell lung carcinoma (EST 2579). Cancer Treat Rep 1984; 68:1183–1184.

100. Pedersen ASG, Bork E, Osterlind K, Dombernowsky P, Hansen HH. Phase II study of teniposide in small cell carcinoma of the lung. Cancer Treat Rep 1984; 68:1289–1291.

101. Wolff SN, Birch R, Sarma P, Greco FA. Randomized dose-response evaluation of etoposide in small cell carcinoma of the lung: a Southeastern Cancer Study Group trial. Cancer Treat Rep 1986; 70:583–587.
102. Evans WK, Feld R, Osoba D, Shepherd FA, Dill J, Deboer G. VP-16 alone and in combination with cisplatin in previously treated patients with small cell lung cancer. Cancer 1984; 53:1461–1466.
103. Harper PG, Dally MB, Geddes DM, Spiro SG, Smyth JF, Souhami RL. Epipodophyllotoxin (VP16-213) in small cell carcinoma of the bronchus resistant to initial combination chemotherapy. Cancer Chemother Pharmacol 1982; 7:179–180.
104. Smit EF, Carney DN, Harford P, Sleijfer DT, Postmus PE. A phase II study of oral etoposide in elderly patients with small cell lung cancer. Thorax 1989; 44:631–633.
105. Slevin ML, Clark PI, Joel SP, et al. A randomized trial to evaluate the effect of schedule on the activity of etoposide in small-cell lung cancer. J Clin Oncol 1989; 7:1333–1340.
106. Smith IE, Harland SJ, Robinson BA, et al. Carboplatin: a very active new cisplatin analog in the treatment of small cell lung cancer. Cancer Treat Rep 1985; 69:43–46.
107. Pallares C, Izquierdo MA, Paredes A, Sagarra AF, De Andrés L, López López JJ. A phase II trial of carboplatin in untreated patients with extensive stage small cell lung cancer. Cancer 1991; 68:40–43.
108. Jacobs RH, Bitran JD, Deutsch M, et al. Phase II study of carboplatin in previously untreated patients with metastatic small cell lung carcinoma. Cancer Treat Rep 1987; 71:311–312.
109. Groen HJM, Smit EF, Haaxma-Reiche H, Postmus PE. Carboplatin as second line treatment for recurrent or progressive brain metastases from small cell lung cancer. Eur J Cancer 1993; 29A:1696–1699.
110. Ettinger D, Finkelstein D, Ritch P, Bonomi P, Blum R. Randomized trial of single agents vs combination chemotherapy in extensive stage small cell lung cancer (SCLC). Proc Am Soc Clin Oncol 1992; 11:295.
111. Blackstein M, Eisenhauer FA, Wierzbicki R, Yoshida S. Epirubicin in extensive small-cell lung cancer: a phase II study in previously untreated patients: a National Cancer Institute of Canada clinical trials group study. J Clin Oncol 1990; 8:385–389.
112. Quoix EA, Giaccone G, Jassem J, et al. Epirubicin in previously untreated patients with small cell lung cancer: a phase II study by the EORTC lung cancer cooperative group. Eur J Cancer 1992; 28A:1667–1670.
113. Macchiarini P, Danesi R, Mariotti R, et al. Phase II study of high-dose epirubicin in untreated patients with small-cell lung cancer. Am J Clin Oncol 1990; 13:302–307.
114. Eckhardt S, Kolaric K, Vukas D, et al. Phase II study of 4′-epi-doxorubicin in patients with untreated, extensive small cell lung cancer. Med Oncol 1990; 7:19–23.
115. Banham SW, Henderson AF, Bicknell S, Hughes J, Milroy R, Monie RD. High dose epirubicin chemotherapy in untreated poorer prognosis small cell lung cancer. Resp Med 1990; 84:241–244.
116. Rosenthal M, Kefford R, Raghavan D, Stuart-Harris R. Epirubicin: a phase II study in recurrent small-cell lung cancer. Cancer Chemother Pharmacol 1991; 28:220–222.
117. Masuda N, Fukuoka M, Kusunoki Y, et al. CPT-11: a new derivative of camptothecin for the treatment of refractory or relapsed small-cell lung cancer. J Clin Oncol 1992; 10:1225–1229.
118. Ardizzoni A, Hansen HH, Dombernowsky P, et al. Topotecan, a new active drug in the second-line treatment of small-cell lung cancer (SCLC): a EORTC phase II study in patients with refractory and sensitive disease. Clin Oncol (in press).
119. Schiff PB, Horowitz SB. Tubulin: a target for chemotherapeutic agents. In: Sartorelli A, ed. Molecular Actions and Targets for Cancer Chemotherapeutic Agents. New York: Academic Press, 1981:483–507.

120. Einzig AI, Wiernik PH, Sasloff J, Runowicz CD, Goldberg GL. Phase II study and long-term follow-up of patients treated with Taxol for advanced ovarian adenocarcinoma. J Clin Oncol 1992; 10:1748–1753.

121. Holmes FA, Walters RS, Theriault RL, et al. Phase II trial of Taxol, an active drug in the treatment of metastatic breast cancer. J Natl Cancer Inst 1991; 83:1797–1805.

122. Murphy WK, Fossella FV, Winn RJ, et al. Phase II study of Taxol in patients with untreated advanced non-small-cell lung cancer. J Natl Cancer Inst 1993; 85:384–388.

123. Ettinger DS, Finkelstein DM, Sarma RP, Johnson DH. Phase II study of paclitaxel in patients with extensive-disease small-cell lung cancer: an Eastern Cooperative Oncology Group study. J Clin Oncol 1995; 13:1430–1435.

124. Cullen MH, Holton C, Stuart NSA. Evaluating new drugs as first treatment in patients with small-cell carcinoma: guidelines for an ethical approach with implications for other chemotherapy-sensitive tumours (letter). J Clin Oncol 1988; 6:1356–1357.

125. Aisner J. Identification of new drugs in small cell lung cancer: phase II agents first? Cancer Treat Rep 1987; 71:1131–1133.

126. Malik STA, Rayner H, Fletcher J, Slevin ML. Phase II trial of mitoxantrone as first-line chemotherapy for extensive small cell lung cancer. Cancer Treat Rep 1987; 71:1291–1292.

127. Cullen MH, Smith SR, Benfield GFA, Woodroffe CM. Testing new drugs in untreated small cell lung cancer may prejudice the results of standard treatment: a phase II study of oral idarubicin in extensive disease. Cancer Treat Rep 1987; 71:1227–1230.

128. Ettinger DS, Finkelstein DM, Abeloff MD, et al. Justification for evaluating new anticancer drugs in selected untreated patients with extensive-stage small-cell lung cancer: an Eastern Cooperative Oncology Group randomized study. J Natl Cancer Inst 1992; 84:1077–1084.

129. Smit EF, de Vries EGE, Meijer C, Mulder NH, Postmus PE. Limitations of the fast green assay for chemosensitivity testing in human lung cancer. Chest 1991; 100:1358–1364.

130. Gazdar AF, Steinberg SM, Russell EK, et al. Correlation of in vitro drug-sensitivity testing results with response to chemotherapy and survival in extensive-stage small cell lung cancer: a prospective clinical trial. J Natl Cancer Inst 1990; 82:117–124.

131. Carmichael J, Mitchell JB, DeGraff WG, et al. Chemosensitivity testing of human lung cancer cell lines using the MTT assay. Br J Cancer 1985; 57:540–547.

132. Cole SPC. Rapid chemosensitivity testing of human lung tumour cells using the MTT assay. Cancer Chemother Pharmacol 1986; 17:259–263.

133. Doyle LA. Mechanisms of drug resistance in human lung cancer cells. Semin Oncol 1993; 20:326–337.

134. Smit EF, de Vries EGE, de Ley LFHM, et al. In vitro response of human small cell lung cancer cell lines to chemotherapeutic drugs: no correlation with clinical data. Int J Cancer 1992; 51:72–78.

135. Milroy R, et al. A randomised clinical study of verapamil in addition to combination chemotherapy in small cell lung cancer. Br J Cancer 1993; 68:813–818.

136. Figueredo A, Arnold A, Goodyear M, et al. Addition of verapamil and tamoxifen to the initial chemotherapy of small cell lung cancer. A phase I/II study. Cancer 1990; 65:1895–1902.

# 2

## Multidrug Resistance in Small Cell Lung Cancer

**Shelagh E. L. Mirski and Susan P. C. Cole**
*Queen's University, Kingston, Ontario, Canada*

### INTRODUCTION

The refinement of combination chemotherapy over the past two decades has significantly increased the median survival time of patients with small cell lung cancer (SCLC) (1). However, acquired resistance to multiple drugs is a major obstacle to successful treatment, and despite improvements in survival, chemotherapy is responsible for the cure of less than 10% of patients. Drug resistance in the clinical setting encompasses a broad range of chemotherapeutic agents including alkylating agents, antimetabolites, platinum-containing drugs, hormones, and natural products. In experimental systems, multidrug resistance refers to a phenotype in which tumor cells exposed to a single agent acquire resistance to that agent and become cross-resistant to an extensive group of natural products and their semisynthetic congeners. However, the spectrum of drugs involved in experimental multidrug resistance is narrower than in clinical drug resistance. Nevertheless, the experimental phenotype is relevant in that it includes many clinically useful drugs such as VP-16 (etoposide), doxorubicin, mitoxantrone, and amsacrine (*m*AMSA).

Two types of multidrug resistance in experimental systems may be defined on the basis of the cellular drug targets involved. In the first, cells are resistant to natural-product drugs that interact with multiple cellular targets (e.g., DNA, membranes, cytoskeletal proteins). Such multidrug resistance is known to be conferred by at least two proteins, the extensively studied 170-kD P-glycoprotein (encoded by the *MDR*1 gene) (2–4) and the more recently discovered 190-kD multidrug resistance protein, MRP (encoded by the *MRP* gene) (5–9). A second type of multidrug resistance is mediated by alterations in a single cellular target, the nuclear enzyme topoisomerase II. This form of resistance includes a more limited range of natural product drugs than the multidrug resistance mediated by MRP or P-glycoprotein. In this chapter, multidrug resistance mediated both by increases in MRP and P-glycoprotein, and by alterations in topoisomerase II will be reviewed, with particular emphasis on the potential role of these mechanisms in the acquired drug resistance of SCLC.

## RESISTANCE TO NATURAL-PRODUCT DRUGS
## WITH MULTIPLE CELLULAR TARGETS

A large body of work over the past 20 years has culminated in the proof, by cDNA transfection experiments, that the increased expression of the 170-kD plasma membrane P-glycoprotein can confer a multidrug resistance phenotype by actively extruding drug from the cell (2,3). Many excellent reviews on this protein and its cognate genes have been published (10–20). Nevertheless, much remains to be learned about how this molecule mediates drug resistance.

Despite the frequency with which P-glycoprotein is overexpressed in multidrug-resistant cell lines, there are many cell lines that display a multidrug resistance phenotype but do not overexpress P-glycoprotein (21–27). Interestingly, a significant proportion of the non–P-glycoprotein resistant cell lines are derived from small cell and non–small cell lung tumors (21,24,25,28–30). Non–P-glycoprotein drug resistance has been attributed to multifactorial processes (31–33). However, in 1992 the 6.5-kb mRNA encoding the 190-kD integral membrane phosphoglycoprotein MRP was described (5), which, when transfected into previously sensitive cells, produced resistance to multiple chemotherapeutic agents (7,34). These studies established that, like P-glycoprotein, MRP overexpression was sufficient to cause multidrug resistance to anthracyclines, *vinca* alkaloids, and epipodophyllotoxins. In addition, MRP conferred resistance to arsenical and antimonial oxyanions (34).

The study of MRP is in its infancy and so, compared to P-glycoprotein, relatively little is known at present about its structure and function. Because so much is known about P-glycoprotein, it is instructive to compare and contrast these two molecules, which are each capable of conferring multidrug resistance. However, it is important to bear in mind that despite some similarities in the drug-resistance phenotypes associated with their overexpression, these two molecules differ significantly in their structure, physiological function, and possibly their modes of action.

### Multidrug Resistance and the ATP-Binding
### Cassette Superfamily

Both P-glycoprotein and MRP are members of the ATP-binding cassette (ABC) superfamily of transport proteins that are involved in the transport of molecules or ions across cellular membranes (5,35). All members of the ABC superfamily contain a multi-spanning transmembrane region and a cytoplasmic nucleotide (ATP)-binding domain (36). The fact that MRP and P-glycoprotein are both members of this family does not imply that they function in a similar manner, because substrates for the ABC proteins are extremely varied. In mammalian systems alone, substrates range from simple ions such as chloride transported by the cystic fibrosis transmembrane conductance regulator (CFTR) (37,38) to relatively complex peptides conveyed by the TAP1 and TAP2 transporters involved in antigen processing (39–42).

### *P-Glycoprotein*

The P-glycoproteins make up a relatively small gene family within the ABC superfamily of transport proteins. There are two human P-glycoproteins, encoded by the *MDR*1 and *MDR*3 (also known as *MDR*2) (43) genes, which have been mapped to chromosome 7 on band q21.1 (44,45). Only the product of the *MDR*1 gene has been shown to confer drug resistance (2). Despite the 80% sequence similarity of the mRNAs encoded by the two human *MDR* genes, there is no evidence that the *MDR*3 gene product can transport cytotoxic drugs; transfection does not confer resistance; and it is rarely detected in multidrug resistant cell lines (46,47). Knowledge of the structure and organization of the analogous mouse P-glycoprotein genes has allowed the generation of gene "knock-out" mice that have provided in vivo models for elucidating the physiological functions of these proteins. Mice in which the *mdr*2 gene (analogous to human *MDR*3) has been knocked out display a defect in phosphatidylcholine transport in hepatocanalicular membranes, suggesting that this P-glycoprotein isoform functions to transport phospholipid into bile (48,49). Mice in which the *mdr*1a (analogous to human *MDR*1) has been knocked out exhibit increased neurosensitivity, indicating a role for this P-glycoprotein isoform in maintaining the blood-brain barrier (50).

A model of P-glycoprotein topology has been derived from computer-assisted hydropathy and consensus motif analyses of its nucleotide and deduced amino acid sequences (Fig. 1) (35,51–56). P-glycoprotein is most likely composed of two very similar halves, each containing a nucleotide-binding domain (NBD), connected by a linker sequence. This tandemly duplicated structure contains 12 transmembrane (TM) segments organized in a "6 + 6" configuration. The validity of this structural model has been examined by confirming the predicted cytoplasmic or extracellular location of the epitopes of several different P-glycoprotein–specific monoclonal antibodies (MAbs) (57–59) and by analyzing the susceptibility of in vitro synthesized P-glycoprotein peptides in membranes to protease digestion or glycosylation (60–62). These studies indicate that the peptide sequences linking the predicted TM1 and TM2, and linking TM7 and TM8, are extracellular. However, the data suggest that in a significant proportion of newly synthesized P-glycoprotein molecules, some of the predicted TM segments are not integrated into the membrane. In contrast to the conventional model of P-glycoprotein (Fig. 1), an alternate model has been proposed in which the two halves are mirror images of each other, and the peptides linking TM4 and TM5, and TM8 and TM9, are extracellular (61,62). In addition, it has recently been proposed that TM7 may be two transmembrane segments, leading to a significant change in the model of the COOH-terminal half of P-glycoprotein (63). Which model best reflects the topology of the majority of P-glycoprotein in the plasma membrane is still undetermined. The functional form of P-glycoprotein in its native state is not known but it may occur as dimers in the plasma membrane (59,64) or in several oligomeric forms (65). Whether or not P-glycoprotein oligomer formation is important for its activity is unknown.

*MRP*

The human *MRP* gene has been mapped to chromosome 16 at band p13.1 (5,66,67). The predicted sequence and domain organization of MRP indicates that, like P-glycoprotein, it belongs to the ABC transporter superfamily (5). However, MRP shares less than 15% amino acid identity with human P-glycoprotein and this similarity occurs almost exclusively within the highly conserved nucleotide binding domains, NBD1 and NBD2. Somewhat unexpectedly, MRP shares much greater homology with other members of the ABC superfamily (5,68), which do not confer resistance to anticancer drugs: CFTR (19% identity), which mediates chloride conductance (37); the sulfonylurea receptor SUR (29%), believed to be involved in insulin secretion (69); the leishmania *ltpgpA* (32%), which confers resistance to arsenic and antimony oxyanions (70,71); and the yeast *YCF1* (43%), which mediates cadmium resistance (68).

P-glycoprotein

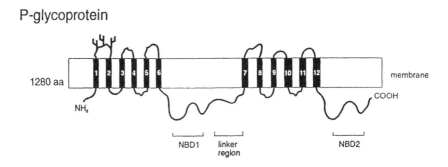

MRP

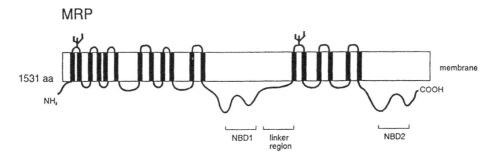

**Figure 1** Predicted secondary structure of human P-glycoprotein and MRP. P-glycoprotein and MRP both have the domain organization common to many human ATP-binding cassette transport proteins—they contain a hydrophobic membrane-spanning domain followed by a hydrophilic cytoplasmic nucleotide-binding domain (NBD). P-glycoprotein is a 170-kD plasma membrane protein of 1280 amino acids, which is encoded by the *MDR*1 gene located on chromosome 7. P-glycoprotein is symmetrically duplicated, and its 12 transmembrane (TM) segments are probably in a "6+6" configuration as shown. MRP is a 190-kD integral membrane protein of 1531 amino acids, which is encoded by the *MRP* gene located on chromosome 16. In contrast to P-glycoprotein, the two halves of the MRP molecule are not symmetrically duplicated. Hydropathy analyses and comparisons of human and murine MRP and other members of a subfamily of ABC proteins indicate that the TM segments of MRP may be in a "11–12+6" configuration as shown (unpublished observations). Potential N-glycosylation sites predicted to be on the noncytoplasmic side of a membrane are indicated.

The deduced amino acid sequence of MRP suggested that it was an ATP-binding, integral membrane N-glycosylated phosphoprotein with a minimum molecular weight of 171 kD. Experimental evidence supporting these predicted structural features has been obtained (8,72,73). In marked contrast to the 6 + 6 topological model of P-glycoprotein, MRP was originally predicted to contain eight transmembrane domains in the NH$_2$-proximal half of the molecule and four in the COOH-proximal half (Fig. 1) (5,72). Recently, a different model—with 11 to 12 transmembrane segments in the NH$_2$-proximal half and six in the COOH-proximal half—has been suggested by comparative analyses of the deduced amino acid sequences of the human and murine *MRP* mRNAs (B.D. Stride et al., unpublished observations). Elucidation of the correct topology of MRP in vivo will require experimental studies similar to those carried out previously with P-glycoprotein.

## Mechanisms of Overexpression of P-glycoprotein and MRP

Elevated protein levels resulting from increased gene expression may be achieved by a number of mechanisms, including gene amplification, transcriptional activation, or a post-transcriptional event such as stabilization of the mRNA or increased translational efficiency. *MDR*1 gene amplification is rarely observed in human cancers (30,74), suggesting that other mechanisms of increased gene expression may be important clinically. In experimental systems, induction of *MDR*1 mRNA expression has been observed in response to cytotoxic drugs (75–78), environmental stresses such as heat shock (79), serum deprivation (80), and UV irradiation (77). *MDR*1 expression has also been reported to be influenced by genes involved in cell proliferation or apoptosis, such as c-Ha-*ras*, *p53*, and c-*raf* (81–83). However, only a few of the endogenous *trans*-activating factors that interact with the *cis*-regulatory elements of the *MDR*1 proximal promoter have been identified or characterized (84–88). In contrast to *MDR*1, *MRP* is amplified in many drug-selected cell lines (5,66,89 and others). The repetitive sequences flanking *MRP* might contribute to the ease with which this gene is amplified (67,90). Increased MRP expression has occasionally been observed in the absence of gene amplification (5,90,91), suggesting that transcriptional regulation may also be important. The 5' end of the human *MRP* gene has recently been isolated, sequenced, and partially characterized (91,92), and the factors involved in *MRP* gene regulation are currently under investigation.

## Transport Functions of P-glycoprotein and MRP

Reduced drug accumulation and enhanced drug efflux are invariably found in cell lines that overexpress P-glycoprotein but less consistently in cell lines that overexpress MRP (93–98). Reduced drug accumulation can be demonstrated using relatively simple methodology that is based on assumptions that may not always be valid (11,99,100). Processes such as drug binding, sequestration, and metabolism (which will vary with each individual drug) complicate the study of drug transport in intact cells. All of these processes can influence the intracellular "free" drug concentration, which in turn will influence rates of drug efflux. In most cases, the degree of reduced accumulation is far less than the degree of resistance observed and the reason for this discrepancy is not fully understood. The methods commonly used to measure drug accumulation and efflux presume that the intracellular distribution of drug in resistant and sensitive cells is the same with respect to location and exchangeability (11). They also assume that active transport is mediated exclusively by the plasma membrane. Particularly in the case of MRP-mediated drug resistance, neither assumption may be valid. Studies with membrane vesicles from MRP-overexpressing cells have not yet demonstrated active transport of drugs, in contrast to membrane vesicles containing P-glycoprotein (see below). In some cells that overexpress either P-glycoprotein or MRP, altered intracellular distribution of a fluorescent anthracycline has been observed (101–103). This observation suggests that MRP or P-glycoprotein participates in a process that sequesters drug away from its nuclear target, although direct experimental evidence that these proteins are involved is lacking. Altered intracellular drug distribution may be responsible for some of the apparent discrepancy between levels of resistance and alterations in total cellular drug accumulation (104,105).

*ATP-Dependent Drug Transport by P-glycoprotein and MRP*

P-glycoprotein is believed to mediate multidrug resistance by binding cytotoxic drugs and exporting them to the outside of the cell in an ATP-dependent process. Biochemical evidence that supports this mode of action includes the labeling of P-glycoprotein with analogues of cytotoxic drugs (106–11), chemosensitizing agents (111–118), and ATP (119–121). Furthermore, ATP-dependent drug binding and transport have been measured in membrane vesicles from cells that overexpress P-glycoprotein (122–125) and in reconstituted systems using an artificial lipid bilayer and partially purified (126,127) or purified (128–131) P-glycoprotein. The question as to whether drug transport is directly coupled to ATP hydrolysis by P-glycoprotein still remains unsettled (131). Similarly, reduced drug accumulation in cells transfected with MRP cDNA has been shown to be ATP-dependent (34,132). MRP has also been shown to bind ATP (72), although it has not yet been formally demonstrated that it is capable of ATP hydrolysis.

Although all cells that overexpress P-glycoprotein are multidrug resistant, the relative levels of resistance to individual cytotoxic drugs can be highly variable. When P-glycoprotein overexpression is induced by in vitro drug selection, the cell line is frequently, but not always, most resistant to the agent used in selection. However, the cross-resistance pattern of the resulting cell line cannot be predicted (27), and it has been postulated that this is caused by the presence of P-glycoprotein mutants that vary in their substrate preferences. Photoaffinity labeling studies with analogues of cytotoxic drugs indicate that there is a direct interaction of P-glycoprotein with its substrates and there is considerable evidence that the predicted membrane-spanning segments (Fig. 1) are important in substrate binding (36). Spontaneous (133–135) and site-directed (136,137) mutations within or in close proximity to these transmembrane regions appear to modulate the activity and substrate specificity of P-glycoprotein. The functional importance of specific amino acids in the predicted cytoplasmic loops of P-glycoprotein (138) and of a small segment in the first intracytoplasmic loop between TM2 and TM3 (139) have also been demonstrated. Thus the substrate preference of P-glycoprotein appears to be the result of many interacting structural determinants, only some of which have been identified.

Precisely how MRP confers multidrug resistance is not known. Although MRP overexpression is usually associated with reduced drug accumulation and ATP-dependent enhanced drug efflux (8,94,97,98,140,141), this association is less consistent than it is with the overexpression of P-glycoprotein (93–98). However, drug accumulation is reduced in an ATP-dependent manner in HeLa cells transfected with MRP cDNA expression vectors, and the rate of drug efflux is enhanced (34,72). As with P-glycoprotein–expressing cell lines, an altered intracellular distribution of fluorescent anthracyclines has been observed in many drug-selected MRP-overexpressing cell lines (5,32, 98,140–143), suggesting that MRP may participate, directly or indirectly, in sequestering drugs away from their intracellular targets (5). Many pharmacokinetic studies have been carried out in drug-selected cell lines that express more than one mechanism of resistance, making comparisons among different cell lines problematic. Furthermore, the predominant location of MRP has been reported to be the endoplasmic reticulum in some cell lines (144) but the plasma membrane in others (72,145). Differences in the localization of MRP might explain part of the variation in drug transport because it is possible that in cell lines with significant levels of MRP on intracellular membranes, the protein functions to sequester drugs, whereas MRP on the plasma membrane might be expected to function in the export of drugs from the cell. The factors governing the apparent variation in membrane localization of MRP remain to be elucidated but likely involve some membrane-trafficking processes.

To establish whether MRP functions as a drug efflux pump analogous to P-glycoprotein, purification and reconstitution studies are required. At present, several observations suggest that the mechanism of MRP function differs from that of P-glycoprotein in some respects. For example, significant ATP-dependent transport of unmodified drugs has not yet been demonstrated in membrane vesicles from cells that overexpress MRP (146) (Loe et al., unpublished results). Furthermore, in contrast to cell lines that overexpress P-glycoprotein, membrane proteins of a doxorubicin-selected leukemia cell line (which is now known to overexpress MRP), could not be labeled with photoaffinity analogues of vinblastine (8,147). Similarly, membranes from the highly MRP-expressing H69AR cell line could not be labeled with a photoaffinity analogue of doxorubicin (72). Thus, there is as yet no direct evidence that MRP functions in the same fashion as P-glycoprotein, and much work remains to be done to understand precisely how MRP confers resistance.

*Physiological Functions of P-glycoprotein and MRP*

Examination of the normal tissue distribution of P-glycoprotein has provided clues to its normal physiological function. Immunohistochemical studies have revealed that P-glycoprotein is frequently localized to the epical or luminal regions of cells in such tissues as jejunum and colon (58,148), hepatocytes (148), pancreatic small ductule epithelia (148), renal proximal tubular epithelia (148–151), adult adrenal cortex (58,150, 152), and in endothelial cells of the blood-brain and other blood-tissue barrier sites (151,153,154). Studies of P-glycoprotein expression in the placenta (150,155) and in peripheral blood and bone marrow cells (150,156–161) appear contradictory, probably because of different methodologies used for measuring *MDR*1 expression. Earlier studies of the tissue distribution of P-glycoprotein suggested that it might have a physiological role in the maintenance of blood-tissue barriers, in the transport of steroids, and/or in the secretion of both metabolites and toxic substances for excretion from the body. Although gene knock-out experiments (see above) suggest that P-glycoprotein probably does function in this manner, the endogenous physiological substrates of P-glycoprotein remain to be identified.

The physiological function of MRP is beginning to be investigated. Initial reports indicate that human and murine *MRP* mRNAs share a markedly different pattern of tissue expression than P-glycoprotein, suggesting that MRP has a different physiological function. *MRP* mRNA is expressed at low levels in many tissues but at a somewhat higher level in lung, testes, and muscle (5,89,162) (unpublished observations). Immunohistochemical studies are in progress that, by identifying the normal cell types in which MRP is expressed, are expected to suggest physiological functions for MRP. It has recently been observed that in membrane vesicle systems, MRP is an ATP-dependent transporter of the leukotriene $C_4$ (146,163,164) and that an inhibitor of leukotriene $C_4$ transport can suppress the photoaffinity binding of leukotriene $C_4$ to MRP (163).

Leukotriene $C_4$ is an arachidonic acid derivative involved in controlling vascular permeability and smooth muscle contraction and may play a role in the pathogenesis of asthma (164). Because leukotriene $C_4$ is a glutathione conjugate, it has been speculated that MRP may be the so-called "GS-X pump" responsible for glutathione conjugate export (165,166) as well as an oxyanion transporter (167). However, there is little evidence that conjugation to glutathione or other endogenous small molecules is an important pathway for biotransformation of chemotherapeutic agents to which MRP confers resistance, particularly the anthracycline antibiotics (168). Investigations are ongoing to identify other endogenous substrates of MRP. In addition, recent cloning of the murine *MRP* mRNA (unpublished observations) will facilitate the generation of mice in which the *MRP* gene has been "knocked-out," an approach that should further our understanding of the normal physiological function(s) of MRP.

### Post-Translational Modifications of P-glycoprotein and MRP

P-glycoprotein and MRP are both modified post-translationally by glycosylation and phosphorylation (72,73). Studies using inhibitors of glycosylation (169,170), or using site-directed mutagenesis to construct *N*-glycosylation deficient P-glycoprotein mutants (171), indicate that drug transport by P-glycoprotein is unaffected by *N*-glycosylation although this has been disputed recently (172). Furthermore, non-glycosylated human P-glycoprotein expressed in insect cells (173), in bacteria (174), and in yeast (175) is fully functional. However, it remains possible that *N*-glycosylation of P-glycoprotein may have effects on its subcellular compartmentalization (173), correct folding, and/or susceptibility to proteolytic degradation (176).

Although P-glycoproteins are known to be phosphorylated in vivo (177–182), it has not been firmly established whether their function or activity is regulated by phosphorylation/dephosphorylation (183–185). Moreover, the specific protein kinases responsible for the in vivo phosphorylation of P-glycoprotein have not been unequivocally identified. However, recent transfection-based studies have provided more direct evidence that phosphorylation by protein kinase isoform $C\alpha$ (186,187), but not isoform $C\gamma$ (188), may be involved in augmenting P-glycoprotein–mediated drug resistance. P-glycoprotein may also be regulated by other kinases that have been studied to a lesser degree (189). Human P-glycoprotein appears to be phosphorylated by protein kinase C on serine residues clustered in the linker or connector region located between the two halves of the molecule (190). Thus it has been suggested that the linker region may be a regulatory domain of P-glycoprotein function (190,191), analogous to the regulatory ("R") domain in CFTR (37,192–194). This idea is attractive, but there is no direct evidence to support this hypothesis at present.

MRP is also *N*-glycosylated with complex oligosaccharides, and when deglycosylated, the electrophoretic mobility of the 190-kD protein is reduced to 170 kD, the minimum molecular weight predicted from its cDNA sequence (8,72). MRP is phosphorylated in vivo, primarily on serine residues, but the kinases responsible are unknown (72,73). Treatment of the drug-selected MRP-overexpressing HL60/Adr cells with protein kinase C inhibitors has been reported to alter the rates of drug accumulation and efflux such that they resemble those of the sensitive parent cells (73). However, these data must be interpreted with caution because of the broad, nonspecific effects of the inhibitors used (185) and because these studies were carried out with drug-selected rather than MRP-transfected cells. What significance post-translational modifications of MRP have with respect to its function remains to be determined.

### Detection of P-glycoprotein and MRP

Methods of determining the levels of P-glycoprotein and MRP in cell lines and clinical samples are described below. These methods have been used widely to detect the presence of P-glycoprotein in tumors in order that this protein can be evaluated as a prognostic indicator and its potential as a therapeutic target for chemosensitizing agents. Because the discovery of MRP is more recent, there are only a limited number of studies measuring levels of this protein in clinical samples (9). Despite considerable expenditure of time and resources, a consensus as to the most useful, relevant, and standardized method of P-glycoprotein measurement has still not been reached. Nevertheless, as discussed below, there have been lessons learned from the large number of clinical investigations of P-glycoprotein that should facilitate similar studies of MRP.

### Measurement of MDR1 and MRP mRNA

In clinical tumor samples and in human tumor cell lines, increased *MDR*1 expression is frequently observed in the absence of, or with only minimal, gene amplification. Consequently, measurement of *MDR*1 mRNA levels, rather than gene amplification, is a more appropriate method of detection. In contrast, increased MRP expression is frequently associated with gene amplification, at least in drug-selected cell lines. Nevertheless, the measurement of *MRP* mRNA levels is still important because increased expression caused by regulatory changes in the transcription or stability of the mRNA may yet prove to be as important for this gene as it is for *MDR*1. Levels of expression of *MDR*1 or *MRP* mRNA in clinical samples have been measured primarily using one of three techniques: slot blot or Northern blot analysis (5,195); RNAse protection assay (89,196,197); or primer-directed reverse transcription (RT) of mRNA into cDNA, followed by polymerase chain reaction (RT-PCR) (158,162,197–212). The major disadvantage of these techniques is that they do not indicate the heterogeneity of expression within a tissue or tumor. mRNA can also be measured in situ (213) and individual cells expressing the mRNA identified, but this technique is labor-intensive and results are difficult to quantify, precluding it from routine laboratory use. RT-PCR has become a very popular method because it is relatively simple, does not require expensive equipment, and offers the greatest sensitivity and therefore requires the least amount of cells or tissue. However, the extreme sensitivity of PCR results in difficulties in accurate quantification of mRNA levels and requires that strict controls be included to eliminate false positives and negatives. The results of many published studies can only be considered semiquantitative at best. Some reports of *MDR*1 or *MRP* expression using an RT-PCR assay are based on normalization to the mRNA levels of a co-amplified constitutively expressed, so-called "housekeeping" gene (e.g., $\beta_2$-microglobulin) (200,201). This approach presumes that the mRNA level of the housekeeping gene is constant among the samples being tested, which may not always be the case. For example, levels of $\beta_2$-microglobulin mRNA would probably not be the best choice with which to normalize *MRP* or *MDR*1 mRNA levels in SCLC cells because expression of this molecule is usually low in this tumor type (214). Recently, more rigorous quantitative RT-PCR methods have been developed using in vitro generated RNA molecules (199,215,216) or competitive DNA fragments (217) as internal standards. Because of their greater reliability, these methods are certain to be used more frequently in future. For example, the challenge of accurately quantitating MRP using RT-PCR has been met by developing a technique based on titration of a competitive DNA fragment that co-amplifies with the target cDNA (218).

*Immunological Measurement of P-glycoprotein and MRP*

A good correlation often exists between mRNA and protein levels in cultured cells, but exceptions have been reported. Therefore, the direct measurement of protein using immunological methods may be a more reliable indicator of P-glycoprotein or MRP levels (219–223). However, concerns about this approach include its insensitivity compared to methods based on measurement of mRNA, problems with antibody specificity (224–226), and inadequately controlled experiments. Nevertheless, immunohistochemical methods have the advantage of being readily adaptable to most laboratories and efforts are under way to develop standardized experimental protocols for detection of both MRP and P-glycoprotein.

The numerous specific polyclonal antibodies (57,227,228) and monoclonal antibodies (MoAbs) (229–239) against P-glycoprotein have played a critical role in furthering our knowledge of the biology of P-glycoprotein and its clinical relevance (220,221, 238–240 and others). Many of the P-glycoprotein–specific MoAbs (Table 1) have been particularly useful because of their commercial availability and because polyclonal antisera are unsuitable for many experimental applications. A number of studies have been published comparing the performance of P-glycoprotein–specific MoAbs in flow cytometric and immunohistochemical assays (223,224,241–243).

P-glycoprotein–specific MoAbs or their derivatives (244–246) that are directed against cell surface epitopes have been considered as potential immunotherapeutic agents. MoAbs may be cytotoxic or growth inhibitory by themselves (235,236) or participate in complement-dependent or antibody-dependent cell-mediated cytotoxicity (233,237,247–249). For example, MoAbs MRK-16, 4E3, and UIC2 can reverse resistance by interfering with P-glycoprotein function (233–235,250,251). In addition, toxic agents have been targeted at P-glycoprotein–expressing cells by conjugation to MoAb MRK-16 (252,253).

**Table 1**  Murine Monoclonal Antibodies Specific for Human P-glycoprotein or MRP

| Name | Isotype | Epitope | Ref. |
|------|---------|---------|------|
| P-glycoprotein specific | | | |
|   C219 | $IgG_{2a}$ | Linear cytoplasmic | 58, 230 |
|   C494 | $IgG_{2a}$ | Linear cytoplasmic | 58, 226, 230 |
|   MRK-16 | $IgG_{2a}$ | Conformation-dependent extracellular | 59, 505 |
|   JSB-1 | $IgG_1$ | Cytoplasmic | 232 |
|   UIC-2 | $IgG_{2a}$ | Conformation-dependent extracellular | 233 |
|   HYB-241 | $IgG_1$ | Conformation-dependent extracellular | 229, 235 |
| MRP specific | | | |
|   QCRL-1 | $IgG_1$ | Linear cytoplasmic | 255 |
|   QCRL-2 | $IgG_{2b}$ | Conformation-dependent cytoplasmic | 255 |
|   QCRL-3 | $IgG_{2a}$ | Conformation-dependent cytoplasmic | 255 |
|   QCRL-4 | $IgG_1$ | Conformation-dependent cytoplasmic | 255 |
|   MRPm6 | $IgG_1$ | Linear cytoplasmic | 145 |

Direct measurement of MRP using immunological methods is desirable for the same reasons as listed above for P-glycoprotein, but also because there is some indication that levels of *MRP* mRNA may not always correlate well with levels of the 190-kD protein (7). Polyclonal antisera raised against MRP-derived synthetic peptides were used in early studies of MRP (7,8,34,72,254) and, more recently, MRP-specific MoAbs have been generated (145,255) that promise to be extremely useful in future investigations (Table 2). None of these MoAbs are against extracellular epitopes, so they cannot be used in flow cytometric studies of live cells and are not obvious candidates for immunotherapeutic agents. The currently available MRP-specific MoAbs are directed against both linear and conformational epitopes, and some are sensitive enough to detect the very low levels of MRP in peripheral blood mononuclear cells (Almquist et al., unpublished).

**Table 2** Resistance Mechanisms in Small Cell Lung Cancer Cell Lines Selected in Natural Product Chemotherapeutic Agents

| Cell line | Selecting drug | P-glycoprotein overexpression | MRP overexpression | Other resistance mechanisms | Laboratory of origin (Refs.) |
|---|---|---|---|---|---|
| H69AR | DOX | No | Yes | Reduced topo IIα and β | Cole (21,31,95, 454,506,507) |
| GLC4/ADR | DOX | No | Yes | Topo II | deVries (89,508) |
| POGB/DX | DOX | No | Yes | Topo II | Zunino (273,286) |
| N592/DX | DOX | No | No | Possibly topo II | Zunino (29) |
| H69/LX4 | DOX | Yes | No | Not topo II | Twentyman (281, 509) |
| POVD/DX | DOX | Yes | No | Topo II | Zunino (286) |
| SBC-3/ADM100 | DOX | Yes | Unk | Decreased topo II | Kiura (284) |
| H69/DAU | DNR | Yes | No | Unk | Jensen (283) |
| H209/V6 | VP-16 | No | No | Topo IIα localization mutant and decreased levels | Cole (382, 466, 467) |
| H69/VP | VP-16 | Yes | Unk | Topo II | Saijo (282) |
| H69/VP | VP-16 | Yes | Yes | Unk | Jensen/Sehested (280,287) |
| VPR-2 | VP-16 | Yes | Unk | Possibly topo II | Glisson (285) |
| SBC-3/ETP | VP-16 | Yes | Unk | Decreased topo II | Kiura (284) |
| OC-NYM/VM | VM-26 | No | Unk | Topo II | Jensen (287,426) |
| H69/VDS | Vindesine | No | Unk | Alterations in tubulin | Saijo (28) |

DOX, doxorubicin; DNR, daunorubicin; topo II, topoisomerase II; Unk, unknown.

*Measurement of Functional Transporter Activity*

It is important to assess the activity of P-glycoprotein or MRP because their presence in a sample does not necessarily indicate functional activity. As discussed above, reduced drug accumulation is relatively simple to measure, but results must be interpreted with care because assumptions that are inherent in the use of these techniques may not always be valid. Flow cytometry and fluorescent microscopic studies of P-glycoprotein–mediated accumulation or efflux activity have employed such compounds as daunorubicin (256,257) and rhodamine 123 (256,258–262). However, rhodamine 123 is not suitable for MRP functional analysis because its accumulation is not reduced in some MRP-overexpressing cell lines (263–265). Other dyes such as calcein acetoxymethylester may be more useful for the evaluation of MRP activity because MRP (but not P-glycoprotein) appears capable of ATP-dependent transport of calcein from the cytoplasm (264,266) (Lautier et al., unpublished). Accumulation has often been measured in the presence and absence of a chemosensitizing agent (such as verapamil or cyclosporin A), which appear to interact directly with P-glycoprotein to interfere with its function, and the difference attributed to P-glycoprotein activity (267,268). However it must be borne in mind that in some cells, chemosensitizers may enhance accumulation through a mechanism(s) unrelated to a direct interaction with P-glycoprotein (269–271). Most of the chemosensitizing compounds available are less effective at reversing MRP-associated resistance (140,272) and the results of attempts to reverse MRP-associated resistance have been somewhat variable, in part because of the use of cell lines that, in addition to elevated levels of MRP, co-overexpress P-glycoprotein or have alterations in topoisomerase II (9). Studies in MRP-transfected cells suggest that, unlike P-glycoprotein, MRP activity is not directly inhibited by verapamil or cyclosporin A (34,132). Therefore, the approach of measuring drug accumulation in the presence or absence of these agents is inappropriate for the measurement of MRP activity. Finally, alterations in intracellular drug distribution may contribute to resistance in either MRP (5,32,98,140–143,273–275) or P-glycoprotein (105,274,276–279) expressing cells and are best detected by the time-consuming and expensive technique of confocal fluorescence microscopy. Thus simple, reliable, and specific functional assays that can discriminate between MRP and P-glycoprotein activities still need to be developed to conclusively establish the clinical significance of these drug resistance proteins. At present, the combined use of methods to measure mRNA, protein, and functional activity is probably the best approach.

## Relevance of P-glycoprotein and MRP to Small Cell Lung Cancer

Drug resistance in SCLC has been investigated both in experimental systems and in clinical samples (31,32,131). The most common experimental approach has been to study drug-resistant SCLC cell lines (Table 3) that have been derived by in vitro drug selection. P-glycoprotein has been found to be overexpressed in relatively few of these cell lines (273,280–287) and, in several instances, has been shown to be coexpressed with other mechanisms of resistance (e.g., alterations in topoisomerase II or overexpression of MRP).

The view has been expressed that the mechanisms of resistance in in vitro selected cell lines may not be clinically relevant because the selective pressure exerted in vitro to develop drug-resistant cell lines is considerably higher than that exerted in the clinical setting (288). For this reason, some investigators have examined and compared lung

**Table 3** Cytotoxic Drugs That Interact with Topoisomerase II

| Chemical class | Example | Intercalates DNA | Stabilizes cleavable complexes | Inhibits catalytic activity[a] | Refs. |
|---|---|---|---|---|---|
| Anthracyclines | Doxorubicin, daunorubicin | Yes | Yes | Yes | 331 |
| Acridines | Amsacrine | Yes | Yes | Unknown | 412, 510 |
| Anthracenediones | Mitoxantrone | Yes | Yes | Unknown | 331 |
| Ellipticines | 2-Methyl-9-hydroxyellipticine | Yes | Yes | Yes | 409, 510 |
| Benzisoquinolinediones | Amonafide | Yes | Yes | Unknown | 511 |
| Quinoline-5,8-diones | Streptonigrin | No | Yes | Yes | 512 |
| Demethylepipodophyllotoxins | VP-16, VM-26 | No | Yes | Yes | 405, 406 |
| Terpenoides | Terpentecin, clerocidin | No | Yes | Unknown | 513 |
| Isoflavanoid | Genistein | No | Yes | Yes | 514, 515 |
| Thiobarbiturates | Merbarone | No | No | Yes | 420 |
| Bisdioxopiperazines | ICRF-193, ICRF-187 | No | No | Yes | 422, 424 |
| Anthracyclines | Aclarubicin | No | No | Yes | 425, 426 |
| | Fostriecin | No | No | Yes | 427 |
| Naphthylurea | Suramin | No | No | Yes | 356 |
| Quinobenoxazines | A-62176, A-74932 | No | No | Yes | 516 |

[a]Some drugs have been shown to inhibit topoisomerase II catalytic activity; however, their cytotoxicity is believed to be caused by stabilization of the cleavable complex. In contrast, other drugs do not stabilize the cleavable complex and appear to act primarily by inhibiting catalytic activity.

cancer cell lines that have not undergone in vitro selection but display different patterns and levels of chemosensitivity in culture or as xenografts in athymic nude mice (289–316, and others). P-glycoprotein or its mRNA has been measured in only a few of these panels of cell lines (290,310,312,317), and a correlation between chemosensitivity and levels of expression has been found in only one (312), again indicating that P-glycoprotein may not be an important resistance mechanism in cultured lung tumor cells.

A number of studies have reported the measurement of P-glycoprotein or its mRNA in samples taken directly from lung cancer patients. These studies should yield the most clinically relevant information but, unfortunately, they are the most difficult to carry out in a rigorous and comprehensive manner, and there is still no consensus regarding the optimal method for detecting and quantifying levels of P-glycoprotein in human tumor samples (318,319). Reports in the literature regarding the prevalence of this protein in various cancers are not always in agreement, and the use of different P-glycoprotein detection methods is probably the major contributing factor to these apparent discrepancies. Some studies have concluded that elevated expression of P-glycoprotein is rarely found in lung tumors (290,320–325); others detected P-glycoprotein in a relatively high proportion of the tumor samples (326–329). There is no obvious explanation for these discordant results; however, only five of these studies examined SCLC tumor samples (290,320,325,326,328) and each used different methodologies, making the results difficult to compare. Roninson and colleagues (326) found that three of three *MDR*1 mRNA-negative SCLC tumors responded to chemotherapy whereas four of four *MDR*1-positive tumors did not, suggesting that P-glycoprotein may be active in a subpopulation of SCLC tumors. When the studies are considered together, it is clear that the importance of P-glycoprotein in SCLC is still uncertain.

Investigations of the clinical relevance of MRP are in their infancy, and there are no published reports of MRP expression in human lung cancer specimens as yet. Several clinical studies indicate that MRP expression may play a role in resistance in some forms of leukemia (67,197,207–209,212,330), in neuroblastoma (206), and in anaplastic thyroid carcinomas (205). With the recent development of probes and methods for detection of *MRP* mRNA and protein, progress in determining the significance of this recently discovered drug resistance protein in lung cancer and other human malignancies should be rapid.

## RESISTANCE MEDIATED BY ALTERATIONS IN TOPOISOMERASE II

### Topoisomerase II Modulates DNA Topology

The finding that type II topoisomerases are targets for a number of clinically important antineoplastic drugs (331) has generated a great deal of interest in these enzymes, and consequently, much has recently been learned about their structure and biological function(s). Type II topoisomerases modulate DNA topology by binding covalently with DNA and thereby generating a transient double-strand break in one double helix through which a second double helix is passed (Fig. 2). There is no one simple consensus recognition/cleavage sequence to topoisomerase II binding, but rather a number of putative sequences have been described, all of which have an asymmetric primary structure (332–336). Binding of topoisomerase II to DNA also appears to be influenced by DNA tertiary structure, occurring preferentially at DNA crossovers (337–339), in intergenic sequences, and at the 5' and 3' boundaries of transcription units (340–342).

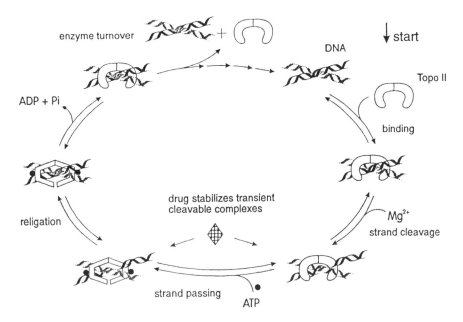

**Figure 2** Catalytic cycle of topoisomerase II and generation of drug-stabilized complexes (363). The topoisomerase II homodimer, represented by the horseshoe-shaped structure, preferentially binds to DNA at points where two duplexes cross. The enzyme cleaves both strands of the DNA and forms a transient $O^4$-phosphotyrosyl covalent bond with the 5'-DNA termini. Topoisomerase II undergoes an ATP-induced conformational change that results in the movement of an intact DNA helix through the double-stranded DNA break created by the enzyme. Topoisomerase II then religates the broken DNA, thereby fixing the DNA helices in their new topological conformation. Topoisomerase II hydrolyzes ATP, regenerating its pre-strand passage conformation and allowing it to dissociate from the DNA. Some chemotherapeutic drugs (see Table 3) appear to stabilize the transient DNA–topoisomerase II cleavable complexes by two distinct mechanisms; increasing the forward rate of DNA cleavage or inhibiting DNA religation. Other drugs inhibit DNA strand passage or ATP hydrolysis.

Two isoforms of the enzyme, designated α and β, are present in mammalian cells (for more detail, see below). Both isoforms are homodimers, and in each subunit there is an active-site tyrosine residue that binds covalently to a 5'-phosphoryl end of the cleaved DNA. In topoisomerase II α, this tyrosine is located at amino acid position 804 (343); in topoisomerase II β, it is at position 821 (344). Precisely how a second double-stranded segment of DNA is transported through the cleaved DNA is unknown (345, 346) but it appears that binding of ATP controls the opening of the protein gate formed across the break by topoisomerase II (337,347–349). The catalytic cycle of topoisomerase II is completed with the rejoining of the cleaved DNA strands, followed by enzyme turnover that is dependent on ATP hydrolysis (337,350). Both before and after strand passage, the religation reaction is in equilibrium with the cleavage reaction; however, the respective "forward" reactions are strongly favored. The enzyme may remain attached and begin a new round of cleavage and strand passage at the same site (processive reaction), or it may dissociate and move to a new location (distributive reaction).

Topoisomerase II is essential for cell survival because it is required for chromosome condensation and chromatid separation by segregating the intertwined daughter DNA molecules that are present at the completion of chromosomal DNA replication (351–360). Topoisomerases also relieve the torsional stress in DNA that is generated during transcription and replication (361–363). In addition to its catalytic functions, topoisomerase II is a component of the nuclear matrix at the base of chromosomal loops and is believed to play a role in chromosome structure (364–367), although the latter function has been questioned recently as the result of studies using *Xenopus* egg extracts (368). A number of excellent reviews on the biology of topoisomerase II and its importance as a target for antitumor drugs have been published in recent years (363, 369–373).

Studies of lower eukaryotes, particularly yeast and *Drosophila*, have led to much of the current understanding of topoisomerase II and its interaction with drugs. However, caution should be exercised in extrapolating this information to mammalian enzymes because significant species differences are known to exist. For example, lower eukaryotes have only one isoform of topoisomerase II (344), in contrast to humans and rodents, which have two isoforms: the 170-kD topoisomerase II α and the 180-kD topoisomerase II β (344,374–378). Although similar in structure and catalytic mechanism, these two isoforms differ in a number of respects, and it is important to bear in mind that most of the published data on human topoisomerase II concerns only the 170-kD α isoform.

## Topoisomerase II Structure and Regulation of Activity

### Topoisomerase II α and β

The human topoisomerase II α 6.1-kb mRNA is predicted to encode a protein of 1531 amino acids, consistent with its molecular mass of 170 kDa (344,379–382). The 180-kD topoisomerase II β was originally distinguished from the previously described 170-kD topoisomerase II α by differences in a number of biochemical and molecular properties (375,383). For example, topoisomerase II β requires a different ionic environment for catalytic activity, may have differences in sequence specificity for DNA binding, and is more heat labile (375). The relative levels of topoisomerase II α and β vary among different cell lines and they may be differentially regulated during the cell cycle (344, 384,385). Moreover, the intranuclear localization of topoisomerase II α and β appear to differ: in a number of cell types examined, topoisomerase II α is in the nucleoplasm whereas topoisomerase II β is restricted to the nucleolus (386,387). The β isoform mRNA is predicted to encode a protein of 1621 amino acids, which is consistent with its larger molecular mass compared to topoisomerase II α (377). However, the mRNAs for the two topoisomerase II isoforms cannot be distinguished in size by RNA blot analysis. Finally, the topoisomerase II α gene has been mapped to chromosome 17, band q21-22 (379,388); the gene for topoisomerase II β is on chromosome 3 at band 3p24 (344,388).

The amino acid identity of topoisomerase II α and β is high at 72% (83% when conservative amino acid changes are included). Studies with purified enzyme and comparisons of the deduced amino acid sequence with the sequence of prokaryotic DNA gyrase (389) have suggested that each subunit of the topoisomerase II homodimer has three functional domains: a NH$_2$-proximal ATPase domain; a central DNA breakage-rejoining domain, which contains the active site tyrosine; and a hydrophilic COOH-proximal domain. The $NH_2$- and COOH-proximal domains are not essential for in vitro catalytic activity and display the most divergence among different species, as well as between topoisomerase II $\alpha$ and $\beta$ (377,390,391). At present, however, the significance of these regions for the properties in which the two isoforms differ is unknown (377, 392).

Current evidence suggests that the two isoforms also differ in their sensitivity to certain drugs. For example, topoisomerase II $\beta$ is more resistant to inhibition by VM-26 (teniposide) and merbarone than is topoisomerase II $\alpha$ (375,393). The two isoforms are thus also likely to differ in the roles they play in sensitivity and resistance to the various drugs with which they interact (393).

*Modulation of Topoisomerase II Levels and Activity*

Regulation of gene transcription is likely the most important mechanism controlling topoisomerase II levels. In some cell types, but not all (394), levels of topoisomerase II $\alpha$ protein, and hence topoisomerase II activity, vary throughout the cell cycle (384, 385,395,396). Synthesis of topoisomerase II $\alpha$ occurs as cells progress from $G_1$ to S phase, with a maximal level of protein at late $G_2$ and mitosis. After mitosis, a significant portion of the protein is degraded. Thus, topoisomerase II activity in some cells may be regulated by protein turnover as well as by transcription. The fact that synthesis of topoisomerase II $\alpha$ is coordinated with the cell cycle indicates that its transcription is tightly regulated. Genomic DNA clones encompassing the 5' end of the topoisomerase II $\alpha$ gene have been isolated and partially characterized (397,398). The *trans*-activating factors that interact with the topoisomerase II promoter region and regulate expression are currently being investigated. In contrast to topoisomerase II $\alpha$, levels of topoisomerase II $\beta$ appear to remain constant throughout the cell cycle (384,385).

Topoisomerase II activity may also be regulated by modification of the polypeptide after translation. In vitro studies of phosphorylation of yeast or *Drosophila* topoisomerase II by protein kinases have usually, but not always, shown that catalytic and/or cleavage activity of the enzyme is increased by phosphorylation (399,400). In vivo, levels of phosphorylation are very low in quiescent cells (395) and vary throughout the cell cycle, having been reported to be highest in $G_2$/M (395,401) or in M-phase cells (402). Thus, phosphorylation of topoisomerase II may provide a second mechanism for the regulation of topoisomerase II activity because phosphorylation may be controlled in a different manner than the level of enzyme expressed (402,403). Alternatively, topoisomerase II may be maintained in a relatively permanent phosphorylation state, as has been demonstrated in HeLa cells where the phosphorylation half-life of topoisomerase II is similar to the half-life of the protein itself (394). It is not yet known which kinase is involved in phosphorylation of topoisomerase II in human cells or whether the sites and regulation of phosphorylation of topoisomerase II $\alpha$ and $\beta$ are similar. Thus the exact role of phosphorylation/dephosphorylation in the regulation of the activity or localization of the human topoisomerase II isoforms is yet to be fully elucidated.

## Topoisomerase II as a Target for Chemotherapeutic Drugs

Many drugs used in cancer chemotherapy exert their cytotoxicity, at least in part, through their interaction with topoisomerase II (Table 3). These drugs have been shown to interact with topoisomerase II in at least one of two ways. Many anthracyclines (e.g., doxorubicin), epipodophyllotoxins (e.g., VP-16 and VM-26), anthracenediones (e.g., mitoxantrone), ellipticines (e.g., 9-hydroxyellipticine), and aminoacridines (e.g., amsacrine) stabilize the normally transient topoisomerase II/DNA cleavage complexes, thus inhibiting the religation of DNA (331,404–414). These topoisomerase II-mediated DNA strand breaks, although often repaired, constitute a signal for apoptotic cell death through a pathway that is still not completely understood (415–418). The interaction domains on topoisomerase II for specific drug classes are poorly defined at present. Furthermore, the drugs appear to influence the enzyme's DNA sequence specificity, allowing the enzyme to cleave DNA at novel sites or sites infrequently utilized in the absence of drugs (419).

Other drugs do not stabilize the cleavable complex but are cytotoxic presumably because they act more like typical inhibitors of this essential enzyme. Such drugs include merbarone (420), bis(2,6-dioxopiperazine) derivatives (360,421–424) (e.g., ICRF-193 and ICRF-187), certain anthracyclines (e.g., aclarubicin) (425,426), and fostriecin (427,428). The exact manner in which these agents inhibit topoisomerase II activity is largely unknown; however, it appears that they may interact with topoisomerase II in a variety of ways (360,424). Cells resistant to drugs that act by stabilizing DNA/topoisomerase II complexes may not be cross-resistant to the second group of topoisomerase inhibitors, making these compounds of potential clinical interest. The two types of drugs may not be useful concurrently because some of these agents antagonize the effect of topoisomerase II/DNA stabilizing drugs, apparently by inhibiting the initial noncovalent DNA-binding reaction of the enzyme and drug (425,429–434).

## Mechanisms of Resistance to Cleavable Complex-Stabilizing Drugs

In contrast to resistance mediated by P-glycoprotein and MRP, which is nearly always associated with reduced drug accumulation, resistance to chemotherapeutic agents that target topoisomerase II occurs through several mechanisms. In cell lines that are resistant to drugs that stabilize the cleavable complex, all of the alterations in topoisomerase II result in a reduced number of cleaved complexes formed. Thus, reduced levels of intranuclear topoisomerase II and/or a mutation in the enzyme that alters its interaction with either the drug or DNA have been observed in numerous drug-selected cell lines.

### Reduced Levels of Topoisomerase II

If levels of topoisomerase II are decreased, then fewer cleaved complexes can be formed and drug resistance may result. Cell lines selected in a variety of drugs, including epipodophyllotoxins (435–436), anthracyclines (95,438–441), mitoxantrone (442–444), amsacrine (383), and 9-hydroxyellipticine (445–447), have reduced levels of topoisomerase II $\alpha$. Many drug-selected cell lines express multiple potential resistance mechanisms (448), and it is not possible to assess the relative importance of reduced topoisomerase II levels in the resistance of such cell lines. However, reduced levels of topoisomerase II $\alpha$ are likely sufficient to cause resistance because in the VP-16–selected hamster cell line, CHO-SMR$_5$, the level of resistance correlates directly with the decrease in topoisomerase II $\alpha$ mRNA and protein, which in turn correlates with the degree of reduced cleavage and strand-passing activities (449). Conversely, an increase in nuclear topoisomerase II levels can result in a drug-hypersensitive phenotype (450,451). Topoisomerase II levels have been measured in panels of unselected lung cancer cell lines to determine whether this enzyme is an important determinant of relative levels of drug sensitivity (289,292,452,453). In general, correlations of enzyme levels with drug sensitivity have been moderate, and the power of such studies to determine whether the level of topoisomerase II is an important contributor to the sensitivity/resistance of some of these cell lines is limited by the likelihood that multiple resistance mechanisms are expressed.

Reduced levels of topoisomerase II β have also been observed in drug-selected cell lines, although this is a less frequent observation than reductions in levels of topoisomerase II α (437,442,454,455). As mentioned previously, purified topoisomerase II α has been reported to be more sensitive than the β isoform to VM-26 and merbarone (375,393). However, more studies are needed to determine whether topoisomerase II α and β differ in their sensitivity to other drugs and whether the isoforms differ in their drug interactions in vivo. A mitoxantrone-selected human leukemia cell line, HL-60/MX2, has been described in which topoisomerase II β is undetectable (442). This observation suggests that levels of the β isoform may be an important determinant of cellular sensitivity to mitoxantrone. Therefore, it is predicted that different relative levels of topoisomerase II α and β will result in different cross-resistance patterns.

A number of drug-selected cell lines have been characterized that express reduced levels of topoisomerase II compared to their parental cell lines, but assays of cleavage and/or strand-passing activities have also revealed that the resistant cells possess topoisomerase II with abnormal biochemical properties. Other drug-selected cell lines have been described that contain an abnormal topoisomerase II, but the levels of immunoreactive enzyme are equivalent to those of their parental cell line. Taken together, these cell lines illustrate the importance of measuring both the levels and activities of this enzyme to obtain an accurate assessment of the contribution of topoisomerase II alterations to drug resistance.

*Altered Topoisomerase II Activity Associated with Point Mutations*

In several cell lines with aberrant topoisomerase II activities, point mutations of topoisomerase II α mRNA have been identified. These mutations have tended to cluster near the ATP-binding region (380,456–460) or in the regions adjacent to the active site tyrosine (459–461). However, in only a few cases has the functional significance of the point mutations in resistance been rigorously assessed. For example, when an arginine-to-glutamien substitution at position 450 (originally identified in the VM-26–selected human leukemia cell line, CEM/VM-1) (459,460) was recreated in the yeast topoisomerase II gene, the mutant enzyme was less sensitive to VP-16 and amsacrine (462). In contrast, although a change in arginine at position 486 to lysine was identified in two amsacrine-selected human cell lines, HL-60/AMSA (463,464) and KBM-3/AMSA (458), the cross-resistance profiles of the two cell lines differed and reconstruction of the amino acid substitution in the corresponding position of yeast topoisomerase II did not result in a drug-resistant enzyme (458). These results call into question the importance of the arginine-to-lysine substitution at position 486. Much work remains to be done to determine which point mutations have functional consequences with respect to drug resistance and which are of clinical significance. Preliminary studies of tumor cells from patients with acute myelogenous leukemia and relapsed acute lymphocytic leukemia did not detect mutations in the ATP-binding or DNA binding domains of topoisomerase II α, suggesting that these mutations may not be frequent causes of drug resistance in these tumor types (460,465).

*Cytoplasmic Localization of Topoisomerase II*

A third mechanism of altered-topoisomerase II resistance, which involves cytoplasmic localization of the enzyme, has recently been described in a mitoxantrone-selected human leukemia cell line (442) and in a VP-16–selected human SCLC cell line, H209/ V6 (466,467). Both of these cell lines express a topoisomerase II α-related protein that is smaller (160 kd) than the normal (170 kD) protein found in parental cells. In contrast to the normal nuclear distribution of topoisomerase II, the smaller topoisomerase is located predominantly in the cytoplasm (442,467). In addition, both cell lines express two topoisomerase II α-related mRNAs: an apparently normal-sized 6.1-kb mRNA and a similar level of a shorter 4.8-kb mRNA (466,468). When the 160-kD topoisomerase II α-related protein of H209/V6 cells and the 170-kD topoisomerase II α from the parental cell line were purified, they were found to possess similar enzymatic properties (467). These data suggested that an alteration had occurred in the normal topoisomerase II α, resulting in a 160-kd protein that is less efficient in localizing to the nucleus but still capable of catalytic function in vitro.

Topoisomerase II proteins with deletions in the COOH-proximal region (which would correspond to the 3′ proximal region of the mRNA) have been expressed in yeast (469,470) and *Drosophila* (471,472) and shown to be enzymatically active in vitro but not in vivo (470–472). This is likely because they localize predominantly in the cytoplasm (470–473). Similar alterations were revealed by RT-PCR analysis of the 4.8-kb mRNA in the resistant SCLC cell line, H209/V6 (382). This mRNA is missing 988 consecutive nucleotides of normal topoisomerase II α sequence corresponding to both coding and noncoding sequences. The absence of this sequence is predicted to result in the net loss of 75 amino acids at the COOH-terminus of the protein. This region of the molecule contains multiple potential nuclear targeting sequences, some of which are almost certain to be essential for the efficient transport of the protein into the nucleus (474–476). Therefore, the protein product of this 4.8-kb mRNA is predicted to contain fewer than normal nuclear localization sequences, which in turn is probably responsible for its predominantly cytoplasmic localization. The cytoplasmic localization of the 160-kD topoisomerase II α provides an explanation for why the protein is resistant to the formation of cleaved complexes in intact H209/V6 cells (466), but not when purified and assayed in vitro with exogenous DNA (467).

There has been insufficient opportunity to assess the prevalence of this resistance mechanism in cell lines or clinical samples. Nuclear localization motifs have been identified throughout the topoisomerase II molecule but their relative importance has not been determined. Consequently, it remains possible that other mutations, including smaller deletions, could have a similar effect on enzyme localization. For this reason screening cells by scanning immunoblots for smaller topoisomerases or for the absence of the COOH-terminal region may not be sufficient to determine whether resistance is occurring through this mechanism. Ideally, immunoblots of nuclear and cytosolic lysates together with immunocytochemistry should be performed to allow the relative amounts of topoisomerase II in the different subcellular compartments to be determined.

## Detection of Topoisomerase II

Sensitive, reliable, and quantitative assays are required to assess the involvement of topoisomerase II in clinical drug resistance. The use of these assays is complicated by the fact that levels of topoisomerase II may vary throughout the cell cycle, and cell cycle analyses are difficult to perform on clinical samples (465). In addition, for reasons discussed above, it is important that both α and β isoforms are measured and that nuclear topoisomerase is distinguished from cytoplasmic topoisomerase II.

*Quantitation of Topoisomerase II Protein and mRNA*

Measurement of topoisomerase II mRNA or protein is technically the most straightforward of the available assays and, for this reason, has been used most commonly in clinical samples (477–483). Isoform-specific cDNAs can be used for Northern blotting (376), and primers for RT-PCR or probes for RNAse protection assays may be designed to allow the measurement of both topoisomerase II α and β mRNAs. However, as has been discussed previously in reference to P-glycoprotein and MRP, technical challenges currently exclude these procedures from routine use in clinical laboratories. Quantitative RT-PCR–based assays for topoisomerase II α have recently been designed that attempt to overcome some of the technical difficulties (484), and such advances may lead to the more common use of RT-PCR. It must be borne in mind that these methods yield no information about the heterogeneity of topoisomerase II expression within any given sample (465). Finally, it is not known whether cellular levels of topoisomerase II mRNA and protein invariably correlate well or whether there might be some post-transcriptional regulation of the amount of protein ultimately expressed.

Point mutations in topoisomerase II mRNAs can be revealed by single-strand conformational polymorphism (SSCP) analysis. SSCP analysis is based on unidirectional RT-PCR followed by electrophoresis in agarose gels. Differences of a single nucleotide can in many cases produce a detectable difference in gel migration (485). Several regions of the topoisomerase II α gene in drug-resistant cell lines and in samples from leukemia patients have been studied using SSCP, but no mutations were detected (460). Nevertheless, the SSCP method may be useful for screening large numbers of tumor samples for specific topoisomerase II mutations.

Immunohistochemical detection methods avoid some of the technical difficulties inherent in measuring mRNA. However, the supply of topoisomerase II isoform-specific anti-peptide polyclonal antibodies is limited (375,376). Recently reported isoform-specific MoAbs may overcome this problem but require further characterization and commercialization before they can be used routinely (386).

*Measurement of Topoisomerase II Catalytic and Cleavage Activities*

Resistant cell lines selected in vitro with drugs that target topoisomerase II often display abnormal cleavage and/or strand-passing activities without detectable changes in the levels of immunoreactive topoisomerase II or its mRNA. Consequently, it may be important to measure the activity of topoisomerase II in clinical samples in addition to simply measuring the enzyme levels. Methods have been developed to measure the ability of topoisomerase II to knot/unknot double-strand circular DNA (486–488), relax supercoiled DNA (337), and catenate/decatenate double-strand DNA circles (489–494). These assays are based on ATP-dependent topoisomerase II–mediated changes in the topology of a DNA substrate that alter its electrophoretic mobility through agarose gels. The DNA products can be visualized by staining with ethidium bromide or more precisely quantitated using radiolabeled DNA substrates. Cleavage activity in the presence of topoisomerase II–interactive drugs can be quantitated when a strong protein denaturant (usually sodium dodecyl sulfate) is used to convert the

DNA/topoisomerase II/drug complexes to protein-linked DNA breaks. The DNA that is bound covalently to topoisomerase II can be recovered and quantitated by filter elution (495) or precipitated with KCl (the SDS-KCl assay) (496). Modifications, including radiolabeling of DNA and protein, have improved the accuracy of quantitation (497). These assays may be carried out in intact cells or in vitro, using nuclear extracts or purified enzymes with a plasmid or viral DNA substrate.

A semiquantitative estimate of the relative cleavage activities of topoisomerase II α and β can be obtained using an immunoblotting band depletion assay that employs isoform-specific antibodies (497–499). In this assay, cells are incubated with or without drug, lysed, and the lysate subjected to polyacrylamide gel electrophoresis. DNA, and any topoisomerase II molecules that are covalently bound to it as a cleaved complex, is unable to enter the gel. As the DNA/topoisomerase complexes are stabilized by increasing concentrations of drug, there will be a dose-dependent decrease in topoisomerase II α and β able to enter the gel and, consequently, a depletion of the bands of topoisomerase II α and/or β detected on an immunoblot.

Assays for measuring the enzymatic and cleavage activities of topoisomerase II generally are not easy to adapt for assessment of large numbers of small tissue samples and at present have been used in only a few studies of clinical samples (465,483,494, 500). Thus, more studies are needed to define the relevance of topoisomerase II alterations in clinical drug resistance—and with improved methodologies, these should be forthcoming.

### Relevance of Alterations in Topoisomerase II to Drug Resistance in Lung Cancer

Clinical studies of topoisomerase II are likely to be even more difficult with solid tumors than they have been with hematological malignancies (465,477). It can be anticipated that such studies will be particularly difficult in SCLC because surgery is rarely clinically indicated and samples are in short supply. There have been only a few studies of the topoisomerase II mRNA or protein levels in human lung cancer specimens (469, 480,481,501), and topoisomerase II activities have been measured in one of these (501). Consequently, the importance of topoisomerase II alterations in the clinical resistance of SCLC and non-SCLC is still largely undetermined (502). The role of topoisomerase II alterations in cultured lung tumor cells has been examined using both unselected SCLC and non-SCLC cell lines (289,292,452,453) as well as xenografts (291) and cell lines selected in vitro with topoisomerase II targeting drugs, such as doxorubicin, VP-16, or VM-26. In a panel of four unselected SCLC and non-SCLC tumor cell lines, Long et al. (289) found that levels of DNA breakage correlated with relative levels of resistance to VM-26 and VP-16. Using larger panels of SCLC and non-SCLC cell lines, levels of topoisomerase II α (mRNA or protein) and activity were measured, as well as drug sensitivity (453,503). In these studies, correlations were found between topoisomerase II content and sensitivity to VP-16 and doxorubicin. Furthermore, topoisomerase II content and activity and VP-16 net accumulation were higher in the SCLC cell lines than in non-SCLC cell lines, consistent with the generally greater chemosensitivity of SCLC (503).

Drug-selected SCLC cell lines that exhibit alterations in topoisomerase II levels and/or activities are described in Table 2. Many of these cell lines also have a drug transport defect and, in some cases, overexpress MRP or P-glycoprotein in addition to alterations in topoisomerase II (5,89,282,285,504). Others do not have a drug transport defect and their resistance seems to be directly attributable to alterations in topoisomerase II. For example, the VP-16–selected H209/V6 cell line does not overexpress P-glycoprotein or MRP but expresses a mutant 160-kD cytoplasmic topoisomerase II α (see above). This resistant SCLC cell line has been a particularly useful model system for characterizing the molecular events underlying cytoplasmic localization of topoisomerase II as a novel resistance mechanism (382,467).

When taken together, the data from both unselected and drug-selected cell lines support a role for alterations in topoisomerase II as determinants of drug sensitivity in SCLC cells. However, the studies on panels of cell lines were reported before the identification of MRP, and before inefficient nuclear localization of topoisomerase II was identified as a resistance mechanism. Multiple resistance mechanisms have been identified in lung cancer cell lines selected in vitro; therefore, it would be interesting to determine whether the expression of MRP or P-glycoprotein along with alterations in topoisomerase II in unselected cell lines would provide a rationalization of their sensitivity levels and cross-resistance profiles. There is also clearly a great need for more studies of samples from SCLC patients to establish clinical relevance. It is important, however, that the design of such studies takes into account the potential multifactorial nature of drug resistance in this disease.

## REFERENCES

1. Ihde DC, Pass HI, Glatstein EJ. Cancer of the lung. In: DeVita Jr VT, Hellman S, Rosenberg SA, eds. Cancer: Principles & Practice of Oncology. 4th ed. Philadelphia: Lippincott, 1993: 23–758.
2. Ueda K, Cardarelli C, Gottesman MM, Pastan I. Expression of a full-length cDNA for the human "*MDR1*" gene confers resistance to colchicine, doxorubicin, and vinblastine. Proc Natl Acad Sci USA 1987; 84:3004–3008.
3. Gros P, Neriah YB, Croop JM, Housman DE. Isolation and expression of a complementary DNA that confers multidrug resistance. Nature 1986; 323:728–731.
4. Gerlach JH, Endicott JA, Juranka PF, Henderson G, Sarangi F, Deuchars KL, Ling V. Homology between P-glycoprotein and a bacterial haemolysin transport protein suggests a model for multidrug resistance. Nature 1986; 324:485–489.
5. Cole SPC, Bhardwaj G, Gerlach JH, et al. Overexpression of a transporter gene in a multidrug-resistant human lung cancer cell line. Science 1992; 258:1650–1654.
6. Cole SPC, Deeley RG. Multidrug resistance-associated protein: sequence correction. Science 1993; 260:879.
7. Grant CE, Valdimarsson G, Hipfner DR, Almquist KC, Cole SPC, Deeley RG. Overexpression of multidrug resistance-associated protein (MRP) increased resistance to natural product drugs. Cancer Res 1994; 54:357–361.
8. Krishnamachary N, Center MS. The MRP gene associated with a non-P-glycoprotein multidrug resistance encodes a 190-kDa membrane bound glycoprotein. Cancer Res 1993; 53: 3658–3661.
9. Cole SPC, Deeley RG. Multidrug resistance associated with overexpression of MRP. In: Hait WN, ed. Drug Resistance. Norwell, MA: Kluwer Academic Press, 1996:39–62.
10. Bradley G, Juranka PF, Ling V. Mechanism of multidrug resistance. Biochim Biophys Acta 1988; 948:87–128.
11. Gerlach JH, Kartner N, Bell DR, Ling V. Multidrug resistance. Cancer Surv 1986; 5:25–46.

12. Gottesman MM, Pastan I. The multidrug transporter, a double-edged sword. J Biol Chem 1988; 263:12163–12166.
13. Juranka PF, Zastawny RL, Ling V. P-glycoprotein: multidrug-resistance and a superfamily of membrane-associated transport proteins. FASEB J 1989; 3:2583–2592.
14. Georges E, Sharom FJ, Ling V. Multidrug resistance and chemosensitization: therapeutic implications for cancer chemotherapy. Adv Pharmacol 1990; 21:185–220.
15. Roninson IB. From amplification to function: the case of the MDR1 gene. Mutation Res 1992; 276:151–161.
16. Tsuruo T. Mechanisms of multidrug resistance and implications for therapy. Jpn J Cancer Res 1988; 79:285–296.
17. Endicott JA, Ling V. The biochemistry of P-glycoprotein-mediated multidrug resistance. Annu Rev Biochem 1989; 58:137–171.
18. Gerlach JH. Structure and function of P-glycoprotein. In: Ozols RF, ed. Drug Resistance in Cancer Therapy. Norwell, MA: Kluwer Academic, 1989:37–53.
19. Gottesman MM, Pastan I. Biochemistry of multidrug resistance mediated by the multidrug transporter. Annu Rev Biochem 1993; 62:385–427.
20. Chin K-V, Pastan I, Gottesman MM. Function and regulation of the human multidrug resistance gene. Adv Cancer Res 1993; 60:157–180.
21. Mirski SEL, Gerlach JH, Cole SPC. Multidrug resistance in a human small cell lung cancer cell line selected in adriamycin. Cancer Res 1987; 47:2594–2598.
22. McGrath T, Center MS. Adriamycin resistance in HL60 cells in the absence of detectable P-glycoprotein. Biochem Biophys Res Commun 1987; 145:1171–1176.
23. Slovak ML, Hoeltge DA, Dalton WS, Trent JM. Pharmacological and biological evidence for differing mechanisms of doxorubicin resistance in two human tumor cell lines. Cancer Res 1988; 48:2793–2797.
24. de Jong S, Zijlstra JG, de Vries EGE, Mulder NH. Reduced DNA topoisomerase II activity and drug-induced DNA cleavage activity in an adriamycin-resistant human small cell lung carcinoma cell line. Cancer Res 1990; 50:304–309.
25. Reeve JG, Rabbitts PH, Twentyman PR. Non-P-glycoprotein-mediated multidrug resistance with reduced EGF receptor expression in a human large cell lung cancer cell line. Br J Cancer 1990; 61:851–855.
26. Nielsen D, Skovsgaard T. P-Glycoprotein as multidrug transporter: a critical review of current multidrug resistant cell lines. Biochim Biophys Acta 1992; 1139:169–183.
27. Hill BT. Differing patterns of cross-resistance resulting from exposures to specific antitumour drugs or to radiation in vitro. Cytotechnology 1993; 12:265–288.
28. Ohta S, Nishio K, Kubo S, et al. Characterisation of a vindesine-resistant human small-cell lung cancer cell line. Br J Cancer 1993; 68:74–79.
29. Supino R, Binaschi M, Capranico G, et al. A study of cross-resistance pattern and expression of molecular markers of multidrug resistance in a human small-cell lung-cancer cell line selected with doxorubicin. Int J Cancer 1993; 54:309–314.
30. Baas F, Jongsma APM, Broxterman HJ, et al. Non-P-glycoprotein mediated mechanism for multidrug resistance precedes P-glycoprotein expression during in vitro selection for doxorubicin resistance in a human lung cancer cell line. Cancer Res 1990; 50:5392–5398.
31. Cole SPC. The 1991 Merck Frosst Award. Multidrug resistance in small cell lung cancer. Can J Physiol Pharmacol 1992; 70:313–329.
32. Cole SPC. Drug resistance and lung cancer. In: Wood J, ed. Cancer: Concept to Clinic. Fairlawn, NJ: Medical Publishing Enterprises, 1992:15–21.
33. Eijdems EWH, Borst P, Jongsma APM, et al. Genetic transfer of non-P-glycoprotein-mediated multidrug resistance (MDR) in somatic cell fusion: dissection of a compound MDR phenotype. Proc Natl Acad Sci USA 1992; 89:3498–3502.
34. Cole SPC, Sparks KE, Fraser K, et al. Pharmacological characterization of multidrug resistant MRP-transfected human tumor cells. Cancer Res 1994; 54:5902–5910.

35. Gerlach JH, Endicott JA, Juranka PF, et al. Homology between P-glycoprotein and a bacterial haemolysin transport protein suggests a model for multidrug resistance. Nature 1986; 324:485–489.

36. Higgins CF. ABC transporters: from microorganisms to man. Ann Rev Cell Biol 1992; 8: 67–113.

37. Riordan JR, Rommens JM, Kerem B-S, et al. Identification of the cystic fibrosis gene: cloning and characterization of complementary DNA. Science 1989; 245:1066–1073.

38. Welsh MJ, Smith AE. Molecular mechanisms of CFTR chloride channel dysfunction in cystic fibrosis. Cell 1993; 73:1251–1254.

39. Kelly A, Powis SH, Kerr L-A, et al. Assembly and function of the two ABC transporter proteins encoded in the human major histocompatibility complex. Nature 1992; 355:641–644.

40. Neefjes JJ, Momburg F, Hammerling GJ. Selective and ATP-dependent translocation of peptides by the MHC-encoded transporter. Science 1993; 261:769–771.

41. Androlewicz MJ, Anderson KS, Cresswell P. Evidence that transporters associated with antigen processing translocate a major histocompatibility complex class I-binding peptide into the endoplasmic reticulum in an ATP-dependent manner. Proc Natl Acad Sci USA 1993; 90:9130–9134.

42. Heemels M-T, Schumacher TNM, Wonigeit K, Ploegh HL. Peptide translocation by variants of the transporter associated with antigen processing. Science 1993; 262:2059–2063.

43. Roninson IB, Chin JE, Choi K, et al. Isolation of human *mdr* DNA sequences amplified in multidrug-resistant KB carcinoma cells. Proc Natl Acad Sci USA 1986; 83:4538–4542.

44. Callen DF, Baker E, Simmers RN, Seshadri R, Roninson IB. Localization of the human multiple drug resistance gene, MDR1, to 7q21.1. Hum Genet 1987; 77:142–144.

45. Fojo A, Lebo R, Shimizu N, et al. Localization of multidrug resistance-associated DNA sequences to human chromosome 7. Somat Cell Mol Genet 1986; 12:415–420.

46. Van der Bliek AM, Baas F, Van der Velde-Koerts T, et al. Genes amplified and overexpressed in human multidrug-resistant cell lines. Cancer Res 1988; 48:5927–5932.

47. Schinkel AH, Roelofs MEM, Borst P. Characterization of the human *MDR*3 P-glycoprotein and its recognition by P-glycoprotein-specific monoclonal antibodies. Cancer Res 1991; 51: 2628–2635.

48. Smit JJM, Schinkel AH, Oude Elferink RPJ, et al. Homozygous disruption of the murine *mdr*2 P-glycoprotein gene leads to a complete absence of phospholipid from bile and to liver disease. Cell 1993; 75:451–462.

49. Ruetz S, Gros P. Phosphatidylcholine translocase: a physiological role for the *mdr*2 gene. Cell 1994; 77:1071–1081.

50. Schinkel AH, Smit JJM, van Tellingen O, et al. Disruption of the mouse *mdr1a* P-glycoprotein gene leads to a deficiency in the blood-brain barrier and to increased sensitivity to drugs. Cell 1994; 77:491–502.

51. Kyte J, Doolittle RF. A simple method for displaying the hydropathic character of a protein. J Mol Biol 1982; 157:105–132.

52. Klein P, Kanehisa M, DeLisi C. The detection and classification of membrane-spanning proteins. Biochim Biophys Acta 1985; 815:468–476.

53. Eisenberg D, Schwarz E, Komaromy M, Wall R. Analysis of membrane and surface protein sequences with the hydrophobic moment plot. J Mol Biol 1984; 179:125–142.

54. Jones DT, Taylor WR, Thornton JM. A model recognition approach to the prediction of all-helical membrane protein structure and topology. Biochemistry 1994; 33:3038–3049.

55. Gros P, Croop J, Housman D. Mammalian multidrug resistance gene: complete cDNA sequence indicates strong homology to bacterial transport proteins. Cell 1986; 47:371–380.

56. Chen C-J, Chin JE, Ueda K, et al. Internal duplication and homology with bacterial transport proteins in the mdr1 (P-glycoprotein) gene from multidrug-resistant human cells. Cell 1986; 47:381–389.

57. Yoshimura A, Kuwazuru Y, Sumizawa T, et al. Cytoplasmic orientation and two-domain structure of the multidrug transporter, P-glycoprotein, demonstrated with sequence-specific antibodies. J Biol Chem 1989; 264:16282–16291.

58. Georges E, Bradley G, Gariepy J, Ling V. Detection of P-glycoprotein isoforms by gene-specific monoclonal antibodies. Proc Natl Acad Sci USA 1990; 87:152–156.

59. Georges E, Tsuruo T, Ling V. Topology of P-glycoprotein as determined by epitope mapping of MRK-16 monoclonal antibody. J Biol Chem 1993; 268:1792–1798.

60. Skach WR, Calayag MC, Lingappa VR. Evidence for an alternate model of human P-glycoprotein structure and biogenesis. J Biol Chem 1993; 268:6903–6908.

61. Zhang J-T, Duthie M, Ling V. Membrane topology of the N-terminal half of the hamster P-glycoprotein molecule. J Biol Chem 1993; 268:15101–15110.

62. Zhang J-T, Ling V. Study of membrane orientation and glycosylated extracellular loops of mouse P-glycoprotein by *in vitro* translation. J Biol Chem 1991; 266:18224–18232.

63. Beja O, Bibi E. Multidrug resistance protein (Mdr)-alkaline phosphatase hybrids in *Escherichia coli* suggest a major revision in the topology of the C-terminal half of Mdr. J Biol Chem 1995; 270:12351–12354.

64. Boscoboinik D, Debanne MT, Stafford AR, Jung CY, Gupta RS, Epand RM. Dimerization of the P-glycoprotein in membranes. Biochim Biophys Acta 1990; 1027:225–228.

65. Poruchynsky MS, Ling V. Detection of oligomeric and monomeric forms of P-glycoprotein in multidrug resistant cells. Biochemistry 1994; 33:4163–4174.

66. Slovak ML, Ho JP, Bhardwaj G, Kurz EU, Deeley RG, Cole SPC. Localization of a novel multidrug resistance-associated gene in the HT1080/DR4 and H69AR human tumor cell lines. Cancer Res 1993; 53:3221–3225.

67. Kuss BJ, Deeley RG, Cole SPC, et al. Deletion of gene for multidrug resistance in acute myeloid leukaemia with inversion in chromosome 16: prognostic implications. Lancet 1994; 343:1531–1534.

68. Szczypka MS, Wemmie JA, Moye-Rowley WS, Thiele DJ. A yeast metal resistance protein similar to human cystic fibrosis transmembrane conductance regulator (CFTR) and multidrug resistance-associated protein. J Biol Chem 1994; 269:22853–22857.

69. Aguilar-Bryan L, Nichols CG, Wechsler SW, et al. Cloning of the β cell high-affinity sulfonylurea receptor: a regulator of insulin secretion. Science 1995; 268:423–426.

70. Callahan HL, Beverley SM. Heavy metal resistance: A new role for P-glycoproteins in *Leishmania*. J Biol Chem 1991; 266:18427–18430.

71. Papadopoulou B, Roy G, Dey S, Rosen BP, Ouellette M. Contribution of the *Leishmania* P-glycoprotein-related gene *lipgpA* to oxyanion resistance. J Biol Chem 1994; 269:11980–11986.

72. Almquist KC, Loe DW, Hipfner DR, Mackie JE, Cole SPC, Deeley RG. Characterization of the 190 kDa multidrug resistance protein (MRP) in drug-selected and transfected human tumor cells. Cancer Res 1995; 55:102–110.

73. Ma L, Krishnamachary N, Center MS. Phosphorylation of the multidrug resistance associated protein gene encoded protein P190. Biochemistry 1995; 34:3338–3343.

74. Shen D-W, Fojo A, Chin JE, et al. Human multidrug-resistant cell lines: Increased *mdr1* expression can precede gene amplification. Science 1986; 232:643–645.

75. Kohno K, Sato S-I, Uchiumi T, et al. Activation of the human multidrug resistance 1 (MDR1) gene promoter in response to inhibitors of DNA topoisomerases. Int J Oncol 1992; 1:73–77.

76. Chaudhary PM, Roninson IB. Induction of multidrug resistance in human cells by transient exposure to different chemotherapeutic drugs. J Natl Cancer Inst 1993; 85:632–639.

77. Uchiumi T, Kohno K, Tanimura H, et al. Involvement of protein kinase in environmental stress-induced activation of human multidrug resistance 1 (MDR1) gene promoter. FEBS Lett 1993; 326:11–16.

78. Kohno K, Sato S-I, Takano H, Matsuo K-I, Kuwano M. The direct activation of human multidrug resistance gene (MDR1) by anticancer agents. Biochem Biophys Res Commun 1989; 165:1415–1421.

79. Miyazaki M, Kohno K, Uchiumi T, et al. Activation of human multidrug resistance-1 gene promoter in response to heat shock stress. Biochem Biophys Res Commun 1992; 187:677–684.

80. Tanimura H, Kohno K, Sato S-I, et al. The human multidrug resistance 1 promoter has an element that responds to serum starvation. Biochem Biophys Res Commun 1992; 183:917–924.

81. Zastawny RL, Salvino R, Chen J, Benchimol S, Ling V. The core promoter region of the P-glycoprotein gene is sufficient to confer differential responsiveness to wild-type and mutant p53. Oncogene 1993; 8:1529–1535.

82. Chin K-V, Ueda K, Pastan I, Gottesman MM. Modulation of activity of the promoter of the human *MDR*1 gene by ras and p53. Science 1992; 255:459–462.

83. Cornwell MM, Smith DE. A signal transduction pathway for activation of the *mdr1* promoter involves the proto-oncogene c-*raf* kinase. J Biol Chem 1993; 268:15347–15350.

84. Ogura M, Takatori T, Tsuruo T. Purification and characterization of NF-R1 that regulates the expression of the human multidrug resistance (MDR1) gene. Nucleic Acids Res 1992; 20:5811–5817.

85. Asakuno K, Kohno K, Uchiumi T, et al. Involvement of a DNA binding protein, MDR-NF1/YB-1, in human MDR1 gene expression by actinomycin D. Biochem Biophys Res Commun 1994; 199:1428–1435.

86. Takatori T, Ogura M, Tsuruo T. Purification and characterization of NF-R2 that regulates the expression of the human multidrug resistance (MDR1) gene. Jpn J Cancer Res 1993; 84:298–303.

87. Ogura M, Takatori T, Sugimoto Y, Tsuruo T. Identification and characterization of three DNA-binding proteins on the promoter of the human *MDR*1 gene in drug-sensitive and -resistant cells. Jpn J Cancer Res 1991; 82:1151–1159.

88. Cornwell MM, Smith DE. SP1 activates the MDR1 promoter through one of two distinct G-rich regions that modulate promoter activity. J Biol Chem 1993; 268:19505–19511.

89. Zaman GJR, Versantvoort CHM, Smit JJM, et al. Analysis of the expression of *MRP*, the gene for a new putative transmembrane drug transporter, in human multidrug resistant lung cancer cell lines. Cancer Res 1993; 53:1747–1750.

90. Eijdems EWHM, de Haas M, Coco-Martin JM, et al. Mechanisms of *MRP* over-expression in four human lung-cancer cell lines and analysis of the *MRP* amplicon. Int J Cancer 1995; 60:676–684.

91. Kurz EU, Grant CE, Vasa MZ, Burtch-Wright RA, Cole SPC, Deeley RG. Analysis of the proximal promoter region of the muiltidrug resistance protein (MRP) gene in three small cell lung cancer cell lines (abstr). Proc AACR 1995; 36:1917.

92. Zhu Q, Center MS. Cloning and sequence analysis of the promoter region of the *MRP* gene of HL60 cells isolated for resistance to Adriamycin. Cancer Res 1994; 54:4488–4492.

93. Schneider E, Horton JK, Yang C-H, Nakagawa M, Cowan KH. Multidrug resistance-associated protein gene overexpression and reduced drug sensitivity of topoisomerase II in a human breast carcinoma MCF7 cell line selected for etoposide resistance. Cancer Res 1994; 54:152–158.

94. Coley HM, Workman P, Twentyman PR. Retention of activity by selected anthracyclines in a multidrug resistant human large cell lung carcinoma line without P-glycoprotein hyperexpression. Br J Cancer 1991; 63:351–357.

95. Cole SPC, Chanda ER, Dicke FP, Gerlach JH, Mirski SEL. Non-P-glycoprotein-mediated multidrug resistance in a small cell lung cancer cell line: evidence for decreased susceptibility to drug-induced DNA damage and reduced levels of topoisomerase II. Cancer Res 1991; 51:3345–3352.

96. McGrath T, Center MS. Mechanisms of multidrug resistance in HL60 cells: Evidence that a surface membrane protein distinct from P-glycoprotein contributes to reduced cellular accumulation of drug. Cancer Res 1988; 48:3959–3963.

97. Marsh W, Sicheri D, Center MS. Isolation and characterization of adriamycin-resistant HL-60 cells which are not defective in the initial intracellular accumulation of drug. Cancer Res 1986; 46:4053–4057.

98. Marquardt D, Center MS. Drug transport mechanisms in HL60 cells isolated for resistance to Adriamycin: evidence for nuclear drug accumulation and redistribution in resistant cells. Cancer Res 1992; 52:3157–3163.

99. Spoelstra EC, Westerhoff HV, Dekker H, Lankelma J. Kinetics of daunorubicin transport by P-glycoprotein of intact cancer cells. Eur J Biochem 1992; 207:567–579.

100. Demant EJF, Sehested M, Jensen PB. A model for computer simulation of P-glycoprotein and transmembrtane Delta pH-mediated anthracycline transport in multidrug-resistant tumor cells. Biochim Biophys Acta 1990; 1055:117–125.

101. Hindenburg AA, Baker MA, Gleyzer E, Stewart VJ, Case N, Taub RN. Effect of verapamil and other agents on the distribution of anthracyclines and on reversal of drug resistance. Cancer Res 1987; 47:1421–1425.

102. Gervasoni Jr, JE, Fields SZ, Krishna S, Baker MA, Rosado M, Thuraisamy K, Hindenburg AA, Taub RN. Subcellular distribution of daunorubicin in P-glycoprotein-positive and -negative drug-resistant cell lines using laser-associated confocal microscopy. Cancer Res 1991; 51:4955–4963.

103. Rutherford AV, Willingham MC. Ultrastructural localization of daunomycin in multidrug-resistant cultured cells with modulation of the multidrug transporter. J Histochem Cytochem 1993; 41:1573–1577.

104. Lankelma J, Mulder HS, van Mourik F, Wong Fong Sang HW, Kraayenhof R, van Grondelle R. Cellular daunomycin fluorescence in multidrug resistant 2780$^{AD}$ cells and its relation to cellular drug localisation. Biochim Biophys Acta 1991; 1093:147–152.

105. Schuurhuis GJ, Broxterman HJ, Cervantes A, et al. Quantitative determination of factors contributing to doxorubicin resistance in multidrug-resistant cells. J Natl Cancer Inst 1989; 81:1887–1892.

106. Safa AR, Glover CJ, Meyers MB, Biedler JL, Felsted RL. Vinblastine photoaffinity labeling of a high molecular weight surface membrane glycoprotein specific for multidrug-resistant cells. J Biol Chem 1986; 261:6137–6140.

107. Safa AR, Mehta ND, Agresti M. Photoaffinity labeling of P-glycoprotein in multidrug resistant cells with photoactive analogs of colchicine. Biochem Biophys Res Commun 1989; 162:1402–1408.

108. Beck WT, Cirtain MC, Glover CJ, Felsted RL, Safa AR. Effects of indole alkaloids on multidrug resistance and labeling of P-glycoprotein by a photoaffinity analog of vinblastine. Biochem Biophys Res Commun 1988; 153:959–966.

109. Safa AR. Photoaffinity labeling of P-glycoprotein in multidrug-resistant cells. Cancer Investigation 1992; 10:295–306.

110. Busche R, Tummler B, Riordan JR, Cano-Gauci DF. Preparation and utility of a radioiodinated analogue of daunomycin in the study of multidrug resistance. Mol Pharmacol 1989; 35:414–421.

111. Kamiwatari M, Nagata Y, Kikuchi H, et al. Correlation between reversing of multidrug resistance and inhibiting of [$^3$H] azidopine photolabeling of P-glycoprotein by newly synthesized dihydropyridine analogues in a human cell line. Cancer Res 1989; 49:3190–3195.

112. Yang C-PH, Mellado W, Horwitz SB. Azidopine photoaffinity labeling of multidrug resistance-associated glycoproteins. Biochem Pharmacol 1988; 37:1417–1421.

113. Bruggemann EP, Germann UA, Gottesman MM, Pastan I. Two different regions of phosphoglycoprotein are photoaffinity-labeled by azidopine. J Biol Chem 1989; 264:15483–15488.

114. Bruggemann EP, Currier SJ, Gottesman MM, Pastan I. Characterization of the azidopine and vinblastine binding site of P-glycoprotein. J Biol Chem 1992; 267:21020–21026.

115. Safa AR, Agresti M, Bryk D, Tamai I. N-(p-Azido-3-[$^{125}$I]iodophenethyl)spiperone binds to specific regions of P-glycoprotein and another multidrug binding protein, spiperophilin, in human neuroblastoma cells. Biochemistry 1994; 33:256–265.

116. Safa AR. Photoaffinity labeling of the multidrug-resistance-related P-glycoprotein with photoactive analogs of verapamil. Proc Natl Acad Sci USA 1988; 85:7187–7191.

117. Foxwell BMJ, Mackie A, Ling V, Ryffel B. Identification of the multidrug resistance-related P-glycoprotein as a cyclosporine binding protein. Mol Pharmacol 1989; 36:543–546.

118. Safa AR, Glover CJ, Sewell JL, Meyers MB, Biedler JL, Felsted RL. Identification of the multidrug resistance-related membrane glycoprotein as an acceptor for calcium channel blockers. J Biol Chem 1987; 262:7884–7888.

119. Cornwell MM, Tsuruo T, Gottesman MM, Pastan I. ATP-binding properties of P-glycoprotein from multidrug-resistant KB cells. FASEB J 1987; 1:51–54.

120. Schurr E, Raymond M, Bell JC, Gros P. Characterization of the multidrug resistance protein expressed in cell clones stably transfected with the mouse mdr1 cDNA. Cancer Res 1989; 49:2729–2734.

121. Georges E, Zhang J-T, Ling V. Modulation of ATP and drug binding by monoclonal antibodies against P-glycoprotein. J Cell Physiol 1991; 148:479–484.

122. Horio M, Gottesman MM, Pastan I. ATP-dependent transport of vinblastine in vesicles from human multidrug-resistant cells. Proc Natl Acad Sci USA 1988; 85:3580–3584.

123. Doige CA, Sharom FJ. Transport properties of P-glycoprotein in plasma membrane vesicles from multidrug-resistant Chinese hamster ovary cells. Biochim Biophys Acta 1992; 1109:161–171.

124. Sehested M, Bindslev N, Demant EJF, Skovsgaard T, Jensen PB. Daunorubicin and vincristine binding to plasma membrane vesicles from daunorubicin-resistant and wild type Ehrlich ascites tumor cells. Biochem Pharmacol 1989; 38:3017–3027.

125. Naito M, Hamada H, Tsuruo T. ATP/Mg$^{2+}$-dependent binding of vincristine to the plasma membrane of multidrug-resistant K562 cells. J Biol Chem 1988; 263:11887–11891.

126. Ambudkar SV, Lelong IH, Zhang J, Cardarelli CO, Gottesman MM, Pastan I. Partial purification and reconstitution of the human multidrug-resistance pump: characterization of the drug-stimulatable ATP hydrolysis. Proc Natl Acad Sci USA 1992; 89:8472–8476.

127. Sharom FJ, Yu X, Doige CA. Functional reconstitution of drug transport and ATPase activity in proteoliposomes containing partially purified P-glycoprotein. J Biol Chem 1993; 268:24197–24202.

128. Shapiro A, Ling V. ATPase activity of purified and reconstituted P-glycoprotein from Chinese hamster ovary cells. J Biol Chem 1994; 269:3745–3754.

129. Sharom FJ. Characterization and functional reconstitution of the multidrug transporter. J Bioenerg Biomem 1995; 27:15–22.

130. Shapiro AB, Ling V. Using purified P-glycoprotein to understand multidrug resistance. J Bioenerg Biomem 1995; 27:7–13.

131. Cole SPC. Multidrug resistance in human lung cancer. In: Pass HI, Mitchell J, Johnson DH, Turrisi AT, eds. Lung Cancer: Principles and Practice. Philadelphia: Lippincott, 1995.

132. Zaman GJR, Flens MJ, Van Leusden MR, et al. The human multidrug resistance-associated protein MRP is a plasma membrane drug-efflux pump. Proc Natl Acad Sci USA 1994; 91:8822–8826.

133. Choi KH, Chen C-J, Kriegler M, Roninson IB. An altered pattern of cross-resistance in multidrug-resistant human cells results from spontaneous mutations in the mdr1 (P-glycoprotein) gene. Cell 1988; 53:519–529.

134. Safa AR, Stern RK, Choi K, et al. Molecular basis of preferential resistance to colchicine in multidrug-resistant human cells conferred by Gly-185 -> Val-185 substitution in P-glycoprotein. Proc Natl Acad Sci USA 1990; 87:7225–7229.

135. Devine SE, Ling V, Melera PW. Amino acid substitutions in the sixth transmembrane domain of P-glycoprotein alter multidrug resistance. Proc Natl Acad Sci USA 1992; 89:4564–4568.

136. Loo TW, Clarke DM. Functional consequences of proline mutations in the predicted transmembrane domain of P-glycoprotein. J Biol Chem 1993; 268:3143–3149.

137. Loo TW, Clarke DM. Functional consequences of phenylalanine mutations in the predicted transmembrane domain of P-glycoprotein. J Biol Chem 1993; 268:19965–19972.

138. Loo TW, Clarke DM. Functional consequences of glycine mutations in the predicted cytoplasmic loops of P-glycoprotein. J Biol Chem 1994; 269:7243–7248.

139. Currier SJ, Kane SE, Willingham MC, Cardarelli CO, Pastan I, Gottesman MM. Identification of residues in the first cytoplasmic loop of P-glycoprotein involved in the function of chimeric human *MDR1-MDR2* transporters. J Biol Chem 1992; 267:25153–25159.

140. Barrand MA, Rhodes T, Center MS, Twentyman PR. Chemosensitisation and drug accumulation effects of cyclosporin A, PSC-833 and verapamil in human MDR large cell lung cancer cells expressing a 190k membrane protein distinct from P-glycoprotein. Eur J Cancer 1993; 29:408–415.

141. Coley HM, Amos WB, Twentyman PR, Workman P. Examination by laser scanning confocal fluorescence imaging microscopy of the subcellular localisation of anthracyclines in parent and multidrug resistant cell lines. Br J Cancer 1993; 67:1316–1323.

142. Cole SPC, Bhardwaj G, Gerlach HJ, Almquist KC, Deeley RG. A novel ATP-binding cassette transporter gene overexpressed in multidrug-resistant human lung tumour cells (abstr). Proc AACR 1993; 34:579.

143. Slapak CA, Mizunuma N, Kufe DW. Expression of the multidrug resistance associated protein and P-glycoprotein in doxorubicin-selected human myeloid leukemia cells. Blood 1994; 84:3113–3121.

144. Marquardt D, McCrone S, Center MS. Mechanisms of multidrug resistance in HL60 cells: detection of resistance-associated proteins with antibodies against synthetic peptides that correspond to the deduced sequence of P-glycoprotein. Cancer Res 1990; 50:1426–1430.

145. Flens MJ, Izquierdo MA, Scheffer GL, et al. Immunochemical detection of the multidrug resistance-associated protein MRP in human multidrug-resistant tumor cells by monoclonal antibodies. Cancer Res 1994; 54:4557–4563.

146. Muller M, Meijer C, Zaman GJR, et al. Overexpression of the gene encoding the multidrug resistance-associated protein results in increased ATP-dependent glutathione S-conjugate transport. Proc Natl Acad Sci USA 1994; 91:13033–13037.

147. McGrath T, Latoud C, Arnold ST, Safa AR, Felsted RL, Center MS. Mechanisms of multidrug resistance in HL60 cells: analysis of resistance associated membrane proteins and levels of *mdr* gene expression. Biochem Pharmacol 1989; 38:3611–3619.

148. Thiebaut F, Tsuruo T, Hamada H, Gottesman MM, Pastan I, Willingham MC. Cellular localization of the multidrug-resistance gene product P-glycoprotein in normal human tissues. Proc Natl Acad Sci USA 1987; 84:7735–7738.

149. Lieberman DM, Reithmeier RAF, Ling V, Charuk JHM, Goldberg H, Skorecki KL. Identification of P-glycoprotein in renal brush border membranes. Biochem Biophys Res Commun 1989; 162:244–252.

150. Sugawara I, Kataoka I, Morishita Y, et al. Tissue distribution of P-glycoprotein encoded by a multidrug-resistant gene as revealed by a monoclonal antibody, MRK 16. Cancer Res 1988; 48:1926–1929.

151. Cordon-Cardo C, O'Brien JP, Boccia J, Casals D, Bertino JR, Melamed MR. Expression of the multidrug resistance gene product (P-glycoprotein) in human normal and tumor tissues. J Histochem Cytochem 1990; 38:1277–1287.

152. Sugawara I, Nakahama M, Hamada H, Tsuruo T, Mori S. Apparent stronger expression in the human adrenal cortex than in the human adrenal medulla of $M_r$ 170,000-180,000 P-glycoprotein. Cancer Res 1988; 48:4611–4614.

153. Cordon-Cardo C, O'Brien JP, Casals D, et al. Multidrug-resistance gene (P-glycoprotein) is expressed by endothelial cells at blood-brain barrier sites. Proc Natl Acad Sci USA 1989; 86:695–698.

154. Thiebaut F, Tsuruo T, Hamada H, Gottesman MM, Pastan I, Willingham MC. Immuno-histochemical localization in normal tissues of different epitopes in the multidrug transport protein P170: evidence for localization in brain capillaries and crossreactivity of one anti-body with a muscle protein. J Histochem Cytochem 1989; 37:159–164.

155. Danks MK, Yalowich JC, Beck WT. Atypical multiple drug resistance in a human leukemic cell line selected for resistance to teniposide (VM-26). Cancer Res 1987; 47:1297–1301.

156. Fojo AT, Ueda K, Slamon DJ, Poplack DG, Gottesman MM, Pastan I. Expression of a multidrug-resistance gene in human tumors and tissues. Proc Natl Acad Sci USA 1987; 84:265–269.

157. Chaudhary PM, Roninson IB. Expression and activity of P-glycoprotein, a multidrug efflux pump, in human hematopoietic stem cells. Cell 1991; 66:85–94.

158. Drach D, Zhao S, Drach J, et al. Subpopulations of normal peripheral blood and bone marrow cells express a functional multidrug resistant phenotype. Blood 1992; 80:2729–2734.

159. Chaudhary PM, Mechetner EB, Roninson IB. Expression and activity of the multidrug resistance P-glycoprotein in human peripheral blood lymphocytes. Blood 1992; 80:2735–2739.

160. Hegewisch-Becker S, Fliegner M, Tsuruo T, Zander A, Zeller W, Hossfeld DK. P-glyco-protein expression in normal and reactive bone marrows. Br J Cancer 1993; 67:430–435.

161. Marie J-P, Brophy NA, Ehsan MN, et al. Expression of multidrug resistance gene *mdr*1 mRNA in a subset of normal bone marrow cells. Br J Haematol 1992; 81:145–152.

162. Abbaszadegan MR, Futscher BW, Klimecki WT, List A, Dalton WS. Analysis of multidrug resistance-associated protein (MRP) messenger RNA in normal and malignant hemato-poietic cells. Cancer Res 1994; 54:4676–4679.

163. Leier I, Jedlitschky G, Buchholz U, Cole SPC, Deeley RG, Keppler D. The *MRP* gene encodes an ATP-dependent export pump for leukotriene C4 and structurally related con-jugates. J Biol Chem 1994; 269:27807–27810.

164. Keppler D. Leukotrienes: Biosynthesis, transport, inactivation and analysis. Rev Physiol Biochem Pharmacol 1992; 121:2–30.

165. Ishikawa T. The ATP-dependent glutathione S-conjugate export pump. TIBS 1992; 17: 463–468.

166. Ishikawa T, Wright CD, Ishizuka H. *GS-X* pump is functionally overexpressed in *cis*-diam-minedichloroplatinum (II)-resistant human leukemia HL-60 cells and down-regulated by cell differentiation. J Biol Chem 1994; 269:29085–29093.

167. Oude Elferink RPJ, Jansen PLM. The role of the canalicular multispecific organic anion transporter in the disposal of endo- and xenobiotics. Pharmacol Ther 1994; 64:77–97.

168. Tew KD. Glutathione-associated enzymes in anticancer drug resistance. Cancer Res 1994; 54:4313–4320.

169. Beck WT, Cirtain MC. Continued expression of vinca alkaloid resistance by CCRF-CEM cells after treatment with tunicamycin or pronase. Cancer Res 1982; 42:184–189.

170. Ichikawa M, Yoshimura A, Furukawa T, Sumizawa T, Nakazima Y, Akiyama S-I. Glyco-sylation of P-glycoprotein in a multidrug-resistant KB cell line, and in the human tissues. Biochim Biophys Acta 1991; 1073:309–315.

171. Schinkel AH, Kemp S, Dolle M, Rudenko G, Wagenaar E. *N*-Glycosylation and deletion mutants of the human *MDR*1 P-glycoprotein. J Biol Chem 1993; 268:7474–7481.

172. Kramer R, Weber TK, Arceci R, et al. Inhibition of *N*-linked glycosylation of P-glycoprotein by tunicamycin results in a reduced multidrug resistance phenotype. Br J Cancer 1995; 71: 670–675.

173. Germann UA, Willingham MC, Pastan I, Gottesman MM. Expression of the human mul-tidrug transporter in insect cells by a recombinant baculovirus. Biochemistry 1990; 29:2295–2303.

174. Bibi E, Gros P, Kaback HR. Functional expression of mouse mdr1 in *Escherichia coli*. Proc Natl Acad Sci USA 1993; 90:9209–9213.

175. Kuchler K, Thorner J. Functional expression of human *mdr1* in the yeast *Saccharomyces cerevisiae*. Proc Natl Acad Sci USA 1992; 89:2302–2306.

176. Lis H, Sharon N. Protein glycosylation. Structural and functional aspects. Eur J Biochem 1993; 218:1–27.

177. Roy SN, Horwitz SB. A phosphoglycoprotein associated with Taxol resistance in J774.2 cells. Cancer Res 1985; 45:3856–3863.

178. Garman D, Albers L, Center MS. Identification and characterization of a plasma membrane phosphoprotein which is present in Chinese hamster lung cells resistant to Adriamycin. Biochem Pharmacol 1983; 32:3633–3637.

179. Hamada H, Hagiwara K, Nakajima T, Tsuruo T. Phosphorylation of the Mr 170,000 to 180,000 glycoprotein specific to multidrug-resistant tumor cells: effects of verapamil, trifluoperazine, and phorbol esters. Cancer Res 1987; 47:2860–2865.

180. Meyers MB. Protein phosphorylation in multidrug resistant Chinese hamster cells. Cancer Commun 1989; 1:233–241.

181. Chambers TC, McAvoy EM, Jacobs JW, Eilon G. Protein kinase C phosphorylates P-glycoprotein in multidrug resistant human KB carcinoma cells. J Biol Chem 1990; 265:7679–7686.

182. Ma L, Marquardt D, Takemoto L, Center MS. Analysis of P-glycoprotein phosphorylation in HL60 cells isolated for resistance to vincristine. J Biol Chem 1991; 266:5593–5599.

183. Carlsen SA, Till JE, Ling V. Modulation of drug permeability in Chinese hamster ovary cells. Possible role for phosphorylation of surface glycoproteins. Biochim Biophys Acta 1977; 467:238–250.

184. Center MS. Evidence that Adriamycin resistance in Chinese hamster lung cells is regulated by phosphorylation of a plasma membrane glycoprotein. Biochem Biophys Res Commun 1983; 115:159–166.

185. Epand RM, Stafford AR. Protein kinases and multidrug resistance. Cancer J 1993; 6:154–158.

186. Yu G, Ahmad S, Aquino A, et al. Transfection with protein kinase Cα confers increased multidrug resistance to MCF-7 cells expressing P-glycoprotein. Cancer Common 1991; 3:181–189.

187. Ahmad S, Glazer RI. Expression of the antisense cDNA for protein kinase Cα attenuates resistance in doxorubicin-resistant MCF-7 breast carcinoma cells. Mol Pharmacol 1993; 43:858–862.

188. Ahmad S, Trepel JB, Ohno S, Suzuki K, Tsuruo T, Glazer RI. Role of protein kinase C in the modulation of multidrug resistance: expression of the atypical γ isoform of protein kinase C does not confer increased resistance to doxorubicin. Mol Pharmacol 1992; 42:1004–1009.

189. Staats J, Marguardt D, Center MS. Characterization of a membrane-associated protein kinase of multidrug-resistant HL60 cells which phosphorylates P-glycoprotein. J Biol Chem 1990; 265:4084–4090.

190. Chambers TC, Pohl J, Raynor RL, Kuo JF. Identification of specific sites in human P-glycoprotein phosphorylated by protein kinase C. J Biol Chem 1993; 268:4592–4595.

191. Orr GA, Han EK-H, Browne PC, et al. Identification of the major phosphorylation domain of murine *mdr*1b P-glycoprotein. Analysis of the protein kinase A and protein kinase C phosphorylation sites. J Biol Chem 1993; 268:25054–25062.

192. Picciotto MR, Cohn JA, Bertuzzi G, Greengard P, Nairn AC. Phosphorylation of the cystic fibrosis transmembrane conductance regulator. J Biol Chem 1992; 267:12742–12752.

193. Chang X-B, Tabcharani JA, Hou Y-X, et al. Protein kinase A (PKA) still activates CFTR chloride channel after mutagenesis of all 10 PKA consensus phosphorylation sites. J Biol Chem 1993; 268:11304–11311.

194. Cheng SH, Rich DP, Marshall J, Gregory RJ, Welsh MJ, Smith AE. Phosphorylation of the R domain by cAMP-dependent protein kinase regulates the CFTR chloride channel. Cell 1991; 66:1027–1036.

195. Goldstein LJ, Galski H, Fojo A, et al. Expression of a multidrug resistance gene in human cancers. J Natl Cancer Inst 1989; 81:116–124.

196. Ueda K, Yamano Y, Kioka N, et al. Detection of multidrug resistance (*MDR*1) gene RNA expression in human tumors by a sensitive ribonuclease protein assay. Jpn J Cancer Res (Gann) 1989; 80:1127–1132.

197. Burger H, Nooter K, Zaman GJR, et al. Expression of the multidrug resistance-associated protein (*MRP*) in acute and chronic leukemias. Leukemia 1994; 8:990–997.

198. Doherty PJ, Huesca-Contreras M, Dosch HM, Pan S. Rapid amplification of complementary DNA from small amounts of unfractionated RNA. Analyt Biochem 1989; 177: 7–10.

199. Futscher BW, Blake LL, Gerlach JH, Grogan TM, Dalton WS. Quantitative polymerase chain reaction analysis of mdr1 mRNA in multiple myeloma cell lines and clinical specimens. Anal Biochem 1993; 213:414–421.

200. Noonan KE, Beck C, Holzmayer TA, et al. Quantitative analysis of *MDR1* (multidrug resistance) gene expression in human tumors by polymerase chain reaction. Proc Natl Acad Sci USA 1990; 87:7160–7164.

201. Murphy LD, Herzog CE, Rudick JB, Fojo AT, Bates SE. Use of the polymerase chain reaction in the quantitation of *mdr*-1 gene expression. Biochemistry 1990; 29:10351–10356.

202. Scanlon KJ, Kashani-Sabet M. Utility of the polymerase chain reaction in detection of gene expression in drug-resistant human tumors. J Clin Lab Anal 1989; 3:323–329.

203. Hoof T, Riordan JR, Tummler B. Quantitation of mRNA by the kinetic polymerase chain reaction assay: a tool for monitoring P-glycoprotein gene expression. Analyt Biochem 1991; 196:161–169.

204. Futscher BW, Abbaszadegan MR, Domann F, Dalton WS. Analysis of *MRP* mRNA in mitoxantrone-selected, multidrug-resistant human tumor cells. Biochem Pharmacol 1994; 47:1601–1606.

205. Sugawara I, Arai T, Yamashita T, Yoshida A, Masunaga S, Itoyama S. Expression of multidrug resistance-associated protein (MRP) in anaplastic carcinoma of the thyroid. Cancer Lett 1994; 82:185–188.

206. Bordow SB, Haber M, Madafiglio J, Cheung B, Marshall GM, Norris MD. Expression of the multidrug resistance-associated protein (MRP) gene correlates with amplification and overexpression of the N-myc oncogene in childhood neuroblastoma. Cancer Res 1994; 54: 5036–5040.

207. Burger H, Nooter K, Sonneveld P, van Wingerden KE, Zaman GJR, Stoter G. High expression of the multidrug resistance-associated protein (MRP) in chronic and prolymphocytic leukaemia. Br J Haematol 1994; 88:348–356.

208. Beck J, Niethammer D, Gekeler V. High mdr1- and mrp-, but low topoisomerase IIα-gene expression in B-cell chronic lymphocytic leukaemias. Cancer Lett 1994; 86:135–142.

209. Hart SM, Ganeshaguru K, Hoffbrand AV, Prentice HG, Mehta AB. Expression of the multidrug resistance-associated protein (MRP) in acute leukemia. Leukemia 1994; 8:2163–2168.

210. Tsuruo T, Iida H, Nojiri M, Tsukagoshi S, Sakurai Y. Potentiation of chemotherapeutic effect of vincristine in vincristine resistant tumor bearing mice by calmodulin inhibitor clomipramine. J Pharm Dyn 1983; 6:145–147.

211. Arceci RJ, Croop JM, Horwitz SB, Housman D. The gene encoding multidrug resistance is induced and expressed at high levels during pregnancy in the secretory epithelium of the uterus. Proc Natl Acad Sci USA 1988; 85:4350–4354.

212. Beck J. Handgretinger R, Dopfer R, Klingebiel T, Niethammer D, Gekeler V. Expression of mdr1, mrp, topoisomerase IIα/β, and cyclin A in primary or relapsed states of acute lymphoblastic leukaemias. Br J Haematol 1995; 89:356–363.

213. Shen D-W, Pastan I, Gottesman MM. *in situ* hybridization analysis of acquisition and loss of the human multidrug-resistance gene. Cancer Res 1988; 48:4334–4339.

214. Doyle A, Martin WJ, Funa K, et al. Markedly decreased expression of class I histocompatibility antigens, protein, and mRNA in human small-cell lung cancer. J Exp Med 1985; 161:1135–1151.

215. Wang AM, Doyle MV, Mark DF. Quantitation of mRNA by the polymerase chain reaction. Proc Natl Acad Sci USA 1989; 86:9717–9721.

216. Vanden Heuvel JP, Tyson FL, Bell DA. Construction of recombinant RNA templates for use as internal standards in quantitative RT-PCR. BioTechniques 1993; 14:395–398.

217. Siebert PD, Larrick JW. PCR mimics: competitive DNA fragments for use as internal standards in quantiative PCR. BioTechniques 1993; 14:244–249.

218. Lazaruk LC, Campling BG, Baer KA, et al. Drug resistance and expression of MRP and MDR1 in small cell lung cancer cell lines (abstr). Proc AACR 1995; 36:1953.

219. Chan HSL, Bradley G, Thorner G, Haddad G, Gallie BL, Ling V. A sensitive method for immunocytochemical detection of P-glycoprotein in multidrug-resistant human ovarian carcinoma cell lines. Lab Invest 1988; 59:870–875.

220. Chan HSL, Thorner PS, Haddad G, Ling V. Immunohistochemical detection of P-glycoprotein: prognostic correlation in soft tissue sarcoma of childhood. J Clin Oncol 1990; 8:689–704.

221. Chan HSL, Haddad G, Thorner PS, et al. P-glycoprotein expression as a predictor of the outcome of therapy for neuroblastoma. N Engl J Med 1991; 325:1608–1614.

222. Dalton WS, Grogan TM, Rybski JA, et al. Immunohistochemical detection and quantitation of P-glycoprotein in multiple drug-resistant human myeloma cells: association with level of drug resistance and drug accumulation. Blood 1989; 73:747–752.

223. Grogan T, Dalton W, Rybski J, et al. Optimization of immunocytochemical P-glycoprotein assessment in multidrug-resistant plasma cell myeloma using three antibodies. Lab Invest 1990; 63:815–824.

224. Finstad CL, Yin BWT, Gordon CM, Federici MG, Welt S, Lloyd KO. Some monoclonal antibody reagents (C219 and JSB-1) to P-glycoprotein contain antibodies to blood group A carbohydrate determinants: a problem of quality control for immunohistochemical analysis. J Histochem Cytochem 1991; 39:1603–1610.

225. Elias JM, Gown AM, Nakamura RM, et al. Special report: quality control in immunohistochemistry. Am J Clin Pathol 1989; 92:836–843.

226. Rao VV, Anthony DC, Piwnica-Worms D. *MDR1* gene-specific monoclonal antibody C494 cross-reacts with pyruvate carboxylase. Cancer Res 1994; 54:1536–1541.

227. Tanaka S, Currier SJ, Bruggemann EP, et al. Use of recombinant P-glycoprotein fragments to produce antibodies to the multidrug transporter. Biochem Biophys Res Commun 1990; 166:180–186.

228. Kartner N, Riordan JR, Ling V. Cell surface P-glycoprotein associated with multidrug resistance in mammalian cell lines. Science 1983; 221:1285–1288.

229. Meyers MB, Rittmann-Grauer L, O'Brien JP, Safa AR. Characterization of monoclonal antibodies recognizing a $M_r$ 180,000 P-glycoprotein: differential expression of the $M_r$ 180,000 and $M_r$ 170,000 P-glycoproteins in multidrug-resistant human tumor cells. Cancer Res 1989; 49:3209–3214.

230. Kartner N, Evernden-Porelle D, Bradley G, Ling V. Detection of P-glycoprotein in multidrug-resistant cell lines by monoclonal antibodies. Nature 1985; 316:820–823.

231. Lathan B, Edwards DP, Dressler LG, Von Hoff DD, McGuire WL. Immunological detection of Chinese hamster ovary cells expressing a multidrug resistance phenotype. Cancer Res 1985; 45:5064–5069.

232. Scheper RJ, Bulte JWM, Brakkee JGP, et al. Monoclonal antibody JSB-1 detects a highly conserved epitope on the P-glycoprotein associated with multi-drug-resistance. Int J Cancer 1988; 42:389–394.

233. Mechetner EB, Roninson IB. Efficient inhibition of P-glycoprotein-mediated multidrug resistance with a monoclonal antibody. Proc Natl Acad Sci USA 1992; 89:5824–5828.

234. Arceci RJ, Stieglitz K, Bras J, Schinkel A, Baas F, Croop J. Monoclonal antibody to an external epitope of the human *mdr1* P-glycoprotein. Cancer Res 1993; 53:310–317.

235. Rittmann-Grauer LS, Yong MA, Sanders V, Mackensen DG. Reversal of *Vinca* alkaloid resistance by anti-P-glycoprotein monoclonal antibody HYB-241 in a human tumor xenograft. Cancer Res 1992; 52:1810–1816.

236. Hamada H, Tsuruo T. Functional role for the 170- to 180-kDa glycoprotein specific to drug-resistant tumor cells as revealed by monoclonal antibodies. Proc Natl Acad Sci USA 1986; 83:7785–7789.

237. Cenciarelli C, Currier SJ, Willingham MC, et al. Characterization by somatic cell genetics of a monoclonal antibody to the *MDR*1 gene product (P-glycoprotein): determination of P-glycoprotein expression in multi-drug resistant KB and CEM cell variants. Int J Cancer 1991; 47:533–543.

238. Deffie AM, Alam T, Seneviratne C, et al. Multifactorial resistance to Adriamycin: relationship of DNA repair, glutathione transferase activity, drug efflux, and P-glycoprotein in cloned cell lines of Adriamycin-sensitive and resistant P388 leukemia. Cancer Res 1988; 48:3595–3602.

239. Miller TP, Grogan TM, Dalton WS, Spier CM, Scheper RJ, Salmon SE. P-Glycoprotein expression in malignant lymphoma and reversal of clinical drug resistance with chemotherapy plus high-dose verapamil. J Clin Oncol 1991; 9:17–24.

240. List AF, Spier C, Greer J, et al. Phase I/II trial of cyclosporine as a chemotherapy-resistance modifier in acute leukemia. J Clin Oncol 1993; 11:1652–1660.

241. Lincke CR, Smit JJM, Van der Velde-Koerts T, Borst P. Structure of the *MDR*3 gene and physical mapping of the human *MDR* locus. J Biol Chem 1991; 266:5303–5310.

242. Krishan A, Sauerteig A, Stein JH. Comparison of three commercially available antibodies for flow cytometric monitoring of P-glycoprotein expression in tumor cells. Cytometry 1991; 12:731–742.

243. van der Valk P, van Kalken CK, Ketelaars H, et al. Distribution of multi-drug resistance-associated P-glycoprotein in normal and neoplastic human tissues. Analysis with 3 monoclonal antibodies recognizing different epitopes of the P-glycoprotein molecule. Ann Oncol 1990; 1:56–64.

244. Hamada H, Miura K, Ariyoshi K, et al. Mouse-human chimeric antibody against the multidrug transporter P-glycoprotein. Cancer Res 1990; 50:3167–3171.

245. Nishioka Y, Sone S, Heike Y, et al. Effector cell analysis of human multidrug-resistant cell killing by mouse-human chimeric antibody against P-glycoprotein. Jpn J Cancer Res 1992; 83:644–649.

246. van Dijk J, Tsuruo T, Segal DM, et al. Bispecific antibodies reactive with the multidrug-resistance-related glycoprotein and cd3 induce lysis of multidrug-resistant tumor cells. Int J Cancer 1989; 44:738–743.

247. Tsuruo T, Hamada H, Sato S, Heike Y. Inhibition of multidrug-resistant human tumor growth in athymic mice by anti-P-glycoprotein monoclonal antibodies. Jpn J Cancer Res (Gann) 1989; 80:627–631.

248. Heike Y, Hamada H, Inamura N, Sone S, Ogura T, Tsuruo T. Monoclonal anti-P-glycoprotein antibody-dependent killing of multidrug-resistant tumor cells by human mononuclear cells. Jpn J Cancer Res (Gann) 1990; 81:1155–1161.

249. Heike Y, Sone S, Yano S, Seimiya H, Tsuruo T, Ogura T. M-CSF gene transduction in multidrug-resistant human cancer cells to enhance anti-P-glycoprotein antibody-dependent macrophage-mediated cytotoxicity. Int J Cancer 1993; 54:851–857.

250. Broxterman HJ, Kuiper CM, Schuurhuis GJ, Tsuruo T, Pinedo HM, Lankelma J. Increase of daunorubicin and vincristine accumulation in multidrug resistant human ovarian carcinoma cells by a monoclonal antibody reacting with P-glycoprotein. Biochem Pharmacol 1988; 37:2389–2393.

251. Pearson JW, Fogler WE, Volker K, et al. Reversal of drug resistance in a human colon cancer xenograft expressing MDR1 complementary DNA by in vivo administration of MRK-16 monoclonal antibody. J Natl Cancer Inst 1991; 83:1386–1391.

252. FitzGerald DJ, Willingham MC, Cardarelli CO, et al. A monoclonal antibody-*Pseudomonas* toxin conjugate that specifically kills multidrug-resistant cells. Proc Natl Acad Sci USA 1987; 84:4288–4292.

253. Dinota A, Tazzari PL, Michieli M, et al. *in vitro* bone marrow purging of multidrug-resistant cells with a mouse monoclonal antibody directed against $M_r$ 170,000 glycoprotein and a saporin-conjugated anti-mouse antibody. Cancer Res 1990; 50:4291–4294.

254. Barrand MA, Heppell-Parton AC, Wright KA, Rabbitts PH, Twentyman PR. A 190-kilodalton protein overexpressed in non-P-glycoprotein-containing multidrug-resistant cells and its relationship to the MRP gene. J Natl Cancer Inst 1994; 86:110–117.

255. Hipfner DR, Gauldie SD, Deeley RG, Cole SPC. Detection of the $M_r$ 190,000 multidrug resistance protein, MRP, with monoclonal antibodies. Cancer Res 1994; 54:5788–5792.

256. Weaver JL, Pine PS, Aszalos A, et al. Laser scanning and confocal microscopy of daunorubicin, doxorubicin, and rhodamine 123 in multidrug-resistant cells. Exp Cell Res 1991; 196: 323–329.

257. Ross DD, Thompson BW, Ordonez JV, Joneckis CC. Improvement of flow-cytometric detection of multidrug-resistant cells by cell-volume normalization of intracellular daunorubicin content. Cytometry 1989; 10:185–191.

258. Tapiero H, Munck J-N, Fourcade A, Lampidis TJ. Cross-resistance to rhodamine 123 in Adriamycin- and daunorubicin-resistant Friend leukemia cell variants. Cancer Res 1994; 44:5544–5549.

259. Kessel D. Exploring multidrug resistance using rhodamine 123. Cancer Commun 1989; 1: 145–149.

260. Ludescher C, Thaler J, Drach D, et al. Detection of activity of P-glycoprotein in human tumour samples using rhodamine 123. Br J Haematol 1992; 82:161–168.

261. Canitrot Y, Lautier D, Lahmy S, Vigo J, Viallet P, Salmon J-M. Nile red labeling of single living cells for contour delineation to quantify and evaluate the distribution of rhodamine 123 with fluorescence image cytometry. J Histochem Cytochem 1993; 41:1785–1793.

262. Lahmy S, Lautier D, Canitrot Y, Laurent G, Salmon J-M. Staining with Hoechst 33342 and rhodamine 123: an attempt to detect multidrug resistant phenotype cells in leukemia. Leukemia Res 1993; 17:1021–1029.

263. de Jong S, Holtrop M, de Vries H, de Vries EGE, Mulder NH. Increased sensitivity of an Adriamycin-resistant human small cell lung carcinoma cell line to mitochondrial inhibitors. Biochem Biophys Res Common 1992; 182:877–885.

264. Feller N, Kuiper CM, Lankelma J, et al. Functional detection of *MDR*1/P170 and *MRP*/P190 mediated multidrug resistance in tumor cells by flow cytometry. Br J Cancer 1995; 72:543–549.

265. Twentyman PR, Rhodes T, Rayner S. A comparison of rhodamine 123 accumulation and efflux in cells with P-glycoprotein-mediated and MRP-associated multidrug resistance phenotypes. Eur J Cancer 1994; 30A:1360–1369.

266. Feller N, Broxterman HJ, Wahrer DCR, Pinedo HM. ATP-dependent efflux of calcein by the multidrug resistance protein (MRP): no inhibition by intracellular glutathione depletion. FEBS Lett 1995; 368:385–388.

267. Nooter K, Sonneveld P, Oostrum R, Herweijer H, Hagenbeek T, Valerio D. Overexpression of the *mdr1* gene in blast cells from patients with acute myelocytic leukemia is associated with decreased anthracycline accumulation that can be restored by cyclosporin-A. Int J Cancer 1990; 45:263–268.

268. Ross DD, Wooten PJ, Tong Y, et al. Synergistic reversal of multidrug-resistance phenotype in acute myeloid leukemia cells by cyclosporin A and Cremophor EL. Blood 1994; 83: 1337–1347.

269. Broxterman HJ, Pinedo HM, Kuiper CM, Kaptein LC, Schuurhuis GJ, Lankelma J. Induction by verapamil of a rapid increase in ATP consumption in multidrug-resistant tumor cells. FASEB J 1988; 2:2278–2282.

270. Vayuvegula B, Slater L, Meador J, Gupta S. Correction of altered plasma membrane potentials. A possible mechanism of cyclosporin A and verapamil reversal of pleiotropic drug resistance in neoplasia. Cancer Chemother Pharmacol 1988; 22:163–168.

271. Hamilton G, Cosentini EP, Teleky B, et al. The multidrug-resistance modifiers verapamil, cyclosporin A and tamoxifen induce an intracellular acidification in colon carcinoma cell lines *in vitro*. Anticancer Res 1993; 13:2059–2064.

272. Cole SPC, Downes HF, Slovak ML. Effect of calcium antagonists on the chemosensitivity of two multidrug resistant human tumour cell lines which do not overexpress P-glycoprotein. Br J Cancer 1989; 59:42–46.

273. Binaschi M, Supino R, Gambetta RA, et al. MRP gene overexpression is a human doxorubicin-resistant SCLC cell line: alterations in cellular pharmacokinetics and in pattern of cross-resistance. Int J Cancer 1995; 62:84–89.

274. Gervasoni Jr, JE, Fields SZ, Krishna S, et al. Subcellular distribution of daunorubicin in P-glycoprotein-positive and -negative drug-resistant cell lines using laser-assisted confocal microscopy. Cancer Res 1991; 51:4955–4963.

275. Hindenburg AA, Gervasoni Jr, JE, Krishna S, et al. Intracellular distribution and pharmacokinetics of daunorubicin in anthracycline-sensitive and -resistant HL-60 cells. Cancer Res 1989; 49:4607–4614.

276. Willingham MC, Cornwell MM, Cardarelli CO, Gottesman MM, Pastan I. Single cell analysis of daunomycin uptake and efflux in multidrug-resistant and -sensitive KB cells: effects of verapamil and other drugs. Cancer Res 1986; 46:5941–5946.

277. Rutherford AV, Willingham MC. Ultrastructural localization of daunomycin in multidrug-resistant cultured cells with modulation of the multidrug transporter. J Histochem Cytochem 1993; 41:1573–1577.

278. Hindenburg AA, Baker MA, Gleyzer E, Stewart VJ, Case N, Taub RN. Effect of verapamil and other agents on the distribution of anthracyclines and on reversal of drug resistance. Cancer Res 1987; 47:1421–1425.

279. Thiebaut F, Currier SJ, Whitaker J, et al. Activity of the multidrug transporter results in alkalinization of the cytosol: measurement of cytosolic pH by microinjection of a pH-sensitive dye. J Histochem Cytochem 1990; 38:685–690.

280. Brock I, Hipfner DR, Nielsen BE, et al. Sequential co-expression of the multidrug resistance genes, MRP and mdr1 and their products in VP-16 (etoposide) selected H69 small cell lung cancer cells. Cancer Res 1995; 55:459–462.

281. Reeve JG, Rabbitts PH, Twentyman PR. Amplification and expression of mdr1 gene in a multidrug resistant variant of small cell lung cancer cell line NCI-H69. Br J Cancer 1989; 60:339–342.

282. Minato K, Kanazawa F, Nishio K, Nakagawa K, Fujiwara Y, Saijo N. Characterization of an etoposide-resistant human small-cell lung cancer cell line. Cancer Chemother Pharmacol 1990; 26:313–317.

283. Jensen PB, Vindelov L, Roed H, et al. *in vitro* evaluation of the potential of aclarubicin in the treatment of small cell carcinoma of the lung (SCCL). Br J Cancer 1989; 60:838–844.

284. Kiura K, Ohnoshi T, Ueoka H, et al. An Adriamycin-resistant subline is more sensitive than the parent human small cell lung cancer cell line to lonidamine. Anti-Cancer Drug Design 1992; 7:463–470.

285. Glisson BS, Alpeter MD. Multidrug resistance in a small cell lung cancer line: rapid selection with etoposide and differential chemosensitization with cyclosporin A. Anticancer Drugs 1992; 3:359–366.

286. Capranico G, Supino R, Binaschi M, et al. Influence of structural modifications at the 3' and 4' positions of doxorubicin on the drug ability to trap topoisomerase II and to overcome multidrug resistance. Mol Pharmacol 1994; 45:908–915.

287. Jensen PB, Roed H, Sehested M, et al. Doxorubicin sensitivity pattern in a panel of small-cell lung-cancer cell lines: correlation to etoposide and vincristine and inverse correlation to carmustine sensitivity. Cancer Chemother Pharmacol 1992; 31:46–52.

288. Zunino F, Binaschi M, Capranico G, De Isabella P, Pratesi G, Supino R. The mechanisms of multiple drug resistance in small cell lung cancer. Cancer Ther Control 1991; 2:45–51.

289. Long BH, Musial ST, Brattain MG. DNA breakage in human lung carcinoma cells and nuclei that are naturally sensitive or resistant to etoposide and teniposide. Cancer Res 1986; 46:3809–3816.

290. Lai S-L, Goldstein LJ, Gottesman MM, et al. MDR1 gene expression in lung cancer. J Natl Cancer Inst 1989; 81:1144–1150.

291. Pratesi G, Capranico G, Binaschi M, et al. Relationships among tumor responsiveness, cell sensitivity, doxorubicin cellular pharmacokinetics and drug-induced DNA alterations in two human small-cell lung cancer xenografts. Int J Cancer 1990; 46:669–674.

292. Binaschi M, Capranico G, De Isabella P, et al. Comparison of DNA cleavage induced by etoposide and doxorubicin in two human small-cell lung cancer lines with different sensitivities to topoisomerase II inhibitors. Int J Cancer 1990; 45:347–352.

293. Carmichael J, Mitchell JB, DeGraff WG, et al. Chemosensitivity testing of human lung cancer cell lines using the MTT assay. Br J Cancer 1988; 57:540–547.

294. Campling BG, Pym J, Baker HM, Cole SPC, Lam Y-M. Chemosensitivity testing of small cell lung cancer using the MTT assay. Br J Cancer 1991; 63:75–83.

295. Carney DN, Mitchell JB, Kinsella TJ. *in vitro* radiation and chemotherapy sensitivity of established cell lines of human small cell lung cancer and its large cell morphological variants. Cancer Res 1983; 43:2806–2811.

296. Tanio Y, Watanabe M, Inoue T, et al. Chemo-radioresistance of small cell lung cancer cell lines derived from untreated primary tumors obtained by diagnostic bronchofiberscopy. Jpn J Cancer Res 1990; 81:289–297.

297. Cole SPC, Campling BG, Dexter DF, Holden JJA, Roder JC. Establishment of a human large cell lung tumor line (QU-DB) with metastatic properties in athymic mice. Cancer 1986; 58:917–923.

298. Pettengill OS, Faulkner CS, Wurster-Hill DH, et al. Isolation and characterization of a hormone producing cell line from human small cell anaplastic carcinoma of the lung. J Natl Cancer Inst 1977; 58:511–518.

299. Pettengill OS, Sorenson GD, Wurster-Hill DH, et al. Isolation and growth characteristics of continuous cell lines from small-cell carcinoma of the lung. Cancer 1980; 45:906–918.

300. Gazdar AF, Carney DN, Russell EK, et al. Establishment of continuous, clonable cultures of small-cell carcinoma of the lung which have amine precursor uptake and decarboxylation cell properties. Cancer Res 1980; 40:3502–3507.

301. Postmus PE, de Ley L, van der Veen AY, Mesander G, Buys CHCM, Elema JD. Two small cell lung cancer cell lines established from rigid bronchoscope biopsies. Eur J Cancer Clin Oncol 1988; 24:753–763.

302. Baillie-Johnson H, Twentyman PR, Fox NE, et al. Establishment and characterisation of cell lines from patients with lung cancer (predominantly small cell carcinoma). Br J Cancer 1985; 52:494–504.

303. Carney DN, Gazdar AF, Bepler G, et al. Establishment and identification of small cell lung cancer cell lines having classic and variant features. Cancer Res 1985; 45:2913–2923.

304. Bepler G, Jaques G, Neumann K, Aumuller G, Gropp C, Havemann K. Establishment, growth properties, and morphological characteristics of permanent human small cell lung cancer cell lines. J Cancer Res Clin Oncol 1987; 113:31–40.

305. Longdon SP, Rabiasz GJ, Anderson L, et al. Characterisation and properties of a small cell lung cancer cell line and xenograft WX322 with marked sensitivity to alpha-interferon. Br J Cancer 1991; 63:909–915.

306. De Leij L, Postmus PE, Buys CHCM, et al. Characterization of three new variant type cell lines derived from small cell carcinoma of the lung. Cancer Res 1985; 45:6024–6033.

307. Campling BG, Haworth AC, Baker HM, et al. Establishment and characterization of a panel of human lung cancer cell lines. Cancer 1992; 69:2064–2074.

308. Bepler G, Jaques G, Havemann K, Koehler A, Johnson BE, Gazdar AF. Characterization of two cell lines with distinct phenotypes established from a patient with small cell lung cancer. Cancer Res 1987; 47:1883–1891.

309. Berendsen HH, De Leij L, de Vries EGE, et al. Characterization of three small cell lung cancer cell lines established from one patient during longitudinal follow-up. Cancer Res 1988; 48:6891–6899.

310. Smit EF, de Vries EGE, Timmer-Bosscha H, et al. *In vitro* response of human small-cell lung-cancer cell lines to chemotherapeutic drugs; no correlation with clinical data. Int J Cancer 1992; 51:72–78.

311. Hand A, Pelin K, Halme M, et al. Interferon-α and interferon-γ combined with chemotherapy: *in vitro* sensitivity studies in non-small cell lung cancer cell lines. Anticancer Drugs 1993; 4:365–368.

312. Poupon MF, Arvelo F, Guguel AF, et al. Response of small-cell lung cancer xenografts to chemotherapy: multidrug resistance and direct clinical correlates. J Natl Cancer Inst 1993; 85:2023–2029.

313. Tsai C-M. Chang K-T, Perng R-P, et al. Correlation of intrinsic chemoresistance of non-small cell lung cancer cell lines with HER-2/neu gene expression but not with ras gene mutations. J Natl Cancer Inst 1993; 85:897–901.

314. Kruczynski A, Kiss R. Evidence of a direct relationship between the increase in the *in vitro* passage number of human non-small cell lung cancer primocultures and their chemosensitivity. Anticancer Res 1993; 13:507–514.

315. Shaw GL, Gazdar AF, Phelps R, et al. Individualized chemotherapy for patients with non-small cell lung cancer determined by prospective identification of neuroendocrine markers and *in vitro* drug sensitivity testing. Cancer Res 1993; 53:5181–5187.

316. Arvelo F, Poupon MF, Le Chevalier T. Establishment and characterization of five human small cell lung cancer cell lines from early tumor xenografts. Anticancer Res 1994; 14: 1893–1902.

317. Milroy R, Plumb JA, Batstone P, et al. Lack of expression of P-glycoprotein in 7 small cell lung cancer cell lines established both from untreated and from treated patients. Anticancer Res 1992; 12:193–200.

318. Arceci RJ. Clinical significance of P-glycoprotein in multidrug resistance malignancies. Blood 1993; 81:2215–2222.

319. Brophy NA, Marie JP, Rojas VA, et al. *Mdr*1 gene expression in childhood acute lymphoblastic leukemias and lymphomas: a critical evaluation by four techniques. Leukemia 1994; 8:327–335.

320. Brambilla E, Moro D, Gazzeri S, et al. Cytotoxic chemotherapy induces cell differentiation in small-cell lung carcinoma. J Clin Oncol 1991; 9:50–61.

321. Sugawara I, Watanabe M, Masunaga A, Itoyama S, Ueda K. Primer-dependent amplification of *mdr*1 mRNA by polymerase chain reaction. Jpn J Cancer Res 1992; 83:131–133.

322. Shin HJC, Lee JS, Hong WK, Shin DM. Study of multidrug resistance (mdr1) gene in non-small-cell lung cancer. Anticancer Res 1992; 12:367–370.

323. Schlaifer D, Laurent G, Chittal S, et al. Immunohistochemical detection of multidrug resistance associated P-glycoprotein in tumour and stromal cells of human cancers. Br J Cancer 1990; 62:177–182.

324. Abe Y, Nakamura M, Ota E, et al. Expression of the multidrug resistance gene (*MDR1*) in non-small cell lung cancer. Jpn J Cancer Res 1994; 85:536–541.

325. Oberli-Schrammli AE, Joncourt F, Stadler M, et al. Parallel assessment of glutathione-based detoxifying enzymes, O$^6$-alkylguanine-DNA alkyltransferase and P-glycoprotein as indicators of drug resistance in tumor and normal lung of patients with lung cancer. Int J Cancer 1994; 59:619–626.

326. Holzmayer TA, Hilsenbeck S, Von Hoff DD, Roninson IB. Clinical correlates of MDR1 (P-glycoprotein) gene expression in ovarian and small-cell lung carcinomas. J Natl Cancer Inst 1992; 84:1486–1491.

327. Volm M, Mattern J, Efferth T, Pommerenke EW. Expression of several resistance mechanisms in untreated human kidney and lung carcinomas. Anticancer Res 1992; 12:1063–1068.

328. Radosevich JA, Robinson PG, Rittmann-Grauer LS, et al. Immunohistochemical analysis of pulmonary and pleural tumors with the monoclonal antibody HYB-612 directed against the multidrug resistance (MDR-1) gene product, P-glycoprotein. Tumor Biol 1989; 10: 252–257.

329. Scagliotti GV, Michelotto F, Kalikatzaros G, et al. Detection of multidrug resistance associated P-170 glycoprotein in previously untreated non small cell lung cancer. Anticancer Res 1991; 11:2207–2210.

330. Schuurhuis GJ, Broxterman HJ, Ossenkoppele GJ, et al. Functional multidrug resistance phenotype associated with combined overexpression of Pgp/*MDR1* and *MRP* together with 1-β-D-arabinofuranosylcytosine sensitivity may predict clinical response in acute myeloid leukemia. Clin Cancer Res 1995; 1:81–3.

331. Tewey KM, Rowe TC, Yang L, Halligan BD, Liu LF. Adriamycin-induced DNA damage mediated by mammalian DNA topoisomerase II. Science 1984; 226:466–468.

332. Sander M, Hsieh T-S. Double strand DNA cleavage by type II DNA topoisomerase from *Drosophila melanogaster*. J Biol Chem 1983; 258:8421–8428.

333. Spitzner JR, Muller MT. A consensus sequence for cleavage by vertebrate DNA topoisomerase II. Nucleic Acids Res 1988; 16:5533–5556.

334. Sander M, Hsieh T-S. *Drosophila* topoisomerase II double-strand DNA cleavage: analysis of DNA sequence homology at the cleavage site. Nucleic Acids Res 1985; 13:1057–1072.

335. Muller MT, Spitzner JR, DiDonato JA, Mehta VB, Tsutsui K. Single-strand DNA cleavages by eukaryotic topoisomerase II. Biochemistry 1988; 27:8369–8379.

336. Andersen AH, Christiansen K, Zechiedrich EL, Jensen PS, Osheroff N, Westergaard O. Strand specificity of the topoisomerase II mediated double-stranded DNA cleavage reaction. Biochemistry 1989; 28:6237–6244.

337. Osheroff N, Shelton ER, Brutlag DL. DNA topoisomerase II from *Drosophila melanogaster*. J Biol Chem 1983; 258:9536–9543.

338. Zechiedrich EL, Osheroff N. Eukaryotic topoisomerases recognize nucleic acid topology by preferentially interacting with DNA crossovers. EMBO J 1990; 9:4555–4562.

339. Howard MT, Lee MP, Hsieh T-S, Griffith JD. *Drosophila* topoisomerase II-DNA interactions are affected by DNA structure. J Mol Biol 1991; 217:53–62.

340. Riou J-F, Gabillot M, Riou G. Analysis of topoisomerase II-mediated DNA cleavage of the *c-myc* gene during HL60 differentiation. FEBS Lett 1993; 334:369–372.

341. Bunch RT, Gewirtz DA, Povirk LF. A combined alkaline unwinding/Southern blotting assay for measuring low levels of cellular DNA breakage within specific genomic regions. Oncol Res 1992; 4:7–15.

342. Webb CF, Eneff KL, Drake FH. A topoisomerase II-like protein is part of an inducible DNA-binding protein complex that binds 5' of an immunoglobulin promoter. Nucleic Acids Res 1993; 21:4363–4368.

343. Wyckoff E, Natalie D, Nolan JM, Lee M, Hsieh T-S. Structure of the *Drosophila* DNA topoisomerase II gene. Nucleotide sequence and homology among topoisomerases II. J Mol Biol 1989; 205:1–13.

344. Jenkins JR, Ayton P, Jones T, et al. Isolation of cDNA clones encoding the β isozyme of human DNA topoisomerase II and localisation of the gene to chromosome 3p24. Nucleic Acids Res 1992; 20:5587–5592.

345. Pommier Y, Kerrigan D, Kohn K. Topological complexes between DNA and topoisomerase II and effects of polyamines. Biochemistry 1989; 28:995–1002.

346. Roca J, Wang JC. DNA transport by a type II DNA topoisomerase: evidence in favor of a two-gate mechanism. Cell 1994; 77:609–616.

347. Roca J, Wang JC. The capture of a DNA double helix by an ATP-dependent protein clamp: a key step in DNA transport by type II DNA topoisomerases. Cell 1992; 71:833–840.

348. Lindsley JE, Wang JC. Proteolysis patterns of epitopically labeled yeast DNA topoisomerase II suggest an allosteric transition in the enzyme induced by ATP binding. Proc Natl Acad Sci USA 1991; 88:10485–10489.

349. Lindsley JE, Wang JC. On the coupling between ATP usage and DNA transport by yeast DNA topoisomerase II. J Biol Chem 1993; 268:8096–8104.

350. Osheroff N. Eukaryotic topoisomerase II. Characterization of enzyme turnover. J Biol Chem 1986; 261:9944–9950.

351. Adachi Y, Luke M, Laemmli UK. Chromosome assembly in vitro: topoisomerase II is required for condensation. Cell 1991; 64:137–148.

352. Downes CS, Mullinger AM, Johnson RT. Inhibitors of DNA topoisomerase II prevent chromatid separation in mammalian cells but do not prevent exit from mitosis. Proc Natl Acad Sci USA 1991; 88:8895–8899.

353. Uemura T, Ohkura H, Adachi Y, Morino K, Shiozaki K, Yanagida M. DNA topoisomerase II is required for condensation and separation of mitotic chromosomes in S. pombe. Cell 1987; 50:917–925.

354. Uemura T, Yanagida M. Isolation of type I and II DNA topoisomerase mutants from fission yeast: single and double mutants show different phenotypes in cell growth and chromatin organization. EMBO J 1984; 3:1737–1744.

355. Uemura T, Yanagida M. Mitotic spindle pulls but fails to separate chromosomes in type II DNA topoisomerase mutants: uncoordinated mitosis. EMBO J 1986; 5:1003–1010.

356. Goto T, Wang JC. Yeast DNA topoisomerase II is encoded by a single-copy, essential gene. Cell 1984; 36:1073–1080.

357. Holm C, Stearns T, Botstein D. DNA topoisomerase II must act at mitosis to prevent nondisjunction and chromosome breakage. Mol Cell Biol 1989; 9:159–168.

358. Clarke DJ, Johnson RT, Downes CS. Topoisomerase II inhibition prevents anaphase chromatid segregation in mammalian cells independently of the generation of DNA strand breaks. J Cell Sci 1993; 105:563–569.

359. DiNardo S, Voelkel K, Sternglanz R. DNA topoisomerase II mutant of Saccharomyces cerevisiae: topoisomerase II is required for segregation of daughter molecules at the termination of DNA replication. Proc Natl Acad Sci USA 1984; 81:2616–2620.

360. Ishida R, Hamatake M, Wasserman RA, Nitiss JL, Wang JC, Andoh T. DNA topoisomerase II is the molecular target of bisdioxopiperazine derivatives ICRF-159 and ICRF-193 in Saccharomyces cerevisiae. Cancer Res 1995; 55:2299–2303.

361. Wang JC. DNA topoisomerases. Annu Rev Biochem 1985; 54:665–697.

362. Osheroff N. Biochemical basis for the interactions of type I and type II topoisomerases with DNA. Pharmacol Ther 1989; 41:223–241.

363. Corbett AH, Osheroff N. When good enzymes go bad: conversion of topoisomerase II to a cellular toxin by antineoplastic drugs. Chem Res Toxicol 1993; 6:585–597.

364. Adachi Y, Kas E, Laemmli UK. Preferential, cooperative binding of DNA topoisomerase II to scaffold-associated regions. EMBO J 1989; 8:3997–4006.

365. Earnshaw WC, Heck MMS. Localization of topoisomerase II in mitotic chromosomes. J Cell Biol 1985; 100:1716–1725.

366. Earnshaw WC, Halligan B, Cooke CA, Heck MMS, Liu LF. Topoisomerase II is a structural component of mitotic chromosome scaffolds. J Cell Biol 1985; 100:1706–1715.

367. Berrios M, Osheroff N, Fisher PA. *In situ* localization of DNA topoisomerase II, a major polypeptide component of the *Drosophila* nuclear matrix fraction. Proc Natl Acad Sci USA 1985; 82:4142–4146.

368. Hirano T, Mitchison TJ. Topoisomerase II does not play a scaffolding role in the organization of mitotic chromosomes assembled in *Xenopus* egg extracts. J Cell Biol 1993; 120: 601–612.

369. Sullivan DM, Ross WE. Resistance to inhibitors of DNA topoisomerases. In: Ozols RF, ed. Molecular and Clinical Advances in Anticancer Drug Resistance. Boston: Kluwer Academic, 1991:57–99.

370. Chen AY, Liu LF. DNA topoisomerases: essential enzymes and lethal targets. Annu Rev Pharmacol Toxicol 1994; 34:191–218.

371. Watt PM, Hickson ID. Structure and function of type II DNA topoisomerases. Biochem J 1994; 303:681–695.

372. Osheroff N, Zechiedrich EL, Gale KC. Catalytic function of DNA topoisomerase II. BioEssays 1991; 13:269–275.

373. Schneider E, Hsiang Y-H, Liu LF. DNA topoisomerases as anticancer drug targets. Adv Pharmacol 1990; 21:149–183.

374. Drake FH, Zimmerman JP, McCabe FL, et al. Purification of topoisomerase II from amsacrine-resistant P388 leukemia cells. Evidence for two forms of the enzyme. J Biol Chem 1987; 262:16739–16747.

375. Drake FH, Hofmann GA, Bartus HF, Mattern MR, Crooke ST, Mirabelli CK. Biochemical and pharmacological properties of p170 and p180 forms of topoisomerase II. Biochemistry 1989; 28:8154–8160.

376. Chung TDY, Drake FH, Tank KB, Per SR, Crooke ST, Mirabelli CK. Characterization and immunological identification of cDNA clones encoding two human DNA topoisomerase II isozymes. Proc Natl Acad Sci USA 1989; 86:9431–9435.

377. Austin CA, Sng J-H, Patel S, Fisher LM. Novel HeLa topoisomerase II is the IIβ isoform: complete coding sequence and homology with other type II topoisomerases. Biochim Biophys Acta 1993; 1172:283–291.

378. Tsutsui K, Okada S, Watanabe M, Shohmori T, Seki S, Inoue Y. Molecular cloning of partial cDNAs for rat DNA topoisomerase II isoforms and their differential expression in brain development. J Biol Chem 1993; 268:19076–19083.

379. Tsai-Pflugfelder M, Liu LF, Liu AA, et al. Cloning and sequencing of cDNA encoding human DNA topoisomerase II and localization of the gene to chromosome region 17q21-22. Proc Natl Acad Sci USA 1988; 85:7177–7181.

380. Hinds M, Deisseroth K, Mayes J, et al. Identification of a point mutation in the topoisomerase II gene from a human leukemia cell line containing an amsacrine-resistant form of topoisomerase II. Cancer Res 1991; 51:4729–4731.

381. Campain JA, Gottesman MM, Pastan I. A novel mutant topoisomerase IIα present in VP-16-resistant human melanoma cell lines has a deletion of alanine 429. Biochemistry 1994; 33:11327–11332.

382. Mirski SEL, Cole SPC. Cytoplasmic localization of a mutant $M_r$ 160,000 topoisomerase IIα is associated with the loss of putative bipartite nuclear localization signals in a drug resistant human lung cancer cell line. Cancer Res 1995; 55:2129–2134.

383. Per SR, Mattern MR, Mirabelli CK, Drake FH, Johnson RK, Crooke ST. Characterization of a subline of P388 leukemia resistant to amsacrine: evidence of altered topoisomerase II function. Mol Pharmacol 1987; 32:17–25.

384. Woessner RD, Mattern MR, Mirabelli CK, Johnson RK, Drake FH. Proliferation- and cell cycle-dependent differences in expression of the 170 kilodalton and 180 kilodalton forms of topoisomerase II in NIH-3T3 cells. Cell Growth Diff 1991; 2:209–214.

385. Kimura K, Saijo M, Ui M, Enomoto T. Growth state- and cell cycle-dependent fluctuation in the expression of two forms of DNA topoisomerase II and possible specific modification of the higher molecular weight form in the M phase. J Biol Chem 1994; 269:1173–1176.

386. Negri C, Chiesa R, Cerino A, et al. Monoclonal antibodies to human DNA topoisomerase I and the two isoforms of DNA topoisomerase II: 170- and 180-kDa isozymes. Exp Cell Res 1992; 200:452–459.

387. Zini N, Martelli AM, Sabatelli P, et al. The 180-kDa isoform of topoisomerase II is localized in the nucleolus and belongs to the structural elements of the nucleolar remnant. Exp Cell Res 1993; 200:460–466.

388. Tan KB, Dorman TE, Falls KM, et al. Topoisomerase IIα and topoisomerase IIβ genes: characterization and mapping to human chromosomes 17 and 3, respectively. Cancer Res 1992; 52:231–234.

389. Lynn R, Giaever G, Swanberg SL, Wang JC. Tandem regions of yeast DNA topoisomerase II share homology with different subunits of bacterial gyrase. Science 1986; 233:647–649.

390. Shiozaki K, Yanagida M. A functional 125-kDa core polypeptide of fission yeast DNA topoisomerase II. Mol Cell Biol 1991; 11:6093–6102.

391. Austin CA, Barot HA, Margerrison EEC, et al. Structure and partial amino acid sequence of calf thymus DNA topoisomerase II: comparison with other type II enzymes. Biochem Biophys Res Commun 1990; 170:763–768.

392. Davies SL, Jenkins JR, Hickson ID. Human cells express two differentially spliced forms of topoisomerase IIβ mRNA. Nucleic Acids Res 1993; 21:3719–3723.

393. Woessner RD, Chung TDY, Hofmann GA, et al. Differences between normal and *ras*-transformed NIH-3T3 cells in expression of the 170kD and 180kD forms of topoisomerase II. Cancer Res 1990; 50:2901–2908.

394. Kroll DJ, Rowe TC. Phosphorylation of topoisomerase II in a human tumor cell line. J Biol Chem 1991; 266:7957–7961.

395. Saijo M, Ui M, Enomoto T. Growth state and cell cycle dependent phosphorylation of DNA topoisomerase II in Swiss 3T3 cells. Biochemistry 1992; 31:359–363.

396. Heck MMS, Hittleman WN, Earnshaw WC. Differential expression of DNA topoisomerases I and II during the eukaryotic cell cycle. Proc Natl Acad Sci USA 1988; 85:1086–1090.

397. Hochhauser D, Stanway CA, Harris AL, Hickson ID. Cloning and characterization of the 5'-flanking region of the human topoisomerase IIα gene. J Biol Chem 1992; 267:18961–18965.

398. Fraser DJ, Brandt TL, Kroll DJ. Topoisomerase IIα promoter *trans*-activation early in monocytic differentiation of HL-60 human leukemia cells. Mol Pharmacol 1995; 47:696–706.

399. Ackerman P, Glover CVC, Osheroff N. Phosphorylation of DNA topoisomerase II by casein kinase II: modulation of eukaryotic topoisomerase II activity *in vitro*. Proc Natl Acad Sci USA 1985; 82:3164–3168.

400. Sayhoun N, Wolf M, Besterman J, et al. Protein kinase C phosphorylates topoisomerase II: topoisomerase activation and its possible role in phorbol ester-induced differentiation of HL-60 cells. Proc Natl Acad Sci USA 1986; 83:1603–1607.

401. Heck MMS, Hittelman WN, Earnshaw WC. *In vivo* phosphorylation of the 170-kDa form of eukaryotic DNA topoisomerase II. Cell cycle analysis. J Biol Chem 1989; 264:15161–15164.

402. Burden DA, Goldsmith LJ, Sullivan DM. Cell-cycle-dependent phosphorylation and activity of Chinese-hamster ovary topoisomerase II. Biochem J 1993; 293:297–304.

403. Bahram S, Arnold D, Bresnahan M, Strominger JL, Spies T. Two putative subunits of a peptide pump encoded in the major histocompatibility complex class II region. Proc Natl Acad Sci USA 1991; 88:10094–10098.

404. Zunino F, Capranico G. DNA topoisomerase II as the primary target of anti-tumor anthracyclines. Anti-Cancer Drug Design 1990; 5:307–317.

405. Osheroff N. Effect of antineoplastic agents on the DNA cleavage-religation reaction of eukaryotic topoisomerase II: inhibition of DNA religation by etoposide. Biochemistry 1989; 28:6157–6160.

406. Ross W, Rowe T, Glisson B, Yalowich J, Liu L. Role of topoisomerase II in mediating epipodophyllotoxin-induced DNA cleavage. Cancer Res 1984; 44:5857–5860.

407. Robinson MJ, Osheroff N. Effects of antineoplastic drugs on the post-strand-passage DNA cleavage/religation equilibrium of topoisomerase II. Biochemistry 1991; 30:1807–1813.

408. Fox ME, Smith PJ. Long-term inhibition of DNA synthesis and the persistence of trapped topoisomerase II complexes in determining the toxicity of the antitumor DNA intercalators mAMSA and mitoxantrone. Cancer Res 1990; 50:5813–5818.

409. Tewey KM, Chen GL, Nelson EM, Liu LF. Intercalative antitumor drugs interfere with the breakage-reunion reaction of mammalian DNA topoisomerase II. J Biol Chem 1984; 259:9182–9187.

410. Fosse P, Rene B, Charra M, Paoletti C, Saucier J-M. Stimulation of topoisomerase II-mediated DNA cleavage by ellipticine derivatives: structure-activity relationship. J Pharmacol Exp Ther 1992; 42:590–595.

411. Monnot M, Mauffret O, Simon V, et al. DNA-drug recognition and effects on topoisomerase II-mediated cytotoxicity. J Biol Chem 1991; 266:1820–1829.

412. Nelson EM, Tewey KM, Liu LF. Mechanism of antitumor drug action: poisoning of mammalian DNA topoisomerase II on DNA by 4'-(9-acridinylamino)-methanesulfon-m-anisidide. Proc Natl Acad Sci USA 1984; 81:1361–1365.

413. Robinson MJ, Osheroff N. Stabilization of the topoisomerase II-DNA cleavage complex by antineoplastic drugs: inhibition of enzyme-mediated DNA religation by 4'-(9-acridinylamino)methanesulfon-m-anisidide. Biochemistry 1990; 29:2511–2515.

414. Rowe TC, Chen GL, Hsiang Y-H, Liu LF. DNA damage by antitumor acridines mediated by mammalian DNA topoisomerase II. Cancer Res 1986; 46:2021–2026.

415. Walker PR, Smith C, Youdale T, Leblanc J, Whitfield JF, Sikorska M. Topoisomerase II-reactive chemotherapeutic drugs induce apoptosis in thymocytes. Cancer Res 1991; 51:1078–1085.

416. Hickman JA. Apoptosis induced by anticancer drugs. Cancer Met Rev 1992; 11:121–139.

417. Bertrand R, Kerrigan D, Sarang M, Pommier Y. Cell death induced by topoisomerase inhibitors. Role of calcium in mammalian cells. Biochem Pharmacol 1991; 42:77–85.

418. Kamesaki S, Kamesaki H, Jorgensen TJ, Tanizawa A, Pommier Y, Cossman J. bcl-2 protein inhibits etoposide-induced apoptosis through its effects on events subsequent to topoisomerase II-induced DNA strand breaks and their repair. Cancer Res 1993; 53:4251–4256.

419. Glisson BS, Ross WE. DNA topoisomerase II: a primer on the enzyme and its unique role as a multidrug target in cancer chemotherapy. Pharmacol Ther 1987; 32:89–106.

420. Drake FH, Hofmann GA, Mong S-M, et al. In vitro and intracellular inhibition of topoisomerase II by the antitumor agent merbarone. Cancer Res 1989; 49:2578–2583.

421. Tanabe K, Ikegami Y, Ishida R, Andoh T. Inhibition of topoisomerase II by antitumor agents bis(2,6-dioxopiperazine) derivatives. Cancer Res 1991; 51:4903–4908.

422. Ishida R, Miki T, Narita T, et al. Inhibition of intracellular topoisomerase II by antitumor bis(2,6-dioxopiperazine) derivatives: mode of cell growth inhibition distinct from that of cleavable complex-forming type inhibitors. Cancer Res 1991; 51:4909–4916.

423. Ishimi Y, Ishida R, Andoh T. Effect of ICRF-193, a novel DNA topoisomerase II inhibitor, on simian virus 40 DNA and chromosome replication in vitro. Mol Cell Biol 1992; 12:4007–4014.

424. Roca J, Ishida R, Berger JM, Andoh T, Wang JC. Antitumor bisdioxopiperazines inhibit yeast DNA topoisomerase II by trapping the enzyme in the form of a closed protein clamp. Proc Natl Acad Sci USA 1994; 91:1781–1785.

425. Jensen PB, Jensen , Demant EJF, et al. Antagonistic effect of aclarubicin on daunorubicin-induced cytotoxicity in human small cell lung cancer cells: relationship to DNA integrity and topoisomerase II. Cancer Res 1991; 51:5903–5909.

426. Jensen PB, Sorensen BS, Sehested M, et al. Different modes of anthracycline interaction with topoisomerase II. Separate structures critical for DNA-cleavage, and for overcoming topoisomerase II-related drug resistance. Biochem Pharmacol 1993; 45:2025–2035.

427. Boritzki TJ, Wofard TS, Besserer JA, Jackson RC, Fry DW. Inhibition of type II topoisomerase by fostriecin. Biochem Pharmacol 1988; 37:4063–4068.

428. de Jong S, Zijlstra JG, Mulder NH, de Vries EGE. Lack of cross-resistance to fostriecin in a human small-cell lung carcinoma cell line showing topoisomerase II-related drug resistance. Cancer Chemother Pharmacol 1991; 28:461–464.

429. Sorensen BS, Sindling J, Andersen AH, Alsner J, Jensen PB, Westergaard O. Mode of action of topoisomerase II-targeting agents at a specific DNA sequence. Uncoupling the DNA binding, cleavage and religation events. J Mol Biol 1992; 228:778–786.

430. Jensen PB, Sorensen BS, Demant EJF, et al. Antagonistic effect of aclarubicin on the cytotoxicity of etoposide and 4′-(9-acridinylamino)methanesulfon-m-anisidide in human small cell lung cancer cell lines and on topoisomerase II-mediated DNA cleavage. Cancer Res 1990; 50:3311–3316.

431. Rowe T, Kupfer G, Ross W. Inhibition of epipodophyllotoxin cytotoxicity by interference with topoisomerase-mediated DNA cleavage. Biochem Pharmacol 1985; 34:2438–2487.

432. Sehested M, Jensen PB, Sorensen BS, Holm B, Friche E, Demant EJF. Antagonistic effect of the cardioprotector (+)-1,2-bis(3,5-dioxopiperazinyl-1-yl)propane (ICRF-187) on DNA breaks and cytotoxicity induced by the topoisomerase II directed drugs daunorubicin and etoposide (VP-16). Biochem Pharmacol 1993; 46:389–393.

433. Woynarowski JM, Sigmund RD, Beerman TA. DNA minor groove binding agents interfere with topoisomerase II mediated lesions induced by epipodophyllotoxin derivative VM-26 and acridine derivative m-AMSA in nuclei from L1210 cells. Biochemistry 1989; 28:2850–3855.

434. Kaufmann SH. Antagonism between camptothecin and topoisomerase II-directed chemotherapeutic agents in a human leukemia cell line. Cancer Res 1991; 51:1129–1136.

435. Ferguson PJ, Fisher MH, Stephenson J, Li D-H, Zhou B-S, Cheng Y-C. Combined modalities of resistance in etoposide-resistant human KB cell lines. Cancer Res 1988; 48: 5956–5964.

436. Matsuo K-I, Kohno K, Takano H, Sato S-I, Kiue A, Kuwano M. Reduction of drug accumulation and DNA topoisomerase II activity in acquired teniposide-resistant human cancer KB cell lines. Cancer Res 1990; 50:5819–5824.

437. Ritke MK, Roberts D, Allan WP, Raymond J, Bergoltz VV, Yalowich JC. Altered stability of etoposide-induced topoisomerase II-DNA complexes in resistant human leukaemia K562 cells. Br J Cancer 1994; 69:687–697.

438. Friche E, Danks MK, Schmidt CA, Beck WT. Decreased DNA topoisomerase II in daunorubicin-resistant Ehrlich ascites tumor cells. Cancer Res 1991; 51:4213–4218.

439. Deffie AM, Batra JK, Goldenberg GJ. Direct correlation between DNA topoisomerase II activity and cytotoxicity in Adriamycin-sensitive and -resistant P388 leukemia cell lines. Cancer Res 1989; 49:58–62.

440. Deffie AM, Bosman DJ, Goldenberg GJ. Evidence for a mutant allele of the gene for DNA topoisomerase II in Adriamycin-resistant P388 murine leukemia cells. Cancer Res 1989; 49:6879–6882.

441. Zwelling LA, Slovak ML, Hinds M, et al. HT1080/DR4: a P-glycoprotein-negative human fibrosarcoma cell line exhibiting resistance to topoisomerase II-reactive drugs despite the presence of a drug-sensitive topoisomerase II. J Natl Cancer Inst 1990; 82:1553–1561.

442. Harker WG, Slade DL, Drake FH, Parr RL. Mitoxantrone resistance in HL-60 leukemia cells: reduced linear topoisomerase II catalytic activity and drug-induced DNA cleavage in association with reduced expression of the topoisomerase II β isoform. Biochemistry 1991; 30:9953–9961.

443. Harker WG, Slade DL, Dalton WS, Meltzer PS, Trent JM. Multidrug resistance in mitoxantrone-selected HL-60 leukemia cells in the absence of p-glycoprotein overexpression. Cancer Res 1989; 49:4552–4549.

444. Kamath N, Grabowski D, Ford J, Kerrigan D, Pommier Y, Ganapathi R. Overexpression of P-glycoprotein and alterations in topoisomerase II in P388 mouse leukemia cells selected *in vivo* for resistance to mitoxantrone. Biochem Pharmacol 1992; 44:937–945.

445. Pommier Y, Schwartz RE, Zwelling LA, et al. Reduced formation of protein-associated DNA strand breaks in Chinese hamster cells resistant to topoisomerase II inhibitors. Cancer Res 1986; 46:611–616.

446. Charcosset J-Y, Saucier J-M, Jacquemin-Sablon A. Reduced DNA topoisomerase II activity and drug-stimulated DNA cleavage in 9-hydroxyellipticine resistant cells. Biochem Pharmacol 1988; 37:2145–2149.

447. Charcosset J-Y, Salles B, Jacquemin-Sablon A. Uptake and cytofluorescence localization of ellipticine derivatives in sensitive and resistant Chinese hamster lung cells. Biochem Pharmacol 1983; 32:1037–1044.

448. Deffie AM, McPherson JP, Gupta RS, Hedley DW, Goldenberg GJ. Multifactorial resistance to antineoplastic agents in drug-resistant P388 murine leukemia, Chinese hamster ovary, and human HeLa cells, with emphasis on the role of DNA topoisomerase II. Biochem Cell Biol 1992; 70:354–364.

449. Webb CD, Latham MD, Lock RB, Sullivan DM. Attenuated topoisomerase II content directly correlates with a low level of drug resistance in a Chinese hamster ovary cell line. Cancer Res 1991; 51:6543–6549.

450. Robson CN, Hoban PR, Harris AL, Hickson ID. Cross-sensitivity to topoisomerase II inhibitors in cytotoxic drug-hypersensitive Chinese hamster ovary cell lines. Cancer Res 1987; 47:1560–1565.

451. Davies SM, Robson CN, Davies SL, Hickson ID. Nuclear topoisomerase II levels correlate with the sensitivity of mammalian cells to intercalating agents and epipodophyllotoxins. J Biol Chem 1988; 263:17724–17729.

452. Giaccone G, Gazdar AF, Beck H, Zunino F, Capranico G. Multidrug sensitivity phenotype of human lung cancer cells associated with topoisomerase II expression. Cancer Res 1992; 52:1666–1674.

453. Kasahara K, Fujiwara Y, Sugimoto Y, et al. Determinants of response to the DNA topoisomerase II inhibitors doxorubicin and etoposide in human lung cancer cell lines. J Natl Cancer Inst 1992; 84:113–118.

454. Evans CD, Mirski SEL, Danks MK, Cole SPC. Reduced levels of topoisomerase II α and β in a multidrug resistant small cell lung cancer cell line. Cancer Chemother Pharmacol 1994; 34:242–248.

455. Beck WT, Danks MK, Wolverton JS, Kim R, Chen M. Drug resistance associated with altered DNA topoisomerase II. Adv Enzyme Reg 1993; 33:113–127.

456. Sullivan DM, Latham MD, Rowe TC, Ross WE. Purification and characterization of an altered topoisomerase II from a drug-resistant Chinese hamster ovary cell line. Biochemistry 1989; 28:5680–5687.

457. Chan VTW, Ng S-W, Eder JP, Schnipper LE. Molecular cloning and identification of a point mutation in the topoisomerase II cDNA from an etoposide-resistant Chinese hamster ovary cell line. J Biol Chem 1993; 268:2160–2165.

458. Lee M-S, Wang JC, Beran M. Two independent amsacrine-resistant human myeloid leukemia cell lines share an identical point mutation in the 170 kDa form of topoisomerase II. J Mol Biol 1992; 223:837–843.

459. Bugg BY, Danks MK, Beck WT, Suttle DP. Expression of a mutant DNA topoisomerase II in CCRF-CEM human leukemic cells selected for resistance to teniposide. Proc Natl Acad Sci USA 1991; 88:7654–7658.

460. Danks MK, Warmoth MR, Friche E, et al. Single-strand conformational polymorphism analysis of the $M_r$ 170,000 isozyme of DNA topoisomerase II in human tumor cells. Cancer Res 1993; 53:1373–1379.

461. Patel S, Fisher LM. Novel selection and genetic characterisation of an etoposide-resistant human leukaemic CCRF-CEM cell line. Br J Cancer 1993; 67:456–463.

462. Nitiss JL, Vilalta PM, Wu H, McMahon J. Mutations in the *gyrB* domain of eukaryotic topoisomerase II can lead to partially dominant resistance to etoposide and amsacrine. Mol Pharmacol 1994; 46:773–777.

463. Odaimi M, Andersson BS, McCredie KB, Beran M. Drug sensitivity and cross-resistance of the 4'-(9-acridinylamino)methanesulfon-*m*-anisidide-resistant subline of HL-60 human leukemia. Cancer Res 1986; 46:3330–3333.

464. Beran M, Andersson BS. Development and characterization of a human myelogenous leukemia cell line resistant to 4'-(9-acridinylamino)-3-methanesulfon-*m*-anisidide. Cancer Res 1987; 47:1897–1904.

465. Kaufmann SH, Karp JE, Jones RJ, et al. Topoisomerase II levels and drug sensitivity in adult acute myelogenous leukemia. Blood 1994; 83:517–530.

466. Mirski SEL, Evans CD, Almquist KC, Slovak ML, Cole SPC. Altered topoisomerase IIα in a drug-resistant small cell lung cancer cell line selected in VP-16. Cancer Res 1993; 53: 4866–4873.

467. Feldhoff PW, Mirski SEL, Cole SPC. Sullivan DMM. Altered subcellular distribution of topoisomerase IIα in a drug resistant human small cell lung cancer cell line. Cancer Res 1994; 54:756–762.

468. Harker WG, Slade DL, Parr RL, Feldhoff PW, Sullivan DM, Holguin MH. Alterations in the topoisomerase IIα gene, messenger RNA, and subcellular protein distribution as well as reduced expression of the DNA topoisomerase IIβ enzyme in a mitoxantrone-resistant HL-60 human leukemia cell line. Cancer Res 1985; 55:1707–1716.

469. Caron PR, Watt P, Wang JC. The C-terminal domain of *Saccharomyces cerevisiae* DNA topoisomerase II. Mol Cell Biol 1994; 14:3197–3207.

470. Shiozaki K, Yanagida M. Functional dissection of the phosphorylated termini of fission yeast DNA topoisomerase II. J Cell Biol 1992; 119:1023–1036.

471. Crenshaw DG, Hsieh T-S. Function of the hydrophilic carboxyl terminus of type II DNA topoisomerase from *Drosophila melanogaster*. I. In vitro studies. J Biol Chem 1993; 268: 21328–21334.

472. Crenshaw DG, Tsieh T-S. Function of the hydrophilic carboxyl terminus of type II DNA topoisomerase from *Drosophila melanogaster*. II. *In vivo* studies. J Biol Chem 1993; 268: 21335–21343.

473. Palayoor ST, Stein JM, Hait WN. Inhibition of protein kinase C by antineoplastic agents: implications for drug resistance. Biochem Biophys Res Commun 1987; 148:718–725.

474. Robbins J, Dilworth SM, Laskey RA, Dingwall C. Two interdependent basic domains in nucleoplasmin nuclear targeting sequence: identification of a class of bipartite nuclear targeting sequence. Cell 1991; 64:615–623.

475. Dingwall C, Laskey RA. Nuclear targeting sequences—a consensus? TIBS 1991; 16:478–481.

476. Hanover JA. The nuclear pore: at the crossroads. FASEB J 1992; 6:2288–2295.

477. McKenna SL, Whittaker JA, Padua RA, Holmes JA. Topoisomerase II expression in normal haemopoietic cells and chronic lymphocytic leukaemia: drug sensitivity or resistance? Leukemia 1993; 7:1199–1203.

478. Kim R, Hirabayashi N, Nishiyama M, Saeki S, Toge T, Okada K. Expression of MDR1, GST-π and topoisomerase II as an indicator of clinical response to Adriamycin. Anticancer Res 1991; 11:429–432.

479. Efferth T, Mattern J, Volm M. Immunohistochemical detection of P glycoprotein, glutathione S transferase and DNA topoisomerase II in human tumors. Oncology 1992; 49: 368–375.

480. Volm M, Mattern J. Expression of topoisomerase II, catalase, metallothionein and thy-midylate-synthase in human squamous cell lung carcinomas and their correlation with dox-orubicin resistance and with patients' smoking habits. Carcinogenesis 1992; 13:1947–1950.

481. Hasegawa T, Isobe K-I, Nakashima I, Shimokata K. Higher expression of topoisomerase II in lung cancers than normal lung tissues: different expression pattern from topoisom-erase I. Biochem Biophys Res Commun 1993; 195:409–414.

482. Gekeler V, Frese G, Noller A, et al. Mdr1/P-glycoprotein, topoisomerase, and glutathione-S-transferase π gene expression in primary and relapsed state adult and childhood leukae-mias. Br J Cancer 1992; 66:507–517.

483. Potmesil M, Hsiang Y-H, Liu LF, et al. Resistance of human leukemic and normal lym-phocytes to drug-induced DNA cleavage and low levels of DNA topoisomerase II. Cancer Res 1988; 48:3537–3543.

484. Withoff S, Smit EG, Meersma GJ, et al. Quantitation of DNA topoisomerase IIα messen-ger ribonucleic acid levels in a small cell cancer cell line and two drug resistant sublines using a polymerase chain reaction-aided transcript titration assay. Lab Invest 1994; 71: 61–66.

485. Orita M, Iwahana H, Kanazawa H, Hayashi K, Sekiya T. Detection of polymorphisms of human DNA by gel electrophoresis as single-strand conformation polymorphisms. Proc Natl Acad Sci USA 1989; 86:2766–2770.

486. Liu LF, Davis JL, Calendar R. Novel topologically knotted DNA from bacteriophage P4 capsids: studies with DNA topoisomerases. Nucleic Acids Res 1981; 9:3979–3989.

487. Danks MK, Schmidt CA, Cirtain MC, Suttle DP, Beck WT. Altered catalytic activity of and DNA cleavage by DNA topoisomerase II from human leukemic cells selected for resistance to VM-26. Biochemistry 1988; 27:8861–8869.

488. Hofmann GA, Mirabelli CK, Drake FH. Quantitative adaptation of the bacteriophage P4 DNA unknotting assay for use in the biochemical and pharmacological characterization of topoisomerase II. Anticancer Drug De 1990; 5:273–282.

489. Schomburg C, Grosse F. Purification and characterization of DNA topoisomerase II from calf thymus associated with polypeptides of 175 and 150 kDa. Eur J Biochem 1986; 160: 451–457.

490. Marini JC, Miller KG, Englund PT. Decatenation of kinetoplast DNA by topoisomerases. J Biol Chem 1980; 255:4976–4979.

491. Hsieh T-S, Brutlag D. ATP-dependent DNA topoisomerase from D. melanogaster revers-ibily catenates duplex DNA rings. Cell 1980; 21:114–125.

492. Krasnow MA, Cozzarelli NR. Catenation of DNA rings by topoisomerases. Mechanism of control by spermidine. J Biol Chem 1982; 257:2687–2693.

493. Sahai BM, Kaplan JG. A quantitative decatenation assay for type II topoisomerases. Analyt Biochem 1986; 156:364–379.

494. Holden JA, Rolfson DH, Wittwer CT. Human DNA topoisomerase II: evaluation of en-zyme activity in normal and neoplastic tissues. Biochemistry 1990; 29:2127–2134.

495. Kohn KW, Ewig RAG, Erickson LC, Zwelling LA. Measurement of strand breaks and cross-links by alkaline elution. In: Friedberg EC, Hanawalt PC, eds. DNA Repair. A Labo-ratory Manual of Research Procedures. New York: Marcel Dekker, 1981:379–401.

496. Trask DK, DiDonato JA, Muller MT. Rapid detection and isolation of covalent DNA/pro-tein complexes: application to topoisomerase I and II. EMBO J 1984; 3:671–676.

497. Zwelling LA, Hinds M, Chan D, et al. Characterization of an amsacrine-resistant line of human leukemia cells. Evidence for a drug-resistant form of topoisomerase II. J Biol Chem 1989; 264:16411–16420.

498. Kaufmann SH, McLaughlin SJ, Kastan MB, Liu LF, Karp JE, Burke PJ. Topoisomerase II levels during granulocytic maturation in vitro and in vivo. Cancer Res 1991; 51:3534–3543.

499. Mayes J, Hinds M, Soares L, Altschuler E, Kim P, Zwelling LA. Further characterization of an amsacrine-resistant line of HL-60 human leukemia cells and its topoisomerase II.

Effects of ATP concentration, anion concentration, and the three-dimensional structure of the DNA target. Biochem Pharmacol 1993; 46:699–707.

500. van der Zee AGJ, Hollema H, de Jong S, et al. P-Glycoprotein expression and DNA topoisomerase I and II activity in benign tumors of the ovary and in malignant tumors of the ovary, before and after platinum/cyclophosphamide chemotherapy. Cancer Res 1991; 51: 5915–5920.

501. McLeod HL, Douglas F, Oates M, et al. Topoisomerase I and II activity in human breast, cervix, lung and colon cancer. Int J Cancer 1994; 59:607–611.

502. Doyle LA. Mechanisms of drug resistance in human lung cancer cells. Semin Oncol 1993; 20:326–337.

503. Cantwell BMJ, Bozzino JM, Corris P, Harris AL. The multidrug resistant phenotype in clinical practice; evaluation of cross resistance to ifosfamide and mesna after VP16-213, doxorubicin and vincristine (VPAV) for small cell lung cancer. Eur J Cancer Clin Oncol 1988; 24:123–129.

504. Keizer HG, Schuurhuis GJ, Broxterman HJ, et al. Correlation of multidrug research with decreased drug accumulation, altered subcellular drug distribution, and increased P-glycoprotein expression in cultured SW-1573 human lung tumor cells. Cancer Res 1989; 49: 2988–2993.

505. Broxterman HJ, Pinedo HM, Schuurhuis GJ, Lankelma J. Cyclosporin A and verapamil have different effects on energy metabolism in multidrug-resistant tumour cells. Br J Cancer 1990; 62:85–88.

506. Cole SPC. Rapid chemosensitivity testing of human lung tumor cells using the MTT assay. Cancer Chemother Pharmacol 1986; 17:259–263.

507. Cole SPC. Patterns of cross-resistance in a multidrug-resistant small-cell lung carcinoma cell line. Cancer Chemother Pharmacol 1990; 26:250–256.

508. Zijlstra JG, de Vries EGE, Mulder NH. Multifactorial drug resistance in an Adriamycin-resistant human small cell lung carcinoma cell line. Cancer Res 1987; 47:1780–1784.

509. Smith PJ, Morgan SA, Fox ME, Watson JV. Mitoxantrone-DNA binding and the induction of topoisomerase II associated DNA damage in multi-drug resistant small cell lung cancer cells. Biochem Pharmacol 1990; 40:2069–2078.

510. Pommier Y, Schwartz RE, Zwelling LA, Kohn KW. Effects of DNA intercalating agents on topoisomerase II induced DNA strand cleavage in isolated mammalian cell nuclei. Biochemistry 1985; 24:6406–6410.

511. Hsiang Y-H, Jiang JB, Liu LF. Topoisomerase II-mediated DNA cleavage by amonafide and its structural analogs. Mol Pharmacol 1989; 36:371–376.

512. Yamashita Y, Kawada S-Z, Fujii N, Nakano H. Induction of mammalian DNA topoisomerase II dependent DNA cleavage by antitumor antibiotic streptonigrin. Cancer Res 1990; 50:5841–5844.

513. Kawada S-Z, Yamashita Y, Fujii N, Nakano H. Induction of a heat-stable topoisomerase II-DNA cleavable complex by nonintercalative terpenoides, terpentecin and clerocidin. Cancer Res 1991; 51:2922–2925.

514. Markovits J, Linassier C, Fosse P, et al. Inhibitory effects of the tyrosine kinase inhibitor genistein on mammalian DNA topoisomerase II. Cancer Res 1989; 49:5111–5117.

515. Yamashita Y, Kawada S-Z, Nakano H. Induction of mammalian topoisomerase II dependent DNA cleavage by nonintercalative flavonoids, genistein and orobol. Biochem Pharmacol 1990; 39:737–744.

516. Permana PA, Snapka RM, Shen LI, Chu DTW, Clement JJ, Plattner JJ. Quinobenoxazines: a class of novel antitumor quinolones and potent mammalian DNA topoisomerase II catalytic inhibitors. Biochemistry 1994; 33:11333–11339.

# 3

## Correlations Between Clinical Outcomes and In Vitro Chemosensitivity Testing in Non–Small Cell Lung Cancer

**David W. Wilbur**
*Loma Linda University School of Medicine and J.L. Pettis Memorial Veterans Medical Center, Loma Linda, California*

### IMPORTANCE OF THE CLINICAL PROBLEM

New lung cancer cases for 1997 are estimated at 178,100 by the American Cancer Society with 160,400 deaths from this disease (1). Most of these (75–80%) are caused by non–small cell lung cancer (NSCLC). The majority of the patients who die of this disease are at some point candidates for palliative chemotherapy, but this chemotherapy is toxic, expensive, and of limited benefit. A recent review including results from 4 meta-analyses suggests a median survival improvement of only 1–3 months for treated compared with untreated control patients (2). Most tumors respond only partially to chemotherapy, and the chances of such responses range from less than 30% in most large multi-institutional trials to over 60% in some large single-institution trials, where the treated population is probably made up of patients with better prognosis. An ideal in vitro test would allow us to select for treatment patients with a 100% response rate. In reality, however, any approach that would allow the reliable prediction of a significant number of the nonresponders—sparing the expense of their treatment and at the same time increasing the probability of response for the treated population—would seem worthy of consideration in an era in which cost control has become a major focus of attention. We will present evidence that in vitro chemosensitivity testing might play such a role.

### HISTORICAL NOTES

The idea of testing cellular material in culture for sensitivity/toxicity to various chemicals probably goes back to Ehrlich and Pasteur in the 1870s (3). An attempt to apply such ideas to human cancer cells and their treatment using an in vitro viability assay was first reported in the 1950s (4). Studies of a clonogenic human tumor assay by Hamburger and Salmon (5) and of its clinical application (6) were received with considerable enthusiasm in the late 1970s. This test was limited by its long time to completion and low success rate in solid tumors. Since that time, refinements using both clonogenic and nonclonogenic assays have been published (7,8). NSCLC has been one of the commonly studied tumor types, but only a few papers have provided enough data to make some judgment about the effectiveness of in vitro testing in this tumor.

## SUMMARY INFORMATION ABOUT ASSAY TECHNIQUES

Table 1 contains pertinent information about in vitro assay techniques used in studies of NSCLC (7–13). The area remains one of research and evolving technology, with no general agreement that one assay scheme is preferred. Assays that take only a few days to complete and ones with a high success rate are obviously advantageous, especially for symptomatic patients. To implement any of these requires a substantial investment, particularly in training. Commercial services are available; many have come and gone in the last 15 years. Theoretical arguments can be presented for preferring either clonogenic or total cell kill assays (7), but so far neither has demonstrated a clear superiority in clinical application. The size of tumor sample needed is a function of the number of viable tumor cells per unit volume. A 1-g specimen will usually allow testing of a large panel of drugs, but a smaller specimen will sometimes be useful. The shortest tests with reported clinical correlations require at least 4 days and the slower ones may take several weeks. The Kern assay, with a tritiated thymidine end point evaluated with scintigraphy, is probably the least labor intensive. The DISC assay, with its microscopic evaluation of each counted cell, allows the best separation of malignant and nonmalignant cells. At this time, an acceptable in vitro assay should reach a successful quality-controlled result at least 70–80% of the time when used initially with an apparently adequate-sized tumor sample.

Table 1  Some Properties of In Vitro Chemosensitivity Assays as Applied to the Study of NSCLC

| Name | Time to complete | Critical parameter | Typical assay success rate[a] | Comments | Ref. |
|---|---|---|---|---|---|
| Salmon assay | 14+ days | Colony growth | 35–70% | Low success in solid tumors | 6, 9 |
| Capillary cloning | 10–14 days | Colony growth | 70% | More successful version of above | 10 |
| Kern assay | 5–6 days | Thymidine incorporation | >80%[b] | Least labor of current assays | 11 |
| DISC assay | 5–6 days | Dye exclusion (viability) | >80%[c] | Identifiable cells, labor intensive | 12 |
| Cytoprint (FCA) assay | 5–7 days | Nontoxic dye uptake | >90% | High success for solid tumors | 13 |

[a]Assuming adequate numbers of tumor cells submitted.
[b]Reported for large study of solid tumors, no separate data for lung cancer.
[c]Studies requiring subculturing or using bronchoscopic specimens had less success.

## PROBLEMS RELATED TO IN VITRO TESTING

A variety of factors have contributed to limiting both investigation and application of in vitro assays in NSCLC. These include cost of getting a tumor sample, cost of the assay, uncertainty about how to interpret the assay when done, and lack of a good alternative therapy if the assay indicates the usual preferred treatment is not likely to work. The latter represents a problem for physicians who are reluctant to offer no treatment and are uncomfortable not using a standard treatment for first-line administration. Oncologists spend much of their professional time treating patients with chemotherapy that has only a 15–40% chance of significant benefit. If an assay is set to maximize its accuracy, it may lead to a significant false-negative rate—i.e., a response rate greater than 10% in patients whose tumor sample is judged negative by assay. The result of this may be a willingness on the part of some treating physicians to ignore the assay.

One group of investigators (14) has reported that obtaining tissue for in vitro chemosensitivity testing is a new indication for thoracotomy, but most investigators or users have only sought samples from major surgery when the surgery was otherwise indicated. Obtaining the sample was then a no-cost extra benefit. Sampling with minor surgery under local anesthesia has seemed reasonable and appropriate. Such sources have included superficial lymph nodes and subcutaneous and cutaneous metastases. Malignant effusions and sometimes bone marrow have also furnished safe and reasonable specimen sources. In my experience and that of others (15,16), one disappointment has been that bronchoscopy specimens are frequently inadequate. Mediastinoscopy with node sampling has been a good source for some patients, particularly when the procedure was otherwise indicated for staging. Specimens from the primary tumor may be collected at the time of potentially curative surgery, especially in high-risk patients. Using the above sources carefully and thoroughly, we estimate that more than half of patients with advanced lung cancer might have the results of an in vitro assay available to aid treatment selection.

The philosophy underlying the testing has turned out to be very important, especially in the design of the test. Originally, it was hoped that in vitro tests would allow selection of a group of patients who would almost all respond to treatment. Under this assumption, cut points for the tests were typically set to optimize accuracy and to keep sensitivity and specificity about the same. Because of a perceived clinical inadequacy of this approach, an alternate philosophy has been advocated (11). This philosophy has been to isolate a group of patients who are very unlikely to respond to treatment. This is a response to the clinical dilemma of the oncologist mentioned above. Tests arranged for this goal have been called "highly specific drug resistance assays." Such tests use high (concentration) times (time) drug exposures and cut points on the test set to readily identify very resistant cells. It should be noted, however, that a "highly specific drug resistance assay" is the same thing as a "highly sensitive drug sensitivity assay." These are just two different ways of describing the same test, and some of us may find it easier to conceptualize the sensitivity test. The goal is to include all sensitive patients in the sensitive group and to enrich that group by excluding a smaller group of patients with highly resistant tumors. Table 2 gives post-test probabilities of response to chemotherapy for patients with pretest response expectations of 20–60% using an in vitro chemosensitivity assay with a range of sensitivities and specificities. Also given are the number of patients per hundred who would not be treated if a strategy of not treating

**Table 2**  Post-Test Probabilities (percent true positive/percent false negative) for NSCLC Response to Chemotherapy as a Function of Assay Outcome (test positive/test negative) of In Vitro Test Sensitivity and Specificity and of Pretest Response Expectation

| Pretest response expectation | Sensitivity/Specificity | | | | |
|---|---|---|---|---|---|
| | 0.80/0.80 | 0.90/0.70 | 0.95/0.65 | 0.99/0.60 | 0.99/0.40 |
| 20% | 50/6 (68)[a] | 43/3 (58) | 40/2 (53) | 38/0.4 (48) | 29/0.6 (32) |
| 30% | 63/10 (62) | 56/6 (52) | 54/3 (47) | 51/0.7 (42) | 41/1.1 (28) |
| 40% | 73/14 (56) | 67/9 (46) | 46/5 (41) | 62/1.1 (36) | 52/1.6 (24) |
| 50% | 80/20 (50) | 75/12 (40) | 73/7 (35) | 71/1.6 (30) | 62/2.4 (20) |
| 60% | 86/27 (44) | 82/18 (34) | 80/10 (29) | 79/2.4 (25) | 71/3.6 (17) |

[a]Percentage response if test positive/percentage response if test negative (percentage of patients who would not be treated if test-negative patients are spared chemotherapy).

test-negative patients was used. As one can see, at essentially all levels a significant number of patients would be spared treatment. This seems satisfactory if the excluded patients have a low chance of benefit. How low that chance must be to make such a strategy acceptable is a philosophical question without a unique obvious answer. One can note that there are essentially no widely used chemotherapy programs for malignant disease with response rates less than 10%. It would thus seem highly reasonable to exclude from treatment patients with a chance of response of less than 5%. For an expected response rate of 20%, a 90%-sensitive test will allow this level of discrimination, but a 99%-sensitive test will work acceptably even for a population with a pretest response expectation of 60%.

## CORRELATIONS OF IN VITRO CHEMOSENSITIVITY AND CHEMOTHERAPY RESPONSE IN NSCLC

Table 3 gives summary data on published correlations for NSCLC. In a few cases the authors included some small cell lung cancer cases along with those of NSCLC. Because most lung cancer is NSCLC, this should not be a major concern. One group (17) did report about the same success in doing the assay on small cell and NSCLC, but the tumors from patients with small cell lung cancer were more sensitive to the drugs in the in vitro assay, just as the clinical data would suggest. We were able to find data for 251 clinical correlations. These were from four different assay systems over about 10 years. The largest number were done using the clonogenic-type assay, with the DISC-type viability assay second. The individual studies are discussed below.

### Prospective Trials Restricted to Lung Cancer

Shimizu et al. (18) reported a trial using a standard clonogenic assay for patients with lung cancer. This was a retrospective correlation and had a very high success rate for a clonogenic assay (71%). Using a cut point of 50% colony suppression gave the test a sensitivity of only 50% but a much higher specificity of 88%.

In 1991, Smit et al. (16) reported an attempt to use a dye exclusion assay for chemosensitivity testing for human lung cancer. They tested only vincristine and car-

**Table 3** Summary of Reported Attempts to Correlate In Vitro Chemosensitivity Assays and Clinical Data in NSCLC

| Author (Ref.) | Technique | Assay success rate | Assays used to direct treatment | Response rate assayed patients | Sensitivity/Specificity (approximate) | |
|---|---|---|---|---|---|---|
| Weisenthal (12) | DISC | (67%)[a] | No | 0/7 | — | 100% |
| Shimizu (18)[b] | Cloning | (71%)[a] | No | 8/34 (24%) | 50% | 88% |
| Hanauske (17)[b] | Cloning | 552/1464 (38%) | Yes | 11/112 (20%) | 82% | 87% |
| Von Hoff (10) | Cloning | (71%)[a] | Yes | 1/4 (25%) | — | — |
| Kern (11) | Mixed | (71%)[a] | No | 10/35 (28%) | 90% | 44% |
| Leone (13)[b] | FCA | (96%)[a] | No | 5/8 (62%) | 100% | 67% |
| Smit (16) | DISC | 7/29 (24%) | No | 0/5 | — | 100% |
| Wilbur (19) | DISC | 35/45 (78%) | Yes | 9/25 (36%) | 67% | 75% |
| Shaw (20) | DISC | 37/161 (23%) | Yes | 2/21 (9%) | — | — |

[a]Success rate only reported overall for a range of solid tumors.
[b]Reported for lung cancer including some unspecified number of small cell tumors.

boplatin and their combination. They used (concentration) times (time) drug exposures about twice those usually achieved clinically and defined sensitivity as less than 30% survival of drug-treated cells. They obtained specimens from 29 patients with NSCLC, but only seven assays were successful. The poor yield largely had to do with the fact that 24 of the specimens were from bronchoscopy, and only five of these were successful. None of the assays showed sensitivity, as the lowest survival rate was 40% for the two-drug combination. Five patients were treated with combination vincristine and carboplatin with no responses. The investigators felt their problems were related to poor yield from the bronchoscopy specimens and to poor survival of the cells in the 4-day culture. No conclusions about sensitivity or specificity of their test can be made, but the technical problems of testing are illustrated.

A prospective trial of chemotherapy selected by an in vitro sensitivity assay was published by Wilbur et al. (19) in 1992. Of 45 assays attempted, 35 (78%) were successful. A dye exclusion assay similar to the one described above was used on fresh tumor tissue that had been sent by overnight mail from the referring hospital. For the 25 patients accepting therapy, a regimen was selected consisting of the three most active drugs from the in vitro assay. Nine (36%) of the patients treated had a response, and survival was longer in responders. The most important pretreatment prognostic parameter for these patients was the in vitro chemosensitivity. It correlated positively with response to treatment and with survival when studied as sensitivity to the best three drugs, all 10 drugs, etoposide alone, or various other subsets of the tested drugs. Sensitivity and specificity were 67% and 75%, respectively, for the treatment scheme used if 31% in vitro survival was used as the cut point. Using a scheme (11) previously published (sensitivity set at the median of the 10-drug set plus one standard deviation), it was noted that none of five test-negative ("highly resistant") tumors responded and nine of 20 sensitive tumors responded. This corresponds to 100% sensitivity and a specificity of 31%. This was done as a pilot study to show feasibility. An attempt was made to do a similar study in a major trials group, but inadequate accrual led to cancellation of that study.

Shaw et al. (20) published a report of individualized chemotherapy for NSCLC using prospective studies of neuroendocrine markers and in vitro chemosensitivity testing. They used a dye exclusion assay for the in vitro testing and attempted to test 12 drugs at concentrations of 10%, 100%, and 1000% of suggested clinically equivalent exposures (12). Drugs were considered active if they had resulted in less than 50% survival at the central or reference concentration. About half the specimens had only enough cells to test at this concentration. The assay was applied to 161 tumor-containing specimens, with success in only 37 (from 36 patients) for a 23% success rate. The success rate was only 7% in the 69 specimens from lung tissue, but the authors don't state whether any of these were bronchoscopic specimens. To eliminate nontumor cells, Shaw et al. subcultured their specimens before doing the assay. This delayed the time to results as much as 3 weeks and probably significantly decreased the yield. Of the 36 patients supplying in vitro data, 21 were treated with a chemotherapy regimen chosen on the basis of these data and 2 (9%) responded. The treatment was chosen from a panel of eight published chemotherapy regimens for NSCLC, but the details of selection were not given. Shaw et al. also treated 69 of the patients with empiric cisplatin and etoposide, with 10 (14%) responders. This was an essentially negative study with no improvement in response rate or survival for the patients with therapy selected by in vitro assay. The clinical interpretation of the study is limited by certain concerns. The assay success rate was remarkably low. More importantly, we find from a previous report from the same research group that NSCLC patients had a worse prognosis if cell lines could be established from their tumors (21). In the current study, Shaw et al. established immortalized cell lines in 62% of the 37 successful assays and in only 12% of another 128 unsuccessful assay attempts. This would suggest that any attempt to compare outcome for assay-successful and assay-unsuccessful patients would be uninterpretable. The investigators did not offer data allowing an estimate of the sensitivity or specificity of their test.

## Correlations for NSCLC Reported as Parts of Broader Trials

Weisenthal et al. (12) first reported clinical correlations for the DISC assay in 1983 and included seven patients with NSCLC. All were judged resistant by the assay and none of them responded to a clinical trial of chemotherapy. Treatment was not selected by reference to the assay. Kitten et al. (22) reported the application of the clonogenic assay to lung cancer in 1983, but their patients appear to have been included in a later report from the same laboratory by Hanauske et al. (17). These authors did not separate small cell from NSCLC, though presumably the majority of their patients had the latter. From 1464 specimens, the investigators successfully cultured 552, with a significantly higher success rate for metastases (48%) than primary sites (31%). Some of the patients had assay-directed therapy and some had only retrospective correlation. The authors presented 112 correlations with test settings such that the sensitivity was 82% and the specificity 87%. A third report, also in 1983 (23), from the same laboratory included a subgroup of the lung cancer patients treated with the best single agent selected from the assay. Some detailed data are given on the in vitro sensitivity and the clinical outcome. Using the 50%-inhibition definition of sensitivity proposed in their paper gives a sensitivity of 88% and a specificity of 75%. Changing the definition of sensitivity to

**Table 4** Data for Assays Utilizing a Threshold Intended to Create a Highly Sensitive Sensitivity Assay or a Highly Specific Resistance Assay

| Author (Ref.) | Assay | Assay success rate | Directed treatment | Response rate | Sensitivity/Specificity (approximate) | |
|---|---|---|---|---|---|---|
| Von Hoff (23) | Cloning | 64% | Yes | 8/40 (20%) | 100% | 53% |
| Kern (11) | Mixed | 71% | No | 10/35 (28%) | 90% | 44% |
| Wilbur (19) | DISC | 78% | Yes | 9/25 (36%) | 100% | 31% |
| Combined data | | | | 26/100 (26%) | 96% | 45% |

a 20% inhibition of colony growth changes the sensitivity to 100% and the specificity to 53%, as shown in Table 4.

Volm et al. (24) reported the use of a short-term tritiated thymidine uptake assay for evaluating sensitivity of NSCLC to drugs in vitro. They did not give any data allowing an estimate of assay success rate, sensitivity, or specificity. They did, however, provide survival curves for chemotherapy-treated patients: five patients judged sensitive by assay and 11 judged resistant. These curves suggested substantially better survival for sensitive patients, but no statistics were provided to support this conclusion.

In 1990, Von Hoff et al. (10) reported a randomized trial comparing physician-selected versus in vitro sensitivity test selected single-drug therapy for patients with advanced tumors (usually solid) having no standard therapy option. A modified clonogenic assay was used that took about 2 weeks to run and had a 71% success rate in this study. The trial collected 65 patients on the physician-selection arm and 68 on the assay-selection arm but only 36 and 19, respectively, received treatment. The response rate was significantly higher for the assay-directed arm (21% vs. 3%) but survival was not significantly affected for the groups overall. The assay-selection arm included 18 NSCLC patients, but only four actually received treatment and one had a partial response. A variety of factors contributed to the low number of evaluable patients; the two most important were test failure and failure to be treated. There was some concern that the 2-week delay from biopsy to assay results might have exacerbated factors leading to the latter. No sensitivity or specificity data were given, but the study illustrates the difficulties of applying such testing in the clinical setting.

Kern and Weisenthal (11) published one of the larger collections of data correlating clinical outcome with in vitro chemosensitivity testing. Data initially from a clonogenic assay and later from a thymidine incorporation assay were lumped together to get 450 clinical correlations. Over many years, 3575 successful assays (71%) had been done on 5059 fresh tumor specimens. It was asserted that the assay success rate had been greater than 80% after changing to the thymidine incorporation scheme. Most of the assays were done for investigational purposes unrelated to patient care, and they were not used to guide treatment. Correlations were studied only when the patients were treated exclusively with assayed drugs. Data from 35 patients with NSCLC were included in the report. The authors defined in vitro sensitivity as cell survival of less than the median plus one standard deviation. The median was determined from all successful assays on all tumor types. Using this definition led to a sensitivity of 90% and a specificity of 44% for NSCLC. Using the same definitions for their whole population, the investigators found a sensitivity of 99.2% and a specificity of 39.6%. The only responder missed by this assay among the 450 patients (132 responses) was one of the NSCLC patients.

Clinical correlations for another variation on the in vitro chemosensitivity theme were reported by Leone et al. (13) in 1991. They reported an assay success rate of 96% for solid tumors, with an overall sensitivity of 98% and a specificity of 81%. They gave separate data for eight lung cancer patients (type not specified). Six of these had clinical responses to chemotherapy, and for them the test had sensitivity of 100% and specificity of 67%. As reported, this test seemed to be a highly sensitive sensitivity assay or a highly specific resistance assay.

## The Highly Sensitive Test Orientation

In Table 4 are data derived from using the in vitro assay as a highly specific resistance assay or highly sensitive sensitivity assay. Kern and Weisenthal (11) presented their data specifically in this way. Their standards were applied to the data collected in the study of Wilbur et al. (19). The third entry comes from the analysis of data published by Von Hoff et al. (23) as described above. Lumping these data together would give a sensitivity of 96% and a specificity of 45% from data on 100 correlations. Considering that these data are from different laboratories and assay techniques, this result suggests the potential for such testing.

## DISCUSSION

We have presented over 10 years of published work with over 250 clinical correlations from a variety of research laboratories using several assay techniques. On this basis, we feel confident in asserting that the in vitro assay contains significant predictive clinical information. It is probably not possible to apply the assay to all patients with lung cancer because of problems obtaining an adequate study sample. More sensitive assay techniques might allow broader application in the future. Currently, the test can be optimally utilized if the physician plans ahead—getting a sample at the time of any surgery for diagnostic or therapeutic purposes.

Test philosophy is also important in the use of this information. If the test is set up as a highly sensitive test so that essentially all responders are identified, practitioners would be comfortable recommending no standard therapy for the resistant patients. This could save a significant number of patients from toxic and expensive therapy that may actually shorten their lives. Alternatively, some of these patients might be given the opportunity to enter phase I trials looking for new non-cross-resistant drugs.

Use of the test to select therapy has been attempted in several small trials in NSCLC but has not been remarkably successful (10,19,20,23). These trials have not ruled out such use, but they suggest that we need a larger panel of non-cross-resistant drugs to be studied in the assay. There is a high degree of clinical cross-resistance in the panel of drugs currently considered active in NSCLC and even in small cell lung cancer, as shown by the fact that responses to second-line treatment in these diseases are much less frequent and usually shorter than responses to first-line treatment.

Further motivation for applying this assay to NSCLC might come from the application of cost-benefit analysis and quality-of-life studies. Sparing a significant number of patients therapy might lead to improvements in both areas.

## ACKNOWLEDGMENTS

The author wishes to thank Dr. Larry Weisenthal for helpful discussions and suggestions and for review of the manuscript, and Lercy Rubin for preparing the manuscript.

## REFERENCES

1. Wingo PA, Tong T, Bolden S. Cancer statistics, 1995. CA Cancer J Clin 1995; 45:8–30.
2. Vokes EE. Integration of vinorelbine into chemotherapy strategies for non-small-cell lung cancer. Oncology 1995; 9:565–577.
3. Albert A. Selective Toxicity. 3rd ed. New York: John Wiley and Sons, 1965.
4. Black MM, Speer FD. Further observations on the effects of cancer chemotherapeutic agents on the in vitro dehydrogenase activity of cancer tissue. J Natl Cancer Inst 1954; 14: 1147–1158.
5. Hamburger AW, Salmon SE. Primary bioassay of human tumor stem cells. Science 1977; 197:461–463.
6. Salmon SE, Hamburger AW, Soehnlen B, et al. Quantitation of differential sensitivity of humor tumor stem cells to anticancer drugs. N Engl J Med 1978; 298:1321–1327.
7. Weisenthal LM. Predictive assays for drug and radiation resistance. In: Masters JRW, ed. Human Cancer in Primary Culture, a Handbook. The Netherlands: Kluwer Academic Publishers, 1991:103–147.
8. Fruehauf JP, Bosanquet AG. In vitro determination of drug response: a discussion of clinical applications. PPO Updates 1993; 7(12):1–16.
9. Von Hoff DD. He's not going to talk about in vitro predictive assays again is he? J Natl Cancer Inst 1990; 82:96–101.
10. Von Hoff DD, Sandbach JF, Clark GM, et al. Selection of cancer chemotherapy for a patient by an in vitro assay versus a clinician. J Natl Cancer Inst 1990; 82:110–116.
11. Kern DH, Weisenthal LM. Highly specific prediction of antineoplastic drug resistance with an in vitro assay using suprapharmacologic drug exposures. J Natl Cancer Inst 1990; 82: 582–588.
12. Weisenthal LM, Marsden JA, Dill PL, Macaluso CK. A novel dye exclusion method for testing in vitro chemosensitivity of human tumors. Cancer Res 1983; 43:749–757.
13. Leone LA, Meitner PA, Myers TJ, et al. Predictive value of the fluorescent cytoprint assay (FCA): a retrospective correlation study of in vitro chemosensitivity and individual responses to chemotherapy. Cancer Invest 1991; 9:491–503.
14. Bertelsen CA, Kern DH, Kaiser LR, et al. Biopsy of thoracic neoplasms for assay of chemosensitivity. New indication for thoracotomy. Arch Surg 1983; 118:1074–1076.
15. Von Hoff DD, Weisenthal LM, Ihde DC, et al. Growth of lung cancer colonies from bronchoscopy washings. Cancer 1981; 48:400–403.
16. Smit EF, de Vries EGE, Meijer C, et al. Limitations of the fast green assay for chemosensitivity testing in human lung cancer. Chest 1991; 100:1358–1363.
17. Hanauske AR, Von Hoff DD. Clinical correlations with the human tumor cloning assay. Cancer Invest 1985; 3:541–551.
18. Shimizu E, Saijo N, Kanzawa F, et al. Correlation between drug sensitivity determined by clonogenic cell assay and clinical effect of chemotherapy in patients with primary lung cancer. Jpn J Cancer Res 1984; 75:1030–1035.
19. Wilbur DW, Camacho ES, Hilliard DA, et al. Chemotherapy of non-small cell lung carcinoma guided by an in vitro drug resistance assay measuring total tumour cell kill. Br J Cancer 1992; 65:27–32.

20. Shaw GL, Gazdar AF, Phelps R, et al. Individualized chemotherapy for patients with non-small cell lung cancer determined by prospective identification of neuroendocrine markers and in vitro drug sensitivity testing. Cancer Res 1993; 53:5181–5187.
21. Stevenson H, Gazdar AF, Phelps R, et al. Tumor cell lines established in vitro: an independent prognostic factor for survival in non-small-cell lung cancer. Ann Intern Med 1990; 113:764–770.
22. Kitten CM, Von Hoff DD, Bennett EV, et al. The human tumor clonogenic assay in the treatment of patients with lung cancer. Ann Thorac Surg 1983; 36:408–410.
23. Von Hoff DD, Clark GM, Stogdill BJ, et al. Prospective clinical trial of a human tumor cloning system. Cancer Res 1983; 43:1926–1931.
24. Volm M, Drings P, Mattern J, et al. Relevance of DNA-fluorimetry and short-term resistance testing for adjuvant treatment of non-small cell lung carcinomas. Anticancer Res 1986; 6:931–934.

# 4

## Liposomal Formulations of Chemotherapeutic Drugs

**Samuel D. Bernal and Yuk-Chor Wong**
*UCLA San Fernando Valley Program, Sepulveda Veterans Administration Medical Center, Sepulveda, California*

**Romulo de Villa**
*UCLA San Fernando Valley Program, Sepulveda Veterans Administration Medical Center, Sepulveda, California, and Far Eastern University, Manila, Philippines*

**Gloria Bernas**
*UCLA San Fernando Valley Program, Sepulveda Veterans Administration Medical Center, Sepulveda, California, and University of Santo Tomas, Manila, Philippines*

### INTRODUCTION

Liposomal formulations of chemotherapeutic agents have great potential for selective delivery of drugs to tumor cells (1). These liposomal constructs offer the possibility of increasing the therapeutic index of various drugs—by decreasing toxicity to normal organs while selectively increasing accumulation in tumor cells. The higher therapeutic index of liposomal drug compared to free drug is the result of many factors; among them, the ability to remain in the circulation with very long half-lives and increased microvascular permeability of tumors. Lipophilic drugs that would otherwise be difficult to administer systemically can be delivered by liposomes (2).

Liposomal drugs also have the potential of overcoming drug resistance of tumors by increasing membrane uptake of drugs and increasing intracellular concentration of drugs. In recent years, many new drugs have been incorporated into liposomal constructs. The liposomal composition has been varied to obtain optimal drug delivery (3). Antibodies have been incorporated to improve tumor targeting. Recently, membrane proteins have been incorporated into liposomes to increase adhesion to tumor cells and increase membrane transport of drug. This chapter reviews these various developments in liposomal formulation for in vitro investigations and in vivo applications in cancer chemotherapy.

### ANTHRACYCLINE-CONTAINING LIPOSOMES

#### In Vitro Studies

Doxorubicin encapsulated in liposomes was observed to have more anticancer toxicity than free doxorubicin and was found to modulate multidrug resistance (MDR) in Chinese hamster LZ cells and human colon cancer cells (4). Vincristine-resistant HL-60/VCR leukemia cells, which express P-glycoprotein, and doxorubicin-resistant HL-60/ADR leukemia cells, which do not express P-glycoprotein, were studied for sensitivity to free doxorubicin and liposome-encapsulated doxorubicin. The concentrations that caused 50% inhibition of growth (IC50) for free doxorubicin were 30 nmol/L for HL-60, 9 $\mu$mol/L for HL-60/ADR, and 0.9 $\mu$mol/L for HL-60/VCR cells. With liposome-encapsulated doxorubicin, the IC50 was 20 nmol/L in parental HL-60 cells and 9 $\mu$mol/L in HL-60/ADR cells, indicating little or no sensitization. However, HL-60/VCR cells were fivefold more sensitive to liposome-encapsulated doxorubicin than to free doxorubicin, with an IC50 that was reduced to 0.17 $\mu$mol/L. HL-60 cells treated with liposome-encapsulated doxorubicin showed less intracellular accumulation of doxorubicin compared to cells treated with free drug. HL-60 VCR cells, on the other hand, accumulated drug twofold to threefold higher with liposomal doxorubicin than that with free doxorubicin.

Liposome-encapsulated doxorubicin appeared to circumvent MDR by specific interaction with P-glycoprotein, as suggested by the complete inhibition of the photo-affinity labeling of P-glycoprotein by azidopine in membrane vesicles of HL-60 VCR cells. Thus, the liposome-encapsulated doxorubicin may be effective in overcoming resistance in the multidrug-resistant phenotype of HL-60/VCR cells by direct interaction with P-glycoprotein.

The effect of liposomal doxorubicin in circumventing drug resistance was also studied in several multidrug-resistant (MDR) cell lines, including CH LZ, MCF-7/ADR cell line, and the ovarian carcinoma SKVLB cell line (5). The effect was specific to MDR cells, as liposomally encapsulated doxorubicin did not enhance cell sensitivity to the drug in the parental cell lines. The empty liposomes in the presence of free doxorubicin (Dox) reversed resistance to the drug at a higher level than that observed when liposome-encapsulated Dox was used. Doxorubicin appeared to have a high affinity for cardiolipin, one of the liposome components, leading to the association of the drug and the cardiolipin-containing liposomes in the culture medium before entry of the drug into cells. However, pretreatment of cells with empty liposomes before drug treatment or with combined incubation of vincristine and empty liposomes did not overcome MDR in CH LZ cells, indicating that doxorubicin must be encapsulated in liposomes to overcome MDR. The MDR in CH LZ cells and its modulation by liposome-encapsulated Dox did not appear to be related to GSH function. The enhanced sensitivity of MDR cells to liposomal doxorubicin seemed to be caused by increased drug accumulation in the cells and intracellular drug redistribution. Using fluorescence confocal microscopy, doxorubicin was observed to be transported and distributed mainly in intracytoplasmic vesicles in SKVLB and MCF-7/ADR cells, whereas in parental cells the drug localized mainly in the nucleus. However, when liposomal doxorubicin was used, the drug distribution pattern in MDR cells was changed by partially shifting the drug to the nuclear compartment. Liposomal doxorubicin may bypass the vesicular transport in MDR cells, with increased nuclear localization and enhancement of the drug effect.

Lecithin or lecithin-cholesterol mixtures modified cell membrane fluidity in a high proportion of cells of AKR lymphoma variants (of varying aggressiveness and drug resistance) and induced higher accumulation of ADR (6). However, the cholesterol-lecithin mixture also induced in some of the variants the emergence of small subpopulations with very low ADR permeability. Modification of cell membrane fluidity may expose tumor cell antigens but also induce low drug permeability when used in conjunction with chemotherapy.

Preformed or lyophilized cardiolipin-containing liposomes were also used to complex doxorubicin (7). Complex formation was performed by vigorous vortexing. As much as 96.8% of the initial drug quantity may be bound to those liposomes under optimal incubation conditions (4 h at 37°C). The binding study showed the presence of two levels of specific binding (dissociation constants, $28 \pm 8$ $\mu$mol/L and $1.0 \pm 0.3$ mmol/L). The drug is firmly integrated in the liposome-membrane lipid bilayer rather than binding at the surface. Cytotoxicity studies using tumor cells revealed efficient drug delivery using liposome-complexed doxorubicin. This new liposomal doxorubicin preparation reversed multidrug resistance in MCF-7/ADR and CH LZ cells at levels equivalent to that obtained with a previously described liposome-encapsulated doxorubicin preparation, showing that the drug is integrated in the liposome carrier and is transported as well into cells. Increased concentration of liposomes at the subcytotoxic level in liposome-complexed doxorubicin enhances drug cytotoxicity in multidrug-resistant CH LZ cells as compared with liposome-encapsulated drug.

Based on the concept that receptors for the vitamin folic acid are often overexpressed on the surface membrane of epithelial cancer cells, folate-targeted liposomes were used to specifically deliver liposome-encapsulated doxorubicin in vitro (8). The lipopsomes included 0.1 mol% of a folate-polyethyleneglycol-distearoylphatidyleth-anolamine (folate-PEG-DSPE) construct into the lipid bilayer, and were then loaded with doxorubicin (Dox). KB carcinoma cells showed uptake of the folate-PEG-liposomal Dox 45-fold higher than that of nontargeted liposomal Dox, and 1.6-times higher than that of free Dox. The cytotoxicity of folate-targeted liposomes toward KB cells was 86-times higher than nontargeted liposomal Dox and 2.7-times higher than free Dox. Folate-targeting was compatible with PEG-coating of the liposomes, such that incorporation of 4 mol% PEG2000-DSPE did not reduce uptake or cytotoxicity of the folate-PEG-liposomal Dox. Uptake of the folate-PEG-liposomal Dox was inhibited by 1 mmol/L free folic acid but not by physiological concentrations of folate. In co-cultures of HeLa and WI38 cells, the folate-PEG-liposomes with encapsulated calcein (a fluorescent dye) were internalized exclusively by the HeLa cells, which overexpress the folate receptors, but not by other cells. These experiments suggest that folate targeting may improve the anticancer specificity of PEG-coated liposomes.

### Intravenous Injection

The antitumor effect of liposome-encapsulated Adriamycin (doxorubicin) with CA19-9 antibody (lipo-ADM-Ab) against a human pancreatic cancer cell line PK-1 was studied in vitro and in vivo (9). The liposomal compound (lipo-ADM-Ab) showed a stronger cell damaging effect than ADM. The intratumor concentration of ADM in the group given intravenous injection of lipo-ADM-Ab showed the highest value, over twice those of lipo c ADM and free ADM after 120 h. Lipo-ADM-Ab showed greated inhibitory effect on the tumor growth in vivo, with final tumor weight at the 19th day reduced to 27% in the lipo-ADM-Ab and 52% in the free ADM group, compared with the untreated control. In this study, targeted chemotherapy using drug encapsulated in liposomes and antibody was found to have a stronger antitumor effect than the administration of anticancer drug alone, perhaps due to increased tumor accessibility and selective targeting of tumor cells.

Anthracyclines encapsulated in hydrogenated phosphatidylinositol (HPI)-containing liposomes showed long circulation time in plasma (10). The tissue distribution, toxicity, and antitumor activity of anthracycline-containing liposomes were studied in mice, compared with phosphatidylglycerol (PG)-containing liposomes. Doxorubicin (Dox) or epirubicin (Epi) was encapsulated in small (65–100 nm mean diameter) HPI or PG liposomes. The levels of Dox and Epi in intramuscular tumor implants of the J6456 lymphoma were elevated by delivery in HPI liposomes but not by delivery in PG liposomes. Dox encapsulation in either PG- or HPI-containing liposomes reduced the lethal toxicity of the drug in mice. However, only the HPI-Dox formulation was more active than free Dox in the treatment of the ascitic J6456 tumor. Treatment with Epi encapsulated in HPI liposomes also showed greater effect compared to that of free Epi. Anthracyclines delivered in long-circulating liposomes are capable of drug delivery with relative selectivity in tumor areas, with improvement in therapeutic index compared to the free drug.

Standard chemotherapy has little effect in the treatment of liver cancer, prompting the investigation of different methods of drug targeting (11). Liposomes as a method of drug delivery has disadvantages that include short shelf-life and poor drug delivery into tumor tissue. Ion-exchange microspheres were studied as an alternative strategy for targeted drug delivery that may overcome these disadvantages while reducing systemic toxicity and maintaining therapeutic efficacy. Compared to controls, Dox treatment with microspheres reduced tumor growth by 79% ($P < .001$), compared with 51% ($P < .01$) for liposomes and 56% ($P < .001$) for free drug. Drug microspheres seemed to increase the antitumor efficacy compared to either free or liposomal drug while reducing systemic toxicity.

Polybutylcyanoacrylate (PBCA) nanoparticles were prepared and loaded with mitoxantrone and injected into leukemia- or melanoma-bearing mice (12). Efficacy and toxicity of mitoxantrone nanoparticles were compared with free mitoxantrone and with a mitoxantrone-liposome formulation (small unilamellar vesicles with a negative surface charge). PBCA nanoparticles and liposomes had different effects on the two tumor types: liposomes prolonged survival time in P388 leukemia, whereas nanoparticles led to a significant tumor volume reduction at the B16 melanoma. Neither nanoparticles nor liposomes were able to reduce the leukopenia caused by mitoxantrone.

Clinical studies using intravenous administration of liposomal anthracyclines were carried out recently. In a phase I clinical study of liposomally encapsulated daunorubicin (DaunoXome), 32 patients were entered, and 30 were evaluable (13). The initial dose escalation from 10 to 60 mg/m² did not result in toxicity. Doses of 80 mg/m² resulted in grade 2 neutropenia in two patients. Those receiving 120 mg/m² showed grade 3 neutropenia. Alopecia was mild, and cardiotoxicity was not observed except for an episode of arrhythmia. In this group of patients with tumors refractory to other chemotherapy, only one minor objective response was observed with the liposomal daunorubicin.

Clinical studies were also carried out using Doxil, a doxorubicin liposome formulation containing polyethylene glycol (14). After intravenous injection, nearly 100% of the drug detected in plasma was in liposome encapsulated form. Compared to free (Dox) doxorubicin, Doxil had slow plasma clearance (0.1 L/h for Doxil versus 45 L/h for free Dox) and had small volume of distribution (4 L for Doxil versus 254 L for free Dox). Significantly, Doxil showed a four- to 16-fold enhancement of drug levels in malignant effusions, which peaked between 3 and 7 days after injection.

### Intra-Arterial Injection

Liposomal Adriamycin (Lip-ADM) was administered to three patients with metastatic adenocarcinoma of the liver through a catheter located in the hepatic artery (15). Two of the patients had gastric cancer and one had sigmoid colon cancer. Lip-ADM was administered at 10, 20, or 50 mg per dose for total ADM doses of 170, 490, and 760 mg, respectively. The survival time was respectively 6, 15, and 17 months from the start of Lip-ADM administration. One patient had a partial response and another had stable disease. No patients showed severe adverse effects, such as nausea, vomiting, stomatitis, alopecia, or cardiotoxicity. There was mild neutropenia in one patient, but anemia or thrombocytopenia did not occur. Because of its lower toxicity, liposomal ADM made it feasible to deliver higher total doses of ADM directly to the liver.

### Intraperitoneal Injection

Liposomal mitoxantrone was also investigated as treatment of peritoneal carcinomatosis, exploiting the slow resorption of liposomal drugs from serous cavities. Mitoxantrone (MXN)-liposomes with various lipid compositions were examined for their anti-tumor activity on peritoneal carcinomatosis induced by a colon cancer cell injection in BALb/c mice (16). MXN carried in phosphatidylcholine:cholesterol (2:1; G-liposomes) showed lower toxicity in mice compared to the free drug. Nontoxic doses (2 mg/kg) of G-liposomal MXN were as effective as free drug. Higher MXN doses (3 mg/kg) encapsulated in either G-liposomes and phosphatidylcholine:cholesterol:dipalmitoylphosphatidylethanolamine (7:2:1) liposomes increased the life span of tumor-bearing mice compared to the free drug and other liposome formulations of the drug.

### Intramucosal Injection

The delivery of Adriamycin to the regional lymph nodes of the stomach following the gastric submucosal injection of liposomal Adriamycin (Lipo-ADR) was studied in 34 gastric carcinoma patients and compared with intravenous administration of free ADR (F-ADR) in another 18 patients (17). The Lipo-ADR was endoscopically injected into the gastric submucosa adjacent to the primary tumor via a needle-tipped catheter, prior to radical gastrectomy. After injection, the ADR concentration in the primary and secondary drainage lymph nodes was found to be higher than in the other regional lymph nodes. In contrast, the intravenous F-ADR showed much lower ADR concentration in all the nodes. Injection of Lipo-ADR was also compared with delivery to the left gastric artery lymph nodes after intravenous administration of an equal dose of F-ADR. The ADR levels in draining lymph nodes were much higher after gastric submucosal injection than with intravenous injection. The gastric submucosal injection of Lipo-ADR appeared to specifically deliver ADR to the regional lymph nodes at high concentrations. The preoperative adjuvant chemotherapy targeting the regional lymph nodes is a potentially useful strategy for preventing the lymph node recurrence of gastric carcinoma.

### Acquired Immunodeficiency Syndrome—Kaposi's Sarcoma

The use of chemotherapy in AIDS-related Kaposi's sarcoma (AIDS-KS) is difficult because of limited efficacy and substantial toxicity. In a phase I/II clinical study, dose escalation of liposomal encapsulated formulation of doxorubicin (Doxil) was carried out in 15 patients with HIV-related, biopsy-confirmed, cutaneous Kaposi's sarcoma (18). Most patients had poor prognostic disease and six patients had previously received combination chemotherapy. The treatment regimen consisted of a dose of Doxil 10 mg/m$^2$, repeated after 2 weeks. Responding patients received maintenance therapy at the same dose every 2 weeks. Nonresponders were treated with increased doses to 20 mg/m$^2$ for the further two cycles, before proceeding to maintenance therapy. The treatment was continued until other intercurrent disease, lack of further response, patient preference, or toxicity precluded further treatment. Partial responses were observed in 11/15 (73%), with disease stabilization in the remaining patients. Doxil was well tolerated, with mainly hematological toxicity. Doxil seemed to be an effective palliative treatment for AIDS-KS.

In another clinical study, pegylated (Stealth) liposomal doxorubicin hydrochloride (SL-DOX) has been found to deliver high concentrations of doxorubicin to Kaposi's sarcoma lesions (19). The efficacy and safety of SL-DOX in the treatment of moderate to severe AIDS-KS was evaluated in a phase II study. Patients were treated biweekly with 10, 20, or 40 mg/m$^2$ SL-DOX. Out of 238 patients who were evaluated, 15 patients (6.3%) had a complete response to SL-DOX, 177 (74.4%) had a partial response, 44 (18.5%) had stable disease, and 2 (0.8%) had disease progression. Neutropenia occurred in over half of patients but only 4 patients discontinued therapy because of neutropenia. A total of 10 patients discontinued therapy because of adverse reactions. SL-DOX has substantial activity in AIDS-KS, with response noted after fewer than three cycles of chemotherapy.

## Cis-PLATINUM-CONTAINING LIPOSOMES

### Liposomal CDDP

Multilamellar liposomes containing cisplatin (L-CDDP) were tested against L 1210 murine leukemia and NIH OVCAR human ovarian cancer cells (20). In vitro cytotoxicity studies showed C50 values of 0.14 and 0.05 $\mu$g/mL with CDDP or L-CDDP, respectively. In vivo administration of L-CDDP in mice resulted in plasma levels of platinum fourfold higher compared with free CDDP. The plasma half-life of L-CDDP was much longer than free CDDP, with platinum accumulations in liver, spleen, kidneys, lungs, and heart that were higher in L-CDDP–treated compared to CDDP-treated mice. Intraperitoneal injections with 12 mg/kg of L-CDDP resulted in higher antitumor efficacy and increased life span of the mice compared to free CDDP. The nephrotoxicity in rats (blood urea nitrogen and creatinine evaluation) of L-CDDP administered intraperitoneally was significantly less than with CDDP. This study confirms that the liposomal encapsulation of CDDP decreases its nephrotoxicity but increases its antitumor efficacy.

### Lipophilic Cisplatin Derivatives

Lipophilic cisplatin derivatives, cis-bis-neodecanoato-trans-R,R-1,2 diaminocyclohexane platinum(II) (NDDP) have been entrapped in multilamellar liposomes composed of dimyristoylphosphatidyl choline (DMPC) and dimyristoylphosphatidyl glycerol (DMPG) (21). The liposome-entrapped NDDP (L-NDDP) was prepared as a lyophilized powder. However, NDDP was found to be an isomeric mixture with different isomeric neodecanoic moieties as leaving groups. For preparation of homogeneous formulations, single isomers of neodecanoic acid were incorporated into a series of highly lipid-soluble cis-bis(neodecanoato) (trans-(R,R)- and -(S,S)-1,2-diaminocyclohexane) platinum(II) [Pt] complexes, and then incorporated into liposomes. The intravenous LD50 values of the various liposomal Pt preparations were between 62.3 and 104 mg/kg. After a single intraperitoneal injection of the optimal dose, the % T/C obtained against L1210 leukemia was between 150 and 253, compared to 160 for cisplatin. The anticancer activity improved with multiple intraperitoneal injections (days 1, 5, and 9), with some of the liposomal Pt preparations showing % T/C of 257, compared to 220 for cisplatin. The liposomal Pt preparations were also more active than cisplatin against L1210 leukemia cells resistant to cisplatin showing % T/C ranging from 185 to 335 for the liposomal Pt, compared to 112 for cisplatin. Thus, the single isomeric forms of NDDP appeared to have consistent activity against cancer cells and were comparable to the mixed isomeric NDDP preparations in terms of toxicity and biological activity. In addition, the liposomal Pt formulations were more active than cisplatin against L1210 cells, including cells resistant to cisplatin. The liposomal Pt formulation, L-NDDP, was not cross-resistant with cisplatin in different in vitro and in vivo systems. It was more active than cisplatin against murine models of experimental liver metastases and found to be non-nephrotoxic in humans. In contrast, free NDDP showed no significant antitumor activity in vivo at the optimal dose of L-NDDP. Higher doses of NDDP showed minimal activity.

The effect of varying the liposome composition, size of the branched leaving groups of the platinum compound, and pH and composition of the aqueous phase were studied to determine how the liposomal carrier enhanced the biological properties of the Pt drug (22). The different liposomal Pt formulations were evaluated for their entrapment efficiency, drug leakage, drug stability, and in vivo toxicity and antitumor activity. DMPG in the lipid bilayer (with normal saline in the aqueous phase) decreased the stability of NDDP in the liposomes and increased its biological activity. In contrast, DMPC in the liposomes increased the stability of NDDP entrapped in liposomes but the formulation showed no antitumor activity. Longer chains of carbon atoms in the leaving groups increased entrapment efficiency and decreased stability of the Pt compounds. Longer chains in the branched leaving groups also increased in situ degradation of the platinum compound and enhanced biological activity and potency. The liposomal NDDP appears to form active intermediates within the lipid bilayers and this activation is linked to its cytotoxic activity. Moreover, the activation reaction was highly dependent on the presence of DMPG and was influenced by the size of the lipophilic leaving group.

The cytotoxicity, cellular accumulation, and DNA interactions induced by liposome-entrapped NDDP (L-NDDP) and cisplatin was studied in A2780 human ovarian carcinoma cells sensitive (A2780/S) and resistant (A2780/PDD) to cisplatin (23). L-NDDP was found to be twofold more cytotoxic than cisplatin against A2780/S cells with 5-h or 24-h drug exposures. The A2780/PDD cells were fourfold resistant to cisplatin, whereas both the A2780/S and A2780/PDD cell lines were equally sensitive to L-NDDP. With shorter drug exposures (5 h), the cytotoxicity of L-NDDP was directly related to the relative content of DMPG in the liposome carrier. However, with 24-h exposures to the drug, L-NDDP cytotoxicity was independent of the liposome composition. Changes in liposome composition or drug exposure time did not alter the resistance index of L-NDDP. The cellular accumulation of cisplatin was reduced by two- to threefold in A2780/PDD cells. In contrast, the cellular accumulation of L-NDDP was similar in both cell lines and two- to fivefold higher than that of cisplatin in A2780/S cells. DMPG in the lipid bilayer enhanced the cellular accumulation of L-NDDP twofold. Pt/DNA levels were determined at different time points after drug exposure for 1 h. The peak Pt/DNA levels in the target cells were observed at 6 h for cisplatin and at 9 h for L-NDDP. The peak Pt/DNA levels and levels of Pt/DNA over time were higher for L-NDDP than cisplatin for both cell lines, using equimolar concentrations of both drugs. Cisplatin generated DNA interstrand and DNA-protein cross-links, and showed a good correlation with cytotoxicity against both cell lines. In contrast, L-NDDP caused only minimal DNA interstrand cross-links in either cell line.

The effect of cisplatin and L-NDDP on inducing internucleosomal DNA fragmentation and cell death was examined in these same cell lines (24). Both drugs were very effective in inducing DNA fragmentation in A2780 cells, but only L-NDDP produced significant DNA fragmentation in A2780/PDD cells, correlating well with the observed cytotoxicity. The endonuclease inhibitor (ATA) inhibited DNA fragmentation caused by either high (30–60 $\mu$mol/L) or low (3–10 $\mu$mol/L) concentrations of both drugs. However, the protein synthesis inhibitor (CHX) inhibited DNA fragmentation caused by low concentrations of either drug but not that caused by high concentrations, suggesting that there are two different pathways for drug-induced cell death that depends on drug concentrations.

The drug accumulation and DNA damage induced by L-NDDP and cisplatin were studied in LoVo and LoVo/PDD cells (25). The accumulation of L-NDDP in LoVo cells was found to be severalfold higher than that of cisplatin. The accumulation of L-NDDP is similar in both cell lines, whereas that of cisplatin is reduced by two- to threefold in LoVo/PDD cells. The transmembrane transport of cisplatin is highly dependent on temperature, whereas that of L-NDDP is not. The cytotoxicity of both agents correlates with the extent of DNA-protein cross-link formation. DNA interstrand cross-linking does not appear to play a role in the cytotoxicity of L-NDDP, whereas it correlates with cisplatin cytotoxicity.

The toxicity and efficacy of the lipophilic dineodecanoato (trans-R,R- and trans-S,S-1,2-diaminocyclohexane) platinum(II) complexes were studied in mice bearing L1210 leukemia cells (26). The LD50 of L-Pt preparations in the mouse ranged from 60 to 104 mg/kg. Most of the L-Pt preparations did not show significant nephrotoxicity at the LD50 dose. Optimal doses of the L-Pt preparations administered intraperitoneally to mice showed significant in vivo antitumor activity against I.P. L1210 leukemia with % T/C 230–300, compared to 220 for cisplatin. The L-Pt preparations were also active against cisplatin-resistant L1210 leukemia cells with % T/C of 237–355 compared to 112 for cisplatin. The L-Pt preparations administered I.P. showed significant antitumor activity against B16 melanoma with % T/C of 144–155, compared to 161 for cisplatin. However, several of the L-Pt preparations administered I.V. did not show significant antitumor activity against M5076 reticulosarcoma.

The pharmacokinetics of liposome-entrapped cis-bis-neodecanoato-trans-R,R-1,2-diaminocyclohexane platinum(II) (L-NDDP) and cisplatin (CDDP) were studied after I.V. and I.P. administration in the rat (27). Equimolar doses of each drug were used, corresponding to 11 mg/kg for L-NDDP and 5 mg/kg for CDDP. Following I.P. administration, systemic absorption was faster in rats receiving CDDP than those receiving L-NDDP. Peak serum platinum (Pt) levels were observed at 30 min after I.P. administration of CDDP, compared to 12 h after similar administration of L-NDDP. After I.V. administration, serum Pt levels were 2–3 times greater in animals treated with L-NDDP than in those treated with CDDP. I.P. administration of L-NDDP resulted in higher Pt levels in the peritoneal fluid, peritoneal tissue, and intestine measured at

6 h than those after either I.V. L-NDDP or CDDP by either I.P. or I.V. route. L-NDDP resulted in higher Pt levels than CDDP when measured in the liver and spleen of rats, independent of the route of administration. However, L-NDDP resulted in lower kidney Pt levels than CDDP, when administered by either I.P. or I.V. routes. Because the mean retention time of L-NDDP in the peritoneum after I.P. administration was more prolonged than CDDP, this may lead to greated therapeutic efficacy of L-NDDP against tumors in the peritoneal cavity, compared with that of I.P. CDDP.

In early clinical trials, the lipophilic diaminocyclohexane (DACH) platinum complexes, such as NDDP, which contains two branched leaving groups of 10 carbons, showed a favorable toxicity profile in a liposomal formulation (28). However, like many other DACH platinum compounds with branched leaving groups, it is unstable within the liposomes, preventing its widespread clinical evaluation. The effect of the configuration of leaving groups on intraliposomal complex stability was determined by studying several DACH platinum complexes containing linear alkyl carboxylato leaving groups of 5–18 carbons. All liposomal preparations of the complexes showed greater than 90% entrapment efficiency. The efficiency of entrapment was independent of lipid composition and length of the leaving group. Drug leakage from the liposomes was minimal, and it was directly related to the length of the leaving group. Stability of the complexes inside the liposomes was inversely related to the length of the leaving group and the content of DMPG (dimyristoyl phosphatidylglycerol) in the liposomes. The length of the leaving group had little effect on intraliposomal stability of compounds with leaving groups smaller than 10 carbons, but the length had major effects on stability of compounds with longer leaving groups. Some compounds with leaving groups of 6 and 10 carbons formed stable liposomal formulations and had significant in vivo antitumor activity against both L1210/S and L1210/PDD leukemias. Compounds with linear leaving groups appeared to be much more stable within DMPG-containing liposomes than compounds with branched leaving groups. For in vivo antitumor activity, the presence of DMPG seemed to be required.

### Perfluoroalkylated Complexes of Platinum

New perfluoroalkylated side-chain (formed by a perfluoroalkyl tail grafted onto a hydrocarbon spacer) bipyridine complexes of platinum, palladium, and their hydrocarbon analogues were dispersed in aqueous solutions in the presence of egg yolk phospholipids (EYP) and were incorporated into EYP vesicles (29). The complexes retained their chemical and structural integrity when entrapped into liposomes, sterilized, and stored for 3 months at 25°C. All complex/liposome preparations consisted mainly of small unilamellar vesicles (size less than 100 nm) together with a population of larger uni- or multilamellar vesicles (100 to 230 nm). These preparations were stable with respect to particle size and size distribution evolution and complex leakage: no precipitate of drug was detected even after 7 months of storage at 25°C. The impact of the perfluoroalkyl tail and of the other structural features of the complexes on their incorporation efficiency into EYP liposomes was studied. A high fluorophilic character (long perfluoroalkyl tail), when tempered by an equally lipophilic one (long hydrocarbon spacer), was not found to be detrimental to the incorporation efficiency of a perfluoroalkylated drug into hydrocarbon vesicles. This incorporation efficiency was considerably improved by the introduction of a double bond between the perfluoroalkyl tail and the hydrocarbon spacer, forming the bipyridine side chains.

## Carboplatin Liposomes

Carboplatin-liposomal preparations injected intraperitoneally into mice in a single dose of 100 mg/kg were found to increase white blood cell counts, with two peaks (30). The first peak appeared on day 2 after drug administration and showed a maximum 10-fold elevation compared with controls of free carboplatin or empty liposomes. This increase was thought to be due to the release and mobilization of cells from storage compartments. The second peak occurred on day 7–8, showing a sixfold increase in white blood cells; it was thought to be the result of bone marrow stimulation. The number of neutrophils, lymphocytes, and platelets increased. Using combined intraperitoneal treatment of mice with 100 mg/kg of cyclophosphamide followed by carboplatin-liposomes one hour later, leukopenia was avoided. The mechanism of stimulation of hematopoiesis by carboplatin-liposomes is not well understood but the effect of carboplatin-liposomes was hypothesized to be the result of cytokine production by macrophages and the relatively fast uptake of the liposomal drug by macrophages.

The distribution in tissue and antitumor effects of freeze-dried liposome-entrapped carboplatin (Lipo-CBDCA) was studied after intraperitoneal administration to rats carrying AH 130 tumors (31). The liposomes were composed of egg lecithin and cholesterol. After the intraperitoneal administration of Lipo-CBDCA, the serum platinum concentration was lower compared to that following either intraperitoneal or intravenous administration of free carboplatin. Intraperitoneal Lipo-CBDCA increased survival of rats bearing AH 130 tumors, apparently with minimal side effects, based upon biochemical and histological studies in the liver, kidney, spleen, and small intestine. The authors suggest that intraperitoneal chemotherapy with Lipo-CBDCA may be more effective than free CBDCA in treating tumors in the peritoneal cavity.

## Combination of CDDP and Valinomycin

Based on the finding that the activity of CDDP against ovarian cancer cells can be enhanced by liposomal valinomycin (MLV-VM) in vitro, MLV-VM was tested for its ability to increase the cytotoxic effects of other platinum analogues (32). MLV-VM and different platinum drugs were tested against two human ovarian cancer cell lines (OVCAR-3 and CaOV-3) and on Chinese hamster ovary (CHO) cells in vitro. MLV-VM was found to increase the cytotoxic effects of cisplatin, ormaplatin, and carboplatin on human ovarian carcinoma cells. The effect of MLV-VM was found to be synergistic with cisplatin, ormaplatin and carboplatin, by median-effect analysis. The addition of VM with cisplatin resulted in greater accumulation of cells at the $G_2/M$ phase and increased protein kinase C (PKC) activity. The results suggest that the accumulation of cells at $G_2/M$ phases and modulation of PKC activity may be the basis for the cytotoxic synergism observed between cisplatin and VM.

In vivo, the combination of liposomal valinomycin (MLV-VM) with CDDP was also found to have significant antitumor activity against murine P388 leukemia and OVCAR-3 (nude mouse model of human ovarian cancer) (33). The addition of MLV-VM to CDDP resulted in increased life span of P388 leukemia-bearing mice and showed a 4-log increased cell killing over the additive effect of the two drugs, pointing to synergistic interaction between MLV-VM and CDDP. Similar synergy was observed between MLV-VM and CDDP on human ovarian OVCAR-3 tumors. The combined therapy of liposome-incorporated valinomycin and cisplatin was not highly toxic to the mice and did not show overlapping nephrotoxicity. However, decreases in liver enzymes, particularly alkaline phosphatase and alkaline aminotransferase, were observed with MLV-VM. The combination of MLV-VM with CDDP appeared to be effective in the treatment of ovarian cancer disseminated within the peritoneal cavity.

## CDDP in Thermosensitive Liposomes

The cytotoxic effect of CDDP contained in thermosensitive liposomes combined with hyperthermia was tested in human osteosarcoma cells (OST) (34). Three different culture conditions were used: (1) drug treatment alone; (2) hyperthermia after drug treatment; and (3) simultaneous hyperthermia and drug treatment. The antitumor effects were determined by inhibition of DNA synthesis and decrease in cell growth rates. The greatest antitumor effect was observed with simultaneous hyperthermia and drug treatments. Accumulation of cellular platinum from thermosensitive CDDP-liposomes was markedly increased by hyperthermia.

The antitumor effect of cisplatin-(CDDP)-encapsulated thermosensitive large unilamellar liposome (ThLip) administration with hyperthermia (HT) was also examined in mice bearing Meth A fibrosarcoma (35). The tumor Pt levels after ThLip administration were increased by HT. The antitumor activity of ThLip + HT, as measured by tumor growth delay or tumor weight inhibition, was larger than that of ThLip without HT or a solution with or without HT. Approximately 10 $\mu$m/mouse CDDP dose in ThLip + HT gave equivalent tumor growth delay to 40 $\mu$g/mouse of CDDP + HT; therefore, the targeted drug delivery enhancement ratio was about 4. Thus, it appears that the HT-combined-CDDP liposomal delivery system using ThLip is capable of decreasing the dose required for effective cytotoxicity of CDDP and thereby increasing its therapeutic index.

## ALKALOID-CONTAINING LIPOSOMES

### Vinblastine

Preparations of vinblastine (VLB) encapsulated within multilamellar vesicle-liposomes (MLV) were evaluated for their ability to reverse target cell resistance in multidrug-resistant (MDR) variants (ADR-1 and ADR-10) of UV-2237M murine fibrosarcoma, made resistant by exposure to Adriamycin (36). VLB was encapsulated in MLV composed of phosphatidylcholine (PC) and phosphatidylserine (PS), at 7:3 molar ratio. The 50% inhibitory concentrations (IC50) of VLB for the parent, ADR-1, and ADR-10 cell lines were 2, 25, and 70 ng/mL, respectively; by comparison, VLB in MLV enhanced sensitivity of tumor cells to VLB, with IC50s of liposomal VLB at 0.5, 5.7, and 12 ng/mL. VLB entrapped in PC:PS MLV appeared to overcome tumor cell resistance to this drug.

### Vincristine

Vincristine (VCR) encapsulated in sterically stabilized liposomes (SL-VCR) prolonged the drug's distribution phase plasma half-life in rats from 0.22 to 10.5 h (37). The LD50 for SL-VCR was not different from free VCR, but mice given sublethal doses of SL-VCR showed less weight loss compared to those given free drug. SL-VCR was more effective than free drug against intraperitoneally or subcutaneously implanted tumors. However, the liposomal formulation was not more effective than free drug when the tumor was inoculated by the I.V. route. A single I.V. 2 mg/kg dose of SL-VCR increased the life span of I.P. P388 implanted mice by 199% whereas survival of mice bearing I.V. implanted P388 cells was increased by only 44%. SL-VCR produced long-term survivors in mice implanted S.C. with murine colon carcinoma, but free drug had no significant effect on tumor growth. Thus, liposomal VCR was found to be effective against S.C. or I.P. implanted tumors but not against rapidly growing disseminated leukemias induced by I.V. injection.

The colon cancer line HT-29mdrI expresses a high amount of gp 170, and is sixfold to sevenfold resistant to VCR compared with the parent cell line (38). Liposome-encapsulated VCR lowered drug resistance in HT-29mdrI cells fourfold. The combination of MRK-16 monoclonal antibody and free VCR increased toxicity twofold compared to free VCR in pl70-expressing cells. MRK-16 antibody combined with liposome-encapsulated VCR increased antitumor toxicity 10-fold. Nonspecific monoclonal antibody NR-LU-10 did not potentiate antitumor effect on HT-29mdrI cells with free VCR or liposome-encapsulated VCR. The addition of verapamil increased the cytotoxicity of free VCR 10-fold; when verapamil was combined with liposome-encapsulated VCR, the cytotoxicity increased 15- to 17-fold. Drug accumulation in HT-29mdrI cells was not significantly different when treated with liposome-encapsulated VCR or free VCR. Thus, liposome encapsulation of VCR appeared to be effective in overcoming multidrug resistance in human colon cancer cells.

## Vincristine Combined with Doxorubicin

Vincristine was also combined with doxorubicin encapsulated in sterically stabilized long-circulating liposomes, to determine efficacy against the spontaneous development of mammary carcinomas in C3H/He mice (39). Monthly prophylactic intravenous injections of 6 mg/kg doses of liposome-encapsulated doxorubicin (DOX-SL) or 1 mg/kg doses of liposome-encapsulated vincristine (VIN-SL) were initiated when mice were 26 weeks old. Whereas 99% of untreated mice developed mammary carcinomas, the monthly prophylactic injections reduced the incidence of first mammary carcinomas to 57% in DOX-SL–treated mice and to 81% in VIN-SL–treated mice. Mice that developed a mammary carcinoma while on the monthly prophylactic protocols were then given weekly I.V. injections of 6 mg/kg DOX-SL or 1 mg/kg VIN-SL. Of the mice that developed a mammary tumor while on the prophylactic protocols, 12 of 30 were cured by the weekly therapeutic use of DOX-SL, and 3 of 8 were cured by weekly therapeutic use of VIN-SL. Metastases were found in 29 of 54 untreated mice, but in only 3 of 72 mice treated with DOX-SL and VIN-SL. Toxicity of the liposomal treatments consisted of transient weight loss during the weekly treatments. The prophylactic treatments with liposomal doxorubicin and vinblastine did not appear to induce drug resistance to subsequent therapeutic administration of drug.

## PACLITAXEL

Because paclitaxel has low aqueous solubility, it requires formulation with Cremophor EL (polyethoxylated castor oil) and ethanol, agents that themselves can cause side effects, including serious hypersensitvity reactions (40). To circumvent this problem, liposomes were prepared containing paclitaxel and phospholipid in a 1:33 molar ratio and containing phosphatidylglycerol and phosphatidylcholine in a 1:9 molar ratio. The antitumor effect was evaluated against colon-26, a paclitaxel-resistant murine tumor. Treatment with liposomal paclitaxel resulted in significant tumor growth inhibition at 10–45 mg/kg per injection whereas free paclitaxel in Cremophor EL was ineffective at delaying tumor growth at maximum tolerated doses of 30 mg/kg per injection. Liposomal paclitaxel was also better tolerated at doses greater than or equal to the maximum tolerated dose of free paclitaxel. The liposomal formulation was physically and chemically stable for more than 2 months at 4°C, or for 1 month at 20°C (41).

## ANTIBODY TARGETING

### Immunoliposomes

Immunoliposomes were developed by covalently coupling AF-20 antibody to liposomes containing carboxyfluorescein (42). The monoclonal antibody AF-20 is an anti-hepatocellular carcinoma (HCC) monoclonal antibody that binds with high affinity to a rapidly internalized 180-kD homodimeric glycoprotein present in high amounts on the surface membrane of human HCC and other human cancer cell lines. AF-20–immunoliposomes specifically bound to HCC and other human cancer cell lines expressing the AF-20 antigen and were rapidly internalized at 37°C. AF-20–conjugated liposomes bound to HCC with efficiencies between 5 and 200 times greater than that of unconjugated liposomes or control liposomes bearing a nonrelevant antibody. The antibody conferred specificity to the liposome–target cell binding as demonstrated by competitive inhibition assays. The antibody-liposomal construct appeared to provide efficient and specific targeting of immunoliposomes to human HCC in vitro.

For hyperthermia treatment of cancer, magnetoliposomes were prepared by coating phospholipid onto magnetite particles (43). Optimum dispersibility was observed with phospholipid: phosphatidylcholine/phosphatidylethanolamine ratio of 2:1. The average size of the magnetoliposomes was 80 nm, composed of aggregates of 10 nm core magnetite particles. Hydrazide pullulan was used to stabilize the phospholipid capsules and provide an anchor for immobilization of antibodies. Between 90 and 180 molecules of antibody were immobilized onto each magnetoliposomes particle by this method. Cancer cells adsorbed and incorporated the antibody-conjugated magnetoliposomes 12 times more efficiently than control particles. The effect of heat on the magnetoliposomes was influenced by the size of the core magnetite. In this report, mangetoliposomes appeared to be useful for selective targeting of tumor cells with the combination of drug and hyperthermia.

### Antibodies Linked to PEG

Long-circulating liposomes (S-liposomes) that are sterically stabilized with lipid derivatives of polyethylene glycol (PEG) were coupled with antibodies, for use as chemotherapeutic drug carriers (37). A new end-group functionalized PEG-lipid derivative pyridylthiopropionoylamine-PEG-distearoylphosphatidyl ethanolamine (PDP-PEG-DSPE) was synthesized, and a new method for attaching monoclonal antibodies to the terminus of PEG on S-liposomes has been developed. By incorporating PDP-PEG-

DSPE into S-liposomes and mild thiolysis of the PDP groups, reactive thiol groups were formed at the periphery of the lipid vesicles. Maleimide-derivatized antibodies can then be efficiently attached to the liposomes under mild conditions. The S-immuno-liposomes produced by this method were efficient in drug loading, had slow drug release, and survived in the circulation for longer periods compared to liposomes lacking PEG. The antibodies reactive with tumor-associated antigens increased selective binding of liposomes to the target cells in vitro. Daunorubicin-containing S-immunolipo-somes showed increased cytotoxicity to the target tumor cells, compared with liposomes lacking the targeting antibody.

## LIPIDS AND THERMOSENSITIVE LIPOSOMES

### Omega-3 Fatty Acids

Omega-3 fatty acids are associated with reduced growth and incidence of certain cancers, and in experimental systems, a fish oil diet rich in omega-3 fatty acids enhanced the survival of mice bearing the myeloid leukemia T27A (44). The omega-3 fatty acid docosahexaenoic acid (DHA, 22:6 delta 4,7,10,13,16,19) was postulated to induce structural changes in tumor cell plasma membranes and to reduce tumor growth in vitro. When mice were inoculated intraperitoneally with T27A tumor, there was 100% mortality of tumor-bearing mice in less than 2 weeks. Liposomes with small unilamellar vesicles (liposomes) were prepared, composed of phosphatidylcholine (PC) with 18:0 in the sn-1 position and one of the different types of fatty acids in the sn-2 position: 18:0, 18:1 omega 9 (oleic), 18:3 omega 3 (alpha-linolenic), 20:4 omega 6 (arachidonic), 22:6 omega 3 (docosahexaenoic, DHA). Tumor-bearing mice were injected intraperi-toneally with the liposomes at various times. The DHA-containing liposomes (18:0, 22:6 PC) increased survival of the tumor-bearing mice when compared with 18:0 18:1 PC. Liposomes containing a different omega-3 fatty acid, 18:0, 18:3 PC (linolenic), also increased survival of tumor-bearing mice. The greatest increase in survival was observed when the liposome treatments were given throughout the tumor growth period, or if the tumor inoculum was mixed with the liposome preparation, even when no further liposome treatments were given. In contrast, no benefit was observed when the liposomes contained 18:0, 18:0 PC (oleic) or 18:2, 20:4 PC (arachidonic). DHA and linolenic acid did not seem to act through mechanisms involving lipid peroxidation or inflammatory responses, but were thought to act by changing the membrane structure. Thus, the omega-3 fatty acids, especially DHA-docosahexaenoic acid (18:0, 22:6 PC) and omega 3 alpha-linolenic acid (18:0, 18:3) introduced as components of liposomes, were demonstrated to have antitumor effects in vivo, leading to increased survival of the tumor-bearing mice.

### Thermosensitive Liposomes

For selective antitumor drug targeting, thermosensitive liposomes have been prepared using synthetic lipids such as dipalmitoyl phosphatidylcholine, distearoyl phosphatidyl choline, and cholesterol (Ch) that are capable of releasing drug locally in response to hyperthermia (45). Temperature-sensitive liposomes were prepared using natural lipids, egg phosphatidylcholine (PC):Ch (7:1 molar ratio), and ethanol 6% (v/v). These liposomes have a transition temperature of 43°C, within the temperature range achievable by local hyperthermic treatment of tumors. Using the chemotherapeutic drug decarbazine [5-(3,3'-dimethyl-1-triazino)imidazole-4-carboxamide] entrapped in these liposomes, the efficacy of temperature-sensitive unilamellar vesicles in combination with hyperthermia was demonstrated in murine fibrosarcomas. Advantages of the phosphatidylcholine:cholesterol liposomes are their being biodegradable, nontoxic, and more cost-effective in comparison with liposomes prepared from synthetic lipids for use in multimodality cancer therapy.

## Sphingosines

Inhibitory effects on in vivo growth of human tumor cells in nude mice and on metastasis of B16 melanoma cells in syngeneic mice were observed with N,N,N-trimethylsphingosine (TMS) and N,N-dimethylsphingosine (DMS) but not unsubstituted sphingosine. The tumor inhibition was attributed to inhibition by TMS or DMS of protein kinase C activity and tumor cell–dependent platelet activation (46). The dosages of both TMS and DMS needed to produce significant antitumor or antimetastasis effects were high (multiple injections of 0.1–0.3 mg/mouse), which may result in hemolysis and hemoglobinuria. However, a liposomal formulation of TMS with egg phosphatidylcholine and cholesterol had no hemolytic effect but was more effective than free TMS in suppressing B16 melanoma cell growth and metastasis. Liposomal TMS was accumulated in tumor tissue at higher concentrations than free TMS and had longer circulation half-life. Thus, the liposomal formulation carried the advantages of increased antitumor effect and decreased toxicity compared to the free drug.

## ANTIMETABOLITE-CONTAINING LIPOSOMES

### Fluorouracil

The efficacy of 5-FU encapsulated in liposomes for the treatment of leukemia was evaluated using a murine model of gamma radiation–induced transplantable leukemia in ICRC strain of mice (47). The investigators compared multilamellar vesicles (MLVs) or large unilamellar vesicles (REVs), prepared using phosphatidyl choline and cholesterol in a molar ratio of 8:2 for neutral and 7:2:1 for charged vesicles, administered as a single I.P. dose in mice. The 5-FU encapsulated in MLVs had no effect on leukemic cells when used at concentrations ranging from 0.6 to 2.5 mg/kg, whereas REVs at a single I.P. dose of 9 mg/kg increased survival of leukemic mice with T/C = 138% and reduced infiltration of leukemic cells in different tissues. The effect of REVs was observed to be improved, compared with 60 mg/kg of free 5-FU, which had an LD10 of 70 mg/kg.

### Ara-C Derivatives

N4-alkyl-1-beta-D-arabinofuranosyl cytosines, lipophilic derivatives of 1-beta-D-arabinofuranosylcytosine (ara-C), were synthesized and incorporated into unilamellar liposomes, with diameters ranging between 40 and 70 nm (48). The liposomal derivatives showed increased antitumor effect against the murine L1210 lymphoid leukemia at molar concentrations that were 16 times lower than those for free ara-C. The N4-alkyl-ara-C derivatives with alkyl chains containing 14–16 C-atoms were highly active against L1210 leukemia, whereas those with shorter chains were inactive. The liposomal N4-hexadecyl-ara-C (NHAC) derivatives had increased resistance to hydrolysis and improved antitumor effect compared with other known N4-acyl-ara-C prodrugs.

The pharmacology of liposomal N4-hexadecyl-1-beta-D-arabinofuranosylcytosine (NHAC) was also studied in HL-60 cells (49). Compared with ara-C, NHAC in liposomal formulations was highly resistant to deamination. The cytotoxicity of NHAC was independent of both the nucleoside transporter mechanism and the deoxycytidine (dCyd) kinase activity. In ara-C–resistant HL-60 cells, NHAC was still cytotoxic, with activity at drug concentrations only 1.6 times higher than sensitive cells. Uptake of NHAC was 6 times higher than ara-C and its intracellular half-life is 4.8 times longer than that of ara-C. The activity of NHAC in ara-C–resistant cells was attributed to increased stability, transporter-independent uptake, and dCyd-kinase–independent cytotoxicity.

## TARGETING WITH MEMBRANE PROTEINS

Although increased DHFR enzyme and decreased polyglutamylation were found at high (> 100 ×) methotrexate (MTX) resistance in human squamous carcinoma cell lines, these mechanisms were present in minor degrees at low levels of resistance where the primary mechanism was decreased membrane transport, associated with membrane protein changes (50,51). By radioiodination of membrane proteins and $^{35}$S-methionine metabolic labeling of cellular proteins, many proteins decreased or increased with development of MTX resistance, but only a few were altered consistently. Of these, only three proteins (46 kD, 57 kD, and 30 kD) were found to revert back to the parental pattern when reversion to drug sensitivity occurred. The 46-kD, pI 7.0 protein (SQM1) was the most prominent change in the membrane (50,51). Using antibody and cDNA probes for SQM1, decreased SQM1 expression was found to be associated with drug resistance whereas increased SQM1 expression was associated with reversion to drug sensitivity.

Using the cDNA construct coding for SQM1 (52), SQM1 protein was produced in bacteria and was purified. The SQM1 protein was incorporated into liposomes containing MTX. When the liposome preparations were incubated with various cell lines, there was preferential binding to carcinoma cell lines compared with normal human fibroblasts and lymphocytes. After adhesion of SQM1-liposomes to the MTX-resistant cell lines (SCC15R), the MTX uptake increased to rates that were similar to those of the sensitive cell lines (SCC15S). The SQM1-liposomes also reversed the drug resistance of the carcinoma cell lines to levels similar to those of the drug-sensitive parent cell lines. Interestingly, the SQM1-MTX-liposomes increased MTX transport and cell killing of SCC15 cell lines that were resistant because of increased DHFR, as well as those with low MTX transport. Thus, the use of a membrane protein with dual functions—promoting cell adhesion and stimulating drug transport—increased the antitumor toxicity and selectivity of liposomal drug in vitro. Similar strategies are being employed for in vivo studies.

## CONCLUSION

In recent years, the technology for selective delivery of chemotherapeutic drugs using liposomes has advanced rapidly. Improvements in liposomal composition have led to prolonged circulation times and increased permeability to the microvasculature of tumors. The result has been to decrease the toxic effects of chemotherapeutic drugs on normal organs while increasing delivery of drug and toxicity to tumors. Furthermore, the addition of targeting proteins to the liposome may preferentially increase adhesion to tumor cells and increase membrane transport of liposome-encapsulated drugs.

## REFERENCES

1. Szoka FC. Liposomal drug delivery: current status and future prospects. In: Wilshut J, Hoekstra D, eds. Membrane Fusion. New York: Marcel Dekker, Inc., 1991:845–890.
2. Booser DH, Hortobagyi GN. Anthracycline antibiotics in cancer therapy. Focus on drug resistance. Drugs 1994; 47(2):223–258.
3. Woodle MC, Lasic DD. Sterically stabilized liposomes. Biochim Biophys Acta 1992; 113: 171–199.
4. Rahman A, Husain SR, Siddiqui J, Verma M, Agresti M, Center M, Safa AR, Glazer RI. Liposome-mediated modulation of multidrug resistance in human HL-60 leukemia cells. J Natl Cancer Inst 1992; 84(24):1909–1915.
5. Thierry AR, Vige D, Coughlin SS, Belli JA, Dritschilo A, Rahman A. Modulation of doxorubicin resistance in multidrug-resistant cells by liposomes. FASEB J 1993; 7(6):572–579.
6. Leibovici J, Klein O, Wollman Y, Donin N, Mahlin T, Shinitzky M. Cell membrane fluidity and Adriamycin retention in a tumor progression model of AKR lymphoma. Biochim Biophys Acta 1996; 1281(2):182–188.
7. Thierry AR, Rahman A, Dritschilo A. A new procedure for the preparation of liposomal doxorubicin: biological activity in multidrug-resistant tumor cells. Cancer Chemother Pharmacol 1994; 35(1):84–88.
8. Lee RJ, Low PS. Folate-mediated tumor cell targeting of liposome-entrapped doxorubicin in vitro. Biochim Biophys Acta 1995; 1233(2):134–144.
9. Akaishi S, Kobari M, Takeda K, Matsuno S. Targeting chemotherapy using antibody-combined liposome against human pancreatic cancer cell-line. Tohoku J Exp Med 1995; 175(1): 29–42.
10. Gabizon AA. Selective tumor localization and improved therapeutic index of anthracyclines encapsulated in long-circulating liposomes. Cancer Res 1992; 52(4):891–896.
11. Codee JP, Lumsden AJ, Napoli S, Burton MA, Gray BN. A comparative study of the anticancer efficacy of doxorubicin carrying microspheres and liposomes using a rat liver tumour model. Anticancer Res 1993; 13(2):539–543.
12. Beck P, Kreuter J, Reszka R, Fichtner I. Influence of polybutylcyanoacrylate nanoparticles and liposomes on the efficacy and toxicity of the anticancer drug mitoxantrone in murine tumour models. J Microencapsul 1993; 10(1):101–114.
13. Guaglianone P, Chan K, DelaFlor-Weiss E, Hanisch R, Jeffers S, Sharma D, Muggia F. Phase I and pharmacologic study of liposomal daunorubicin (DaunoXome). Invest New Drugs 1994; 12(2):103–110.
14. Gabizon A, Catane R, Uziely B, Kaufman B, Safra T, Cohen R, Martin F, Huang A, Barenholz Y. Prolonged circulation time and enhanced accumulation in malignant exudates of doxorubicin encapsulated in polyethylene-glycol coated liposomes. Cancer Res 1994; 54: 987–992.
15. Konno H, Marno Y, Matsuda I, Nakamura S, Baba S. Intra-arterial liposomal Adriamycin for metastatic adenocarcinoma of the liver. Eur Surg Res 1995; 27(5):301–306.

16. Genne P, Olsson NO, Gutierrez G, Duchamp O, Chauffert B. Liposomal mitoxantrone for the local treatment of peritoneal carcinomatosis induced by colon cancer cells. Anticancer Drug Des 1994; (2):73–84.

17. Akamo Y, Mizuno I, Yotsuyanagi T, Ichino T, Tanimoto N, Yamamoto T, Nagata M, Takeyama H, Shinagawa N, Yura J, et al. Chemotherapy targeting regional lymph nodes by gastric submucosal injectiion of Illl Adriamycin in patients with gastric carcinoma. Jpn J Cancer Res 1994; 85(6):652–658.

18. James ND, Coker RJ, Tomlinson D, Harris JR, Gompels M, Pinching AJ, Stewart JS. Liposomal doxorubicin (Doxil): an effective new treatment for Kaposi's sarcoma in AIDS. Clin Oncol (R Coll Radiol) 1994; 6(5):294–296.

19. Goebel FD, Goldstein D, Goos M, Jablonowski H, Stewart JS. Efficacy and safety of Stealth liposomal doxorubicin in AIDS-related Kaposi's sarcoma. The International SL-DOX Study Group. 1996. Br J Cancer 1996; 73(8):989–994.

20. Gondal JA, Preuss HG, Swartz R, Rahman A. Comparative pharmacological, toxicological and antitumoral evaluation of free and liposome-encapsulated cisplatin in rodents. Eur J Cancer 1993; 29A(11):1536–1542.

21. Khokhar AR, al-Baker S, Brown T, Perez-Soler R. Chemical and biological studies on a series of lipid-soluble (trans-(R,R)- and -(S,S)-1,2-diaminocyclohexane)platinum(II) complexes incorporated in liposomes. J Med Chem 1991; 34(1):325–329.

22. Perez-Soler R, Khokhar AR. Lipophilic cisplatin analogues entrapped in liposomes: role of intraliposomal drug activation in biological activity. Cancer Res 1992; 52(22):6341–6347.

23. Han I, Ling YH, al-Baker S, Khokhar AR, Perez-Soler R. Cellular pharmacology of liposomal cis-bis-neodecanoato-trans-R,R-1,2-diamonocyclohexaneplatinum(II) in A2780/S and A2780/PDD cells. Cancer Res 1993; 53(20):4913–4919.

24. Han I, Ling YH, Khokhar AR, Perez-Soler R. Cell death and DNA fragmentation induced by liposomal platinum(II) complex, L-NDDP in A2780 and A2780/PDD cells. Anticancer Res 1994; 14(2A):421–426.

25. Han I, Hguyen T, Yang LY, Khokhar AR, Perez-Soler R. Cellular accumulation and DNA damage induced by liposomal cis-bis-neodecanoato-trans-R,R-1,2-diaminocyclohexane-platinum+ + +(II) in LoVo and LoVo/PDD cells. Anticancer Drugs 1994; 5(1):64–68.

26. Khokhar AR, al-Baker S, Perez-Soler R. Toxicity and efficacy studies on a series of lipid-soluble dineodecanoato(trans-R,R- and trans-S,S-1,2-diaminocyclohexane) platinum (II) complexes entrapped in liposomes. Anticancer Drugs 1992; 3(2):95–100.

27. Vadiei K, Siddik ZH, Khokhar AR, al-Baker S, Sampedro F, Perez-Soler R. Pharmacokinetics of liposome-entrapped cis-bis-neodecanoato-trans-R,R-1,2-diaminocyclohexane platinum(II) and cisplatin given i.v. and i.p. in the rat. Cancer Chemother Pharmacol 1992; 30(5):365–369.

28. Perez-Soler R, Francis K, al-Baker S, Pilkiewicz F, Kohokhar AR. Preparation and characterization of liposomes containing a lipophilic cisplatin derivative for clinical use. J Microencapsul 1994; 11(1):41–54.

29. Garelli N, Vierling P. Incorporation of new amphiphilic perfluoroalkylated bipyridine platinum and palladium complexes into liposomes: stability and structure-incorporation relationshiips. Biochim Biophys Acta 1992; 1127(1):41–48.

30. Fichtner I, Reszka R, Schutt M, Rudolph M, Becker M, Lemm M, Richter J, Berger I. Carboplatin-liposomes as activators of hematopoiesis. Oncol Res 1993; 5(2):65–74.

31. Yasui T, Mizuno I, Ichino T, Akamo Y, Yamamoto T, Itabashi Y, Saito T, Kurahashi S, Tanimoto N, Yura J, et al. Antitumor effect of liposome-entrapped carboplatin after intraperitoneal administration in rats. Gan To Kagaku Ryoho 1992; 19(10 Suppl):1753–1755.

32. Daoud SS, Sakata MK. In vitro interaction of liposomal valinomycin and platinum analogs: cytotoxic and cytokinetic effects. Anticancer Drugs 1993; 4(4):479–486.

33. Daoud SS. Combination chemotherapy of human ovarian xenografts with intraperitoneal liposome-incorporated valinomycin and cis-diamminedichloroplatinum(II). Cancer Chemother Pharmacol 1994; 33(4):307–312.

34. Hattori M, Matsui N, Ohta H, Otsuka T, Yamada K, Assai K, Kato T. Antitumor effect of thermosensitive CDDP-liposomes on human osteosarcoma cells in culture. Nippon Seikeigeka Gakkai Zasshi 1992; 66(5):476–484.

35. Iga K, Hamaguchi N, Igari Y, Ogawa Y, Gotoh K, Ootsu K, Toguchi H, Shimamoto T. Enhanced antitumor activity in mice after administration of thermosensitive liposome encapsulating cisplatin with hyperthermia. J Pharmacol Exp Ther 1991; 257(3):1203–1207.

36. Seid CA, Fidler IJ, Clyne RK, Earnest LE, Fan D. Overcoming murine tumor cell resistance to vinblastine by presentation of the drug in multilamellar liposomes consisting of phosphatidylcholine and phosphatidylserine. Sel Cancer Ther 1991; 7(3):103–112.

37. Allen TM, Brandeis E, Hansen CB, Kao GY, Zalipsky S. A new strategy for attachment of antibodies to sterically stabilized liposomes resulting in efficient targeting to cancer cells. Biochim Biophys Acta 1995; 1237(2):99–108.

38. Sela S, Husain SR, Pearson JW, Longo DL, Rahman A. Reversal of multidrug resistance in human colon cancer cells expressing the human MDR1 gene by liposomes in combination with monoclonal antibody or verapamil. J Natl Cancer Inst 1995; 87(2):123–128.

39. Vaage J, Donovan D, Loftus T, Uster P, Working P. Prophylaxis and therapy of mouse mammary carcinomas with doxorubicin and vincristine encapsulated in sterically stabilized liposomes. Eur J Cancer 1995; 31A(3):367–372.

40. Sharma A, Mayhew E, Straubinger RM. Antitumor effect of Taxol-containing liposomes in a Taxol-resistant murine tumor model. Cancer Res 1993; 53(24):5877–5881.

41. Sharma A, Straubinger RM. Novel Taxol formulations: preparation and characterization of taxol-containing liposomes. Pharm Res 1994; 11(6):889–896.

42. Moradpour D, Compagnon B, Wilson BE, Nicolau C, Wands JR. Specific targeting of human hepatocellular carcinoma cells by immunoliposomes in vitro. Hepatology 1995; 22(5):1527–1537.

43. Shinkai M, Suzuki M, Iijima S, Kobayashi T. Antibody-conjugated magnetoliposomes for targeting cancer cells and their application in hyperthermia. Biotechnol Appl Biochem 1995; 21(Pt 2):125–137.

44. Jenski LJ, Zerouga M, Stillwell W. Omega-3 fatty acid-containing liposomes in cancer therapy. Proc Soc Exp Biol Med 1995; 210(3):227–233.

45. Chelvi TP, Ralhan R. Designing of thermosensitive liposomes from natural lipids for multimodality cancer therapy. Int J Hyperthermia 1995; 11(5):685–695.

46. Park YS, Hakomori S, Kawa S, Ruan F, Igarashi Y. Liposomal N,N,N-trimethylsphingosine (TMS) as an inhibitor of B 16 melanoma cell growth and metastasis with reduced toxicity and enhanced drug efficacy compared to free TMS: cell membrane signaling as a target in cancer therapy III. Cancer Res 1994; 54(8):2213–2217.

47. Joshi SV, Vaidya SG, Nerurkar VR, Soman C. Treatment of gamma radiation-induced transplanted leukemia in ICRC mice by liposomally encapsulated 5-fluorouracil. Leuk Res 1993; 17(7):601–607.

48. Schwendener RA, Schott H. Treatment of L1210 murine leukemia with liposome-incorporated N4-hexacecyl-1-beta-D-arabinofuranosyl cytosine. Int J Cancer 1992; 51(3):466–469.

49. Horber DH, Schott H, Schwendener RA. Cellular pharmacology of a liposomal preparation of N4-hexadecyl-1-beta-D-arabinofuranosylcytosine, a lipophilic derivative of 1-beta-D-arabinofuranosylcytosine. Br J Cancer 1995; 71(5):957–962.

50. Bernal SD, Speak JA, Boeheim K, Dreyfuss AI, Wright JE, Teicher BA, Rosowsky A, Tsao SW, Wong Y-C. Reduced membrane protein associated with resistance of human

squamous carcinoma cells to methotrexate and cis-platinum. Mol Cell Biochem 1990; 95: 61–70.

51. Bernal SD, DeVilla RS, Wong Y-C. Congruence of SQM1 protein expression with methotrexate sensitivity and transport. Cancer Invest 1995; 12(1):23–30.

52. Wong Y-C, Tsao SW, Kakefuda M, Bernal SD. cDNA cloning of a novel cell adhesion protein expressed in human squamous carcinoma cells. Biochem Biophys Res Commun 1990; 166:984–992.

# 5

## Tamoxifen Resistance and Breast Cancer

**Lin Soe and Michael W. DeGregorio**
*University of California, Davis, California*

### INTRODUCTION

Tamoxifen is a nonsteroidal antiestrogen that was first developed as an oral contraceptive. Although this use was found to be ineffective, it was postulated that an antiestrogen might have an anticancer effect on hormone-dependent malignancies such as breast cancer. The first evidence of tamoxifen's effectiveness in the treatment of breast cancer, presented by Cole et al. in 1971 (1), stimulated numerous preclinical and clinical studies. Mouridsen et al. published the first comprehensive clinical trial in 1978 (2), and tamoxifen has since become the most commonly used hormonal therapy for breast cancer.

A meta-analysis that evaluated the clinical benefits of systemic therapy was presented by the Early Breast Cancer Trialists Collaborative Group, and data from 30,000 women treated with tamoxifen were included (3). Of those women treated with tamoxifen, 51.2% survived disease-free for at least 10 years, compared to 44.7% in the control group. The difference between the two groups was established at 6.6%. Mortality rates of the two groups at 10 years were 58.5% and 52.0%, respectively, with a net difference of 6.2%. Therefore, six of 100 patients treated with tamoxifen will have a survival benefit from tamoxifen versus no therapy.

In patients with or without positive axillary nodes, tamoxifen was beneficial. The disease-free survival and overall survival for the node-positive group were 8.8% and 5.1%, respectively. In the node-negative patients, absolute risk reduction of the disease-free survival and overall survival were 8.2% and 3.5%, respectively. Age also played a role in tumor recurrence among women taking tamoxifen. The reduction in animal odds of recurrence was 12% for women under 50 years of age; this figure rose to 29% for women above the age of 50.

The levels of progesterone and estrogen receptors have a direct relationship to clinical response to tamoxifen therapy. The response rate to tamoxifen therapy among estrogen receptor–positive (ER+) breast cancer patients is approximately 50%, whereas only 5% response rates are seen in estrogen receptor–negative (ER–) breast cancer patients (2). Little or no benefit from treatment with tamoxifen was reported when ER or progesterone receptor (PR) levels were less than 10 fmol per gram of protein (4). A 7% absolute risk difference in 5-year disease-free survival is seen when PR levels are

10 fmol or more per gram of protein, whereas a 5% difference is noted in 5-year disease-free survival when ER levels are 10 fmol or more per gram of protein.

The importance of estrogen receptor levels was also evaluated by the Scottish Breast Cancer Trials Committee (5). In their study, the greatest benefit related to tamoxifen was seen in patients with ER levels of more than 100 fmol/g protein, where the benefit improved from 11% to 25% over 5 years when compared to results from patients with ER levels less than 99 fmol/g protein. A linear increase in the disease-free survival was correlated to ER levels.

Further evidence of the importance of ER levels was presented by the Danish Breast Cancer Cooperative Group (6). In the Danish study, postmenopausal women with ER levels of 100 fmol or more per gram of protein were the only group who benefited from tamoxifen therapy. These findings support the theory that the major cytostatic anticancer activity of tamoxifen occurs through an antiestrogenic mechanism by binding competitively at the estrogen receptor.

Despite the early detection of breast cancer and effective local treatment, distant recurrence has been difficult to control through systemic therapies such as hormonal therapy and chemotherapy. The main reasons for treatment failures have been either innate drug resistance or the development of acquired drug resistance. In the case of tamoxifen resistance, both of these types are commonly encountered in patients with breast cancer. We will devote the remainder of the chapter to a discussion on the possible mechanisms responsible for innate and acquired tamoxifen resistance.

## TAMOXIFEN RESISTANCE

Tamoxifen resistance is a major clinical problem in the treatment of breast cancer. In general, there are two types of tamoxifen resistance—innate and acquired resistance. Innate resistance is seen in 50% of ER-positive patients with metastatic disease. Acquired tamoxifen resistance is typically seen in the majority of patients with metastatic disease who have previously responded to tamoxifen. Notably, in a subset of patients who develop acquired tamoxifen resistance, there is clinical evidence that tamoxifen even stimulates tumor growth.

## CLINICAL ASPECTS OF TAMOXIFEN RESISTANCE

The development of tamoxifen resistance is more clearly seen in metastatic disease, when some patients who respond to tamoxifen eventually develop a response failure. In the data from a collaborative group study in which tamoxifen was used as adjuvant therapy after resectable breast cancers or local disease, approximately 60% of node-positive patients and 30% of node-negative patients experienced a relapse after 10 years of follow-up (3). In metastatic disease, the median duration of response to tamoxifen varied from 5.8 to 20 months in different studies (7). In one study of premenopausal women, the response to tamoxifen was higher among those who developed menopausal symptoms during therapy, such as hot flashes, altered menstruation, or amenorrhea (8). However, this finding has not been supported by other investigators (9). In the same study, women who first responded to tamoxifen—only to have the disease progress later—responded favorably to ovarian ablation, a second line of hormonal therapy.

In a collective series of phase II trials, the response rate to oophorectomy was 40% after resistance to tamoxifen developed. In contrast, the response rate to an oophorectomy was 13% in patients who initially failed to respond to tamoxifen. Interestingly, a positive response to second-line hormonal therapy, such as an oophorectomy, is more dependent on a good initial response to tamoxifen than estrogen receptor status (10,11).

In some patients who experienced disease progression while taking tamoxifen, withdrawal of treatment produced a regression of the disease. In one report, five patients out of 28 who initially responded to tamoxifen and later developed disease progression showed withdrawal responses following discontinuation of tamoxifen therapy (12). Patients who never responded to tamoxifen did not show any signs of a withdrawal response. Tamoxifen withdrawal effects were also reported in a larger group of patients treated with tamoxifen (13). Of 87 patients whose disease progressed on tamoxifen, 23% responded to withdrawal, but none of those without an initial response had any changes on withdrawal of tamoxifen therapy. The difference in the incidence of positive tamoxifen withdrawal effect is probably due to the different length of follow-up after discontinuation of tamoxifen treatment. Because tamoxifen has a long half-life, it was necessary to observe patients for 6 weeks to allow the body to eliminate the drug and its metabolites. Therefore, attention to duration after cessation of therapy was needed when interpreting the presence of a withdrawal response.

## MECHANISMS OF TAMOXIFEN ACTION AND RESISTANCE

Tamoxifen is thought to exert its antitumor effects through the estrogen receptor. The estrogen receptor contains discrete domains involved in hormone binding, DNA binding, and subsequent activation of estrogen-responsive genes. Estrogen receptors are known to have five distinctive functional domains, A/B, C, D, E, and F, which are encoded by eight exons with some overlap between these regions (14). Regions D and E appear to primarily involve hormone (ligand) binding and dimerization. Domain C (DNA-binding domain, DBD) confers a DNA-binding function; domains A/B and E contain two transcription-activating functions. When estrogen binds to the hormone-binding domain (HBD) of estrogen receptors, the receptors dissociate from a heat-labile complex, dimerize, and bind to estrogen-responsive elements (EREs) to stimulate transcription (15) (Fig. 1). Two transcriptional activation functions in the estrogen receptor contribute to this process—AF-1 and AF-2. AF-1 in the amino-terminal domain of the receptor is hormone independent, and AF-2 in the C-terminal domain functions only when an agonist is bound (16).

Tamoxifen competitively binds to estrogen receptors. This inhibits AF-2 activity and prevents transcription, although it does not block estrogen receptor binding to EREs (17). In vitro, tamoxifen was shown to inhibit the incorporation of tritiated thymidine, suppress DNA polymerase activity, and reduce both total DNA content and the total cell number when exposed to a ER+ human breast cancer cell line (MCF-7) (18,19). The cystostatic effects of tamoxifen were reflected in $G_0/G_1$ block and reduced S phase (20). The in vitro effects of tamoxifen in ER+ cells were prevented or reversed by the addition of estradiol (21).

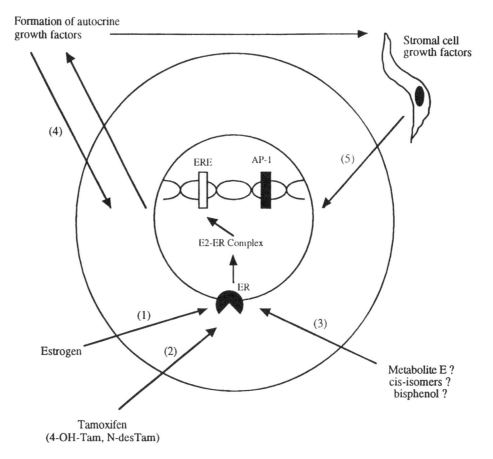

**Figure 1** (1) Estrogen binds to ER and estrogen-ER complex (E2-ER) activates ERE site promoter gene. (2) 4-OH-Tam and N-des-Tam bind to ER, preventing estrogen binding and blocking formation of E2-ER complex. (3) Metabolite E, bisphenol, and *cis*-isomers, mixed estrogenic and antiestrogenic metabolites of estrogen, may bind to ER to form a complex and activate ERE site with increased transcription. (4) Autocrine growth factors stimulate signal transduction and cell growth. (5) Stromal cells, stimulated by growth factors, produce more growth factors that stimulate epithelial cancer cells as paracrine growth factor.

In addition to its antiestrogenic action, tamoxifen also has partial estrogen-agonist effects on uterine tissues. Its weak estrogenic action has been noted in post-menopausal women, in whom it causes changes in gonadotropin levels, plasma protein levels, and vaginal epithelium (22–24).

Interestingly, about 5% of women with ER–, advanced breast cancer appear to have a tumor response to tamoxifen but unfortunately it does not prolong the survival (1). Tamoxifen has also shown a dose-dependent inhibitory action in hormone-independent cell cultures (18). These inhibitory effects of tamoxifen at high concentrations are not reversed by estrogen administration, and, therefore, two spectra of mechanisms related to the effects of tamoxifen on breast cancer cells are believed to be estrogen-reversible and estrogen-irreversible effects (25).

In support of these hormone-independent actions, Reddel et al. suggested that dual mechanisms of tamoxifen may exist (26). In their study, MCF-7 cells were treated with tamoxifen and ICI-145680, an analogue with the identical affinity for estrogen receptors as tamoxifen but without affinity for specific, high-affinity, antiestrogen binding sites (AEBS). The effect of ICI-145680 was significantly less potent than tamoxifen.

## Heterogeneity of Tumor Cells and Tamoxifen Resistance

A breast tumor may consist of a heterogeneous mixture of tumor cells with respect to hormone dependence and independence. Endocrine therapy might only reduce the bulk of hormone-sensitive cells, while it permits rapid growth of the hormone-independent tumor cells. It is possible that cellular heterogeneity leads to the lack of uniformity in response to tamoxifen. Estrogen binding is rarely observed in all cells in a tumor specimen. In one study, 25% of the tumors had no cells with positive, indirect immunofluorescence, while 5% of the tumors were characterized by estrogen binding of all cells (27). The remaining 71% of the tumors had varying numbers of cells with evidence of estradiol binding. Moreover, a study showed the heterogeneity of PR and DNA ploidy in breast cancer cells, suggesting the existence of a mixed subpopulation of breast cancer cells remodeling the phenotype of the tumor while under the influence of tamoxifen (28). Rather than being resistant, different subsets of cells can be inhibited or stimulated by tamoxifen. The speed of emergence of hormone-independent cells also suggests that growth is more likely to be the result of a phenotype modulation rather than the selection of chance mutation (29). Theoretically, this phenotype modulation should develop with the emergence of predominantly ER– and PR– cells. In actuality, phenotype modulation may also be caused by the emergence of cells with mutated estrogen receptors. Therefore, mere demonstrations of the presence of estrogen receptors in these cells alone should not necessarily be used as evidence against this hypothesis. However, this phenomenon cannot explain the underlying mechanism of a significant response to ovarian ablation after the development of tumor resistance to tamoxifen if surviving clones are supposed to be hormone-independent. Clinical studies also suggest that resistance to tamoxifen is not always caused by a selection of hormone-independent and/or ER– clones of tumor cells. Sequential biopsy studies have shown that the early apparent loss of estrogen receptors was common when the second biopsy was performed while the patient was taking tamoxifen or within 2 months of cessation of treatment. Presumably, this is because of receptor occupancy by drugs causing false-negative ligand-binding assay results (30). When the biopsy was performed more than 2 months after cessation of therapy, the tumors frequently remained ER+.

## Estrogenic Action of Tamoxifen and Its Metabolites and the Development of Resistance

Clinical findings have revealed that approximately 40% of the achievable responses with second-line hormonal therapy such as ovarian ablation, which occurred after resistance to tamoxifen or evidence of tamoxifen withdrawal effects, reflect the stimulatory effect of tamoxifen. Stimulated growth of ER+ cell lines has also been described (31,32). In animal models, long-term treatment with tamoxifen in athymic mice eventually resulted in the growth of MCF-7, ER+ breast tumors (33,34). When these tumors were transplanted to other mice, they grew only in the presence of tamoxifen (35).

Interestingly, the growth of these tamoxifen-stimulated tumors could be partially inhibited with pure antiestrogens (36). These findings support the existence of a tamoxifen-specific stimulatory effect.

Tamoxifen is known to possess estrogenic as well as antiestrogenic properties on different tissues of different species of animals. For example, tamoxifen acts as an estrogen in the mouse, a partial agonist in the rat, and a complete antagonist in the chick (37). It also displays estrogenlike activity in dog and human endometrium, causing a thickening of this tissue. An explanation of this phenomenon is the possibility that tamoxifen is metabolized differently in different species and in different tissues, and it may be locally metabolized into potent estrogenic metabolites by tumor cells and stromal cells in cases of tamoxifen resistance or tamoxifen-stimulated growth. *Trans*-tamoxifen undergoes liver metabolism to *N*-desmethyltamoxifen and 4-hydroxytamoxifen, both of which have antiestrogenic properties. *N*-desmethyltamoxifen is the major metabolite found in human serum, and it is further metabolized into metabolite Z (di-desmethyltamoxifen) and metabolite Y, the side-chain alcohol (38,39) (Fig. 2). Besides these four metabolites, at least two estrogenic metabolites of tamoxifen have also been identified: metabolite E (without a di-methylaminoethane side chain) and bisphenol (40). Although this hypothesis is plausible, metabolite E has only a weak potency as an estrogen and a low affinity for estrogen receptors in vivo (39–41). Therefore, large amounts of metabolite E should be detected. However, no significant changes in tamoxifen and its metabolites in the blood of patients treated with tamoxifen have been noted (42). This may be because changes in metabolism may occur inside the cells and, accordingly, changes in the profile of metabolites would not be evident in the blood. In support of this theory, an altered metabolism of tamoxifen, reduced tamoxifen concentrations, and increased ratios of estrogenic *cis*-4-hydroxytamoxifen compared to antiestrogenic *trans*-4-hydroxytamoxifen were evident in tamoxifen-stimulated growth (43). This is in contrast to responding patients who had a high total tumor tamoxifen level and low ratios of *cis*- and *trans*-4-hydroxytamoxifen. A similar metabolite profile has also been described in extracts from a panel of breast cancer tumors from patients with acquired resistance (44). An estrogenic tamoxifen metabolite, E, was again identified in tumors isolated from five patients who underwent an unsuccessful short period of tamoxifen therapy. Metabolite E was identified in both de novo resistant and acquired resistant tumors. Evidence of the presence of the other estrogenic metabolite, bisphenol, was also observed in these tumors, but it could not be confirmed by mass-spectrometry techniques (45). The ability of the pure antiestrogen ICI 164,384 to inhibit tamoxifen-stimulated growth of MCF-7 tumors (32) and also the ability of ICI 182,780 to inhibit tamoxifen-stimulated growth (46) add more strength to this hypothesis. However, fixed-ring nonisomerizable analogues, or other analogues that are resistant to conversion into metabolite E, fail to prevent tamoxifen-stimulated growth. Stimulated growth was still seen without available metabolite E in culture, which raises concerns about additional mechanism(s) related to tamoxifen resistance.

## Hormonal Adaptation

Tamoxifen competitively inhibits the action of estrogen by binding at estrogen receptors, while a rise in the estrogen level reverses the effects of antiestrogens. Resistance to aminoglutethamide therapy has been associated with an elevation of circulating estrogen at the time of relapse (47). Beyond that, premenopausal women are less likely

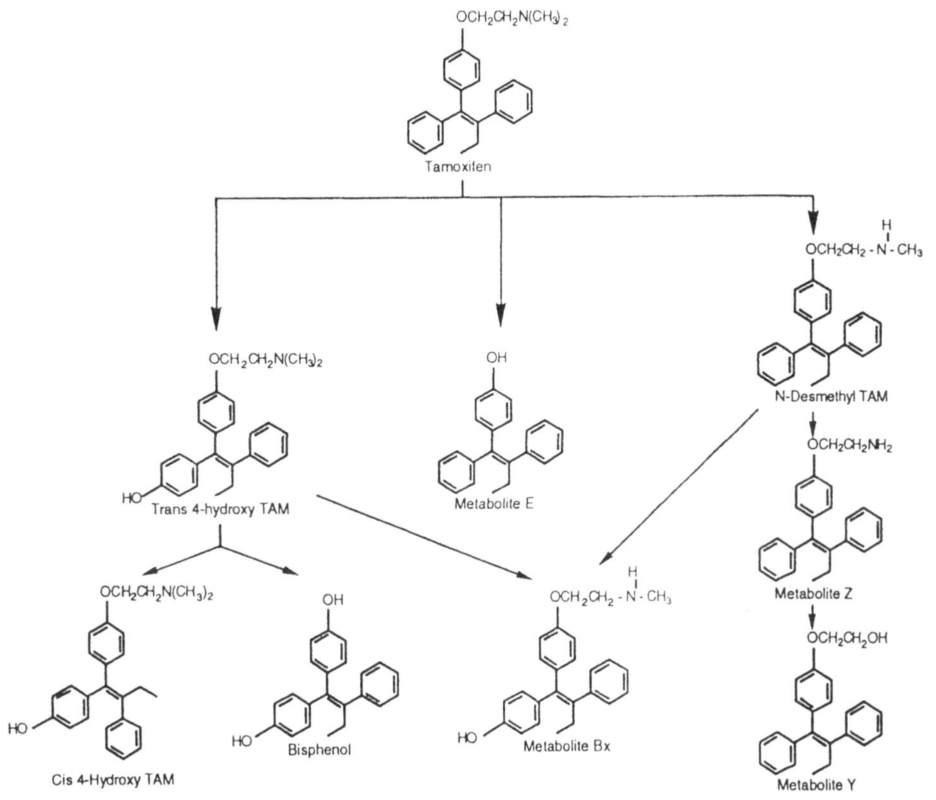

**Figure 2** Chemical structure of tamoxifen and its metabolites.

to respond to tamoxifen, in part because the majority of breast tumors in premenopausal women are ER–. Tamoxifen is also known to raise the circulating levels of estrogen and progesterone significantly above the normal level in premenopausal women who are being treated for breast cancer (48,49). This necessitates a higher concentration of tamoxifen to suppress growth. The success of second-line hormonal therapy may be explained by this mechanism. Ovarian ablation may produce a response in tumor resistance to tamoxifen by removing the adaptive rise in estrogen as a response to tamoxifen therapy. However, the elevated levels of estrogen are not always found to be associated with tamoxifen resistance (50).

## Altered Estrogen Receptor Levels

The binding of tamoxifen to estrogen receptors causes cells to be deprived of estrogen. This deprivation may trigger a feedback mechanism that causes an increase in the synthesis of estrogen receptors in an attempt to form a complex to meet the demand of the cells. This mechanism will result in a failure of tamoxifen to effectively prevent estrogen from binding to estrogen receptors. Up-regulation of estrogen receptor levels was first described in cell lines after exposure to tamoxifen (51), and it was later

noted in 10 postmenopausal patients with ER+ and PR+ diseases who were treated
with tamoxifen. Two fine-needle aspiration biopsies were performed before treatment
and 8 days after initial tamoxifen therapy. The results were compared with those from
a control group that was not treated with tamoxifen. Although no significant changes
in the ER and PR levels were seen in the control group, a significant change developed
in the receptor levels of the treatment group. Both ER and PR levels doubled after
tamoxifen treatment when studied with an enzyme immunoassay (52). Although no
attempt was made in that study to correlate the association between up-regulation of
receptors and estrogen resistance, an in vitro study used an EFM-19 estrogen-sensitive
human breast cancer cell line to show stimulated growth with long-term tamoxifen
treatment in relation to increased estrogen receptor level. This growth was associated
with a 50% increase in the receptor concentration over an untreated parallel cell line
(53).

Resistance to antiestrogens may also be the result of a loss of estrogen receptors.
Mechanisms of methylation, gene mutation, and defective transcription have been postulated. In an earlier study of patients responding to endocrine therapy, mean levels of
estrogen receptors fell from 260 fmol/g to 12 fmol/g (54). A similar observation was
also made of nonresponders: mean levels fell from 155 fmol/g to 32 fmol/g. However,
the study used a dextran-coated charcoal technique, and tamoxifen may have interfered
with the assay, generating falsely low receptor levels (55). In another study of tumors
from patients with tamoxifen resistance, an immunohistochemical technique was used
to detect both bound and free receptors. Estrogen receptors were found in 7 of 13
tumors examined (56). Actually, it is not uncommon that breast tumors in patients with
acquired resistance remain receptor-positive. In vitro studies suggest that after a selection of antiestrogen-resistant cells, many resistant cell lines may remain sensitive to
estrogen, suggesting that these cells still contain estrogen receptors (57,58).

## Variant Forms of Estrogen Receptors

As discussed earlier, maintenance of estrogen receptors in hormone-independent and
hormone-stimulated tumors is well evident both in vitro and in vivo. However, the tests
used to detect the presence of receptors cannot differentiate between wild-type receptors and variant or mutated forms. These variant forms of the receptor may be responsible for hormone-independent growth or tamoxifen resistance in those tumors that
are ER+. Protein structure modifications may also lead to altered affinity of estrogen
receptors for tamoxifen. Site-specific mutations in the gene coding for estrogen receptors may potentially result in various types of functionally abnormal receptors, and
these mutations may render the estrogen receptors entirely nonfunctional or transcrip-
tionally inactive despite maintaining their ability to bind estrogen with a high affinity.
Thus, the tumor would appear clinically as though it were ER−. Alternatively, mutation
may result in transcription in important domains of the receptor, causing a generation
of ER forms that are functionally active but exhibit altered affinities for estrogens and
antiestrogens. Coexpressions of variant estrogen receptors and wild-type estrogen receptors have been shown to be dependent on the level of expression of each type and
may influence the nature of hormone dependence and independence (59).

Early studies failed to demonstrate the presence of variant forms of estrogen
receptors, but several different ER mutations were detected in a later study of com-

plementary DNA prepared from T47D cells by cloning and sequence analysis. This included frame-shift mutations within DNA and the hormone-binding domains of the receptors (60). With immunohistochemical procedures, the presence of estrogen receptors deficient in nuclear binding of ER+ tumors was also described (61). Another remarkable finding related to mutant estrogen receptors was that the lack of a hormone-binding domain could constitutively activate transcription, even in the absence of hormones (62). Patients with constitutive nuclear binding (those with estrogen receptors that can bind nuclei) were refractory to hormone therapy. These results suggest that resistant tumors may contain defective estrogen receptors. This hypothesis has been further substantiated by studies using larger series of human breast tumor specimens. Even though endocrine response data were not available from these later studies, they suggest that truncated forms of estrogen receptors that fail to bind in gel-retardation assays may be present in tumors. The coexpression of deleted exon 5 variant and wild-type estrogen receptors was described in hormone-dependent MCF-7 and hormone-independent BT-20 cell lines. Notably, the level of expression of each estrogen receptor type found varied in MCF-7 and BT-20 cells (59). In BT-20 cell lines, the exon 5 deletion appeared to be a predominant message, as determined by RNase protection assay; MCF-7 cells expressed somewhat more wild-type receptors. Likewise, coexpression of variant receptors with the wild type was seen in primary breast tumors.

Variant forms of estrogen receptor RNA have also been reported in breast tumors classified both as ER/PR+ and ER/PR− by ligand-binding analysis (63,64). RNA-directed polymerase chain reactions were used to detect them. These estrogen-receptor variants have either exon 3, 5, or 7 deleted and were found to be expressed in combination with wild-type estrogen receptor transcripts. Various levels of variant and wild-type estrogen receptors were seen among tumors that were ER− and PgR+, which often expressed high levels of a variant estrogen receptor lacking exon 5 of the hormone-binding domain of the receptor. These deletions resulted in the production of a variant estrogen receptor truncated within the hormone-binding domain that was unable to bind estrogen. However, the receptor appeared to bind DNA and was constitutive for activation of estrogen-responsive genes. When the exon 5 variant was coexpressed with wild-type receptors in MCF-7 cells, tamoxifen-resistant growth was conferred on these cells. Thus, overexpression of the variant, even in the presence of wild-type receptors, may contribute to tamoxifen resistance. Furthermore, ER+ tumors that express wild-type estrogen receptors often coexpress the exon 4 estrogen receptor deletion variant. Tumors with this variant may escape the normal growth dependence of estrogen, and subclones may be selected under conditions where tamoxifen is present, which would inhibit only the wild-type receptor present in these cells.

Murphy et al. initially identified abnormally sized ER mRNA by Northern hybridization, and they have recently cloned these altered estrogen receptors from human breast tumors. Three different ER mRNAs were identified with a divergent sequence from a known estrogen receptor sequence at exon/intron borders. At the point of divergence, non-ER sequences have been inserted. These insertions were either unknown or homologous to long interspersed repetitive line-1 sequences. These three altered estrogen receptors were all missing the hormone-binding domain of the receptor in addition to containing unique non-ER segments. Dotzlaw et al. further elaborated these divergences and showed that the ER mRNA variants expressed normal estrogen receptor sequences through exons 1, 2, and 3 but then showed divergent sequences that were unrelated to ER mRNA (65).

In one study of 20 tamoxifen-resistant and 20 tamoxifen-sensitive tumors, eight exons of ER-complementary DNA were analyzed by single-strand conformation polymorphism (SSCP), and the variant conformers were sequenced to identify the nucleotide changes. Only two mutations in exon 6 of all 20 tamoxifen-resistant tumors were noted, leading to the conclusion that mutations in estrogen receptor occur at a low frequency and do not account for most estrogen-independent, tamoxifen-resistant breast tumors. Possible reasons for the low detection of mutations were either due to the fact that the mutation was present in a very small number of cells and could not be detected by SSCP, or estrogen receptor mutations were rare and occurred at a very low frequency (66).

## Alternative Pathway of Estrogen Receptor Action

In regular pathways, the estrogen-ER complex activates ERE sites on the promoter gene. Recent studies have described the possibility of an alternative pathway that allows tamoxifen to activate transcription (67,68). Instead of stimulating ERE sites on a promoter gene, both estrogen and tamoxifen have been directed to an AP-1 site, causing increased transcription (Fig. 3). AP-1, initially recognized as phorbol-ester–inducible enhancer binding protein, has a nucleic acid sequence similar to the c-*jun* proto-oncogene and DNA-binding domain of the transcription factor in yeast, GCN4 (69). Homodimers of c-*jun* or heterodimers with c-*fos* as a AP-1 transcription factor can modulate gene expression by activating the AP-1 site. In a study by Webb et al., a step-by-step demonstration of estrogen and tamoxifen stimulation of an AP-1 pathway was made. A human collagenase promoter containing an AP-1 site was transfected to HeLa cells and studied with estrogen and tamoxifen. Activation by tamoxifen was found to be more potent than estrogen in cells with intact AP-1 sites, and the pattern was lost when an AP-1 site was deleted, indicating that the potent activation of tamoxifen was related to AP-1 even more than estrogen. When direct substitution of EREs to AP-1 was performed, tamoxifen activation disappeared while the estrogen response was restored. In the absence of estrogen receptors, the tamoxifen response was also lost, showing a requirement of estrogen receptors for this activation. In the study of the endometrial cell line HeLa and the breast cancer cell line MDA453, cell-specific activation of AP-1 pathways was noted. In MDA453 breast cancer cells, the AP-1 driven collagenase promoter was activated efficiently by estrogen but not by tamoxifen. In this study, an observation about deleted estrogen receptors was also made. Deletion of hormone-binding domain (HBD) gave a constitutively active receptor that was able to activate at an ERE in endometrial, breast, and ovarian cancer cell lines. These results support the previous observations of mutated estrogen receptors activating cell growth. When the relationship between deleted estrogen receptors and activity at AP-1 sites was studied, potent activity was seen only in endometrial cell lines and not in breast or ovarian cell lines, again showing tissue-specific AP-1 activation. Intact DBDs were also demonstrated to be necessary for activation of ER-directed AP-1 pathways, but estrogen activation was seen in some cells without intact DBDs. On the other hand, estrogen response was biphasic, and high levels of estrogen receptors can squelch the response; therefore, estrogen receptors can stimulate or repress

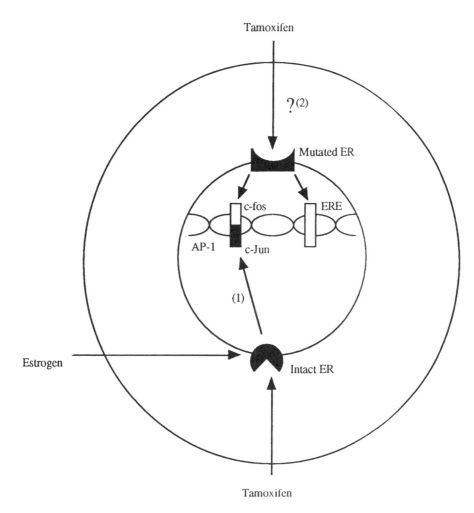

**Figure 3** (1) Activation of AP-1 by estrogen and antiestrogens. This requires ER, and binding of ER to AP-1 is at c-*jun* but not at c-*fos*. (2) Mutated ER with deleted HBD constitutively activates ERE. It also has potent activity at AP-1 site, especially in cells with weak ERE activity, such as HeLa endometrial cells. But its activity at AP-1 site is weak in cells with strong ERE activity, such as MDA-453 breast cancer cells. The role of mutated ER in tamoxifen-resistant and stimulated growth is not known yet but highly possible. The direct relationship between tamoxifen therapy and the development of mutated ER still needs to be clarified.

collagenase expression. Tamoxifen activity at an AP-1 site may be strong in cells where its activity at an ERE is weak, as in HeLa cells; but it remains weak at an AP-1 site in cells where its activity on ERE is strong, as in MDA453 breast cancer cell lines. Therefore, tamoxifen activation of transcription with an alternative pathway is evident, but the question remains whether this happens in tamoxifen-resistant or stimulated breast tumors or whether the tissue specificity of this pathway is overcome by long-term treatment with tamoxifen (70).

## Tamoxifen and Autocrine/Paracrine Growth Factors

Several reports have described the possibility that breast cancer cells might function as small endocrine glands, synthesizing and secreting a wide variety of polypeptide growth factors (71,72). Modulation of breast cancer cell growth and proliferation by these growth factors may be one of the complex antineoplastic mechanisms of antiestrogens. Tamoxifen therapy inhibits the production of transforming growth factor–$\alpha$ (TGF-$\alpha$) and insulinlike growth factor I (IGF-I) in the plasma of patients treated with tamoxifen and induced production of TGF-$\beta$ (68).

Transfection of TGF-$\alpha$ cDNA was shown to cause transformation of normal mammary epithelial cells (72). TGF-$\alpha$ is associated with cell growth activation in general, and its effect is mediated through the epidermal growth factor receptor (EGFR). This activity, as well as the stimulatory activity of insulinlike growth factor I and platelet-derived growth factor (PDGF), were shown to be induced by estradiol in hormone-dependent breast cancer cells and secreted constitutively by estrogen-independent cells (74). Depletion of steroids from MCF-7 estrogen-dependent cell culture media resulted in a marked (70–80%) but transient reduction in TGF-$\alpha$ mRNA and TGF-$\alpha$ protein and is associated with a decrease in growth rate. However, it was followed by a progressive partial rise in TGF-$\alpha$ mRNA and protein levels despite the continued steroid deprivation. Rapid steroid-independent growth was also established later (75).

TGF-$\beta$ acts as an inhibitory growth factor in most cases, but its association with growth stimulation is also reported (76). At least three different isomers of TGF-$\beta$ have been detected: TGF-$\beta$1, TGF-$\beta$2, and TGF-$\beta$3. The precise role of these growth factors in the proliferation of cancer cells is not yet known. When MCF-7 cells were treated with an antiestrogen causing growth inhibition, secretion of TGF-$\beta$ was induced eight- to 27-fold (77). In the same study, when the TGF-$\beta$ produced from MCF-7 cells—estrogen-dependent cells with ER—was introduced to ER– human breast cancer cells, it caused growth inhibition. That growth inhibition was reversed with TGF-$\beta$ antibodies and confirmed the growth-inhibitory effect of TGF-$\beta$. In a different study, the absence of secretion of TGF-$\beta$ was shown in antiestrogen-resistant MCF-7 cells when treated with tamoxifen, but growth inhibition was produced with exogenous TGF-$\beta$ (74). Estrogen has also been shown to decrease the inhibitory activity of TGF-$\beta$ on cell growth (76,77), and the initial increase in TGF-$\beta$1, $\beta$2, and $\beta$3 in MCF-7 cell cultures in continuous deprivation of steroids was associated with a slowed growth rate (75). This was followed by a decrease in TGF-$\beta$ levels and an associated rapid growth rate, without the presence of steroid.

The adaptation of estrogen-dependent cells to survive in the presence of estrogen antagonists may also be related to physiological and biomedical mechanisms or altered signal transduction that help cells to circumvent the inhibitory effects of tamoxifen. The relationship between the growth and proliferation of breast tumor cells and growth factors has been demonstrated both in vitro and in vivo as described earlier, but the precise role and pathway of that association still needs to be elucidated. Transient changes in levels of TGF-$\alpha$ and TGF-$\beta$ have been associated with estrogen deprivation and steroid-independent growth of MCF-7 cells, which were originally estrogen dependent (75). Epidermal growth factor, through which TGF-$\alpha$ mediates the growth-stimulatory effect, can also reverse the inhibitory effects of antiestrogens on estrogen-stimulated growth (78,79). Theoretically, the acquired ability of cells to express TGF-$\alpha$ and IGF-I, which stimulate growth, while simultaneously suppressing the production of inhibitory TGF-β could result in resistance to tamoxifen. In vitro studies have, in fact, shown that growth factors can reverse the inhibitory effects of tamoxifen (80,81). On the other hand, daily injection of human recombinant TGF-β1 was required to maintain the growth of MCF-7 cells in ovariectomized athymic mice (82). In the same study, injection of 2G7 IgG2b antibody, which neutralizes TGF-β1, β2, and β3, was shown to block the formation of MDA-231 (estrogen-independent) tumors at the injection site along with lung metastasis in nude mice. Therefore, further evidence is certainly required to understand the complex effect of these mechanisms in vivo.

## Decreased Intracellular Drug Concentration

Multiple drug resistance associated with the *MDR1* gene and decreased accumulation of drug in the cells secondary to the active efflux of drug is a well-characterized mechanism of drug resistance. Acquisition of the *MDR1* gene caused the overexpression of P-glycoprotein, which behaves like an efflux pump. This form of drug resistance caused resistance to multiple structurally unrelated drugs (83). Again, mixed data exist regarding the efflux as a tamoxifen-resistance mechanism.

Although the decreased level of intracellular drug concentrations in MCF-7 xenografts of immune-deprived mice with tamoxifen-resistant and tamoxifen-stimulated cells has been described (43), the mechanism was secondary to altered metabolism. In a prospective study of 53 patients treated with tamoxifen, the association of acquired resistance with decreased intratumoral drug concentrations was seen. A similar association could not be found in de novo resistant tumors, and no observation of metabolites was made to exclude altered metabolisms (84). Although no efflux pump has been identified with tamoxifen resistance, an increase in P-glycoprotein was noted following estradiol treatment in a rat mammary adenocarcinoma model (85). This increase was evident even in the absence of tamoxifen resistance. Moreover, in a subsequent follow-up study, a reversal of tamoxifen resistance was noted with verapamil, an agent capable of reversing MDR-mediated drug resistance (86).

## Antiestrogen Binding Sites

Both estrogen-dependent and estrogen-independent breast cancer cells have been shown to contain antiestrogen binding sites (AEBS) (87). Antiestrogen binding sites bind only to antiestrogens with high affinity—they do not bind at all to estrogens (88). Their function is not yet clear, and hypotheses of their function as mediators of ER-independent anticancer effects of tamoxifen or as mediators responsible for the development of tamoxifen resistance were made with limited information. Theoretically, if it is assumed that AEBS are not functioning as part of an inhibitory effect on tumor cell growth, their binding of antiestrogens may cause a decreased availability of antiestrogens to estrogen receptors and may impair their effectiveness. In one study, antiestrogen binding was compared in uterine preparations, where estrogen receptor activity exceeded AEBS, and in liver preparations, where AEBS binding predominated. The results suggested that when AEBS activity predominated, tamoxifen was virtually bound to AEBS and only a limited amount was available to estrogen receptors. Furthermore, the AEBS:ER ratio was three times greater in antiestrogen-resistant MCF-7 cells than in antiestrogen-sensitive wild-type MCF-7 cells (89). An excess of AEBS activity over estrogen receptor activity was also shown in 128 human breast tumors.

However, altered or excessive AEBS activity was not always found in estrogen-resistant clones (90–92).

## CONCLUSION

The development of tamoxifen resistance or tamoxifen-stimulated growth is the result of one or more complex mechanisms. For example, an alteration in an intracellular signaling pathway as a direct response to tamoxifen or in response to the modification of the extracellular environment—such as a change in levels of growth and inhibiting factors—may play a major role in development of acquired resistance. Additionally, the appearance of mutated estrogen receptors or the development of ER with constitutive DNA binding capacity may contribute to the development of antiestrogen resistance. Future pharmacogenetic studies of tamoxifen may yield some guidance in recognizing the group of patients who might not benefit from antiestrogen therapy or might develop resistance. Finally, it would be prudent to encourage additional research on the molecular basis of tamoxifen resistance and stimulated growth prior to the testing of tamoxifen as a chemopreventive in healthy women (93).

## ACKNOWLEDGMENTS

We thank Timothy B. Cadman, Gregory T. Wurz, and Frederick J Meyers, MD for their critical appraisal and help in preparing this chapter.

## REFERENCES

1. Cole MP, Jones CTA, Todd IDH. A new antioestrogenic agent in late breast cancer. An early clinical appraisal with ICI 46474. Br J Cancer 1971; 25:270–275.
2. Mouridsen H, Palshof J, Patterson J, et al. Tamoxifen in advanced breast cancer. Cancer Treat Rev 1978; 5:131–141.
3. Early Breast Cancer Trialists' Collaborative Group. Systemic treatment of early breast cancer by hormonal, cytotoxic, or immune therapy. Lancet 1992; 339:71–85.
4. Fisher B, Redmond C, Brown A, Fisher E, Wolmark N, et al. Adjuvant chemotherapy with and without tamoxifen in the treatment of primary breast cancer: 5-year results from the National Surgical Adjuvant Breast and Bowel Project Trial. J Clin Oncol 1986; 4:459–471.
5. Report from the Breast Cancer Trials Committee, Scottish Cancer Trials Office (MRC), Edinburg. Adjuvant tamoxifen in the management of operable breast cancer: the Scottish trial. Lancet 1987; 2:171–175.
6. Rose C, Anderson KW, Mouridsen H, Thorpe S, Pedersen BV, et al. Danish Breast Cancer Cooperative Group. Beneficial effect of adjuvant tamoxifen therapy in primary breast cancer patients with high oestrogen receptor values. Lancet 1985; 1:16–19.
7. Rose C, Mouridsen HT. Treatment of advanced breast cancer with tamoxifen. Recent Results Cancer Res 1984; 91:230–242.
8. Pritchard KI, Thomson DE, Myers RE, Sutherland DJA, et al. Tamoxifen therapy in premenopausal patients with metastatic breast cancer. Cancer Treat Rep 1980; 64:787–796.

9. Herderson IC. Endocrine therapy of metastatic breast cancer. In: Harris JR, Hellman S, Henderson IC, Kinne DW, eds. Breast Dis 1993:559–603.

10. Sawka CA, Pritchard KI, Paterson AHG, et al. Role and mechanism of action of tamoxifen in premenopausal women with metastatic breast carcinoma. Cancer Res 1986; 46:3152–3156.

11. Buchanan RB, Blamey RW, Durrant KR, et al. A randomized comparison of tamoxifen with surgical oophorectomy in premenopausal patients with advanced breast cancer. J Clin Oncol 1986; 4:1326–1330.

12. Canney PA, Griffiths T, Lateif TN, Priestman TJ. Clinical significance of tamoxifen withdrawal response. Lancet 1987; 1:36.

13. Taylor SG, Gelman RS, Falkson G, Cummings FJ. Combination of chemotherapy compared to tamoxifen as initial therapy for stage IV breast cancer in elderly women. Ann Intern Med 1986; 104:455–461.

14. White JH, Metzger D, Chambon P. Expression and Function of the Human Estrogen Receptor in Yeast. Cold Spring Harbor: Cold Spring Harbor Laboratory, 1988:819.

15. Kumar V, Green S, Stack G, Berry M, Jin JR, et al. Functional domains of the human estrogen receptor. Cell 1987; 51:941–951.

16. Dauvios S, Deniellan PS, White R, Parker MG. Antiestrogen ICI 164,384 reduces cellular estrogen receptor content by increasing its turnover. Proc Natl Acad Sci USA 1992; 89:4037–4041.

17. Webster NJ, Green S, Jin JR, Chambon P. The hormone-binding domains of estrogen and glucocorticoid receptors contain an inducible transcription activation function. Cell 1988; 54:199–207.

18. Jordan VC. Biochemical pharmacology of antiestrogen action. Pharmacol Rev 1984; 36:245–276.

19. Sutherland RL, Reddel RR, Green MD. Effect of oestrogen on cell proliferation and cell cycle kinetics: a hypothesis on the cell cycle effects of antioestrogens. Eur J Cancer Clin Oncol 1983; 19:307–318.

20. Osborne CK, Boldt DH, Clark GM, et al. Effect of tamoxifen on human breast cancer cell cycle kinetics: accumulation of cells in early G1 phase. Cancer Res 1983; 43:3583.

21. Lippman M, Bolan G, Huff K. Interactions of antiestrogens with human breast cancer in long-term tissue culture. Cancer Treat Rep 1976; 60:1421–1429.

22. Jordan VC, Fritz NF, Tormey DC. Endocrine effects of adjuvant chemotherapy and long term tamoxifen administration on node positive patients with breast cancer. Cancer Res 1987; 47:624.

23. Fex G, Adielsson G, Mattson W. Oestrogen-like effects of tamoxifen on the concentrations of proteins in plasma. Acta Endocrinol 1981; 97:109.

24. Ferrazzi E, Cartei G, Matarazzo R, et al. Oestrogen-like effects of tamoxifen on vaginal epithelium. Br Med J 1997 1:1335.

25. Sutherland RL, Watts CKW, Hall RE, Ruenitz PC. Mechanisms of growth inhibition by nonsteroidal antioestrogens in human breast cancer cells. J Steroid Biochem 1987; 27:891–897.

26. Reddel RR, Murphy LC, Sutherland RL. Effect of biological active metabolites of tamoxifen on proliferation kinetics of MCF-7 human breast cancer cell in vitro. Cancer Res 1983; 43:4618–4624.

27. Mercer WD, Lippman ME, Todd JH, et al. Histological grade in predicting response to endocrine treatment. Breast Cancer Res Treat 1986; 8:165–166.

28. Horwitz HB. Can hormone "resistant" breast cancer cells be inappropriately stimulated by tamoxifen? Ann NY Acad Sci 1993; 684:63–74.

29. Arteaga CL, Osborn CK. Growth inhibition of human breast cancer cells in vitro with an antibody against the type I somatomedin receptor. Cancer Res 1989; 49:6237–6241.

30. Hull DF, Clark GM, Osborne CK, et al. Multiple estrogen receptor assays in human breast cancer. Cancer Res 1983; 43:413.
31. Simon WE, Albrecht M, Trams G, et al. In vitro growth promotion of human mammary carcinoma cells by steroid hormones, tamoxifen, and prolactin. J Natl Cancer Inst 1984; 73:313–321.
32. Gottardis MM, Wagner RJ, Bordon EC, et al. Differential ability of antiestrogens to stimulate breast cancer cell (MCF-7) growth in vivo and in vitro. Cancer Res 1989; 49:4765–4769.
33. Osborn CK, Coronado EB, Robinson JP. Human breast cancer in athymic nude mouse: cytotoxic effect of long-term tamoxifen therapy. Eur J Cancer 1987; 23:1189–1194.
34. Gottardis MM, Jordan VC. Development of tamoxifen-stimulated growth of MCF-7 tumors in thymic mice after longterm antiestrogen administration. Cancer Res 1988; 48:5183–5187.
35. Gottardis MM, Jiang SY, Jeng MH, Jordan VC. Inhibition of tamoxifen-stimulated growth of an MCF-7 tumor variant in athymic mice by novel steroidal antiestrogens. Cancer Res 1989; 49:4090–4093.
36. Gottardis MM, Richio M, Stuaswaroop PG, et al. Effect of steroidal and nonsteroidal antiestrogens on the growth of a tamoxifen-stimulated human endometrial carcinoma (EnCa 101) in athymic mice. Cancer Res 1990; 50:3189.
37. Furr BJA, Jordan VC. The pharmacology and clinical use of tamoxifen. Pharmacol Ther 1984; 25:127–205.
38. Kemp JV, Adams HK, Wakeling AE, et al. Identification and biological activity of tamoxifen metabolites in human serum. Biochem Pharmacol 1983; 32:2045–2082.
39. Jordan VC, Bain RR, Brown RR, et al. Determination and pharmacology of new hydroxylated metabolite of tamoxifen in observed in patient sera during therapy for advanced breast cancer. Cancer 1983; 43:1446–1450.
40. Lyman SD, Jordan VC. Metabolism of tamoxifen and its uterotrophic activity. Biochem Pharmacol 1985; 34:2787–2794.
41. Liberman ME, Gorski J, Jordan VC. An estrogen receptor model to describe the regulation of prolactin synthesis by antiestrogens in vitro. J Biol Chem 1983; 258:4741–4745.
42. Langan-Fahey SM, Tormey DC, Jordan VC. Tamoxifen metabolites in patients on long-term adjuvant therapy for breast cancer. Eur J Cancer 1990; 26:883–888.
43. Osborn CK, Coranado E, Wiebe VJ, et al. Acquired tamoxifen resistance: Correlation with reduced tumor levels of tamoxifen and isomerization of trans-4-hydroxytamoxifen. J Natl Cancer Inst 1991; 83:1477–1482.
44. Osborne CK, Coronado E, Wiebe VJ, et al. Acquired tamoxifen resistance in breast cancer correlates with reduced accumulation of tamoxifen and trans-4-hydroxytamoxifen. J Clin Oncol 1992; 10:304–310.
45. Wiebe VJ, Osborne CK, McGuire WL, DeGregorio MW. Identification of estrogenic tamoxifen metabolite(s) in tamoxifen resistant human breast tumors. J Clin Oncol 1992; 10:990–994.
46. Osborn CK. Mechanisms for tamoxifen resistance in breast cancer; possible role of tamoxifen metabolism. J Steroid Biochem Mol Biol 1993; 47:83–89.
47. Dowsett M, Harris AL, Smith IE, Jeffcoate SL. Endocrine changes associated with relapse in advanced breast cancer patients on aminoglutathemide therapy. J Clin Endocrinol Metab 1984; 58:99–104.
48. Sherman BM, Chapler FK, Circkard K, Wycoff D. Endocrine consequences of continuous antiestrogen therapy with tamoxifen in pre-menopausal women. J Clin Invest 1979; 64:398.
49. Ravdin PM, Fritz NF, Tormey DC, Jordan VC. Endocrine status of premenopausal node-positive breast cancer patients following adjuvant chemotherapy and long-term tamoxifen. Cancer Res 1988; 48:1026–1029.

50. Taylor RE, Powles TJ, Humphreys J, et al. Effects of endocrine therapy on steroid-receptor content of breast cancer. Br J Cancer 1982; 45:80–85.

51. Kiang DT, Kollander RE, Thomas T, Kennedy BJ. Up-regulation of estrogen receptors by nonsteroidal antiestrogens in human breast cancer. Cancer Res 1989; 49:5312–5316.

52. Noguchi S, Motorama K, Inaji H, Imaoka S, Koyama H. Up-regulation of estrogen receptor by tamoxifen in human breast cancer. Cancer 1993; 72:1266–1272.

53. Simon WE, Trams G, Holzel F. Long-term treatment of estrogen sensitive human breast cancer Cell Line EFM-19 with tamoxifen resulted in tamoxifen-stimulated growth of cells. Arch Gynaecol Obstet 1993; 253:131–141.

54. Osborne CK, Wiebe VI, McGuire WL, et al. Tamoxifen and the isomers of 4-hydroxyta-moxifen in tamoxifen-resistant tumors from breast cancer patients. J Clin Oncol 1992; 10:304.

55. Bronzert DA, Greene GL, Lippman ME. Selection and characterization of a breast cancer cell line resistant to the anti-estrogen LY117018. Endocrinology 1985; 117:1409.

56. Nawata H, Bonzert D, Lippman ME. Isolation and characterization of a tamoxifen resistant cell line derived from MCF-7 human breast cancers. J Biol Chem 1981; 256:5016.

57. Graham ML II, Krent NL, Miller LA, et al. T47Dco Cells, genetically unstable and containing estrogen receptor mutations, are a model for the progression of breast cancer to hormone resistance. Cancer Res 1990; 50:333.

58. Raam S, Robert N, Constantine AP, et al. Defective estrogen receptors in human mammary cancers: their significance in defining hormone dependence. J Natl Cancer Inst 1988; 80:756.

59. Castles CG, Fuqua SAW, Klots DM, Hill SM. Expression of a constitutively active estrogen receptor variant in estrogen receptor-negative BT-20 human breast cancer cell line. Cancere Res 1991; 53:5934–5939.

60. Kumar V, Green MD, Stack G, Berry M, Jin JR, et al. Functional domains of the human estrogen receptor. Cell 1987; 51:941–951.

61. Scott GK, Kushner P, Vigne JL, et al. Truncated forms of DNA binding estrogen receptors in human breast cancer. J Clin Invest 1991; 88:700.

62. Foster BD, Cavner DR, Parl FF. Binding analysis of estrogen receptor to its specific DNA target site in human breast cancer. Cancer Res 1991; 51:3405.

63. Fuqua SAW, Fitzgerald SD, Chamness GC, et al. Variant human breast tumore estrogen receptor with constitutive transcriptional activity. Cancer Res 1991; 51:105.

64. Fuqua SAW, Fitzgerald SW, Allred DC, et al. Inhibition of estrogen receptor action by naturally occurring variant in human breast tumors. Cancer Res 1992; 52:483.

65. Dotzlaw H, Alkhalaf M, Murphy LC. Characterization of estrogen receptor variant mRNAs for human breast cancers. Mol Endocrinol 1992; 6:773–785.

66. Karnik PS, Kulkarni S, Liu X, Budd T, Bukowski RM. Estrogen receptor mutations in tamoxifen-resistant breast cancer. Cancer Res 1994; 54:349–353.

67. Umarayara Y, Kawamori R, Watada H, Imano E, et al. Estrogen regulation of the insulin-like growth factor I gene transcription involves an AP-1 enhancer. J Biol Chem 1994; 269: 16433–16442.

68. Phillips A, Chalbos D, Rochafort H. Estradiol increases and anti-estrogens antagonize the growth factor-induced activator protein-1 activity in MCF-7 breast cancer cells without affecting c-fos and c-jun synthesis. J Biol Chem 1993; 268:14103–14108.

69. Bohmann D, Bos TJ, Admon A, Nishimura T, Vogt PK, Tjian R. Human proto-oncogene c-jun encodes a DNA binding protein with structural and functional properties of transcription factor AP-1. Science 1987; 238:1386–1392.

70. Webb P, Lopez GN, Uht RM, Kushner PJ. Tamoxifen activation of the estrogen receptor/ AP-1 pathway: potential origin for the cell-specific estrogen-like effects of antiestrogens. Mol Endocrinol 1995; 9:443–456.

71. Osborne CK. Polypeptide growth factors: their potential value in the management of breast cancer patients. In: Handerson IC, ed. Adjuvant Therapy of Breast Cancer. Norwell, Mass: Kluwer Academic Publishers, 1992:315–329.

72. Dickson RB, Lippman ME. Molecular determinants of growth, angiogenesis, and metastasis in breast cancer. Semin Oncol 1992; 19:286–289.

73. Shanker V, Ciardiello F, Kim N, et al. Transformation of normal mouse mammary epithelial cells following transfection with a human transforming growth factor cDNA. Mol Carcinog 1989; 2:1–11.

74. Lippman ME, Dickson RB, Gelmann EP, Rosen N, et al. Growth inhibitory peptide production by human breast carcinoma cells. J Steroid Biochem 1988; 30:53–61.

75. Herman HE, Katzenellenbogen BS. Alterations in transforming growth factor-alpha and -beta production and cell responsiveness during the progression of MCF-7 human breast cancer cells to estrogen-autonomous growth. Cancer Res 1994; 54:5867–5874.

76. Osborne CK, Coronado E, Wiebe VJ, et al. Acquired tamoxifen resistance in breast cancer correlates with reduced accumulation of tamoxifen and trans-4-hydroxytamoxifen. J Clin Oncol 1992; 10:304–310.

77. Wiebe VJ, Osborne CK, McGuire WL, DeGregorio MW. Identification of estrogenic tamoxifen metabolite(s) in tamoxifen resistant human breast tumors. J Clin Oncol 1992; 10: 990–994.

78. Konga M, Sutherland RL. Epidermal growth factor partially reverses the inhibitory effects of antiestrogens on T47D human breast cancer growth. Biochem Biophys Res Commun 1987; 146:739–745.

79. Cormler EM, Jordan VC. Contrasting ability of antiestrogens to inhibit MCF-7 growth stimulated by estradiol or epidermal growth factor. Eur J Cancer Clin Oncol 1989; 25:57–63.

80. Fishman JH. Estradiol and tamoxifen interaction at receptor sites at 37°C. Endocrinology 1983; 113:1164.

81. Clark JH, Mitchell WC, Guthrie SC. Triphenylethylene antiestrogen binding sites (TABS) specificity. J Steroid Biochem 1987; 26:433.

82. Areataga CL, Dugger TC, Winnier AR, Forbes JT. Evidence for a positive role of transforming growth factor-beta in human breast cancer cell tumorigenesis. Cell Biochem 1993; 17G:187–193.

83. Gerlach JH, Kartner N, Bek DR, et al. Multidrug resistance in human cancer. N Engl J Med 1987; 316:1388.

84. Johnston SRD, Haynes BP, Smith IE, Jarman M, et al. Acquired tamoxifen resistance in human breast cancer and reduced intra-tumoral drug concentration. Lancet 1993; 342:1521–1522.

85. Kellen JA, Georges E, Ling V. Decreased P-glycoprotein in a tamoxifen-tolerant breast carcinoma model. Anticancer Res 1991; 11:1243.

86. Kellen JA, Wong A, Georges E, et al. R-verapamil decreased antiestrogen resistance in a breast cancer model. Anticancer Res 1991:809.

87. Miller MA, Sheen YY, Mullick A, Katzenellenbogen BS. Anti-oestrogen binding oestrogen receptors and additional anti-oestrogen binding sites in human breast cancer cells. In: Jordan VC, ed. Estrogen/Antioestrogen Action and Breast Cancer Therapy. Madison: University of Wisconsin Press, 1986:127–148.

88. Sutherland AA, Murphy LC, Foo MS, Green MD, et al. High affinity antioestrogen binding site distinct from the oestrogen receptor. Nature 1980; 228:273–275.

89. Pavlik EJ, Nelson K, Srinivasan S, et al. Resistance to tamoxifen with persisting sensitivity to estrogen; Possible mediation by excessive antiestrogen binding site activity. Cancer Res 1992; 52:4106.

90. Nawata H, Chang MJ, Bronzert D, et al. Estradiol independent growth of subline of MCF-7 human breast cancer cells in culture. J Biol Chem 1981; 256:6895.

91. Nawata H, Bronzert D, Lippman ME. Isolation and characterization of a tamoxifen resistance cell line derived from MCF-7 human breast cancer cell. J Biol Chem 1981; 256:5016.
92. Faye JC, Jozan S, Redwilh G, et al. Physicochemical and genetic evidence for specific antiestrogen binding sites. Proc Natl Acad Sci USA 1983; 80:3158.
93. DeGregorio MW, Maenpaa JU, Wiebe VJ. Tamoxifen for the prevention of breast cancer: no. Important Adv Oncol 1995; 175–185.

# 6

## Resistance to Endocrine Therapy in Breast Cancer

**Per E. Lønning**
*Haukeland University Hospital, Bergen, Norway*

## INTRODUCTION

Breast cancer is the most frequent form of cancer in females in the Western world (1). One out of 10 American women will develop breast cancer during her lifetime, and only about 50% of patients treated for breast cancer will experience a permanent cure (2). The reason for therapeutic failure is the development of drug resistance.

The history of endocrine therapy in breast cancer started just a decade ago with the important discovery of Beatson that castration might precipitate tumor regression in premenopausal women (3). The concept of ablative surgery as endocrine treatment of advanced breast cancer was extended to postmenopausal women half a century later by the discoveries of Dao and Huggins (4) and Luft et al. (5) that adrenalectomy as well as hypophysectomy might provoke tumor regression in this group of patients. Although different forms of hormone additive treatment with estrogens, glucocorticoids, or androgens was implemented for breast cancer therapy in the 1940s and 1950s (6–8), contemporary medical endocrine treatment started with the introduction of the anti-estrogen tamoxifen in 1971 (9).

Endocrine therapy plays a pivotal role in breast cancer treatment. Seventy to 80% of all breast cancers contain estrogen receptors (ER), and among these 50–70% may respond to first-line endocrine therapy (10). However, the response is of limited duration: the great majority of patients will relapse because of the development of drug resistance within 2 years.

Endocrine therapy also has a well-established role in the adjuvant treatment of breast cancer. Castration in premenopausal women and tamoxifen in pre- as well as postmenopausal women have been shown to improve long-term disease-free survival and also overall survival (11,12).

Despite a long history of use of endocrine treatment in breast cancer and well-characterized clinical effects, the mechanisms causing resistance to endocrine treatment in vivo is poorly understood. Tumors that lack ER are not able to respond to estrogens as a mitogenic stimulus and therefore may not respond to estrogen deprivation or blocking of estrogen stimulation by antiestrogens. On the other hand, our understanding of the mechanisms of primary as well as acquired resistance in ER-positive tumors is to a large extent limited by the incompleteness in our understanding of the mechanisms by which antiendocrine drugs work in breast cancer. Thus, before we review possible mechanisms of resistance, a brief overview will be given of sex hormone disposition and the different types of endocrine treatment in breast cancer patients.

## THE ENDOCRINOLOGY OF BREAST CANCER

### Estrogen Disposition

Ovarian estrogen synthesis ceases at the menopause, but postmenopausal women still synthesize estrogens by converting circulating androgens into estrogens by the process named aromatization (13). This reaction takes place in different tissues throughout the body such as skin, connective tissue, muscle, and the liver (14–19). The main substrates for this process are androstenedione, which is converted into estrone, and testosterone, which is converted into estradiol (13). The bulk of circulating androstenedione and about 50% of circulating testosterone is thought to be secreted by the adrenal cortex; the residual androgens are believed to have an ovarian origin (20,21). The aromatase enzyme has a higher substrate affinity for androstenedione compared to testosterone; about 1–4% of circulating androstenedione is converted into estrone, whereas only about 0.1–0.5% of testosterone is converted into estradiol (13). Estrone and estradiol are interconvertible, and it has been estimated that about half the amount of plasma estradiol in postmenopausal women may arise by conversion from estrone (13).

Notably, circulating estradiol may not be the only estrogen source for the tumor cells, neither in postmenopausal nor in premenopausal women. Estrogens may be synthesized by fibroblasts in the tumor cell vicinity. In addition, breast cancer cells contain the aromatase enzyme to a variable degree (22–24), and intratumor estradiol may be synthesized from other plasma estrogens. Estradiol, the biologically most active estrogen, is found in the plasma of postmenopausal women at a concentration of 10–50 pM only; the concentration of plasma estrone is about 80–100 pM (25). An estrogen of particular interest in postmenopausal women is estrone sulfate. Although this estrogen has no biological activity on its own, its high plasma concentration (mean concentration of about 400–500 pM) and the fact that breast cancer tissue contains the enzymes required to convert estrone sulfate into estrone and estradiol makes this hormone an interesting source of intratumor estradiol (26–28). The concentration of estradiol in breast cancer tissue obtained from postmenopausal women is above 10-fold the concentration found in the plasma (29–31), with little difference in tissue concentration between pre- and postmenopausal women (30). It is not known whether there may be particular mechanisms concentrating estrogens in cells. Possible pathways contributing to intracellular estradiol are depicted in Figure 1.

### Hormone Receptors in Breast Cancer

Although albative endocrine therapy has been known for a long time to cause regression in breast cancer, the scientific rationale for the mechanisms causing tumor regression in some patients but not in others was provided by the important discovery by Jensen and coworkers of the estrogen receptor (ER) in breast cancer and their finding that expression of this receptor predicted response to ablative endocrine therapy (32).

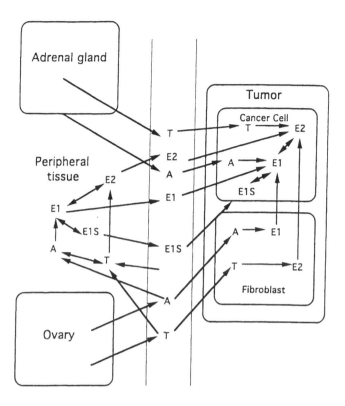

**Figure 1** Pathways contributing to intracellular estrogens in postmenopausal women: A = androstenedione, T = testosterone, $E_1$ = estrone, $E_2$ = estradiol, $E_1S$ = estrone sulfate.

The role of ER in predicting the likelihood of response to endocrine manipulation and its role as a prognostic factor in breast cancer is well documented (10,33–35). In a large study, about 60% of premenopausal and 75% of postmenopausal breast cancers were found to express an ER concentration above 10 fmol/mg protein, the value generally accepted as the threshold value for receptor positivity (10). For patients who express a positive value for ER, the likelihood of achieving a response to first-line endocrine therapy in advanced disease is about 50–75%, with the highest chance of a response observed among patients with high ER values and among those who, in addition to being ER positive, also express the progesterone receptor (PR) (10,35). The reason for this is most probably that synthesis of the PR is stimulated by estrogens, and thus expression of this receptor is considered to be a marker of a functional ER (36).

Over the past years, new insight into the biology of ER has been gained, in particular through research on the effects of different antiestrogens. The ER protein exists as a monomer with three distinctive domains, termed the N-terminal (which contains AF-1, a transcription activation region), a DNA-binding domain, and an estrogen-binding domain with a second transcription activation region, named AF-2 (37,38). After estradiol binding, the ER undergoes a conformational change, after which the ligand/ER complex undergoes dimerization (39). The homodimer binds to specific DNA sequences called estrogen responsive elements (ERE), which in turn promote transcription (40). It is noteworthy that AF-1 seems to function independent of ligand binding as soon as the ER binds to ERE, whereas AF-2 seems to depend on estrogen ligand binding for transcription activity (38,41–43). Interestingly, a receptor variant with a defective hormone-binding domain and AF-2 but with intact AF-1 has recently been isolated from ER-negative PgR-positive human breast carcinomas (44).

In addition to the discovery of different forms of mutant receptors (45–48), several investigators have shown the existence of specific antiestrogen binding sites with no affinity for estradiol (49–51). Of particular interest is the recent observation (52) that the ER itself may contain two different binding sites: the one site binding estradiol as well as antiestrogens may be responsible for the estrogen agonistic effect of all ligands; the other site, binding antiestrogens only, could be responsible for the antiestrogenic effects of these compounds.

Estradiol is a most potent mitogen to ER-positive breast cancer cells. In recent years, endocrine treatment in breast cancer has been synonymous with deprivation of estrogen stimulation of the tumor cells, either by eliminating estrogen hormones or by blocking their action with antiestrogens. However, other hormones may influence breast cancer growth. In vitro studies have revealed that progestins inhibit as well as stimulate (53–55) breast cancer cell growth, depending on the experimental conditions. In vivo, progestins administered in high doses may cause tumor regression in breast cancer patients (56). Recent studies have revealed the progesterone receptor to exist as an A and B form (57). These forms have different biological activity, inasmuch as antiprogestins, under certain conditions, may act as progestin agonists when binding to the B form (but not the A form) of the PR (58). It should also be considered that many breast tumors, in addition to the ER and PR, contain receptors for androgen and glucocorticoids (59,60). Androgens may inhibit breast cancer cell growth in vitro as well as in DMBA-induced mammary carcinomas in rats (61,62). Studies in breast cancer patients indicate that adding progestins (63) as well as androgens (64) or glucocorticoids (65) to tamoxifen treatment may improve the clinical response rate. Yet these observations do not provide a definite proof that any of these receptors are involved in the clinical effect observed. Progestins influence estrogen disposition in vivo (see below), and glucocorticoids and androgens may suppress ACTH stimulation of the adrenals and gonadotropin stimulation of the ovaries, respectively, thereby suppressing synthesis of the androgens androstenedione and testosterone, the major substrates for peripheral estrogen synthesis in postmenopausal women (Fig. 1).

## MECHANISMS OF ACTION OF ENDOCRINE THERAPY IN BREAST CANCER

### Rationale for Endocrine Therapy

The rationale for endocrine therapy is based on empirical data revealing estrogen deprivation as well as treatment with antiestrogens to produce tumor regression in human breast cancer. The theory that these treatment options work by depriving the tumor cells of their estrogen stimulation is supported by in vitro data showing that estrogen withdrawal as well as adding antiestrogens to ER-positive cell lines inhibits their growth. However, it should be stated that additional mechanisms of action that may not be detected in in vitro experiments may be of importance to the antitumor effects of these treatment options in vivo, as paracrine as well as endocrine interactions involving other tissues and organ systems may be involved. To some extent, this may be accounted for by growing the tumor cells in castrated nude mice, which have an endocrine milieu resembling that of postmenopausal women (66,67). The classic example of a drug for which multiple mechanisms of action in vivo has been suggested is the antiestrogen tamoxifen. According to classic wisdom, this drug acts by blocking the ER to mitogenic stimulation by estradiol (68). However, several other mechanisms of action have been proposed, including paracrine as well as endocrine interactions. In vitro, tamoxifen inhibits secretion of insulinlike growth factor II (IGF-II) as well as IGF-binding proteins in ER-positive tumor cells (69–72). In vivo, tamoxifen has been found to suppress plasma levels of IGF-I and to elevate the plasma level of one of the IGF-binding proteins (IGFBP-1), which may further inhibit the endocrine delivery of this growth factor (73–75). In addition, tamoxifen enhances the secretion of transforming growth factor-β (TGF-β) by fibroblasts in tumor cell vicinity (76). The progestin megestrol acetate may influence the disposition of plasma estrogens (77) but also the disposition of IGF-I by inhibiting a protease degrading an IGF-binding protein in plasma (78). On the other hand, it should be noted that responses to all forms of endocrine therapy are found to correlate with expression of the ER (79). Although this observation strongly suggests the ER is directly involved in the antitumor action of these drugs, in particular expression of the ER correlates to expression of receptors for growth factors like IGF-I and IGF-II and the epidermal growth factor (IGF-IR and EGF-R) (80,81). These growth factors may have a significant influence on breast cancer growth (82,83).

In some cases, there may be uncertainties about which organ system is the major target for the drug. Until recently, aromatase inhibitors were thought to exert their antitumor effects by suppressing total body estrogen production. However, the detection of aromatase in breast cancers and recent findings that there may be lack of complete cross-resistance to treatment with different aromatase inhibitors (see below) have raised the possibility that, at least in some patients, influence on intratumor aromatase may be more important than the influence on general estrogen disposition.

## Types of Endocrine Treatment in Breast Cancer

Contemporary endocrine treatment modalities in breast cancer include estrogen deprivation (medical/surgical or radiological castration in premenopausal women or use of aromatase inhibitors in postmenopausal women), antiestrogens, or synthetic progestins (medroxyprogesterone, MPA, and megestrol acetate, MA) administered in high-dose drug regimens. In addition, antiprogestins are being investigated in early clinical trials. Before addressing possible mechanisms of drug resistance, a brief description of the different treatment modalities and their mechanisms of action will be given. For more details on these subjects, the reader may consider contemporary reviews (13,79,84–86).

### Antiestrogens

These drugs belong to two major classes: nonsteroidal antiestrogens, which are all triphenylethylene derivatives, and steroidal antiestrogens, which are all estradiol derivatives modified by a side chain in the 7-position (Figs. 2 and 3).

Of the nonsteroidal antiestrogens, the first in general use, tamoxifen, is the contemporary endocrine treatment option most widely used for breast cancer. The drug is extensively metabolized (85). One of the metabolites, 4-hydroxytamoxifen, is a much more potent estrogen antagonist compared to the mother compound, and this meta-

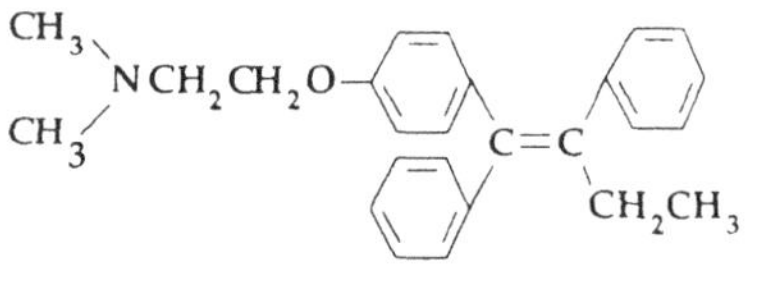

**Tamoxifen**

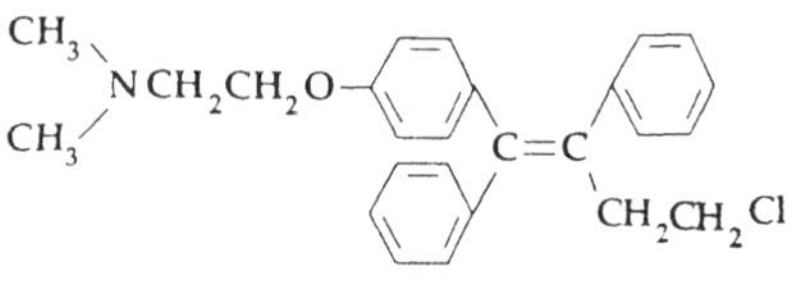

**Toremifene**

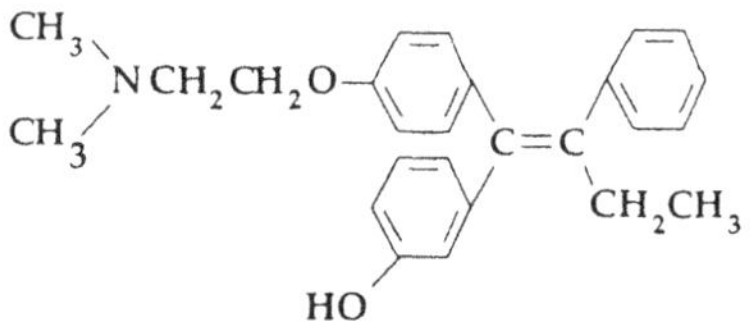

**Droloxifene**

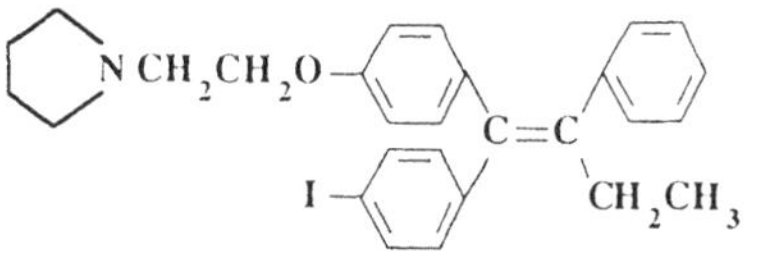

**Idoxifene**

**Figure 2** Antiestrogens belonging to the triethylene (tamoxifen) class.

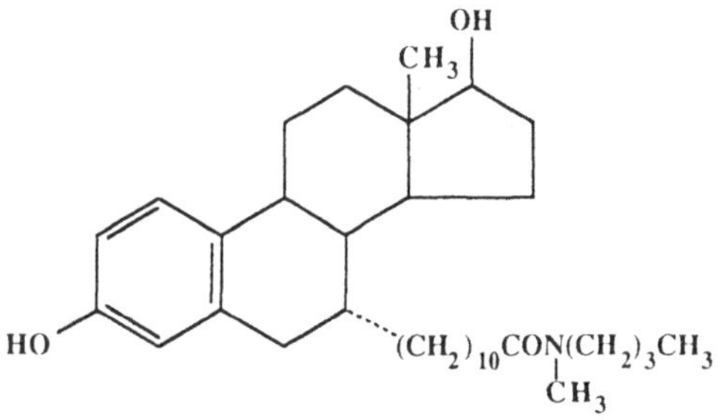

**ICI 164,384**

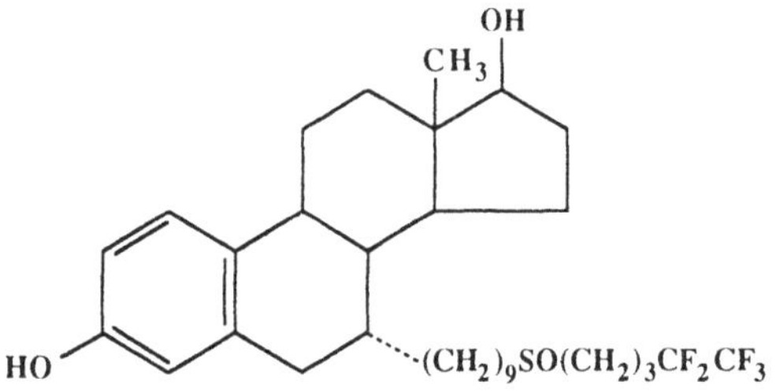

**ICI 182,780**

**Figure 3** Antiestrogens belonging to the steroidal class.

bolite is considered to be responsible for the antitumor effect of tamoxifen in vivo (87,88).

Several new nonsteroidal antiestrogens such as toremifene, droloxifene, and idoxifene have been taken into clinical trials (89–91). Although these drugs may differ somewhat from tamoxifen in regard to estrogen agonistic activities (92,93), observations so far indicate cross-resistance to tamoxifen and these novel drugs in human breast cancer (94–96).

Tamoxifen binds to the estrogen receptor and, like estradiol, produces dimerization and DNA-binding. Unlike estradiol, tamoxifen does not induce transcription, probably because of a defective folding of the ER (40,97). However, despite decades of research, several important questions remain to be answered about the mechanism(s) of action of tamoxifen. A controversial question is why the drug appears not to act as a pure estrogen antagonist but to behave as a partial antagonist/agonist, depending on the test system used (68,84). Some authors (98) have proposed that tamoxifen may inhibit the activation region AF-2 on the ER but not the region AF-1, which might then express estrogen agonistic activity independent of ligand binding when the receptor complex associates with its ERE on the DNA. Others (99) have shown activation of protein kinase A to enhance the estrogen agonistic activity of tamoxifen. In addition, tamoxifen does not bind to the ER alone; several investigations have revealed the existence of specific antiestrogen binding sites with no affinity for estradiol (49–51). It is not clear whether this antiestrogen binding site represents a single or multiple sites. The biological meaning of such antiestrogen binding sites to the mechanism of action or development of resistance to tamoxifen remains unknown, but it has been proposed that these antiestrogen binding site(s) might function as an intracellular "scavenger" preventing antiestrogens from binding to the EAR (100). Interestingly, Jensen and coworkers have provided evidence for a specific antiestrogen binding site with no affinity for estradiol located on the ER itself (52,101). According to their hypothesis, this binding site may be responsible for the antiestrogenic effects of all forms of antiestrogens, while the estrogen-agonistic effects of tamoxifen may be exerted by binding to the estradiol binding site. This finding may be of significance to our understanding of the mechanism of action as well as mechanism(s) of resistance to antiestrogens.

Other effects that may contribute to the antitumor effect of tamoxifen is inhibition of calmodulin and protein kinase C, enhancement of secretion of TGF-β by fibroblasts in tumor cell vicinity, reduction in plasma IGF-I with elevation of the IGF-binding protein IGFBP-1, inhibition of secretion of IGF-II by the tumor cell, downregulation of the IGF-receptor, inhibition of secretion of TGF-α and reduced expression of the epidermal growth factor receptor (EGFR) (70,74,76,102–107). Tamoxifen in general has no effect on ER-negative cells; however, there are examples of tamoxifen inhibiting growth of some ER-negative cell lines (108,109).

Steroidal antiestrogens have been named "pure antiestrogens" because they have been found to be devoid of estrogen agonistic effects in all test systems so far (110). One of these compounds (ICI 182.780) has been evaluated in patients suffering from metastatic breast cancer. This study revealed lack of cross-resistance between tamoxifen and the steroidal antiestrogen, inasmuch as ICI 182.780 caused objective tumor regression in seven of 19 patients and stable disease in six of 19 patients resistant to tamoxifen (111).

The biochemical action of steroidal antiestrogens differs from that of tamoxifen. These drugs reduce the half-life of the ER, thereby reducing its concentration (112).

In addition, they have been found to inhibit ER folding as well as dimerization and DNA binding (95,113).

*Estrogen Deprivation*

Suppression of plasma estrogens may cause tumor regression in pre- as well as postmenopausal women. In premenopausal women, this is achieved by castration (medical/radiological/surgical); in postmenopausal women, it may be achieved by use of aromatase inhibitors. Thus, suppression of plasma estrogens from premenopausal to postmenopausal levels as well as suppression of plasma estrogens from postmenopausal to supra-low levels both may cause a clinical response in breast cancer patients.

Aromatase inhibitors (Figs. 4 and 5) act by inhibiting the conversion of circulating androgens to estrogens (13). Notably, these drugs have little effect in premenopausal women. Although aromatase inhibitors may influence ovarian aromatase, this inhibition is compensated by an increased secretion of gonadotropins (114,115).

Despite two decades of use, there are still some unsolved questions about the mechanisms of action of aromatase inhibitors in breast cancer. A major problem is the internal inconsistency between the results obtained from tracer studies evaluating the ability of different aromatase inhibitors to inhibit the conversion of tracer androstenedione into estrone in vivo and the effect of the same drugs on plasma estrogen levels. Different aromatase inhibitors—such as aminoglutethimide, formestane, fadrazole, and vorozole—have all been reported to inhibit in vivo aromatization by 85–93% (116–120). Despite this, plasma estrogen levels are suppressed by 50–80% only (121–125).

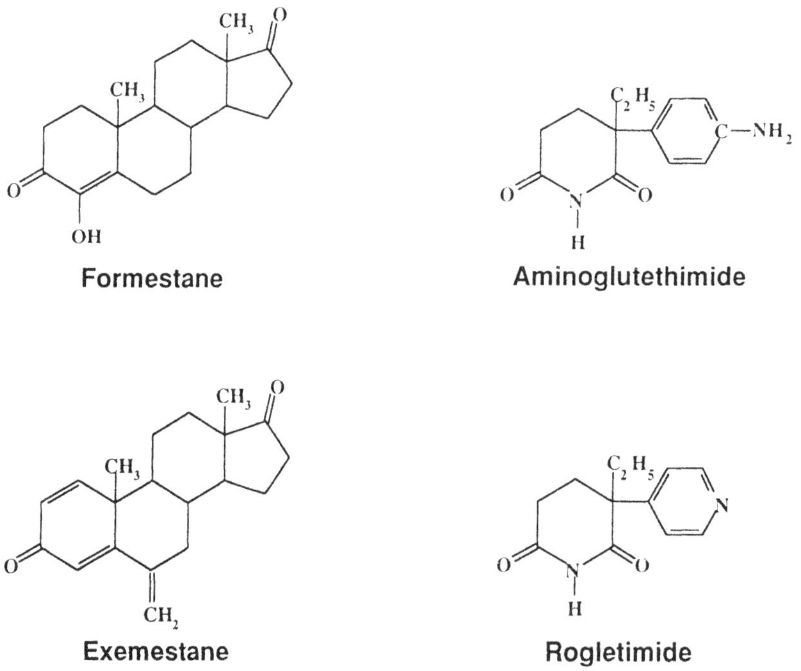

**Formestane**

**Aminoglutethimide**

**Exemestane**

**Rogletimide**

Figure 4   Aromatase inhibitors belonging to the aminoglutethimide class (aminoglutethimide and rogletimide) and steroidal aromatase inhibitors (formestane and exemestane).

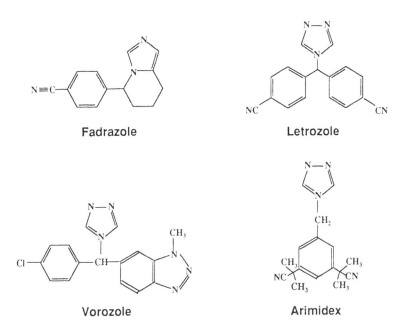

**Figure 5**  Novel aromatase inhibitors belonging to the triazole class.

A recent study showed the triazole drug letrazole inhibited in vivo aromatization by >98% (126), yet plasma estrogen levels were suppressed by about 80%. Whether this is caused by alternative estrogen sources in these patients or lack of sensitivity in the radioimmunoassays is currently not known. Ongoing studies in our department, using a highly sensitive radioimmunoassay to determine plasma estrone sulfate, suggest this inconsistency, at least to some extent, may be the result of method artifacts (127).

As mentioned above, the aromatase enzyme may be detected in different tissues throughout the body and also in breast tumor tissue. Accordingly, estradiol either may be obtained by uptake from the circulation or may be synthesized in cancer cells (or by fibroblasts in tumor cell vicinity) from circulating androgens or from estrone sulfate. Two small studies have evaluated the contribution of plasma estrogens to intratumor estrogens in vivo (128,129); they both suggested a substantial interindividual variation in the contribution from local synthesis. Such a difference may be of relevance to the development of resistance to treatment with aromatase inhibitors. Studies evaluating the endocrine effects and aromatase inhibition with different aromatase inhibitors have assessed plasma and urinary estrogens and measured whole body aromatization. On the other hand, preliminary results from Dr. Miller's group in Edinburgh on human tumor biopsies have revealed that some tumors are less sensitive than others to the inhibitory action of particular aromatase inhibitors (see below).

*Progestins and Antiprogestins*

The exact mechanism by which progestins administered as high-dose regimens exert their antitumor effect is not known. The two drugs most commonly used are medroxy-progesterone acetate and megestrol acetate (Fig. 6) administered in doses of 1000 mg or 160 mg daily, respectively (85).

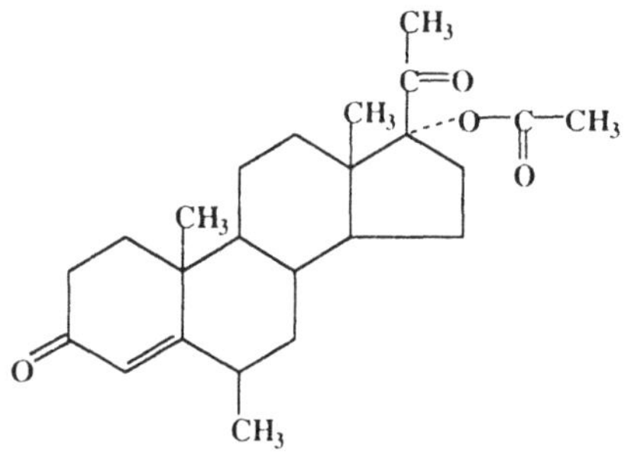

**Medroxyprogesterone acetate**

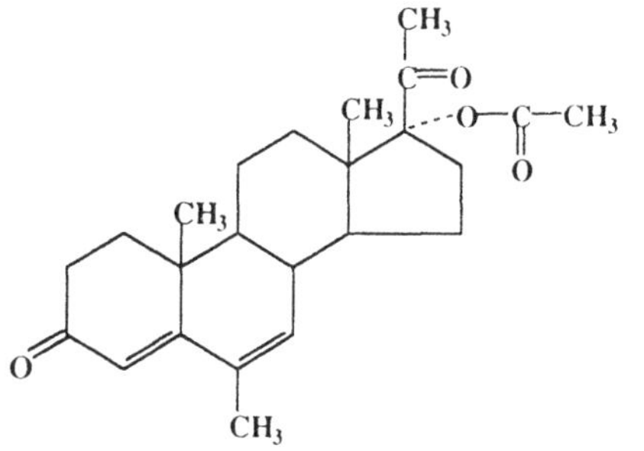

**Megestrol acetate**

**Figure 6**  Synthetic progestins used in breast cancer treatment.

There are several mechanisms by which progestins may cause their antitumor effects. They may act by binding to the PR. It is well known that a positive value of the PR predicts for a response to treatment with progestins. However, as said above, the PR may be considered a marker of a functional ER, and a positive value of PR predicts for a response to all forms of endocrine therapy. As for ER versus PR, the two receptors seem to be of equal value in predicting a response to progestins in breast cancer (56).

Progestins have been found to down-regulate the concentration of ER in the endometrium and in breast cancer cells in culture (130,131), but studies on human breast cancers do not support this hypothesis (132,133). In general, the action of progestins on breast cancer cells in vitro is restricted to cell lines expressing PR (54,134); medroxyprogesterone acetate has also been found to inhibit the growth of human mammary cancer cells lacking ER as well as PR but expressing high levels of the androgen receptor (135). In a recent study evaluating medroxyprogesterone acetate treatment in advanced breast cancer (136), expression of the androgen receptor was found to be the only parameter predicting for a response in multivariate analysis. However, as expression of the androgen receptor correlates to expression of the ER as well as the PR (137), the result needs to be interpreted carefully and should be confirmed in other studies. In vivo, progestins may deprive tumor cells of their estrogen stimulation, as progestins have been found to suppress plasma levels of estrogens in postmenopausal women by suppressing adrenal steroid synthesis. Several studies have shown megestrol acetate as well as megestrol acetate suppresses plasma estrogen levels by about 30% (77,138,139); however, ongoing studies in our department, in which we have measured plasma estrogen levels with highly sensitive radioimmunoassays, suggest medroxyprogesterone acetate 160 mg daily suppresses plasma estrogens by about 70–80%. In the endometrium, progestins inhibit the estradiol dehydrogenase responsible for converting estrone into the biologically more active estradiol (140), and the possibility exists that progestins may have similar effects on local metabolism of estrogens in tumor tissue.

In vivo studies have revealed progestins elevate plasma levels of IGF-I (141). This effect may be secondary to an increased protein binding, as recent data suggest progestins in high doses inhibit a protease degrading IGFBP-3 (78), the major IGF-binding protein in human plasma (142), in breast cancer patients. Thus, the possibility exists that progestins may reduce endocrine delivery of IGF-I (and IGF-II) to breast cancer cells in vivo. In addition, progestins have been found to down-regulate the concentration of the IGF-receptor (IGF-IR) in breast cancer cells (143).

Progestins have also been shown to inhibit P-glycoprotein (144). This effect could explain why progestins have been found to enhance the antitumor effect of chemotherapy in breast cancer patients with hormone-insensitive tumors (145).

Recently, antiprogestins have been synthesized and are currently being investigated in the treatment of breast cancer. The first antiprogestin, mifepristone (RU486, Fig. 7), which also blocks the glycocorticoid receptor (54), binds to the PR with an affinity five times higher than that of natural progesterone (53,146) and inhibits growth of PR-positive breast cancer cells in vitro (54,147). More recently, second-generation antiprogestins, including onapristone (ZK 98299) and ZK 112993, have become available (148). As progestins as well as antiprogestins inhibit cell proliferation, the possibility exists that antiprogestins could act as progesterone agonists. However, although progestins and antiprogestins both seem to inhibit cell growth in the $G_1$ phase of the cell cycle (134,149), they seem to exert their growth inhibition at different time points during this phase (150).

Pilot trials (151,152) have demonstrated antitumor effects of mifepristone in breast cancer patients, and larger studies are under way.

## RESISTANCE TO ENDOCRINE THERAPY IN BREAST CANCER

### Clinical Observations

A well-known clinical observation concerns the lack of cross-resistance to different endocrine treatment options. Several studies have reported a response rate of at least 50% to second-line endocrine treatment among patients with an acquired resistance to tamoxifen following an initial response. In contrast, second-line endocrine therapy is associated with a low (10–20%) response rate in patients not responding to tamoxifen (153–158).

Some critical comments should be made about the figures for second-line response rates. First, most of these observations relate to patients given tamoxifen as first-line therapy. Although there are reports evaluating tamoxifen as second-line therapy to aminoglutethimide (153,158,159), the number of observations is limited. What may be concluded is that the results confirm lack of cross-resistance between aminoglutethimide and tamoxifen also when aminoglutethimide is used as first-line therapy;

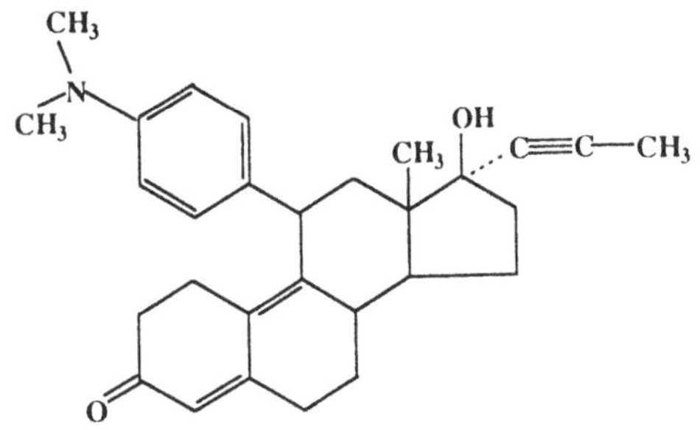

**Mifepristone (RU 3846)**

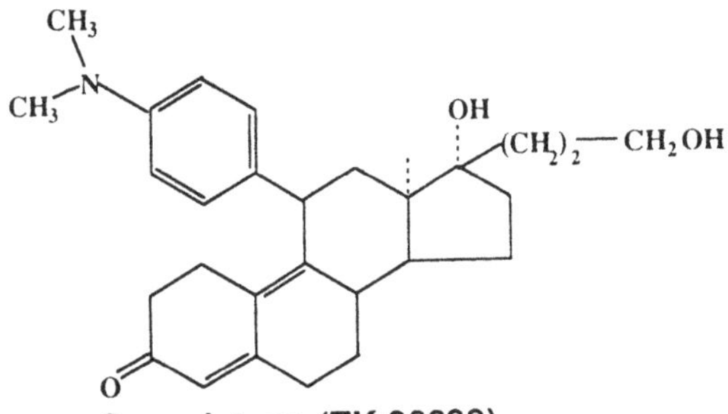

**Onapristone (ZK 98299)**

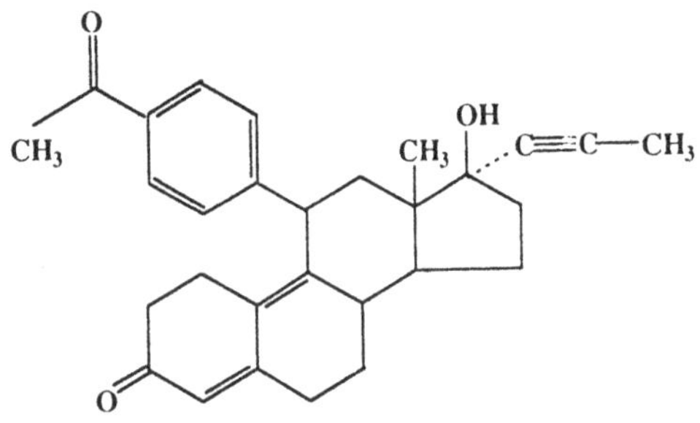

**ZK 112 993**

**Figure 7** Antiprogestins.

but whether the response to tamoxifen after aminoglutethimide is as high as the response to aminoglutethimide after tamoxifen cannot be deduced from the data available. Also, it should be noted that patients treated with second-line hormone treatment are a selected subgroup based on criteria such as slowly progressive disease, locoregional disease, or skeletal deposits that are known to be associated with a favorable response to endocrine manipulation. In the crossover studies conducted, only a limited fraction of the patients were actually crossed over to the alternative treatment option. Most likely, many patients with less favorable clinical characteristics (rapid progressive disease, visceral involvement, etc.) were excluded from second-line endocrine therapy and received chemotherapy instead. Thus, the figures of 50% and 10–20% for response rates to second-line endocrine treatment in tamoxifen responders and failures, respectively, refers to selected patient groups. However, there are reasons to believe that most clinicians are even more restrictive, offering second-line hormone therapy to patients failing on first-line endocrine treatment compared to patients responding to first-line endocrine treatment; accordingly, there is no reason to doubt that a significant difference in response rate to second-line therapy among patients failing and those responding to first-line treatment does exist.

Interestingly, a recent study reported lack of cross-resistance to tamoxifen and a steroidal, "pure" antiestrogen, ICI 182.380 (111). Clearly, some patients may respond to third- and, in some cases, fourth-line endocrine treatment (160–165). However, although acquired resistance often may be drug-specific and does not signal a general endocrine resistance, after each treatment option an increasing number of tumors will become hormone resistant, and, ultimately, all tumors progress to the stage of hormone refractoriness.

## Mechanisms of Resistance to Endocrine Treatment in Breast Cancer

Resistance to endocrine treatment may be classified as primary (or de novo) resistance and acquired resistance.

Primary resistance is characterized by either lack of response to a certain endocrine treatment regimen or an early relapse (for practical purposes, within 2 years) during adjuvant endocrine treatment. Acquired resistance is characterized by progressive disease following an initial response to a certain drug therapy. Some patients develop a late relapse years after terminating adjuvant therapy; therefore, it is not possible to deduce from the clinical behavior of their disease whether they had primary resistance or developed resistance to their adjuvant endocrine therapy, as many patients with an ER-positive breast cancer may have a late relapse as a natural course of their disease (166). If endocrine treatment was terminated some time before emergence of a relapse, patients may still be sensitive to the treatment option applied in the adjuvant setting.

Several mechanisms of resistance to endocrine therapy have been proposed, but except for the type of resistance associated with lack of the ER, there is little hard evidence suggesting any of these mechanisms are responsible for endocrine resistance in human breast carcinomas. Possible mechanisms of resistance are mutated ERs, alterations in post-ER mechanisms, alterations in the endocrine milieu or in tumor sensitivity to estrogens, changes in growth factor disposition or growth factor receptor concentrations, or alterations in the pharmacokinetics of endocrine drugs (general disposition or local metabolism in the tumor).

As for expression of ER and PR in primary breast cancers: as mentioned, 60–75% of the tumors express ER and about 60% express PR (10). Interestingly, the ratio of patients with PR-negative tumors seems to increase following different forms of endocrine therapy (167). Lack of reduction of PR in patients studied by means of sequential biopsies in relation to tamoxifen (168) may be due to induction of the receptor caused by the estrogen-agonistic effect of tamoxifen. There seems to be little reduction in the ratio of patients expressing ER (167). It is tempting to speculate that this may reflect an increased ratio of tumors expressing a biologically inactive ER, a finding that may be of relevance to development of endocrine resistance.

## Different Drugs

*Antiestrogens*

The antiestrogen tamoxifen is by far the endocrine treatment modality for which the mechanisms of endocrine resistance have been most extensively studied. Studies on tamoxifen are complicated by several factors. As mentioned above, the drug itself as well as several of its metabolites express partial estrogen antagonistic and agonistic activities; the balance between the two effects may vary according to species as well as the organ system under consideration. Although explanations of the partial estrogen agonistic activity have been offered (52,98,99), neither the phenomenon itself nor its implications for the mechanism of action or the development of resistance to tamoxifen are fully understood.

Second, tamoxifen has a complicated pharmacokinetic profile. The drug is extensively concentrated in the tissue in general, as manifested by a high steady-state volume of distribution (85), and the drug has been found in high concentrations in different tissues, including metastasis from breast cancers (169,170). The high concentration of tamoxifen in tumor tissue may not be accounted for by binding to the ER, as the molar concentration of tamoxifen by far exceeds the concentration of the receptor (85). In addition, tamoxifen and its metabolites are highly bound to plasma proteins (171,172). Assuming only the unbound fraction of tamoxifen to be biologically active, it is difficult to say which concentration of tamoxifen or its active metabolite 4-hydroxytamoxifen should be used in vitro to correspond to the biological active concentration of tamoxifen in vivo. This may have relevance to our understanding of clinical resistance to tamoxifen. A well-known phenomenon is tumor flare (acceleration of tumor-related symptoms during initiation of tamoxifen therapy) despite later objective response (173). This observation suggests that at a lower concentration, tamoxifen could stimulate the growth of tumor cells in vivo. It is noteworthy that although there is no general evidence suggesting the agonistic effect of tamoxifen dominates at particular drug concentrations, Horwitz et al. (174) found induction of the PgR (an estrogen agonistic effect of tamoxifen) occurs when tamoxifen is added at lower concentrations but not when the concentration of tamoxifen is increased. Recent findings of a lower concentration of tamoxifen in tissue from tamoxifen-resistant tumors compared to sensitive ones (see below) suggest that the concentration of the drug may be of significant importance to its antitumor effect.

Although most breast cancer cell lines lack ER and do not respond to estradiol as a mitogen, cell lines such as MCF-7 and ZR-75-1 express ER and are dependent on estrogens for growth in vitro as well as in nude mice. Stable cell line variants of ZR-75-1 and MCF-7 that still express a normal ER but are resistant to tamoxifen despite being either estrogen dependent or responsive have been characterized [see (175) for references to original works]. In general, such cell lines are sensitive to steroidal antiestrogens (176–179); however, cell lines expressing cross-resistance to tamoxifen and steroidal antiestrogens (180,181) and also cell lines resistant to steroidal antiestrogens but sensitive to tamoxifen (182) have been described. So far, we lack explanations for these observations, but interestingly Lykkesfeldt et al. (179) have shown that tamoxifen did not induce PR in a resistant cell line, contrary to what it did in the mother line, suggesting tamoxifen may not induce transcription in the resistant cell line.

Of particular interest is the observation that tamoxifen, under certain circumstances, may stimulate tumor growth. Such models have been established with growth

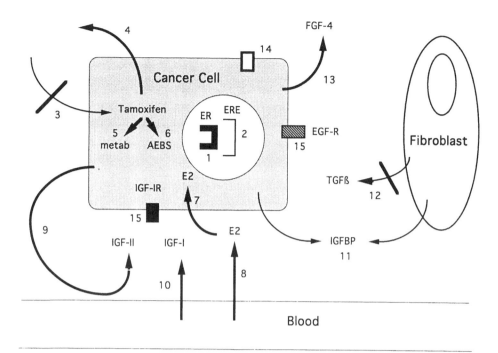

**Figure 8**  Theoretical mechanisms that may confer resistance to tamoxifen in cancer cells: (1) alterations in the ER; (2) alterations in post-ER mechanisms; (3) reduced uptake of tamoxifen in the tumor cell; (4) enhanced extrusion of tamoxifen from the tumor cell; (5) alterations in intracellular metabolism of tamoxifen; (6) an increased binding of tamoxifen to antiestrogen binding sites (AEBS); (7) failure of tamoxifen to inhibit estrogen uptake in the tumor cell; (8) increased endocrine delivery of estradiol ($E_2$) to the tumor cell due to elevation of plasma estradiol (premenopausal women); (9) loss of inhibition of the secretion of IGF-II from tumor cells; (10) escape of plasma IGF-I from the suppressive effect of tamoxifen; (11) modulation of IGF-binding proteins that might enhance the biological activity of IGF-I and -II; (12) loss of enhancement of TGF-$\beta$ secretion from fibroblasts; (13) increased expression of the fibroblast growth factor-4 (FGF-4); (14) increased expression of HER-2/neu; (15) failure of tamoxifen to down-regulate expression of IGF-IR or EGF-R.

of MCF-7 tumors in nude mice exposed over long time periods (>6 months) to treatment with tamoxifen (183,184). These tumors express ER, are stimulated by estradiol as well as by tamoxifen, but are inhibited by steroidal antiestrogens (185,186). It has been known for a long time that postmenopausal breast cancer patients treated with estrogens in pharmacological doses may experience a withdrawal response when terminating treatment (187). Similar responses have been documented in patients terminating tamoxifen treatment (188), but there is uncertainty about the frequency of such responses, as most patients terminating tamoxifen therapy because of relapse will begin a second therapeutic regimen with no time interval in-between to assess whether a withdrawal response occurs or not. Possible mechanisms of resistance to antiestrogens are depicted in Figure 8.

Alterations in the ER or Post-ER Mechanisms.   Although early studies determining ER with use of binding assays reported that tamoxifen reduced the concentration of the ER (189–192), there is now evidence that this observation may be the result of occupancy of the ER by the tamoxifen ligand yielding false-negative results. Recent studies using immunoassays (168,193,194) have not revealed any consistent influence of tamoxifen therapy on expression of the ER. Receptor measurements in human breast cancers resistant to tamoxifen have shown that a large number of these tumors still express ER (194,195), and sequential biopsies do not suggest loss of ER to be a major cause of acquired resistance to tamoxifen (194).

Although point-mutated mouse (196) as well as human (197) ERs that have a reduced sensitivity to estradiol but retain their sensitivity to tamoxifen have been characterized, point-mutated ERs sensitive to estradiol but resistant to tamoxifen have not been characterized so far (198). However, it has been shown that a single point mutation in the ER (199) can make tamoxifen act as an estrogen agonist instead of an antagonist.

Recently, a mutant ER lacking most of the ligand-binding portion of the protein and AF-2 was isolated from an ER-negative but PR-positive human breast cancer (44). In a later study, the same group found this receptor variant to be expressed also in ER+/PR+ tumors (200). Their hypothesis—that expression of this receptor may cause ligand-independent induction of transcription by the AF-1 domain on the ER—is supported by the finding that transfection of this mutant receptor into MCF-7 cells (with intact, wild-type ER) causes estrogen-independent growth and elevated expression of the PR (201). Interestingly, these MCF-7 cells were still sensitive to the steroidal antiestrogen ICI 164.384 (201). Expression of this receptor variant has been studied in a large number of tamoxifen-resistant and primary tumors (202). The mutant receptor was expressed with the same frequency in the two tumor groups. However, in the subgroup of ER-positive tumors that also expressed pS2, a higher expression of the mutant receptor was found in tamoxifen-resistant tumors compared with the primary ones. Accordingly, although this mutant ER may confer resistance to tamoxifen in some tumors, it is not likely to be responsible for resistance in the majority of breast cancers. A truncated ER-form found to inhibit binding of the wild-type ER to its cogent response element was recently identified in ER+/PR– human breast cancers (48). Thus, the possibility exists that mutant receptors may coexist with the normal ER in breast cancer and cause endocrine resistance, either by inhibiting the action of the wild-type receptor or by promoting hormone-independent growth.

Except for the studies mentioned above, few studies have evaluated ER mutations in tamoxifen-resistant breast cancers. Although several studies have reported expression of ER in tumors resistant to tamoxifen (195,203), this finding does not exclude the possibility that mutant and normal ERs may be coexpressed in the same tumor.

Turning to post-receptor mechanisms: One study showed that some tumors expressing immunoreactive ER may fail to demonstrate binding of the receptor to the DNA (204). Several possible candidates for post-receptor mechanisms causing endocrine resistance exist. Recently, Jordan's group reported overexpression of the ER-responsive element (ERE), which caused 4-hydroxytamoxifen to act as an estrogen agonist instead of an antagonist (205). Other possibilities could be alterations in proteins involved in cell cycle control. Estrogens and antiestrogens exert their effects on cell growth in the early part of the $G_1$ phase of the cell cycle (206,207). Cyclin D1, which plays a critical role for cell progression through the $G_1$ phase (208), is frequently over-expressed in breast cancers (209–211), but whether this may be related to tamoxifen resistance is currently not known.

Alterations in the Hormonal Milieu.    Tamoxifen elevates plasma levels of estradiol in premenopausal women as the result of disturbance of ovarian follicle maturation (212,213). In theory, plasma estrogens in high concentrations may compete with tamoxifen for binding to the ER in premenopausal women. However, a recent study comparing treatment with an LHRH-analogue with or without tamoxifen found no difference in response rate in the two treatment arms (214), suggesting that plasma estrogen levels in patients treated with tamoxifen may be of minor importance to the efficacy of the drug. In postmenopausal women, tamoxifen causes a slight suppression of plasma estradiol, most probably secondary to a reduced ovarian secretion of testosterone (26). In contrast, plasma estrone sulfate is slightly elevated in postmenopausal women (26). The mechanism causing this increase is unknown. However, in vitro studies have shown tamoxifen to inhibit the uptake and conversion of estrone sulfate into estradiol in tumor cells (215–218), and the increase in plasma estrone sulfate during treatment may reflect a reduced bioavailability of this estrogen conjugate. If tamoxifen exerts some of its antitumor effect by inhibiting the uptake or conversion of estrogens within the tumor cell, alterations in intratumor disposition of estradiol could make tumor cells resistant to tamoxifen. However, so far no study has addressed alterations in estrogen concentrations or estrogen uptake in tumor cells in relation to tamoxifen resistance.

Alterations in Oncogenes, Growth Factors, or Growth Factor Receptors.    Transfection of MCF-7 cells with fibroblast growth factor-4 (219) or HER-2/neu (220) has been shown to induce resistance to tamoxifen. Tamoxifen has been shown to enhance the expression of HER-2/neu in vitro (221,222). However, short-term treatment with tamoxifen has been found to suppress the expression of HER-2/neu in ER-negative breast cancers but to have no effect on HER-2/neu in ER-positive breast carcinomas (223). Interestingly, amplification or overexpression of the HER-2/neu oncogene has been shown to predict a poor prognosis in patients receiving adjuvant tamoxifen (224, 225) or adjuvant chemotherapy (224) but not in untreated patients, suggesting this growth factor is associated with primary resistance to these treatment options.

Tamoxifen has been shown to influence the disposition of several growth factors of relevance to breast cancer growth. Although the biological implications of these changes are currently not understood, it is likely that such alterations are involved in the antitumor action but also in the development of resistance to therapy. As mentioned earlier, tamoxifen has been shown to down-regulate expression of EGF-R and TGF-$\alpha$ but to enhance the secretion of TGF-$\beta$. Of particular importance could be the influence of tamoxifen on the IGF system. Most human breast cancers contain receptors for IGF (IGF-IR) (80,81) that bind IGF-I as well as IGF-II and are thought to be responsible for the mitogenic stimulus of both growth factors (226). Tamoxifen down-regulates expression of IGF-IR, inhibits secretion of IGF-II and IGF-binding proteins in tumor cells in vitro, and suppresses plasma levels of IGF-I but elevates plasma IGFBP-1. The influence of IGF-binding proteins on the local disposition of IGF-I and IGF-II is not known, as different binding proteins have been found to inhibit as well as to enhance the biological effect of the IGFs in vitro depending on the experimental conditions (142). In theory, therefore, alterations in IGF-binding proteins caused by tamoxifen treatment could enhance the biological activity of the IGFs. On the other hand, if tamoxifen exerts part of its growth-inhibitory effect on tumor cells by interacting with the IGF system, any escape of tumor cells from these effects (such as outgrowth of tumor cell clones overexpressing the IGF-IR or IGF-II) may cause tamoxifen resistance. The contribution of alterations in the IGF system to the antitumor effect as well as to resistance to tamoxifen remains to be elucidated. However, apart from the influences of tamoxifen on the disposition of the IGFs, evidence suggests that IGF-II may be directly involved as a mediator of the mitogenic response to estradiol in ER-positive tumors (227). Although no ER-positive, hormone-insensitive cell lines constitutively expressing IGF-II have been characterized, IGF-II has been found to be constitutively expressed in hormone-insensitive, ER-negative MDA-MB-231 xenografts (227). As for IGF-I, Wiseman et al. (178) have shown that tamoxifen, like estradiol, may enhance binding of IGF-I to its receptor in tamoxifen-resistant MCF-7 cells, whereas only estradiol was able to cause this effect in MCF-7 cells sensitive to the inhibitory effect of tamoxifen. More studies evaluating alterations in the IGF-system in relation to tamoxifen resistance in vitro and in vivo are required to evaluate the role of these growth factors.

Pharmacokinetic Alterations.   Although no study has compared total body pharmacokinetics of tamoxifen in patients responding to therapy and in nonresponders, studies of rodents as well as of humans have reported a lower concentration of tamoxifen in tumors resistant to tamoxifen compared with tumors responding to treatment (228–230). An increased expression of P-glycoprotein in human breast cancers not responding to tamoxifen treatment has been reported (231), but these investigators did not measure the concentration of tamoxifen in the tumors. On the other hand, low concentration of tamoxifen in rodent tumors resistant to tamoxifen has been reported not to be associated with expression of the P-glycoprotein (232).

Another mechanism that could be responsible for tumor resistance is alterations in tamoxifen metabolism, with an increased production of estrogen agonistic metabolites. One study reported an increased concentration of such metabolites (metabolite E and bisphenol) in human breast cancers resistant to tamoxifen therapy (233). Another metabolite of potential interest is 4-hydroxytamoxifen. Similar to tamoxifen, 4-hydroxytamoxifen exists as a *cis*- and a *trans*-optical isomer. *Trans*-4-hydroxytamoxifen is a most potent antiestrogen, considered to be responsible for the antiestrogenic action of tamoxifen in vivo; the *cis*- form is a weak estrogen agonist/antagonist (234,235). One of the groups that reported a reduced concentration of tamoxifen in resistant tumors also found a reduced concentration of *cis*- as well as *trans*-4-hydroxytamoxifen; in addition, they found an increase in the *cis/trans*-4-hydroxytamoxifen ration in MCF-7 xenografts whose growth was stimulated by tamoxifen, as well as in human breast cancers resistant to tamoxifen therapy (228,229). They suggested that an increase in the *cis/trans*- ratio of this metabolite might cause an increase in the estrogen agonistic effect of tamoxifen and that this could be responsible for tamoxifen-stimulated tumor growth. However, Dr. Jordan's group has shown that non-isomerable antiestrogens may also stimulate the growth of tamoxifen-resistant MCF-7 xenografts in nude mice (236), suggesting alterations in the isomerization of metabolites may not be the mechanism responsible for tumor growth in this model. In a recent study, the San Antonio group reported tamoxifen stimulated growth of MCF-7 tumors in nude mice in a dose-dependent manner with no evidence of an increase in the *cis/trans*- ratio for 4-hydroxytamoxifen (237). Accordingly, further studies are required to determine the role of alterations in intracellular drug disposition as possible mechanisms of resistance to antiestrogens.

A third possibility is alterations in intracellular distribution of tamoxifen. Thus, Pavlik et al. (100) reported an exceptionally high concentration of antiestrogen binding sites in a cell line sensitive to estradiol but resistant to tamoxifen. The possibility exists that these binding sites may act as scavengers, preventing tamoxifen from binding to the ER.

*Estrogen Deprivation*

Alterations in Tumor Sensitivity to Estrogen Stimulation.   Cell lines such as MCF-7 and ZR-75-1 are dependent on estrogens to maintain their growth; recently, however, sublines that do not depend on estrogens for their growth but express ER and are still able to respond to estradiol as a mitogenic stimulus have been developed (180, 238). Thus, breast cancer cells are able to adapt to alterations in their endocrine environment in vitro. In vivo, estrogens are known to stimulate tumor growth in pre- as well as postmenopausal women despite a considerable difference in plasma estradiol levels in the two groups. Considering possible mechanisms of primary resistance to estrogen deprivation in ER-positive tumors, two possibilities exist. For unknown reasons, ER-positive tumor cells may be hormone resistant and therefore not dependent on estrogens for their growth. The other possibility is that different tumors need estrogens in different concentrations to sustain their growth and that the estrogen concentration following castration or during treatment with an aromatase inhibitor may still be sufficient to stimulate the growth of some cancers. Regarding acquired resistance, the possibility exists that individual tumors may change their sensitivity to estrogens in response to alterations in their endocrine environment. To evaluate these hypothesis, two questions have to be addressed. First, is there any evidence that patients who do not respond to estrogen deprivation (primary resistant patients) may respond to a further lowering of their plasma estrogen levels? Second, is there evidence that patients who respond to estrogen deprivation may achieve a second response to further estrogen deprivation on relapse?

In answer to the first question, indirect evidence supports a theory of a dose-response relationship between the degree of estrogen deprivation and the chance of achieving a clinical response to therapy. It is well known that treatment with different drugs acting on adrenal or ovarian steroid synthesis—such as LHRH-analogues, ketoconazole, trilostane, glucocorticoids administered in low doses, and low-potent aromatase inhibitors such as testololactone—may all cause a modest suppression of plasma estrogens in postmenopausal women and a low, but significant, response rate [see (239) for references to original works]. Also, there is direct evidence that some patients who have not responded to one type of estrogen deprivation may respond to a more aggressive therapy. Thus, Murray and Pitt (240) found four of 17 patients who did not respond to aminoglutethimide 250 mg daily, a regimen commonly used in breast cancer (241), did achieve an objective response when the dose was escalated to 1000 mg daily. While aminoglutethimide 250 mg daily is effective in inhibiting in vivo aromatization (242), aminoglutethimide also suppresses plasma estrogen levels by enhancing the metabolism of estrone sulfate (243,244), and this effect is dose dependent (245). In a pilot study, we have shown that patients who do not respond to treatment with the steroidal aromatase inhibitor formestane may achieve further suppression of their plasma estrogen levels and, in some cases, a clinical response, by having aminoglutethimide added in concert (246). So far no study has compared response rate and duration of response in premenopausal patients treated with castration plus an aromatase inhibitor with castration alone.

Turning to the second question, many patients treated with aromatase inhibitors have previously undergone castration for their breast cancer. However, the majority of such patients have received other forms of endocrine therapy (mainly antiestrogens, but also progestins) between their castration and treatment with an aromatase inhibitor; therefore, the effect of further estrogen deprivation at the time of progression after castration cannot be assessed. Except for a pilot trial evaluating formestane as second-line therapy after relapse during treatment with an LHRH-analogue (goserelin), the response rate to treatment with an aromatase inhibitor as second-line therapy following castration has not been reported. In this study, four of six patients who progressed after an initial response to treatment with goserelin achieved a second objective response when formestane was added in concert (247). It has also been shown that patients who have previously been treated with adrenalectomy or hypophysectomy may respond to further estrogen suppression with the aromatase inhibitor aminoglutethimide; responses to aminoglutethimide were seen among patients previously responding to the surgical procedures but also among previous nonresponders (248).

Two important conclusions may be drawn from these observations. First, primary resistance to estrogen deprivation seems to some extent to be a dose-related phenomenon. However, it is not known whether there may be any "threshold" value for which the optimal response rate is achieved. Future studies with novel, highly potent aromatase inhibitors will address this question. Second, some patients may achieve a stepwise response to estrogen deprivation with a second response to further estrogen suppression on relapse. This observation supports the hypothesis that progression following an initial response to estrogen deprivation may be the result of adaptation of the tumor to a "new" hormonal environment, probably through selection of cellular clones that may be growth-stimulated by estradiol at a concentration that was not able to stimulate growth of the majority of tumor cells at the time of remission. Little is known about possible mechanisms that could be responsible for such an alteration. No study has evaluated alterations in tumor characteristics after castration. Considering estrogen deprivation with use of aromatase inhibitors, neither short-term (194) nor long-term (249) treatment with such drugs has been shown to produce significant alterations in the ER expression in breast cancers. However, more studies are required to evaluate alterations in biological parameters in breast cancers treated with estrogen deprivation.

On the other hand, there may be alternative explanations for these findings. Patients who progress during treatment with aminoglutethimide have been shown to respond to pituitary ablation (250) but also to treatment with formestane (251); neither of these treatment options is considered to be more effective in suppressing plasma estrogens compared to aminoglutethimide (123,252). Also, it should be recognized that alterations in the endocrine milieu relate to plasma hormone levels. Given the findings (30) that estrogen concentrations do not seem to differ much in tumor tissue obtained from pre- and postmenopausal women, the possibility exists that alterations in plasma estrogen concentrations caused by castration may not be accompanied by similar alterations in the concentration of estrogens in tumor tissue.

Alterations in Hormone Disposition.   For unknown reasons, peripheral aromatization seems to be somewhat higher in postmenopausal women than in premenopausal women (253). Although glucocorticoids as well as growth factors have been shown to influence the aromatase enzyme in fibroblasts in culture (254,255), little is known about mechanisms influencing the aromatase enzyme in vivo. No study has evaluated plasma estrogen levels over time in patients treated with surgical or radiological castration. A recent study reported an increase in plasma estrogen levels over a period of 2 years in patients after initiation of treatment with an LHRH-analogue (247). Although the increase was moderate, and plasma levels did not approach what is seen in premenopausal women, the possibility exists that this could be of importance in stimulating the growth of cancer cells in some patients. One study reported a slight increase in plasma levels of estrone in patients on aminoglutethimide therapy at time of relapse (256). However, this increase is likely to be secondary to a concomitant increase in plasma levels of adrenal steroids, which could be a nonspecific stress response to worsening of their disease. No study has determined in vivo aromatization in patients who progress following an initial response to an aromatase inhibitor. It is noteworthy that although several studies have evaluated total body estrogen synthesis and plasma estrogen levels in patients treated with different aromatase inhibitors, little is known about the influence of hormone treatment on intratumor estrogen levels. Only one study, including six patients (257), has determined tumor estrogen levels in relation to treatment with an aromatase inhibitor. Thus, the possibility of alterations in estrogen disposition within the tumor tissue at the time of progression cannot be ruled out.

Alterations in Local Aromatase Activity in Breast Cancers. A possible explanation of resistance to aromatase inhibitors is mutations in the aromatase gene in tumor cells (Fig. 9). Miller has investigated the influence of different aromatase inhibitors on in vitro aromatization in human breast cancer biopsies. He has shown that the aromatase enzyme in some tumors has a reduced sensitivity to the inhibitory action of formestane despite a normal sensitivity to nonsteroidal aromatase inhibitors such as aminoglutethimide and fadrazole (258). Formestane is a so-called type I inhibitor, binding to the substrate-binding site on the aromatase enzyme, whereas aminoglutethimide and fadrazole are type II inhibitors, binding to the catalytic site (259). Site mutations in the cDNA have been shown to produce aromatase enzyme variants with a reduced sensitivity to formestane but not to aminoglutethimide (260). So far, however, analysis of human breast cancers that have a reduced sensitivity to formestane in vitro has not demonstrated mutations in the aromatase enzyme (249).

Another interesting possibility is overexpression of the normal aromatase enzyme in breast carcinomas. MCF-7 cells following transfection show an increased growth rate in steroid-free medium and a pronounced enhancement of growth in response to androgens (261). This response was inhibited by the nonsteroidal aromatase inhibitor fadrazole. Measurement of aromatase activity in human breast cancer samples obtained before and during treatment with aromatase inhibitors has revealed that treatment with aminoglutethimide (262) but not formestane (128) increases the aromatase activity by a factor of 2 to 75. This phenomenon may not necessarily be related to the enzyme-inhibitory effect of aminoglutethimide. Aminoglutethimide is a well-known inducer of mixed function oxidases (263), and the possibility exists that it may also induce the aromatase enzyme. In addition, aminoglutethimide is usually administered in concert with glucocorticoids (241)—and glucocorticoids have been shown to induce expression of the aromatase in fibroblasts in vitro (254). Treatment with aminoglutethimide plus glucocorticoids is not likely to have a similar influence on the extraglandular aromatase in general, as tracer studies have shown this drug regimen

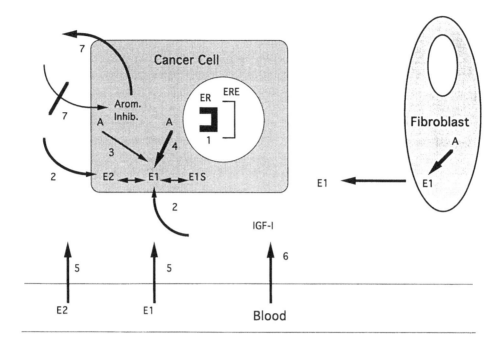

**Figure 9** Possible mechanisms that might cause resistance to aromatase inhibitors in breast cancer cells: (1) alterations in the sensitivity of the tumor cell to estrogens; (2) increased sensitivity of tumor cells to low estrogen concentrations due to enhanced uptake of estrogens in the cells; (3) mutant aromatase enzyme not inhibited by the aromatase inhibitor; (4) increased expression of the normal aromatase enzyme in the tumor cell or in fibroblasts; (5) increase in plasma estrogen levels; (6) increased delivery of IGF-I; (7) reduced uptake or enhanced extrusion of drug from the tumor cell.

inhibits total body aromatization by more than 90% (118,249). This finding, however, does not refute the hypothesis that aminoglutethimide as well as other aromatase inhibitors could influence local aromatase activity in the tumor. Growth factors may influence aromatase activity (255). Tumor cells as well as fibroblasts in the tumor cell vicinity secrete growth factors, and drugs could influence local aromatase activity indirectly by interacting with growth factors. Thus, the finding of O'Neil et al. (264) and Reed et al. (255) that benign breast tissue obtained in the vicinity of breast carcinomas expresses a higher aromatase activity than tissue obtained elsewhere in the breast may be consistent with a hypothesis that tumor cells could modulate aromatase activity in normal tissue. However, others could not confirm this observation (265).

Whatever the mechanisms might be, a differential effect of different aromatase inhibitors on intratumor aromatase is probably the most likely explanation for the findings of Murray and Pitt (251) that patients who become resistant to aminoglutethimide may subsequently respond to treatment with formestane.

*Alterations in Growth Factors or Growth Factor Receptors.* Treatment with aminoglutethimide causes a moderate elevation in plasma levels of IGF-I (78). Two studies (78,141) of formestane found this drug to have no influence on plasma levels of IGF-I. However, one study (266) reported long-term treatment with formestane 500 mg (but not 250 mg) every second week elevated plasma levels of IGF-I. Further studies are warranted to address the influence of different aromatase inhibitors on the IGF system in relation to drug response and emergence of drug resistance.

Pharmacokinetic Alterations. Aminoglutethimide is a well-known inducer of mixed-function oxidases. The drug has been shown to induce its own metabolism (267, 268) as well as the metabolism of several other xenobiotics (269). However, this enzyme induction seems to be fully developed within 2 weeks of treatment (270). Noteworthy, studies of plasma pharmacokinetics of aminoglutethimide in patients on chronic treatment did not reveal any significant alterations in drug disposition over time (268), and alterations in drug metabolism are not likely to be responsible for acquired resistance to aminoglutethimide. On the other hand, aminoglutethimide enhances the metabolism of tamoxifen and progestins (271–273), and it is likely that a suboptimal plasma concentration of these drugs may explain why administration of tamoxifen or a progestin together with aminoglutethimide does not improve the response rate compared to single drug therapy (274–279).

As for other aromatase inhibitors, except for drugs belonging to the "aminoglutethimide class," such as rogletimide (280), there is no evidence suggesting that any of these drugs may stimulate enzymes involved in drug metabolism. However, so far no study has evaluated the pharmacokinetics of any of these drugs over time and in relation to treatment response. Nor has there been any study evaluating tissue concentrations in normal tissue or breast cancer tissue in particular.

Another possibility is local alterations in the disposition of aromatase inhibitors at the tumor level. Thus, a reduced uptake or enhanced extrusion of formestane from the tumor cells could explain the observation of Miller (258), discussed above, that this drug has little effect on the aromatase enzyme in some tumors (258). However, the author did not measure drug concentration in his tissue samples. Except for a pilot study measuring the concentration of formestane in tumor tissue after short-term treatment (257), no study has evaluated the concentration of any aromatase inhibitor in tumor tissue.

*Progestins and Antiprogestins*

As mentioned above, a major problem in studying the influence of progestins on breast cancer is the uncertainties about the mechanism of action of these drugs in vivo. In particular, this relates to the question whether direct PgR-mediated effects are involved in the antitumor action of progestins in vivo or whether they may exert their effect indirectly by influencing the disposition of estrogens or IGF-I.

If depriving the tumor cell of the biologically active estradiol (by suppressing total estrogens or through alterations in local hormone disposition) is pivotal to the antitumor action of progestins, one might anticipate a high degree of cross-resistance to progestins and aromatase inhibitors. However, as mentioned above, there is not complete cross-resistance to treatment with different aromatase inhibitors, and the possibility exists that there may be cross-resistance to treatment with progestins and some aromatase inhibitors but not others. Some authors have suggested cross-resistance to treatment with progestins and the aromatase inhibitor aminoglutethimide (281); others (163,282) have reported lack of cross-resistance. It is well known that some patients may respond to third-line endocrine treatment—which, in most cases, means that they will have either an aromatase inhibitor followed by a progestin or a progestin followed by an aromatase inhibitor as second- and third-line treatment, respectively (162,164). The conclusion that may be drawn at this stage is that there is not complete cross-resistance between aromatase inhibitors and progestins, but data are too sparse to provide a reasonable estimate about the response rate to third-line treatment and to address whether a partial cross-resistance may exist.

So far there are no data available to evaluate cross-resistance between antiprogestins and other endocrine treatment modalities.

Alterations in the Steroid Receptors or Post-Receptor Mechanisms.   The human mammary carcinoma cell line T-47D is much used to study the effects of progestins and antiprogestins on cell growth in vitro. This cell line contains the ER in low concentration but high concentrations of the PR. As mentioned above, progestins are found to inhibit the growth of T-47D cells, although in some experiments they have been found to stimulate growth.

Contrary to what is the case for the ER, up to now no mutant PRs have been identified.

There is little evidence suggesting resistance to progestins may be caused by loss of PR. Down-regulation of PR with retinoic acid has been described to reduce sensitivity to progestins in T-47D cells (283); resistance to progestins has also been described in cell lines still harboring PR at a concentration moderately reduced compared to the mother cell lines (284,285).

Recent studies have brought new insight into the mechanistic action of the PR. It is now clear that PR exists in two normal variants, named A and B (57). The receptor undergoes dimerization, and, in addition to A/A and B/B homodimers, A/B heterodimers are found. Studies of progesterone antagonists have revealed important differences in the physiological action of the different receptor forms. It is now clear that under certain conditions, antiprogestins may behave like progesterone agonists. This ability is restricted to binding to the type B receptor (58,286). Interestingly, this agonistic effect seems to be enhanced by cAMP (286). Although these observations may be of significance in relation to resistance to antiprogestins, and probably also to progestins, further in vitro studies as well as clinical studies are required to assess the biochemical and the clinical profiles of resistance to these drugs.

Alterations in Growth Factors or Growth Factor Receptors.   Progestins have been found to increase the concentration of mRNA for EGF as well as TGF-α but to down-regulate mRNA for TGF-β in T-47D cells (149,287,288). Also, progestins have been found to increase the concentration of the EGF receptor (289). These effects may all be detrimental, as EGF as well as TGF-α may stimulate growth of breast cancer cells through binding to the EGFR. As mentioned earlier, progestins may influence the disposition of IGF-I in vivo but also down-regulate the concentration of IGF-IR, the receptor mediating the growth-stimulating effects of IGF-I and IGF-II on breast cancer cells. So far, alterations in these growth factors have not been compared in patients responding and those not responding to progestin therapy. Neither have they been studied over time in relation to development of acquired resistance.

Pharmacokinetic Alterations.   Progestins—in particular, medroxyprogesterone acetate—are poorly absorbed. Although the exact bioavailability is not known either for medroxyprogesterone acetate or for megestrol acetate, the former, given as a dose of 1000 mg daily, produces plasma concentrations that are only 30–50% of the plasma concentration of megestrol acetate when this drug is administered as a dose of 160 mg daily (271,290,291). Plasma pharmacokinetics suggest a high concentration of the drugs in the tissue (85), and studies in rodents suggest the drug may be concentrated selectively in certain tissues, such as breast cancer tissue (292). The disposition may be critical to the antitumor activity of progestins, inasmuch as a "threshold" level of a mean plasma concentration of 100–150 $\mu$g/L has been suggested as a requirement to achieve optimal antitumor effects of these drugs (293). However, other investigators (294) could not confirm this observation. So far no study has evaluated possible alterations in plasma pharmacokinetics of progestins in relation to the development of drug resistance or measured intratumor concentration of progestins in tumors resistant to progestin therapy.

## SUMMARY AND CONCLUSION

Although recent studies have brought new insight into the biological effects of endocrine therapy, the problem of resistance to endocrine therapy is still poorly understood. The field studied most extensively so far is resistance to antiestrogens. Several possible explanations have been offered during recent years, but as of yet, studies on human breast tumors have not provided an explanation for drug resistance in the majority of ER-positive tumors. Considering possible mechanisms of resistance to estrogen deprivation and to treatment with progestins and antiprogestins, this field suffers from a general lack of information about alterations in tumor biological parameters in relation to treatment. Treatment with progestins has been found to influence growth factors such as EGF and TGF-$\alpha$, but the impact of these alterations on the antitumor effect of the drugs is not known. Clearly, there is a need for more investigations into the effects of these drugs at the molecular level and, in particular, to study cell lines selected for resistance to progestins and antiprogestins to achieve knowledge about the biochemical alterations associated with drug resistance. In addition, clinical studies evaluating cross-resistance to treatment options such as steroidal antiestrogens and aromatase inhibitors, or to progestins versus antiprogestins, may provide important information for a better understanding of the mechanisms of resistance.

## ACKNOWLEDGMENTS

The secretarial assistance of Mrs. H. Hjortung and Mrs. Y. Hornsleth is highly appreciated.

## REFERENCES

1. Muir C, Waterhouse J, Mack T, Powell J, Whelan S. Cancer incidence in five continents. Vol 5. IARC Scientific Publication. Lyon: International Agency for Research on Cancer, 1988.
2. Harris JR, Morrow M, Bonadonna G. Cancer of the breast. In: De Vita, et al., eds. Cancer, Principles and Practice of Oncology. 4th ed. Philadelphia: Lippincott, 1993:1264–1332.

3. Beatson GT. On the treatment of inoperable cases of carcinoma of the mamma. Suggestions for a new method of treatment, with illustrative cases. Lancet 1896; 2:104–107.

4. Dao TL, Huggins C. Bilateral adrenalectomy in the treatment of cancer of the breast. Arch Surg 1955; 71:645–657.

5. Luft R, Olivecrona H, Sjøgren B. Hypophysectomy in man. Nord Med 1953; 47:351.

6. Zondek B. The effect of prolonged administration of estrogen on the uterus and the anterior pituitary of human beings. JAMA 1940; 114:1850–1854.

7. Kofman S, Nagamani D, Buenger RE, Taylor SG. The use of prednisolone in the treatment of disseminated breast carcinoma. Cancer 1958; 11:226–232.

8. De Nosaquo N. Androgens and estrogens in the treatment of disseminated mammary carcinoma. Retrospective study of nine hundred fourty-four patients. JAMA 1960; 172:1271–1283.

9. Cole MP, Jones CTA, Todd IDH. A new anti-oestrogenic agent in late breast cancer. An early clinical appraisal of ICI 146474. Br J Cancer 1971; 25:270–275.

10. McGuire WL. Steroid receptors in human breast cancer. Cancer Res 1978; 38:4289–4291.

11. Early Breast Cancer Trialists' Collaborative Group. Systemic treatment of early breast cancer by hormonal, cytotoxic, or immune therapy—Part 1. Lancet 1992; 339:1–15.

12. Early Breast Cancer Trialists' Collaborative Group. Systemic treatment of early breast cancer by hormonal, cytotoxic, or immune therapy—Part 2. Lancet 1992; 339:71–85.

13. Lønning PE, Dowsett M, Powles TJ. Postmenopausal estrogen synthesis and metabolism: alterations caused by aromatase inhibitors used for the treatment of breast cancer. J Steroid Biochem 1990; 35:355–366.

14. Schweikert HU, Milewich L, Wilson JD. Aromatization of androstenedione by isolated human hairs. J Clin Endocrinol Metab 1975; 40:413–417.

15. Schweikert HU, Milewich L, Wilson JD. Aromatization of androstenedione by cultured human fibroblasts. J Clin Endocrinol Metab 1976; 43:785–795.

16. Smuk M, Schwers J. Aromization of androstenedione by human adult liver in vitro. J Clin Endocrinol Metab 1977; 45:1001–1012.

17. Perel E, Killinger DW. The interconversion and aromatization of androgens by human adipose tissue. J Steroid Biochem 1979; 10:623–627.

18. Matsumine H, Hirato K, Yanaihara T, Tamada T, Yoshida M. Aromatization by skeletal muscle. J Clin Endocrinol Metab 19876; 63:717–720.

19. Frisch RE, Canick JA, Tulchinsky D. Human fatty marrow aromatizes androgen to estrogen. J Clin Endocrinol Metab 1980; 51:395–396.

20. Vermeulen A. The hormonal activity of the postmenopausal ovary. J Clin Endocrinol Metab 1976; 42:247–253.

21. Sluijmer AV, Heineman MA, de Jong FH, Evers JLH. Endocrine activity of the postmenopausal ovary: the effects of pituitary down-regulation and oophorectomy. J Clin Endocrinol Metab 1995; 80:2163–2167.

22. Abul-Haji YJ, Iverson R, Kiand DT. Aromatization of androgens by human breast cancer. Steroids 1979; 33:205–222.

23. Bolufer P, Ricart E, Lluch A, et al. Aromatase activity and estradiol in human breast cancer: its relationship to estradiol and epidermal growth factor receptors and to tumor-node-metastasis staging. J Clin Oncol 1992; 10:438–446.

24. Silva MC, Rowlands MG, Dowsett M, et al. Intratumoral aromatase as a prognostic factor in human breast cancer. Cancer Res 1989; 49:2588–2591.

25. Lønning PE, Helle SI, Johannessen DC, et al. Relations between sex hormones, sex hormone binding globulin, insulin-like growth factor-I and insulin-like growth factor binding protein-1 in postmenopausal breast cancer patients. Clin Endocrinol 1995; 42:23–30.

26. Lønning PE, Johannessen DC, Adlercreutz H, Lien EA, Ekse D. Influence of tamoxifen on sex hormones, gonadotrophins and sex hormone binding globulin, in postmenopausal breast cancer patients. J Steroid Biochem Mol Biol 1995; 52:491–496.

27. Santner SJ, Leszcynski D, Wright C, et al. Estrone sulfate: a potential source of estradiol in human breast cancer tissue. Breast Cancer Res Treat 1986; 7:35–44.

28. Beranek PA, Folkerd EJ, Ghilchik MW, James VHT. 17-beta-hydroxysteroid dehydrogenase and aromatase activity in breast fat from women with benign and malignant breast tumours. Clin Endocrinol 1984; 20:205–212.

29. Millington D, Jenner DA, Jones T, Griffiths K. Endogenous steroid concentration in human breast tumours determined by high-resolution mass fragmentography. Biochem J 1974; 139: 473–475.

30. Van Landeghem AAJ, Poortman J, Nabuurs M, Thijssen JHH. Endogenous concentration and subcellular distribution of estrogens in normal and malignant human breast tissue. Cancer Res 1985; 45:2900–2906.

31. Vermeulen A, Deslypere JP, Paridaens R, Laclercq G, Roy F, Heuson JC. Aromatase, 17β-hydroxysteroid dehydrogenase and intratissular sex hormone concentration in cancerous and normal glandular breast tissue in postmenopausal women. Eur J Cancer Clin Oncol 1986; 22:515–525.

32. Jensen EV, Block GE, Smith S, Kyser K, DeSombre ER. Estrogen receptors and breast cancer response to adrenalectomy. Natl Cancer Inst Monogr 1971; 34:55–70.

33. Block GE, Ellis RS, DeSombre E, Jensen E. Correlation of estrophilin content of primary mammary cancer to eventual endocrine treatment. Ann Surg 1978; 188:372–376.

34. Osborne CK, Yochmowitz MG, Knight WA, McGuire WL. The value of estrogen and progesterone receptors in the treatment of breast cancer. Cancer 1980; 46:2884–2888.

35. Ravdin PM, Green S, Melink Dorr T, et al. Prognostic significance of progesterone receptor levels in estrogen receptor-positive patients with metastatic breast cancer treated with tamoxifen: results of a prospective Southwest Oncology Group study. J Clin Oncol 1992; 10: 1284–1291.

36. Horwitz KB, McGuire WL, Pearson OH, Segaloff A. Predicting response to endocrine therapy in human breast cancer: a hypothesis. Science 1975; 189:726–727.

37. Kumar V, Green S, Staub A, Chambon P. Localisation of the oestradiol-binding and putative DNA-binding domains of the human oestrogen receptor. EMBO Journal 1986; 5:2231–2236.

38. Kumar V, Green S, Stack G, Berry M, Jin JR, Chambon P. Functional domains of the human estrogen receptor. Cell 1987; 51:941–951.

39. Kumar V, Chambon P. The estrogen receptor binds tightly to its responsive elements as a ligand-induced homodimer. Cell 1988; 55:145–156.

40. Klinge CM, Bambara RA, Hilf R. Antiestrogen-liganded estrogen receptor interaction with estrogen responsive element DNA in vitro. J Steroid Biochem Mol Biol 1992; 43:249–262.

41. Webster NJG, Green S, Jin JR, Chambon P. The hormone-binding domains of the estrogen and glucocorticoid receptors contain an inducible transcription activation function. Cell 1988; 54:199–207.

42. Lees JA, Fawell SE, Parker MG. Identification of two transactivation domains in the mouse oestrogen receptor. Nucleic Acids Res 1989; 17:5477–5488.

43. Tora L, White J, Brou C, et al. The human estrogen receptor has two independent nonacidic transcriptional activation functions. Cell 1989; 59:477–487.

44. Fuqua SA, Fitzgerald SD, Chamness GC, et al. Variant human breast tumor estrogen receptor with constitutive transcriptional activity. Cancer Res 1991; 51:105–109.

45. Garcia T, Lehrer S, Bloomer W, Schachter B. A variant estrogen receptor messenger ribonucleic acid is associated with reduced levels of estrogen binding in human mammary tumors. Mol Endocrinol 1988; 2:785–791.

46. Murphy LC, Dotzlaw H. Variant estrogen receptor mRNA species detected in human breast cancer biopsy samples. Mol Endocrinol 1989; 3:687–693.

47. Scott GK, Kushner P, Vigne J-I, Benz CC. Truncated forms of DNA-binding estrogen receptors in human breast cancer. J Clin Invest 1991; 88:700–706.

48. Fuqua SAW, Fitzgerald SD, Allred DC, et al. Inhibition of estrogen receptor action by a naturally occurring variant in human breast tumors. Cancer Res 1992; 52:483–486.

49. Sutherland RL, Murphy LC, Foo MS, Green MD, Whybourne AM. High-affinity antioestrogen binding site distinct from the oestrogen receptor. Nature 1980; 288:273–275.

50. Leo G, Cappiello G, Poltronieri P, et al. Tamoxifen binding sites heterogeneity in breast cancer: a comparative study with steroid hormone receptors. Eur J Cancer 1991; 27:452–456.

51. Brandes LJ, Bogdanovic RP. New evidence that the antiestrogen binding site may be a novel growth-promoting histamine receptor (H3) which mediates the antiestrogenic and antiproliferative effects of tamoxifen. Biochem Biophys Res Commun 1986; 134:601–608.

52. Hedden A, Müller V, Jensen EV. A new interpretation of antiestrogen action. Ann NY Acad Sci. In press.

53. Horwitz KB. The antiprogestin RU 38486: receptor-mediated progestin versus antiprogestin actions screened in the estrogen insensitive T-47Dco human breast cancer cells. Endocrinology 1985; 116:2236–2245.

54. Bardon S, Vignon F, Chalbos D, Rochefort H. RU486, a progestin and glucocorticoid antagonist, inhibits the growth of breast cancer cells via the progesterone receptor. J Clin Endocrinol Metab 1985; 50:692–697.

55. Hissom JR, Moore MR. Progestin effects on growth in the human breast cancer cell line T-47D—possible therapeutic implications. Biochem Biophys Res Commun 1987; 145:706–709.

56. Lundgren S. Progestins in breast cancer treatment. A review. Acta Oncol 1992; 31:709–722.

57. Horwitz KB. The molecular biology of RU486. Is there a role for antiprogestins in the treatment of breast cancer? Endocr Rev 1992; 13:146–163.

58. Tung L, Mohamed KM, Hoeffler JP, Takimoto GS, Horwitz KB. Antagonist-occupied human progesterone B-receptors activate transcription without binding to progesterone response elements, and are dominantly inhibited by A-receptors. Mol Endocrinol 1993; 7:1256–1265.

59. Allegra JC, Lippman ME, Thompson EB, et al. Relationship between the progesterone, androgen, and glucocorticoid receptor and response rate to endocrine therapy in metastatic breast cancer. Cancer Res 1979; 39:1973–1979.

60. Søreide JA, Lea OA, Varhaug JE, Skarstein A, Kvinnsland S. Androgen receptors in operable breast cancer: relation to other steroid hormone receptors, correlations to prognostic factors and predictive value for effect of adjuvant tamoxifen treatment. Eur J Surg Oncol 1992; 18:112–118.

61. Poulin R, Baker D, Labrie F. Androgens inhibit basal and estrogen-induced cell proliferation in the ZR-75-1 human breast cancer cell line. Breast Cancer Res Treat 1988; 12:213–225.

62. Davois S, Li S, Martel C, et al. Inhibitory effect of androgens on DMBA-induced mammary carcinoma in the rat. Breast Cancer Res Treat 1989; 14:299–306.

63. Sedlacek SM. An overview of megestrol acetate for the treatment of advanced breast cancer. Semin Oncol 1988; 15(suppl):3–13.

64. Tormey DC, Lippman ME, Edwards BK, Cassidy JG. Evaluation of tamoxifen doses with and without fluoxymesterone in advanced breast cancer. Ann Intern Med 1983; 98:139–144.

65. Rubens RD, Tinson CL, Coleman RE, et al. Prednisolone improves the response to primary endocrine treatment for advanced breast cancer. Br J Cancer 1988; 58:626–630.

66. Seibert K, Shafie SM, Triche TJ, et al. Clonal variation of MCF-7 breast cancer cells in vitro and in athymic nude mice. Cancer Res 1983; 43:2223–2239.

67. Brünner N, Svenstrup B, Spang-Thomsen M, Bennett P, Nielsen A, Nielsen J. Serum steroid levels in intact and endocrine ablated BALB/c nude mice and their intact littermates. J Steroid Biochem 1986; 25:429–432.

68. Furr BJA, Jordan VC. The pharmacology and clinical uses of tamoxifen. Pharmacol Ther 1984; 25:127–205.

69. Yee D, Cullen KJ, Paik S, et al. Insulin-like growth factor II mRNA expression in human breast cancer. Cancer Res 1988; 48:6691–6696.

70. Cullen KJ, Yee D, Bates SE, et al. Regulation of human breast cancer by secreted growth factors. Acta Oncologica 1989; 28:835–839.

71. McGuire WL Jr, Jackson JG, Figueroa JA, Shimasaki S, Powell DR, Yee D. Regulation of insulin-like growth factor-binding protein (IGFBP) expression by breast cancer cells: use of IGFBP-1 as an inhibitor of insulin-like growth factor action. J Natl Cancer Inst 1992; 84: 1336–1341.

72. Coutts A, Murphy LJ, Murphy LC. Regulation of IGF-binding proteins by progestins and antiestrogens in T-47D human breast cancer cells (abstr). Proc Am Assoc Cancer Res 1993; 34:93.

73. Colletti RB, Roberts JD, Devlin JT, Copeland KC. Effect of tamoxifen on plasma insulin-like growth factor I in patients with breast cancer. Cancer Res 1989; 49:1882–1884.

74. Lønning PE, Hall K, Aakvaag A, Lien EA. Influence of tamoxifen on plasma levels of insulin-like growth factor I and insulin-like growth factor binding protein I in breast cancer patients. Cancer Res 1992; 52:4719–4723.

75. Lahti EI, Knip M, Laatikainen TJ. Plasma insulin-like growth factor I and its binding proteins 1 and 3 in postmenopausal patients with breast cancer receiving long term tamoxifen. Cancer 1994; 74:618–624.

76. Butta A, MacLennan K, Flanders KC, et al. Induction of transforming growth factor $\beta_1$ in human breast cancer in vivo following tamoxifen treatment. Cancer Res 1992; 52:4261–4264.

77. Alexieva-Figusch J, Blankenstein MA, Hop WCJ, et al. Treatment of metastatic breast cancer patients with different dosages of megestrol acetate: dose relations, metabolic and endocrine effects. Eur J Cancer Clin Oncol 1984; 20:33–40.

78. Frost VJ, Helle SI, Lønning PE, van der Stappen JWJ, Holly JMP. Effects of treatment with aminoglutethimide, formestane (4-hydroxyandrostenedione) or megestrol acetate in insulin-like growth factor-I and -II, IGF-binding proteins and insulin-like growth factor binding protein-3 protease status in patients with advanced breast cancer. J Clin Endocrinol Metab. In press.

79. Santen RJ, Manni A, Harvey H, Redmond C. Endocrine treatment of breast cancer in women. Endocr Rev 1990; 11:221–265.

80. Pekonen F, Partanen S, Mäkinen T, Rutanen E-M. Receptors for epidermal growth factor and insulin-like growth factor I and their relation to steroid receptors in human breast cancer. Cancer Res 1988; 48:1343–1347.

81. Foekens JA, Portengen H, van Putten WLJ, et al. Prognostic value of receptors for insulin-like growth factor I, somatostatin, and epidermal growth factor in human breast cancer. Cancer Res 1989; 49:7002–7009.

82. Karey KP, Sirbasku DA. Differential responsiveness of human breast cancer cell lines MCF-7 and T47D to growth factors and 17 B-estradiol. Cancer Res 1988; 48:4083–4092.

83. Sutherland RL, Lee CSL, Feldman RS, Musgrove EA. Regulation of breast cancer cell cycle progression by growth factors, steroids and steroid antagonists. J Steroid Biochem Mol Biol 1992; 41:3–8.

84. Jordan VC, Murphy CS. Endocrine pharmacology of antiestrogens as antitumor agents. Endocr Rev 1990; 11:578–610.

85. Lønning PE, Lien E, Lundgren S, Kvinnsland S. Clinical pharmacokinetics of endocrine agents used in advanced breast cancer. Clin Pharmacokinet 1992; 22:327–358.

86. Lønning PE, Lien EA. Mechanisms of action of endocrine treatment for breast cancer. Crit Rev Oncol Hematol. In press.

87. Allen KE, Clark ER, Jordan VC. Evidence for the metabolic activation of non-steroidal antioestrogens: a study of structure-activity relationships. Br J Pharmacol Chemother 1980; 71:83–91.

88. Borgna JL, Rochefort H. Hydroxylated metabolites of tamoxifen are formed in vivo and bound to estrogen receptor in target tissues. J Biol Chem 1981; 256:859–868.

89. Valavaara R, Pyrhonen S, Heikkinen M, Rissanen P, Blanco G. Toremifene, a new anti-estrogenic compound, for treatment of advanced breast cancer: phase II study. Eur J Cancer Clin Oncol 1988; 24:785–790.

90. Bruning PF. Droloxifene, a new anti-oestrogen in postmenopausal advanced breast cancer: preliminary results of a double-blind dose-finding phase II trial. Eur J Cancer 1992; 28A: 1404–1407.

91. Coombes RC, Haynes BP, Dowsett M, et al. Idoxifene: report of a phase I study in patients with metastatic breast cancer. Cancer Res 1995; 55:1070–1074.

92. Løser R, Seibel K, Roos W, Eppenberger U. In vivo and in vitro anti-estrogenic action of 3-hydroxytamoxifen, tamoxifen and 4-hydroxytamoxifen. Eur J Cancer Clin Oncol 1985; 21:985–990.

93. Kawamura I, Mizota T, Mukumoto S, et al. Antiestrogenic and antitumor effects of droloxifene in experimental breast carcinoma. Arzneimittelforschung 1989; 39:889–893.

94. Stenbygaard LE, Herrstedt J, Thomsen JF, Svendsen KR, Engelholm SA, Dombernowsky P. Toremifene and tamoxifen in advanced breast cancer—a double-blind cross-over trial. Breast Cancer Res Treat 1993; 25:57–63.

95. Buzdar AU, Marcus C, Holmes F, Hug V, Hortobagyi G. Phase II evaluation of Ly156758 in metastatic breast cancer. Oncology 1988; 45:344–345.

96. Vogel CL, Shemano I, Schoenfelder J, Gams RA, Green MR. Multicenter phase-II efficacy trial of toremifene in tamoxifen-refractory patients with advanced breast cancer. J Clin Oncol 1993; 11:345–350.

97. Parker MG. Action of "pure" antiestrogens in inhibiting estrogen receptor action. Breast Cancer Res Treat 1993; 26:131–137.

98. Berry M, Metzger T, Chambon P. Role of the two activating domains of the oestrogen receptor in the cell-type and promoter-context dependent agonistic activity of the anti-oestrogen 4-hydroxytamoxifen. EMBO J 1990; 9:2811–2818.

99. Fujimoto N, Katzenellenbogen BS. Alterations in the agonist/antagonist balance of anti-estrogens by activation of protein kinase A signalling pathways in breast cancer cells: anti-estrogen-selectivity and promoter-dependence. Mol Endocrinol 1994; 8:296–304.

100. Pavlik E, Nelson K, Srinivasan S, et al. Resistance to tamoxifen with persisting sensitivity to estrogen: possible mediation by excessive antiestrogen binding site activity. Cancer Res 1992; 5:4106–4112.

101. Hedden A, Müller V, Jensen EV. A two-site model for the reaction of hormone antagonists with estrogen and progestin receptors. J Steroid Biochem Mol Biol. In press.

102. Lien EA, Johannessen DC, Aakvaag A, Lønning PE. Influence of tamoxifen on human plasma IGF-I levels in breast cancer patients. J Steroid Biochem Mol Biol 1992; 41:541–543.

103. Noguchi S, Motomura K, Inaji H, Imaoka S, Koyama H. Down-regulation of transforming growth factor-alpha by tamoxifen in human breast cancer. Cancer 1993; 72:131–136.

104. Berthois Y, Dong XF, Martin PM. Regulation of epidermal growth factor receptor by estrogen and antiestrogen in the human breast cancer cell line MCF. Biochem Biophys Res Commun 1989; 159:126–131.

105. O'Brian CA, Liskamp RM, Solomon DH, Weinstein IB. Inhibition of protein kinase C by tamoxifen. Cancer Res 1985; 45:2462–2465.

106. Lam HYP. Tamoxifen is a calmodulin antagonist in the activation of cAMP phosphodi-esterase. Biochem Biophys Res Commun 1984; 118:27–32.

107. Freiss G, Rochefort H, Vignon F. Mechanisms of 4-hydroxytamoxifen anti-growth factor activity in breast cancer cells: alterations of growth factor receptor binding sites and tyrosine kinase activity. Biochem Biophys Res Commun 1990; 173:919–926.

108. Croxtall JD, Emmas C, White JO, Choudhary Q, Flower RJ. Tamoxifen inhibits growth of oestrogen receptor-negative A549 cells. Biochem Pharmacol 1994; 47:197–202.

109. Charlier C, Chariot A, Antoine N, Merville MP, Gielen J, Castronovo V. Tamoxifen and its active metabolite inhibit growth of estrogen receptor-negative MDA-MB-435 cells. Biochem Pharmacol 1995; 49:351–358.

110. Wakeling AE. The future of new pure antiestrogens in clinical breast cancer. Breast Cancer Res Treat 1993; 25:1–9.

111. Howell A, DeFriend D, Robertson J, Blamey R, Walton P. Response to a specific antioestrogen (ICI 182780) in tamoxifen-resistant breast cancer. Lancet 1995; 345:29–30.

112. Dauvois S, Danielian PS, White R, Parker MG. Antiestrogen ICI 164,384 reduces cellular estrogen receptor content by increasing its turnover. Proc Natl Acad Sci USA 1992; 89: 4037–4041.

113. Arbuckle ND, Dauvois S, Parker MG. Effects of antioestrogens on the DNA binding activity of oestrogen receptors in vitro. Nucleic Acids Res 1992; 20:3839–3844.

114. Santen RJ, Samojlik E, Wells SA. Resistance of ovary to blockade of aromatization with aminoglutethimide. J Clin Endocrinol Metab 1980; 51:473–477.

115. Harris AL, Dowsett M, Jeffcoate SL, McKinna JA, Morgan M, Smith IE. Endocrine and therapeutic effects of aminoglutethimide in premenopausal patients with breast cancer. J Clin Endocrinol Metab 1982; 55:718–722.

116. Lønning PE, Jacobs S, Jones A, Haynes B, Powles TJ, Dowsett M. The influence of CGS 16949A on peripheral aromatisation in breast cancer patients. Br J Cancer 1991; 63:789–793.

117. Jones AL, MacNeill F, Jacobs S, Lønning PE, Dowsett M, Powles TJ. The influence of intramuscular 4-hydroxyandrostenedione on peripheral aromatisation in breast cancer patients. Eur J Cancer 1992; 28A:1712–1716.

118. MacNeill FA, Jones SL, Jacobs S, Lønning PE, Powles TJ, Dowsett M. The influence of aminoglutethimide and its analogue rogletimide on peripheral aromatisation in breast cancer. Br J Cancer 1992; 66:692–697.

119. Reed MJ, Lai LC, Owen AM, et al. Effect of treatment with 4-hydroxyandrostenedione on the peripheral conversion of androstenedione to estrone and in vitro tumor aromatase activity in postmenopausal women with breast cancer. Cancer Res 1990; 50:193–196.

120. Van der Wall E, Donker TH, de Frankrijker E, Nortier HWR, Thijssen JHH, Blankenstein MA. Inhibition of the in vivo conversion of androstenedione to estrone by the aromatase inhibitor vorozole in healthy postmenopausal women. Cancer Res 1993; 53:4563–4566.

121. Vermeulen A, Paridaens R, Heuson JC. Effects of aminoglutethimide on adrenal steroid secretion. Clin Endocrinol 1983; 19:673–682.

122. Santen RJ, Worgul TJ, Lipton A, Harvey H, Boucher A. Aminoglutethimide as treatment of postmenopausal women with advanced breast carcinoma. Ann Intern Med 1982; 96:94–101.

123. Dowsett M, Cunningham DC, Stein RC, Evans S, Dehenin L. Dose-related endocrine effects and pharmacokinetics of oral and intramuscular 4-hydroxyandrostenedione in postmenopausal breast cancer patients. Cancer Res 1980; 49:1306.

124. Dowsett M, Stein RC, Mehta A, Coombes RC. Potency and selectivity of the non-steroidal aromatase inhibitor CGS 16949A in postmenopausal breast cancer patients. Clin Endocrinol 1990; 32:623–634.

125. Johnston SRD, Smith IE, Doody D, Jacobs S, Robertshaw H, Dowsett M. Clinical and endocrine effects of the oral aromatase inhibitor vorozole in postmenopausal patients with advanced breast cancer. Cancer Res 1994; 54:5875–5881.

126. Dowsett M, Jones A, Johnston SRD, Jacobs S, Trunet P, Smith IE. In vivo measurement of aromatase inhibition by letrozole (CGS 20267) in postmenopausal patients with breast cancer. Clin Cancer Res. In press.

127. Lønning PE, Ekse D. A new sensitive radioimmunoassay for measurement of plasma estrone sulphate in patients on treatment with aromatase inhibitors. J Steroid Biochem Mol Biol. In press.

128. Reed MJ, Owen AM, Lai LC, et al. In situ oestrone synthesis in normal breast and breast tumour tissues: effect of treatment with 4-hydroxyandrostenedione. Int J Cancer 1989; 44:233–237.

129. Miller WR. Importance of intratumoural aromatase, and its susceptibility to inhibitors. In: Dowsett M, ed. Aromatase inhibition—then, now and tomorrow. London: Parthenon Publishing Group, 1994:43–53.

130. Tseng L, Gurpide E. Effect of progestins on estradiol receptor levels in human endometrium. J Clin Endocrinol Metab 1975; 41:402–404.

131. Vignon F, Bardon S, Chalbos D, Rochefort H. Antiestrogenic effect of R5020, a synthetic progestin in human breast cancer cells in culture. J Clin Endocrinol Metab 1983; 56:1124–1130.

132. Noguchi S, Yamamoto H, Inaji H, Imaoka S, Koyama H. Inability of medroxyprogesterone acetate to down regulate estrogen receptor level in human breast cancer. Cancer 1990; 65:1375–1379.

133. Lundgren S, Kvinnsland S, Varhaug JE, Utaaker E. The influence of progestins on receptor levels in breast cancer metastasis. Anticancer Res 1987; 7:119–124.

134. Sutherland RL, Hall RE, Pang GYN, Musgrove EA, Clarke CL. Effect of medroxyprogesterone acetate on proliferation and cell cycle kinetics of human mammary carcinoma cells. Cancer Res 1988; 48:5084–5091.

135. Hackenberg R, Hawighorst T, Filmer A, et al. Medroxyprogesterone acetate inhibits the proliferation of estrogen and progesterone-receptor negative MFM-223 human mammary cancer cells via the androgen receptor. Breast Cancer Res Treat 1993; 25:217–224.

136. Birrell SN, Roder DM, Horsfall DJ, Bentel JM, Tilley WD. Medroxyprogesterone acetate therapy in advanced breast cancer: the predictive value of androgen receptor expression. J Clin Oncol 1995; 13:1572–1577.

137. Lea O, Kvinnsland S, Thorsen T. Improved measurement of androgen receptors in human breast cancer. Cancer Res 1989; 49:7162–7167.

138. Van Veelen H, Willemse PHB, Sleifer DT, et al. Mechanism of adrenal suppression by high-dose medroxyprogesterone acetate in breast cancer patients. Cancer Chemother Pharmacol 1985; 15:167–170.

139. Lundgren S, Lønning PE, Utaaker E, Aakvaag, Kvinnsland S. Influence of progestins on serum hormone levels in postmenopausal women with advanced breast cancer I: general findings. J Steroid Biochem 1990; 36:99–104.

140. Tseng L, Gurpide E. Induction of human endometrial estradiol dehydrogenase by progestins. Endocrinology 1975; 97:825–833.

141. Reed MJ, Christodoulides A, Koistinen R, et al. The effect of endocrine therapy with medroxyprogesterone acetate, 4-hydroxyandrostenedione or tamoxifen on plasma concentrations of insulin-like growth factor (IGF)-I, IGF-II and IGFBP-1 in women with advanced breast cancer. Int J Cancer 1992; 52:208–212.

142. Helle SI, Lønning PE. Insulin-like growth factors in breast and prostatic cancer. Endocrine-Rel Cancer 1995; 2:153–169.

143. Goldfine ID, Papa V, Vigneri R, Siiteri P, Rosenthal S. Progestin regulation of insulin and insulin-like growth factor I receptors in cultured human breast cancer cells. Breast Cancer Res Treat 1992; 22:69–79.

144. Fleming GF, Amato JM, Agresti M, Safa AR. Megestrol acetate reverses multidrug resistance and interacts with P-glycoprotein. Cancer Chemother Pharmacol 1992; 29:445–449.

145. Gundersen S, Kvinnsland S, Klepp O, et al. Chemotherapy with or without high-dose medroxyprogesterone acetate in oestrogen-receptor-negative advanced breast cancer. Eur J Cancer 1992; 28:390–394.

146. Herrmann W, Wyss R, Riondel A, et al. The effect of an antiprogesterone steroid on women: interruption of the menstrual cycle and of early pregnancy. C R Hebd Seances Acad Sci 1982; 284:933–937.

147. Gill PG, Vignon F, Bardon S, et al. Difference between R 5020 and the antiprogestin RU 486 in antiproliferative effects on human breast cancer cells. Breast Cancer Res Treat 1987; 10:37–45.

148. Michna H, Nishino Y, Neef G, McGuire WL, Schneider MR. Progesterone antagonists: tumor-inhibiting potential and mechanism of action. J Steroid Biochem Mol Biol 1992; 41:339–348.

149. Musgrove EA, Lee CSL, Sutherland RL. Progestins both stimulate and inhibit breast cancer cell cycle progression while increasing expression of transforming growth factor a, epidermal growth factor receptor, c-fos and c-myc genes. Mol Cell Biology 1991; 11:5032–5043.

150. Musgrove EA, Sutherland RL. Effects of the progestin antagonist RU 486 on T-47D cell cycle kinetics and cell cycle regulatory genes. Biochem Biophys Res Commun 1993; 195: 1184–1190.

151. Romieu G, Maudelonde T, Uhlmann A, et al. The antiprogestin RU 486 in advanced breast cancer: preliminary clinical trial. Bull Cancer 1987; 74:455–461.

152. Klijn JGM, de Jong FH, Bakker GH, et al. Antiprogestins, a new form of endocrine therapy for human breast cancer. Cancer Res 1989; 49:2851–2856.

153. Harvey HA, Lipton A, White DS, et al. Cross-over comparison of tamoxifen and aminoglutethimide in advanced breast cancer. Cancer Res 1982; 42(suppl: 345):1s–3s.

154. Buzdar AU, Powell KC, Blumenschein GR. Aminoglutethimide after tamoxifen therapy in advanced breast cancer: M. D. Anderson Hospital experience. Cancer Res 1982; 42 (suppl):3448s–3450s.

155. Kvinnsland S, Lønning PE, Dahl O. Treatment of breast carcinoma with aminoglutethimide. Acta Radiol Oncol 1984; 23:421–424.

156. Murray RML, Pitt P. Aminoglutethimide in tamoxifen-resistant patients: the Melbourne experience. Cancer Res 1982; 42(suppl):3437s–3441s.

157. Kaye SB, Woods RL, Fox RM, Coates AS, Tattersall HN. Use of aminoglutethimide as second-line endocrine therapy in metastatic breast cancer. Cancer Res 1982; 42(suppl): 3445s–3447s.

158. Smith IE, Harris AL, Morgan M, et al. Tamoxifen versus aminoglutethimide in advanced breast carcinoma: a randomised cross-over trial. Br Med J 1981; 283:1432–1434.

159. Gale KC, Andersen JW, Tormey DC, et al. Hormonal treatment for metastatic breast cancer. An Eastern Cooperative Oncology Group Phase III Trial comparing aminoglutethimide to tamoxifen. Cancer 1994; 73:354–361.

160. Lønning PE, Wiedemann G, Kvinnsland S, Lundgren S. Welche Hormontherapie bei fortgeschrittenem Mammakarzinom des Mannes (Ger). [Advanced carcinoma of the breast in the male: what is the best hormonal treatment?] Dtsch Med Wschr 1988; 113: 1358–1361.

161. Elomaa I, Blomqvist C, Rissanen P. Aminoglutethimide as second line therapy in advanced breast cancer. Breast Cancer Res Treat 1986; 7(suppl):51–54.

162. Geisler J, Johannessen DC, Anker G, Lønning PE. Treatment with formestane alone and in combination with aminoglutethimide in heavily pretreated breast cancer patients: clinical and endocrine effects. Submitted.

163. Garcia-Giralt E, Ayme Y, Carton M, et al. Second and third line hormonotherapy in advanced post-menopausal breast cancer: a multicenter randomized trial comparing medroxyprogesterone acetate with aminoglutethimide in patients who have become resistant to tamoxifen. Breast Cancer Res Treat 1992; 24:139–145.

164. Iveson TJ, Ahern J, Smith IA. Response to third-line endocrine treatment for advanced breast cancer. Eur J Cancer 1993; 29A:572–574.

165. Zambetti M, Brambilla C, Tancini G, Bonadonna G. Aminoglutethimide in postmeno-pausal breast cancer refractory to multiple hormonal and cytostatic treatments. Tumori 1987; 73:369–373.

166. Brinkley D, Haybittle JL. Long-term survival of women with breast cancer. Lancet 1984; 1:1118.

167. Kvinnsland S. Steroid receptor assay and prognosis. In: Stoll BA, ed. Breast Cancer Treatment and Prognosis. Oxford: Blackwell Scientific Publications, 1986:140–155.

168. Johnston SRD, Saccani-Jotti G, Smith IE, Newby J, Dowsett M. Change in oestrogen receptor expression and function in tamoxifen-resistant breast cancer. Endocrine-Rel Cancer 1995; 2:105–110.

169. Lien EA, Solheim E, Ueland PM. Distribution of tamoxifen and its metabolites in rat and human tissues during steady state treatment. Cancer Res 1991; 51:4837–4844.

170. Lien EA, Wester K, Lønning PE, Solheim E, Ueland PM. Distribution of tamoxifen and metabolites into brain tissue and brain metastases in breast cancer patients. Br J Cancer 1991; 63:641–645.

171. Sjøholm I, Ekman B, Kober A, et al. Binding drugs to human serum albumin XI. Mol Pharmacol 1979; 16:767–777.

172. Lien EA, Solheim E, Lea OA, et al. Distribution of 4-hydroxy-N-desmethyltamoxifen and other tamoxifen metabolites in human biological fluids during tamoxifen treatment. Cancer Res 1989; 49:2175–2183.

173. Plotkin D, Lechner JJ, Jung WE, Rosen PJ. Tamoxifen flare in advanced breast cancer. JAMA 1978; 240:2644–2646.

174. Horwitz KB, Koseki Y, McGuire WL. Estrogen control of progesterone receptor in human breast cancer: role of estradiol and antiestrogen. Endocrinology 1978; 103:1742.

175. Westley BR, May FEB. In vitro development of tamoxifen resistance. Endocrine-Rel Cancer 1995; 2:37–44.

176. Brünner N, Frandsen TL, Holst-Hansen C, et al. MCF-7/LCC2: a 4-hydroxytamoxifen resistant human breast cancer variant that retains sensitivity to the steroidal antiestrogen ICI 182,780. Cancer Res 1993; 53:3229–3232.

177. Hu XF, Veroni M, De Luise M, et al. Circumvention of tamoxifen resistance by the pure anti-estrogen ICI 182,780. Int J Cancer 1993; 55:373–376.

178. Wiseman LR, Johnson MD, Wakeling AE, Lykkesfeldt AE, May FEB, Westley BR. Type I IGF receptor and acquired tamoxifen resistance in oestrogen-responsive human breast cancer cells. Eur J Cancer 1993; 29A:2256–2264.

179. Lykkesfeldt AE, Madsen MW, Briand P. Altered expression of estrogen-regulated genes in a tamoxifen-resistant and ICI 164,384 and ICI 182,780 sensitive human breast cancer cell line, MCF-7/TAM$^R$-1. Cancer Res 1994; 54:1587–1595.

180. Clarke R, Brünner N, Thompson EW, et al. The inter-relationships between ovarian-independent growth, tumorigenicity, invasiveness and antioestrogen resistance in the malignant progression of human breast cancer. J Endocrinol 1989; 122:331–340.

181. Brünner N, Boysen B, Killgaard TL, Frandsen TL, Jirus S, Clarke R. Resistance to 4OH-tamoxifen does not confer resistance to the steroidal antiestrogen ICI 182,780, while acquired resistance to ICI 182,780 results in cross-resistance to 4OH-TAM. Breast Cancer Res Treat 1993; 27:135.

182. Lykkesfeldt AE, Larsen SS, Briand P. Human breast cancer cell lines resistant to pure anti-estrogens are sensitive to tamoxifen treatment. Int J Cancer 1995; 61:529–534.

183. Osborne CK, Coronado EB, Robinson JP. Human breast cancer in the athymic nude mouse: cytostatic effects of long-term antiestrogen therapy. Eur J Cancer Clin Oncol 1987; 23: 1189–1196.

184. Gottardis MM, Jordan VC. Development of tamoxifen-stimulated growth of MCF-7 tumors in athymic mice after long-term antiestrogen administration. Cancer Res 1988; 48: 5783–5787.

185. Gottaradis MM, Wagner RJ, Borden EC, Jordan VC. Differential ability of antiestrogens to stimulate breast cancer cell (MCF-7) growth in vivo and in vitro. Cancer Res 1989; 49:4756–4769.

186. Gottardis MM, Jiang SY, Jeng MJ, Jordan VC. Inhibition of tamoxifen-stimulated growth of an MCF-7 tumor variant in athymic mice by novel steroidal antiestrogens. Cancer Res 1989; 49:4090–4093.

187. Engelsman E. Therapy of advanced breast cancer; a review. Eur J Cancer Clin Oncol 1983; 19:1775–1778.

188. Howell A, Dodwell DJ, Anderson H, Redford J. Response after withdrawal of tamoxifen and progestogens in advanced breast cancer. Ann Oncol 1992; 3:611–617.

189. Allegra JC, Barlock A, Huff KK, Lippman ME. Changes in multiple or sequential estrogen receptor determinations in breast cancer. Cancer 1980; 45:792–794.

190. Taylor RE, Powles TJ, Humphreys J, et al. Effects of endocrine therapy on steroid receptor content of breast cancer. Br J Cancer 1982; 45:80–85.

191. Hull DF, Clark GM, Osborne CK, Chamness GC, Knight WA, McGuire WL. Multiple estrogen receptor assays in human breast cancer. Cancer Res 1983; 43:413–416.

192. Crawford J, Cowan S, Fitch R, Smith DC, Leake RE. Stability of oestrogen receptor status in sequential biopsies from patients with breast cancer. Br J Cancer 1987; 56:137–140.

193. Noguchi S, Motomura K, Inaji H, Imaoka S, Koyama H. Up-regulation of estrogen receptor by tamoxifen in human breast cancer. Cancer 1993; 71:1266–1272.

194. Murray PA, Gomm J, Ricketts D, Powles T, Coombes RC. The effect of endocrine therapy on the levels of oestrogen and progesterone receptor and transforming growth factor-β1 in metastatic human breast cancer: an immunocytochemical study. Eur J Cancer 1994; 30A:1218–1222.

195. Encarnacion CA, Ciocca DR, McGuire WL, Clark GM, Fuqua SAW, Osborne CK. Measurement of steroid hormone receptors in breast cancer patients on tamoxifen. Breast Cancer Res Treat 1993; 26:237–246.

196. Danielian PS, White R, Hoare SA, Fawell SE, Parker MG. Identification of residues in the estrogen receptor which confer differential sensitivity to estrogen and hydroxytamoxifen. Mol Endocrinol 1993; 7:232–240.

197. Pakdel F, Katzenellenbogen BS. Human estrogen receptor mutants with altered estrogen and antiestrogen ligand discrimination. J Biol Chem 1992; 267:3429–3437.

198. Rea DW, Parker MG. Structure and function of the oestrogen receptor in relation to its altered sensitivity to oestradiol and tamoxifen. Endocrine-Rel Cancer 1995; 2:13–17.

199. Jiang SY, Langen-Fahey SM, Stella AL, McCague R, Jordan VC. Point mutation of estrogen receptor (ER) in the ligand-binding domain changes the pharmacology of antiestrogens in ER-negative breast cancer cells stably expressing complementary DNAs for ER. Mol Endocrinol 1992; 6:2167–2174.

200. Zhang Q-X, Borg A, Fuqua SAW. An exon 5 deletion variant of the estrogen receptor frequently coexpressed with wild-type estrogen receptor in human breast cancer. Cancer Res 1993; 53:5882–5884.

201. Fuqua SAW, Wolf DM. Molecular aspects of ED variants in breast cancer. Breast Cancer Res Treat 1995; 35:233–241.

202. Daffada AA, Johnston SR, Smith IE, Detre S, King N, Dowsett M. Exon 5 deletion variant estrogen receptor messenger RNA expression in relation to tamoxifen resistance and progesterone receptor/pS2 status in human breast cancer. Cancer Res 1995; 55:288–293.

203. Karnik PS, Kulkarni S, Liu XP, Budd GT, Bukowski RM. Estrogen-receptor mutations in tamoxifen-resistant breast-cancer. Cancer Res 1994; 54:349–353.

204. Foster BD, Cavener DR, Parl FF. Binding analysis of the estrogen receptor to its specific DNA target site in human breast cancer. Cancer Res 1991; 51:3405–3410.

205. Catherino WH, Jordan VC. Increasing the number of tandem estrogen response elements increases the estrogenic activity of a tamoxifen analogue. Cancer Lett 1995; 92:39–47.

206. Leung BS, Potter AH. Mode of estrogen action on cell proliferation in CAMA-1 cells: II. Sensitivity to G1 phase population. J Cell Biochem 1987; 34:213–225.

207. Musgrove EA, Wakeling AE, Sutherland RL. Points of action of estrogen antagonists and a calmodulin antagonist within the MCF-7 human breast cancer cell cycle. Cancer Res 1989; 49:2398–2404.

208. Sutherland RL, Watts CKW, Musgrove EA. Cell cycle control by steroid hormones in breast cancer: implications for endocrine resistance. Endocrine-Rel Cancer 1995; 2:87–96.

209. Buckley MF, Sweeney KJE, Hamilton JA, et al. Expression and amplification of cyclin genes in human breast cancer. Oncogene 1993; 8:2127–2133.

210. Bartkova J, Lukas M, Müller H, Lützhøft D, Strauss M, Bartek J. Cyclin D1 protein expression and function in human breast cancer. Int J Cancer 1994; 57:353–361.

211. Gillet C, Fantl V, Smit R, et al. Amplification and overexpression of cyclin D1 in breast cancer detected by immunohistochemical staining. Cancer Res 1994; 54:1812–1817.

212. Groom GV, Griffiths K. Effect of the anti-oestrogen tamoxifen on plasma levels of luteinizing hormone, follicle-stimulating hormone, prolactin, oestradiol and progesterone in normal pre-menopausal women. J Endocrinol 1976; 70:421–428.

213. Sherman BM, Chapler FK, Crickard K, Wycoff D. Endocrine consequences of continuous antiestrogen therapy with tamoxifen in premenopausal women. J Clin Invest 1979; 64:368–404.

214. Jonat W, Kaufmann M, Blamey RW, et al. A randomised study to compare the effect of the luteinising hormone releasing hormone (LHRH) analogue goserelin with or without tamoxifen in pre- and perimenopausal patients with advanced breast cancer. Eur J Cancer 1995; 31A:137–142.

215. Gelly C, Pasqualini JR. Effect of tamoxifen and tamoxifen derivatives on the conversion of estrone-sulfate to estradiol in the R-27 cells, a tamoxifen-resistant line derived from MCF-7 human breast cancer cells. J Steroid Biochem 1988; 30:321–324.

216. Pasqualini JR, Gelly C. Effect of tamoxifen and tamoxifen derivatives on the conversion of estrone sulfate to estradiol in the MCF-7 mammary cancer cell line. Cancer Lett 1988; 40:115–121.

217. Evans TRJ, Rowlands MG, Jarman M, Coombes RC. Inhibition of estrone sulfatase enzyme in human placenta and human breast carcinoma. J Steroid Biochem Mol Biol 1991; 39:493–499.

218. Purohit A, Reed MJ. Oestrogen sulphatase activity in hormone-dependent and hormone-independent breast-cancer cells: modulation by steroidal and non-steroidal therapeutic agents. Int J Cancer 1992; 50:901–905.

219. McLeskey SW, Kurebayashi J, Honig SF, et al. Fibroblast growth factor 4 transfection of MCF-7 cells produces cell lines that are tumorigenic and metastatic in ovariectomized or tamoxifen-treated athymic nude mice. Cancer Res 1993; 53:2168–2177.

220. Benz CC, Scott GK, Sarup JC, et al. Estrogen-dependent, tamoxifen-resistant tumorigenic growth of MCF-7 cells transfected with HER2/neu. Breast Cancer Res Treat 1993; 24:85–95.

221. Antoniotti S, Maggiora P, Dati C, De Bortoli M. Tamoxifen upregulates c-erbB-2 expression in estrogen-responsive breast cancer cells in vitro. Eur J Cancer 1992; 28:318–321.

222. Wärri AM, Laine AM, Majasuo KE, Alitalo KK, Härkönen PL. Estrogen suppression of erbB2 expression is associated with increased growth rate of ZR-75-1 human breast cancer cells in vitro and in nude mice. Int J Cancer 1991; 49:616–623.

223. LeRoy X, Escot C, Brouillet J-P, et al. Decrease of c-erbB-2 and c-myc RNA levels in tamoxifen-treated breast cancer. Oncogene 1991; 6:431–437.

224. Têtu B, Brisson J. Prognostic significance of HER-2/neu oncoprotein expression in node-positive breast cancer. Cancer 1994; 73:2359–2365.

225. Borg Å, Baldetorp B, Bernö K, Killander D, Olsson H, Rydén S, Sigurdsson H. ERBB2 amplification is associated with tamoxifen resistance in steroid-receptor positive breast cancer. Cancer Lett 1994; 81:137–144.

226. Arteaga CJ, Kitten LJ, Coronado EB, et al. Blockade of the type I somatomedin receptor inhibits growth of human breast cancer cells in athymic mice. J Clin Invest 1989; 84:1418–1423.

227. Brünner N, Moser C, Clarke R, Cullen K. IGF-1 and IGF-II expression in human breast cancer xenografts: relationship to hormone independence. Breast Cancer Res Treat 1992; 22:39–45.

228. Osborne CK, Coronado E, Allred DC, Wiebe V, DeGregorio M. Acquired tamoxifen resistance: correlation with reduced breast tumor levels of tamoxifen and isomerization of trans-4-hydroxytamoxifen. J Natl Cancer Inst 1991; 83:1477–1482.

229. Osborne CK, Wiebe VJ, McGuire WL, Ciocca DR, DeGregorio MW. Tamoxifen and the isomers of 4-hydroxytamoxifen in tamoxifen-resistant tumors from breast cancer patients. J Clin Oncol 1992; 10:304–310.

230. Johnston SRD, Haynes BP, Smith IE, et al. Acquired tamoxifen resistance in human breast cancer and reduced intra-tumoral drug concentration. Lancet 1993; 342:1521–1522.

231. Keen JC, Miller EP, Bellamy C, Dixon JM, Miller WR. P-glycoprotein and resistance to tamoxifen. Lancet 1994; 343:1047–1048.

232. Osborne CK. Tamoxifen metabolism as a mechanism for resistance. Endocrine-Rel Cancer 1995; 2:53–58.

233. Wiebe VJ, Osborn CK, McGuire WL, DeGregorio MW. Identification of estrogenic tamoxifen metabolite(s) in tamoxifen-resistant human breast tumors. J Clin Oncol 1992; 10:990–994.

234. Katzenellenbogen JA, Carlson KE, Latzenellenbogen BS. Facile geometric isomerization of phenolic non-steroidal estrogens and antiestrogens: limitations to the interpretation of experiments characterizing the activity of individual isomers. J Steroid Biochem 1985; 22: 589–596.

235. Malet C, Gompel A, Spritzer P, et al. Tamoxifen and hydroxytamoxifen isomers versus estradiol effects on normal human breast cells in culture. Cancer Res 1988; 48:7193–7199.

236. Wolf DM, Langan-Fahey SM, Parker CJ, McCague R, Jordan VC. Investigation of the mechanism of tamoxifen-stimulated breast tumor growth with nonisomerizable analogues of tamoxifen and metabolites. J Natl Cancer Inst 1993; 85:806–812.

237. Maenpaa J, Wiebe V, Wurz G, et al. Reduced tamoxifen accumulation is not associated with stimulated growth in tamoxifen resistance. Cancer Chemother Pharmacol 1994; 35: 149–152.

238. Clarke R, Brünner N, Katzenellenbogen BS, et al. Progression of human breast cancer cells from hormone-dependent to hormone-independent growth both in vitro and in vivo. Proc Natl Acad Sci USA 1989; 86:3649–3653.

239. Lønning PE. New endocrine drugs for treatment of advanced breast cancer. Acta Oncol 1990; 29:379–386.

240. Murray R, Pitt P. Low-dose aminoglutethimide without steroid replacement in the treatment of postmenopausal women with advanced breast cancer. Eur J Cancer Clin Oncol 1985; 21:19–22.

241. Lønning PE, Kvinnsland S. Mechanisms of action of aminoglutethimide as endocrine therapy of breast cancer. Drugs 1988; 35:685–710.

242. Dowsett M, Santner SJ, Santen RJ, Jeffcoate SL, Smith IE. Effective inhibition by low dose aminoglutethimide of peripheral aromatisation in postmenopausal breast cancer patients. Br J Cancer 1985; 52:31–35.

243. Lønning PE, Johannessen DC, Thorsen T. Alterations in the production rate and the metabolism of oestrone and oestrone sulfate in breast cancer patients treated with aminoglutethimide. Br J Cancer 1989; 60:107–111.

244. Lønning PE, Johannessen DC, Thorsen T, Ekse D. Effects of aminoglutethimide on plasma estrone sulfate not caused by aromatase inhibition. J Steroid Biochem 1989; 33:541–545.

245. Lønning PE, Kvinnsland S, Thorsen T, Ekse D. Aminoglutethimide as an inducer of microsomal enzymes. Part 2: endocrine aspects. Breast Cancer Res Treat 1986; 7(suppl): 77–82.

246. Lønning PE, Dowsett M, Jones A, et al. Influence of aminoglutethimide on plasma oestrogen levels in breast cancer patients on 4-hydroxyandrostenedione treatment. Breast Cancer Res Treat 1992; 23:57–62.

247. Dowsett M, Stein RC, Coombes RC. Aromatization inhibition alone or in combination with GnRH agonists for the treatment of premenopausal breast cancer patients. J Steroid Biochem Mol Biol 1992; 43:155–159.

248. Samojlik E, Santen RJ, Worgul TJ. Suppression of residual oestrogen production with aminoglutethimide in women following surgical hypophysectomy or adrenalectomy. Clin Endocrinol 1984; 20:43–51.

249. Miller WR, Hawkins RA, Mullen P, Sourdaine P, Telford J. Aromatase inhibition: determinants of response and resistance. Endocrine-Rel Cancer 1995; 2:73–85.

250. Bundred NJ, Eremin O, Stewart HJ, et al. Beneficial response to pituitary ablation following aminoglutethimide. Br J Surg 1986; 73:388–389.

251. Murray R, Pitt P. Aromatase inhibition with 4-OH androstenedione after prior aromatase inhibition with aminoglutethimide in women with advanced breast cancer. Breast Cancer Res Treat 1995; 35:249–253.

252. Santen RJ, Santner S, Davis B, Veldhuis J, Samojlik E, Ruby E. Aminoglutethimide inhibits extraglandular estrogen production in postmenopausal women with breast carcinoma. J Clin Endocrinol Metab 1978; 47:1257–1265.

253. Longcope C, Kato T, Horton R. Conversion of blood androgens to estrogens in normal adult men and women. J Clin Invest 1969; 48:2191–2201.

254. Simpson ER, Ackerman GE, Smith ME, Mendelson CR. Estrogen formation in stromal cells of adipose tissue of women: induction by glucocorticoids. Proc Natl Acad Sci USA 1981; 78:5690–5694.

255. Reed MJ, Topping L, Coldham NG, et al. Control of aromatase activity in breast cancer cells: the role of cytokines and growth factors. J Steroid Biochem Mol Biol 1993; 44:589–596.

256. Dowsett M, Harris AL, Smith IE, Jeffcoate SL. Endocrine changes associated with relapse in advanced breast cancer patients on aminoglutathimide therapy. J Clin Endocrinol Metab 1984; 58:99–104.

257. Reed MJ, Aherne GW, Ghilchik MW, Patel S, Chakraborty J. Concentrations of oestrone and 4-hydroxyandrostenedione in malignant and normal breast tissues. Int J Cancer 1991; 49:562–565.

258. Miller WR. In vitro and in vivo effects of 4-hydroxyandrostenedione on steroid and tumour metabolism. In: Coombes RC, Dowsett M, eds. 4-Hydroxyandrostenedione—A New Approach to Hormone-Dependent Cancer. London–New York: Royal Society of Medicine Services, 1991:45–49.

259. Miller WR. Aromatase inhibitors in the treatment of advanced breast cancer. Cancer Treat Rev 1989; 16:83–93.

260. Kadohama N, Yarborough C, Zhou D, Chen S, Osawa Y. Kinetic properties of aromatase mutants Pro308Phe, Asp309Asn and Asp309Ala and their interactions with aromatase inhibitors. J Steroid Biochem Mol Biol 1992; 43:693–701.

261. Macaulay VM, Nicholls JE, Gledhill J, Rowlands MG, Dowsett M, Ashworth A. Biological effects of stable overexpression of aromatase in human hormone-dependent breast cancer cells. Br J Cancer 19??; 69:77–83.

262. Miller Wr, O'Neill JS. The importance of local synthesis of estrogen within the breast. Steroids 1988; 50:537–548.

263. Lønning PE. Aminoglutethimide enzyme induction: pharmacological and endocrinological implications. Cancer Chemother Pharmacol 1990; 26:241–244.

264. O'Neill JS, Elton RA, Miller WR. Aromatase activity in adipose tissue from breast quadrants: a link with tumour site. Br Med J 1988; 296:741–743.

265. Thijssen JHH, Daroszewski J, Milewicz A, Blankenstein MA. Local aromatase activity in human breast tissues. J Steroid Biochem Mol Biol 1993; 44:577–582.

266. Ferrari L, Zilembo N, Bajetta E, et al. Effect of two-4-hydroxyandrostenedione doses on serum insulin-like growth factor I levels in advanced breast cancer. Breast Cancer Res Treat 1994; 30:127–132.

267. Murray FT, Santner S, Samojlik E, Santen RJ. Serum aminoglutethimide levels: studies of serum half life, clearance, and patient compliance. J Clin Pharmacol 1979; 19:704–711.

268. Lønning PE, Schanche JS, Kvinnsland S, Ueland PM. Single-dose and steady-state pharmacokinetics of aminoglutethimide. Clin Pharmacokinet 1985; 10:353–364.

269. Lønning PE, Kvinnsland S, Bakke OM. Effect of aminoglutethimide on antipyrine, theophylline and digitoxin disposition in breast cancer. Clin Pharmacol Ther 1984; 36:796–802.

270. Lønning PE, Ueland PM, Kvinnsland S. The influence of a graded dose schedule of aminoglutethimide on the disposition of the optical enantiomers of warfarin in patients with breast cancer. Cancer Chemother Pharmacol 1986; 17:177–181.

271. Lien EA, Anker G, Lønning PE, Solheim E, Ueland PM. Decreased serum concentrations of tamoxifen and its metabolites induced by aminoglutethimide. Cancer Res 1990; 50:5851–5857.

272. Lundgren S, Lønning PE, Aakvaag A, Kvinnsland S. Influence of aminoglutethimide on the metabolism of medroxyprogesterone acetate and megestrol acetate in post-menopausal patients with advanced breast cancer. Cancer Chemother Pharmacol 1990; 27:101–105.

273. Van Deijk WA, Blijham GH, Mellink WAM, Meulenberg PMM. Influence of aminoglutethimide on plasma levels of medroxyprogesterone acetate: its correlation with serum cortisol. Cancer Treat Rep 1988; 69:85.

274. Alonso-Munoz MC, Ojeda Gonzales MB, Beltran-Fabregat M, et al. Randomized trial of tamoxifen versus aminoglutethimide and versus combined tamoxifen and aminoglutethimide in advanced postmenopausal breast cancer. Oncology 1988; 45:350–353.

275. Smith IE, Harris AL, Morgan M, Gazet JC, McKinna JA. Tamoxifen versus aminoglutethimide versus combined tamoxifen and aminoglutethimide in the treatment of advanced breast carcinoma. Cancer Res 1982; 42(suppl):3430s–3433s.

276. Corkery J, Leonard RCF, Henderson IC, et al. Tamoxifen and aminoglutethimide in advanced breast cancer. Cancer Res 1982; 42(suppl):3409s–3414s.

277. Milsted R, Habeshaw T, Kaye S, et al. A randomized trial of tamoxifen versus tamoxifen with aminoglutethimide in postmenopausal women with advanced breast cancer. Cancer Chemother Pharmacol 1985; 14:272–273.

278. Ingle JN, Green SJ, Ahmann DL, et al. Randomized trial of tamoxifen alone or combined with aminoglutethimide and hydrocortisone in women with metastatic breast cancer. J Clin Oncol 1986; 4:958–964.

279. Nagel GA, Wander HE, Blossey HC. Phase II study of aminoglutethimide and medroxyprogesterone acetate in the treatment of patients with advanced breast cancer. Cancer Res 1982; 42(suppl):3442s–3444s.

280. Haynes BP, Jarman M, Dowsett M, et al. Pharmacokinetics and pharmacodynamics of the aromatase inhibitor 3-ethyl-3-(4-pyridyl)piperidine-2,6-dione in patients with postmenopausal breast cancer. Cancer Chemother Pharmacol 1991; 27:367–372.

281. Alberto P, Mermillod B, Kaplan E, et al. A clinical trial of aminoglutethimide in advanced postmenopausal breast carcinoma: low response in patients previously treated with medroxyprogesterone. Eur J Cancer Clin Oncol 1985; 21:423–428.

282. Nemoto T, Rosner D, Patel JK, Dao TL. Aminoglutethimide in patients with metastatic breast cancer. Cancer 1989; 63:1673–1675.

283. Clarke CL, Graham J, Roman SD, Sutherland RL. Direct transcriptional regulation of the progesterone receptor by retinoic acid diminishes progestin responsiveness in the breast cancer cell line T-47D. J Biol Chem 1991; 266:18969–18975.

284. Braunsberg H, Coldham HG, Leake RE, Cowan SK, Wong W. Actions of a progestogen on human breast cancer cells: mechanisms of growth stimulation and inhibition. Eur J Cancer Clin Oncol 1987; 23:563–571.

285. Murphy LC, Dotzlaw H, Wong MSJ, Miller T, Murphy LJ. Mechanisms involved in the evolution of progestin resistance in human breast cancer cells. Cancer Res 1991; 51:2051–2057.

286. Sartorius CA, Tung L, Takimoto GS, Horwitz KB. Antagonist-occupied human progesterone receptors bound to DNA are functionally switched to transcriptional agonists by cAMP. J Biol Chem 1993; 268:9262–9266.

287. Murphy LC, Murphy LJ, Dubik D, Bell GI, Shiu RPC. Epidermal growth factor gene expression in human breast cancer cells: regulation of expression by progestins. Cancer Res 1988; 48:4555–4560.

288. Murphy LC, Dotzlaw H. Regulation of transforming growth factor alpha and transforming growth factor beta messenger ribonucleic acid abundance in T-47D human breast cancer cells. Mol Endocrinol 1989; 3:611–617.

289. Murphy LC, Murphy LJ, Shiu RPC. Progestin regulation of EGF-receptor mRNA accumulation in T-47D human breast cancer cells. Biochem Bio0phys Res Commun 1988; 150: 192–196.

290. Lundgren S, Lønning PE. Influence of progestins on serum hormone levels in postmenopausal women with advanced breast cancer II: a differential effect of megestrol acetate and medroxyprogesterone acetate on serum estrone sulfate and sex hormone binding globulin. J Steroid Biochem 1990; 36:105–109.

291. Lundgren S, Kvinnsland S, Utaaker E. Oral high-dose progestins as treatment for advanced breast cancer. Acta Oncol 1989; 28:811–816.

292. Kinci FA, Angee I, Chang CL, Radel HW. Plasma levels and accumulation into various tissues of 6-methyl-17a-acetoxy-4,6-pregnandiene-3,20-dione after oral administration or absorption from polydimethyl-siloxane implants. Acta Endocrinol 1970; 64:508–518.

293. Johnson PA, Bonomi PD, Anderson KM, Wolter JM, Economou SG. Megestrol acetate, first-line therapy for advanced breast cancer. Semin Oncol 1986; 13:15–19.

294. Beex L, Burghouts J, van Turnhout J, et al. Oral versus i.m. administration of high-dose medroxyprogesterone acetate in pretreated patients with advanced breast cancer. Cancer Treat Rep 1987; 71:1151–1156.

# 7

## Heat Shock Proteins and Drug Resistance in Breast Cancer

**Daniel R. Ciocca and Laura M. Vargas Roig**
*Laboratory of Reproduction and Lactation, Regional Center for Scientific and Technological Research (CRICYT), Mendoza, Argentina*

### INTRODUCTION

One of the major unsolved problems in cancer treatment is drug resistance at the time of initial chemotherapy (innate drug resistance) or following an initial period of clinical response to the chemotherapeutic drugs (acquired drug resistance). With the advances in cell and molecular biology, our understanding of the mechanisms involved in drug resistance has broadened considerably. Among the mechanisms used by tumor cells that become resistant to various types of drug treatments are those effective not only against cytotoxic drugs but also to other forms of therapies—e.g., radiotherapies, hormonotherapies, thermotherapies, and gene therapies. This is seen when complex mechanisms regulated through several different pathways are involved, as occurs with those interfering with apoptosis. The heat shock protein (HSP)-regulated mechanisms are also very complex, and it is reasonable to expect that they could be involved with resistance to several forms of cancer treatment. HSPs are synthesized by stressed cells; the list of stressors is very large, and in general the response is useful in defending the cells against the noxa(e) that induced the stress protein response: these proteins participate in the homeostasis of the cell by performing a multiplicity of functions.

On the other hand, there are conditions of cell damage or stress that may induce the expression of genes/proteins that are known to participate in drug resistance such as P170, type II DNA topoisomerase, or p53 (1–4). In this chapter, we restrict our presentation to the family of stress-responsive proteins known as HSPs; in particular, the involvement of HSPs in drug resistance in breast cancer. However, we will review the literature on other cancer cells and tissues as well. We want the clinical oncologist to be aware of the possible roles of HSPs in drug resistance; our aim is to stimulate the study of these proteins both in the laboratory and clinical settings—to confirm whether they indeed play a significant role in drug resistance. If we find that HSPs are involved in drug resistance, then we can design better individualized cancer treatments and also try novel approaches to modify the HSP response and thus avoid drug resistance.

**Table 1** Heat Shock Proteins, Well-Characterized HSP-Associated Proteins, and Roles in Which HSPs Have Been Involved

| HSPs family/members[a,b] | Associated proteins[b,c] | Roles |
|---|---|---|
| hsp110, hsp100 | Actin (6) | May protect heat-sensitive ribosome production (7) |
| hsp90/hsp90α, hsp90β, grp94 | Calmodulin (8)<br>Actin (6)<br>Tubulin (9)<br>Steroid hormone receptors (10)<br>Cellular protein kinases (11)<br>Retroviral transforming proteins (12)<br>hsp70 (13,14)<br>hsp56 (14)<br>p60, p50, . . . (10,14) | Protein folding and unfolding (13,15)<br>Maintenance of certain proteins in inactive form (16)<br>Immunity (17) |
| hsp70/hsp72, hsc73, grp78 (=BiP), PBP74 (18) | hsp90 (13,14)<br>hsp56 (14)<br>hsp40 (19)<br>p53 (20)<br>Steroid hormone receptors (10)<br>Tubulin (21)<br>Intermediate filaments (22)<br>Actin (23)<br>Nucleotides (24)<br>Viral oncogene products (25,26)<br>pRb110 (27) | Protein folding and unfolding (15,28)<br>Assembly and disassembly of multimeric complexes, thermo-tolerance (5,29)<br>Polypeptide translocation (30)<br>Disassembly of clathrin-coated vesicles (31)<br>Protein degradation, cell proliferation and differentiation (32)<br>Class II antigen processing (33)<br>Immunity (17) |
| hsp60 | | Chaperonin (34)<br>Protein folding and unfolding, organelle translocation (15)<br>Assembly of multimeric complexes, immunity (17) |
| hsp56 (immunophilin) | Steroid hormone receptors (35)<br>hsp90 (14)<br>hsp70 (14) | Protein folding and trafficking in the cell (36)<br>Immunity (17) |
| hsp47 | Procollagen, types I-V collagen (37) | Collagen-specific molecular chaperone (37) |
| hsp40 | hsp70 (19)<br>p53 (19) | Protein folding (28) |
| hsp27 and other small hsp/hsp26, αA-crystallin, αB-crystallin (38), hsp32 (39) | Actin (40)<br>Estrogen receptor (41)<br>Platelet factor XIII (42) | Protein folding and unfolding (13,43,44)<br>Inhibition actin polymerization (40)<br>Growth arrest (44,45)<br>Differentiation (44,46) |
| hsp10 | | Cell proliferation (47)<br>Protein folding (48) |
| Ubiquitin | Histones H2A and H2B, denatured globin, platelet-derived growth factor receptor (49) | Protein degradation (50)<br>Immunity (17) |

[a]Some of the HSPs are still under characterization/investigation and for this reason we do not know with certainty if they belong to a specific family (i.e., hsp10).
[b]References are in parentheses.
[c]HSPs acting as molecular chaperones bind several proteins; however, in this list we included those proteins that have been more or less well characterized.

## HEAT SHOCK PROTEINS

### General Considerations

HSPs are produced by cells in response to a variety of insults (5). These proteins may be grouped according to their molecular weight into several families (Table 1). Each family consists of closely related proteins encoded by members of a gene family.

The HSP families have several common features: (a) they are preferentially expressed following heat shock, whereas synthesis of other proteins is repressed; (b) they are found in practically all living organisms/cells (prokaryotic and eukaryotic); (c) their amino acid sequences are highly conserved throughout evolution; and (d) they have in the promoter region of their genes a specific DNA motif called heat shock responsive element (HSRE or HSE), which is activated by specific heat shock transcription factors (HSTF or HSF) (51).

Most HSPs are expressed at rather significant levels in unstressed cells under physiological conditions (constitutive or cognate: HSC) depending on the cell cycle, hormonal influences, differentiation stages of the cells, etc. (Fig. 1). HSPs play important physiological roles—for instance, acting as molecular chaperones in the folding/unfolding, activation/inactivation, oligomerization, transport, and degradation of other proteins. Several excellent reviews on HSPs have been published (5,44,50–53).

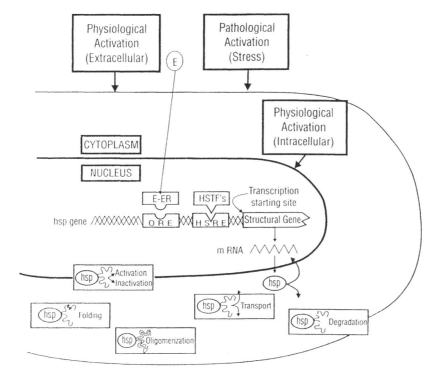

**Figure 1**  Schematic representation of a cell showing HSP-responsive pathways. As an example of physiological activation (extracellular), we find estrogen (E) stimulation, binding to estrogen receptor (ER). This estrogen–estrogen receptor complex then acts on other responsive elements (ORE) in the promoter region of a heat shock gene. HSTF's, heat shock transcription factors; HSRE, heat shock responsive element; hsp, heat shock protein.

The heat shock response is a fundamental cellular defense against conditions that damage the cell, permitting a rapid resumption of normal cellular activities during the recovery period. The cells exposed to a moderate heat shock survive subsequent more extreme temperatures much better than the cells that had not previously been heat shocked. This phenomenon is called thermotolerance (54–56). Several studies have shown that the HSPs are essential in thermotolerance; for example, cells in which the synthesis of HSPs is blocked fail to acquire thermotolerance, and cells injected with antibodies specific against a HSP quickly die following their exposure to a brief heat shock treatment (57). However, not all the studies support a correlation between HSP levels and enhanced resistance against heat and other stresses, suggesting that other proteins/systems may also be important in cell protection (reviewed in Ref. 58). The specific mechanisms of HSP action to protect the cells from heat-induced death are still under investigation (59).

### Presence in Human Cancer Tissues

In humans, HSPs may be expressed in normal and pathological cells and tissues, including neoplastic conditions. Many times these proteins have been studied in cultured tumor cells. Here, however, we review the presence of HSPs in clinical cancer samples, at the same time grouping the different tumors with their general response to cytotoxic drugs (Table 2).

The study of HSPs in cancer tissues is relatively novel; for this reason, the list of HSPs present in different tumor types is incomplete. Future studies are needed to expand our knowledge of HSP expression in tumor tissues—if possible, correlating their expression with anatomopathological and clinical characteristics.

## ON THE MECHANISMS OF ACTION IN DRUG RESISTANCE: AN INCOMPLETE PICTURE

At present, we do not have a clear understanding of the mechanisms of action of HSPs in mediating drug resistance. However, we may advance some speculations based on the interrelations of HSPs with other proteins/mechanisms that are known to be involved in drug resistance, with the aim of challenging further studies relevant to this important research area.

### HSPs and P170

Is it possible that a relationship exists between HSPs and P170? Of special interest here is the presence of heat shock responsive elements in the promoter region of the *MDR*1 gene; the mRNA levels for P170 may increase in some cells in response to heat shock and to other stressful situations (3). Then, HSTFs may regulate *MDR*1 gene expression via the heat shock responsive elements; in addition, there is evidence that HSPs themselves participate in the regulation of the heat shock response, interacting with the HSTFs (91). However, we have evidence that the *MDR*1/P170 system may not be activated by heat shock in some tumor cells. This was seen in two human breast cancer cell lines (MCF-7 and MDA-MB-231) studied for drug resistance following heat shock, a condition that selectively increased cell resistance to doxorubicin without affecting the

**Table 2**  Human Tumors Grouped According to Their General Response to Chemotherapy (the presence of HSPs in these tumors is presented)

| Tumors | HSPs (Ref.) |
| --- | --- |
| Highly responsive tumors | |
|    Acute lymphocytic leukemia | hsp27 (60) |
|    Choriocarcinoma | ? |
|    Ewing's sarcoma | ? |
|    Hodgkin's lymphoma | ? |
|    Osteogenic sarcoma | ? |
|    Embryonal rhabdomyosarcoma | ? |
|    Small-cell lung cancer | ? |
|    Testicular carcinoma | hsp60 (61) |
|    Wilms' tumor | ? |
| Moderately responsive tumors | |
|    Acute myeloid leukemia (HL-60) | hsp27 (62), hsp70 (63), hsp90 (64) |
|    Bladder carcinoma | hsp27 (65) |
|    Brain (meningioma, neuroblastoma, etc.) | hsp27 (66–69) |
|    Breast carcinoma | hsp27 (70,71), hsp70 (72), hsp90 (73) |
|    Carcinoma of the uterine cervix | hsp27 (74,75), hsp70, hsc70, hsp90 (unp. observations) |
|    Colon carcinoma | hsp60 (61), αB-crystallin (76) |
|    Endometrium carcinoma | hsp27 (71,74) |
|    Erythroleukemia | hsp70, hsp90 (77) |
|    Gastric carcinoma | hsp27 (78), hsp70 (79) |
|    Non-Hodgkin's lymphoma | hsp70 (80) |
|    Ovarian carcinoma | hsp27 (81), hsp60 (82), hsp70 (83), hsp90 (84) |
|    Prostate carcinoma | hsp27 (65,70) |
|    Head and neck cancer | ? |
|    Multiple myeloma | ? |
| Unresponsive/poorly responsive tumors | |
|    Non-small-cell lung cancer | hsp27 (unpub. observation), hsp63, hsp72, hsp73, hsp90 (85) |
|    Hepatocellular carcinoma | hsp27 (86,87) |
|    Melanoma | hsp72 (88) |
|    Pancreatic carcinoma | hsp70, hsp90, ubiquitin (89) |
|    Renal cell carcinoma | αB-crystallin (76) |
|    Soft tissue sarcoma (malignant fibrous histiocytoma) | hsp27 (90) |
|    Thyroid carcinoma | αB-crystallin (76) |
|    Esophageal carcinoma | ? |

P170 mRNA levels (92). Moreover, MDA-A$_1^R$ breast cancer cells selected for doxorubicin resistance and expressing a multidrug resistance phenotype did not show a further increase in drug resistance following heat shock (92). In these cancer cells, the *MDR*1/ P170 system was not participating in the heat shock response. In future studies, using clinical cancer samples, it will be important to explore whether the *MDR*1 gene is significantly activated by stressful situations via HSTF/HSPs. Finally, in a preliminary study, one HSP, hsp90, was co-precipitated with P170 in drug-resistant cells, suggesting cooperation between HSPs and the P170 drug efflux pump (93).

## HSPs and p53

There is mounting evidence that p53 is an important protein involved in cancer therapy because cellular resistance to ionizing radiation and to cytotoxic drugs may be dependent on p53 throughout modulation of apoptosis (94–97). Recent studies have linked HSPs with p53. For instance, mutant p53 proteins form complexes with hsp72, hsc73, and hsp40, some of them with prolonged half-life (19,20,98–101). We have to remember that one of the functions of HSPs is recognizing altered proteins; therefore, it is possible that HSPs are binding some p53 mutated forms triggered by the improperly folded nascent p53 proteins. Moreover, using 5' deletion constructs of the hsp70 promoter, researchers have shown transactivation of the hsp70 promoter by mutated p53 species via heat shock responsive elements (102). In contrast, wild-type human p53 may reduce transcription from the human hsp70 promoter (103). Taken together, these data show that hsp70 expression is regulated both by wild-type and some mutated forms of p53, but we do not know whether the p53–HSP interactions are of physiopathological significance mainly in the process of drug resistance mediated by apoptosis. A recent study has shown that the synthesis of hsp70 was inhibited by quercetin administration in tumor cell lines; quercetin exerted cytotoxic activity inducing apoptosis (104). In these experiments, no apoptosis was induced by quercetin when the tumor cells were first exposed to heat shock, suggesting that hsp70 is involved in protecting the cells from apoptosis. So far the evidence indicates that some mutated forms of p53 could stimulate hsp70 expression—an important chaperone that is strongly implicated in making the cells less susceptible to thermal stress, to several cytotoxic agents, and perhaps also to apoptosis. On the one hand, therefore, tumor cells carrying mutated p53 species are unable to direct the cells to apoptosis; and on the other hand, they may be overexpressing the HSPs involved in drug resistance. However, this attractive hypothesis should be taken with caution because recent immunohistochemical studies examining clinical breast cancer samples revealed a lack of association between nuclear p53 accumulation and cytoplasmic or nuclear hsp70 levels (105), or even an inverse correlation between hsp70 and p53 (106).

## HSPs in Cell Proliferation and Differentiation

The responsiveness of tumor cells to several chemotherapeutic drugs depends on the phase of the cell cycle (cell cycle phase–specific agents); chemotherapy-resistant tumors tend to grow more slowly than chemotherapy-sensitive tumors. Is it possible that HSPs are involved in drug resistance modulating cell proliferation? This question makes sense if we consider that besides p53, hsp70 (the most studied HSP) interacts with several gene/protein products that are very important during the processes of cell proliferation and transformation, i.e., c-myc, adenovirus E1A, SV40 large T antigen, and retinoblastoma gene product pRb110 (25,27,107,108). At present, however, the role for HSPs in cell proliferation is controversial; some studies support the theory that certain HSPs, such as hsp72, hsc73, and hsp90, could be related to elevated cellular proliferation, but there are also studies suggesting that these HSPs are involved with cell growth arrest and increased differentiation (109–117). We have been studying more extensively a low-molecular-weight HSP, hsp27, and we believe that this protein is more implicated in cell growth arrest (45,118–121) than in cell proliferation (122). In a preliminary study using human breast cancer biopsy samples, we analyzed on a cell-by-cell basis the expression of hsp27 with that of two proliferation markers (PCNA and AgNOR); the study revealed an inverse correlation between hsp27 overexpression and cell proliferation (123). In addition, hsp27 overexpression has been noted in more differentiated tumors (74,75); and even within a particular tumor, the protein was more expressed in the more differentiated areas (as evaluated by histopathology and by the expression of differentiation markers) (75). Thus, hsp27 may be conferring drug resistance by mechanisms involved with cell growth arrest and increased differentiation.

Besides the mechanisms mentioned above, HSPs are involved in several other important cell functions (activation/inactivation of molecules, signal transduction mechanisms, intracellular transport, cell- and antibody-mediated immunity, microtubule stabilization, etc.); these proteins are still under active investigation. Therefore, the emerging roles of HSPs in cell physiology/pathology will open new avenues of understanding that could be translated to drug resistance studies—to better know if and how HSPs are implicated in chemotherapy treatments.

## LABORATORY EVIDENCES FOR DRUG RESISTANCES

### HSPs and Drug Resistance in Cultured Cells

The first evidence that HSPs could be involved in drug resistance came from the observation that mammalian cells became more resistant to doxorubicin and to actinomycin D if the cells were exposed to nonlethal elevated temperatures *prior* to drug exposure (124,125). The stress induced by ethanol also induced thermotolerance and tolerance to doxorubicin in cultured cells (126). At that time, HSPs were not studied; however, we now know that these proteins are induced by hyperthermia and ethanol. Hyperthermia is used in cancer treatment as an adjuvant to increase the cytotoxicity of certain anticancer drugs and of radiotherapy. The mechanisms of this synergism have been reviewed elsewhere (127,128). When researchers became more aware of the existence of HSPs, several laboratories began to explore the roles of these proteins in drug resistance. Among the strategies used are those correlating drug resistance/sensitivity with HSP levels in cells where the HSPs have been induced/repressed by different experimental conditions. Also, differential screening of cDNAs, transfection of HSP genes, administration of antisense oligonucleotides, and genomic mutations have been used for the study of HSPs in several tumor cell lines with different sensitivities to chemotherapeutic drugs. Table 3 shows a summary of the cell lines tested for drug resistance. Although HSPs seem to be implicated in drug resistance in several cell lines, it is clear that HSPs are not universally associated with drug resistance.

We decided to explore the involvement of HSPs in drug resistance in human breast cancer cells, taking advantage of the finding of a cell line (MCF-7/BK) that constitutively overexpressed a low-molecular-weight HSP (hsp27) (92). The resistance to doxorubicin of this cell line was compared with the resistance to the same drug of another human breast cancer cell line (MDA-MB-231), which under normal (37°C) control conditions did not overexpress hsp27. We found that the resistance to doxorubicin was considerably higher in MCF-7/BK cells. Next, we induced the heat shock

**Table 3** Summary of Cell Lines Tested for Drug Resistance and Where Different HSPs Have Been Studied

| Cell line | HSPs implicated | Drug implicated | Ref. |
|---|---|---|---|
| | Positive correlation with drug resistance | | |
| Chinese hamster | | | |
| HA-1 (ovary fibroblast) | ? | Actinomycin D, doxorubicin | 124–126 |
| HA-1 | hsp70 | Doxorubicin, VM-26 | 129, 130 |
| O23 (lung fibroblast) | hsp27 | Doxorubicin, actinomycin D | 131 |
| V79 (ovary) | grp78 | VP-16 | 132 |
| Breast cancer (human) | | | |
| MCF-7, MDA-MB-231 | hsp27, hsp70 | Doxorubicin | 92, 122, 133 |
| MCF-7 | hsc70, hsp90 | Mitoxantrone | 134 |
| MCF-7 | hsp27 | X-irradiation→vincristine vinblastine, VP-16 | 135 |
| Colon cancer (human) | | | |
| S1-M1-3,2 | hsp70, hsp90 | Mitoxantrone | 134 |
| Cervix (human, squamous) and endothelial cells (bovine, aorta) | | | |
| HeLa, ME-180, and endothelium | hsp27 (phosphor.) | Tumor necrosis factor | 136, 137 |
| Head and neck (squamous) | | | |
| UMSCC5/10b | hsp60 | Cisplatin | 138 |
| Melanoma (murine) | | | |
| B16 | hsp27 | Hydrogen peroxide | 139 |
| Leukemia | | | |
| Leukemic cell lines | hsp90, hsp70 | Glucocorticoid | 140 |
| Fibrosarcoma (murine) | | | |
| WEHI-S | hsp70 | Tumor necrosis factor | 141 |
| Gliosarcoma (rat) | | | |
| 9L | hsp70 | Vincristine | 142 |
| Liver (human) | | | |
| BEL-7404 (also mouse cells) | hsp60 | Cisplatin | 143 |
| Ovarian (human) | | | |
| 2780/CP | hsp60 | Cisplatin | 144 |
| Human and murine | | | |
| Not specified | hsp90 | Not specified | 93 |
| | No correlation with drug resistance | | |
| Colon, testicular carcinoma cells | hsp27, hsp60, hsp72, hsp73, hsp90 | Cisplatin | 145 |
| Ovarian (human, 2008) | hsp60 | Cisplatin | 146 |
| Chinese hamster | hsp70/78 | Doxorubicin | 147 |
| Ovarian, gastric, testicular, etc. | hsp27, hsp60, hsp70 | Cisplatin, doxorubicin | 148 |
| Breast (human, MCF-7) | hsp27 | Drugs and x-ray | 135 |

response in both cell lines by incubating the cells at 42°C for 2 h followed by a resting period of 4 h at 37°C to allow the synthesis of the HSPs. After this, the two cell lines were exposed to doxorubicin: both cell lines were more resistant to doxorubicin after heat shock. Figure 2 shows the survival curves of the cell lines tested. In these cells, heat shock did not induce the P170 and grp78 systems (92).

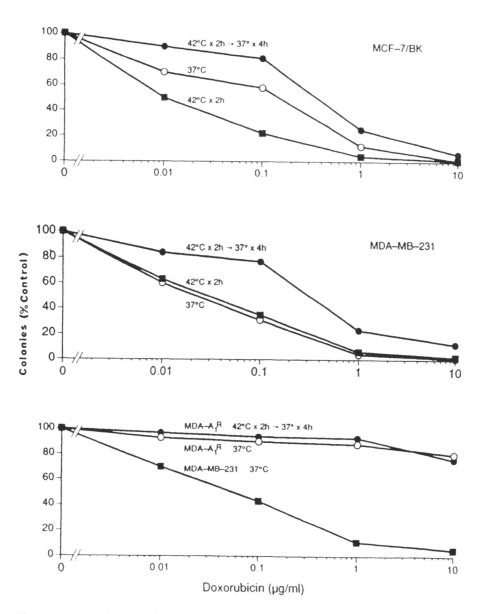

**Figure 2** Survival curves of human breast cancer cells exposed to increasing concentrations of doxorubicin, before (37°C) and after heat shocks (with and without a resting period). Soft agar clonogenic assays. (From Ref. 92.)

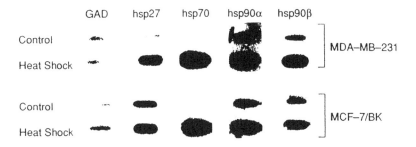

**Figure 3**   Slot blot analyses of mRNA levels for the HSPs before (37°C) and after heat shock (42°C) of two human breast cancer cell lines studied. GAD was used as a control to compare sample loading. Note elevated hsp27 mRNA levels in MCF-7/BK cells growing at 37°C. (From Ref. 92.)

The mRNA expression levels for hsp27, hsp70, and hsp90 in MCF-7/BK and MDA-MB-231 cells before and after heat shock are shown in Figure 3.

Although both cell lines showed increased doxorubicin resistance when they were first exposed to a heat shock, more drug resistance was induced in the cell line showing higher hsp70 and hsp27 expression levels after heat shock (MDA-MB-231, 16-fold resistance). MCF-7/BK cells showed moderate doxorubicin resistance (threefold). In these cells, little hsp27 mRNA levels, total mass of protein, and phosphorylation were obtained after heat shock (92). A competent heat shock response was associated with increased resistance to doxorubicin, and the resistance elicited was even better when hsp27 and hsp70 were coordinately induced. In this study model, the heat shock response did not increase the resistance to other drugs tested (colchicine, 5-fluorouracil, cisplatin, actinomycin D, and methotrexate).

In addition, we explored the doxorubicin resistance before and after heat shock of MDA-A$_1^R$ cells, cells that were selected for doxorubicin resistance and that overexpressed the P170 system (Fig. 2). No additional resistance to doxorubicin was obtained after heat shock. The two-dimensional gel electrophoresis study of these cells showed that hsp27 could not be phosphorylated after heat shock and that these cells were already expressing high hsp70 levels even before heat shock (92).

Of interest is that the levels of resistance conferred by overexpression of the P170 system (MDA-A$_1^R$ cells) was a lot higher than that obtained by the activation of the heat shock system (MCF-7/BK and MDA-MB-231 cells) (Fig. 2). It will be important to correlate these findings with the clinical situation. Is the activation of the HSP system relevant in explaining resistance to certain drugs in human tumors?

### Drugs That Stimulate HSP Expression in Cultured Cells

There are many causes that may stimulate the heat shock protein response in cancer cells and tissues. Among important stressors we find lack of adequate oxygenation, presence of necrotic/toxic cell areas, changes in the pH, cells undergoing starvation—all of them followed by a cascade of metabolic effects. Besides these stressors, another interesting factor that should be taken into consideration is the possibility that the cytotoxic drugs by themselves could participate in the stimulation/repression of the

**Table 4** Effect of Antitumor Agents on the Expression of HSPs in Cultured Cells

| HSP involved | Drug/chemical | Effect | Ref. |
|---|---|---|---|
| hsp70 | Nitrosourea | ↑ | 149, 150 |
| | Chlorambucil, cis-platinum | = | 149 |
| | Herbimycin A | ↑ | 151 |
| | Hemin | ↑ | 152 |
| | Dimethyl sulfoxide | ↓ | 153 |
| | Quercetin | ↓ | 154 |
| | N-methylformamide | ↑ ↓ (dosis related) | 155 |
| hsc70 | N-methylformamide | ↓ | 156 |
| hsp90 | Nitrosourea | ↑ | 150 |
| | N-methylformamide | ↑ ↓ (dosis related) | 155 |
| hsp60 | Nitrosourea | ↑ (little) | 150 |
| | Phorbol esters, γ-interferon, retinoic acid | ↑ | 157 |
| hsp27 | Nitrosourea | ↑ (little) | 150 |
| | Phorbol ester | ↑ (phosphor.) | 118, 119 |
| | Tumor necrosis factor | ↑ (phosphor.) | 158 |
| | Leukemic inhibitory factor | ↑ (phosphor.) | 159 |
| | Retinoic acid | ↑ | 69, 160 |
| | Cisplatin, daunomycin, doxorubicin | ↑ | 161 |
| | Cytosine arabinose, vincristine, colchicine, 5FU, aminopterin, amethopterin, cyclophosphamide, mithramycine | = | 161 |

HSP response. Table 4 lists examples of anticancer agents that may affect the expression of HSPs in cultured cells.

As in other experiments performed on cultured cells, different cell lines may respond differently to the agents tested. For example, we failed to induce increased hsp27 expression in MCF-7/BK human breast cancer cells following cis-platinum administration (unpublished observation). This anticancer drug induced hsp25 (the rodent homologue of human hsp27) expression in Ehrlich ascites tumor cells (160). In any case, it is clear that at least in cultured tumor cells, certain cytotoxic drugs may regulate the HSP response. Further studies are necessary to clarify whether this also happens in clinical cancers and whether this is significant in explaining acquired drug resistance.

## CLINICAL EVIDENCES FOR DRUG RESISTANCE

At present, very few studies have been designed to explore whether HSPs are implicated in drug resistance. hsp27 has been more studied in breast cancer patients because this particular HSP was first described as an estrogen-regulated protein, associated with estrogen receptors (70,71). The presence of estrogen receptors is a good marker

**Table 5**  hsp27 Expression in Breast Cancer Patients: Prognostic Correlations and Response to Treatments

| Authors | Patients | Prognosis | Response to | | |
|---|---|---|---|---|---|
| | | | Hormonotherapy | Chemotherapy | Radiotherapy |
| Cano (162) | 27 | NT[a] | hsp27+:>response | NT | NT |
| Andersen (163) | 103 | NT | No correlation | NT | NT |
| Seymour (164) | 51 | hsp27+:>OS | NT | hsp27+:>response | NT |
| Thor (165) | 300 | OS:No correlation (hsp27+:<DFS in LN+ only) | NT | NT | NT |
| Damstrup (166) | 119 | No correlation | No correlation | NT | NT |
| Hurlimann (167) | 196 | No correlation | No correlation | No correlation | No correlation |
| Love (168) | 361 | No correlation (>hsp27:<DFS in LN- only) | NT | NT | NT |

[a]Abbreviations used: NT, not tested; OS, overall survival; DSF, disease-free survival; LN+/-, axillary lymph node positive or negative patients.

for selecting patients for endocrine therapy; however, not all breast cancer patients with estrogen receptor–positive tumors respond to endocrine manipulations. For this reason, additional estrogen-regulated proteins have been analyzed, among them hsp27. An early report of a few patients tested encouraged this because it was stated that patients with estrogen receptor–positive/hsp27-positive tumors responded better to endocrine therapy than estrogen receptor–positive/hsp27-negative tumor patients (162). Unfortunately, as can be seen in Table 5, this initial finding has not been confirmed by other studies correlating the expression of hsp27 with the response to hormonotherapy, even when in these studies the presence of estrogen receptors was of value in predicting the hormone responsiveness. One possible explanation for this is that although hsp27 is associated with estrogen receptors, there are cases in which these two proteins are not associated; hsp27 expression may be stimulated not only by estrogens but also by many different signals coming from several stressful situations.

Table 5 shows a summary of the clinical studies correlating hsp27 with disease prognosis and response to therapies in breast cancer patients. In one of these studies (164), the presence of hsp27 predicted response to treatment with cyclophosphamide, mitoxantrone, and vincristine (with or without tamoxifen, according to the estrogen receptor status). The authors reported that metastatic breast cancer patients with hsp27-positive tumors showed a higher response rate than those with hsp27-negative tumors, and that hsp27-positive patients had better overall survival. In contrast, another group reported no correlation between hsp27 expression and response to chemotherapy as well as with response to antihormone therapy and radiotherapy (167). In addition, these authors did not find a correlation between hsp27 and survival or recurrence at 5 years (a subgroup of estrogen receptor–negative/hsp27-positive patients showed a better prognosis, but this did not reach statistically significant values). Clearly, we need more carefully designed studies, with homogeneous groups of patients, to draw more conclusions about the value of hsp27 in predicting responsiveness to therapies. We are collaborating with the group at San Antonio (Division of Medical Oncology, University of Texas Health Science Center) evaluating biopsies from metastatic breast cancer patients who were estrogen receptor–positive and who received tamoxifen for several years. We hope to have conclusions from this study soon; its strengths are the number of patients involved, the complete follow-up, and the highly defined clinical end points.

hsp27 has also been evaluated in gastric cancer patients entered in a randomized trial of adjuvant tamoxifen therapy (169). Although the number of patients in this study was small, the hsp27-positive patients treated with tamoxifen showed a statistically significant shorter survival time when compared with the untreated control group. This result might be explained by taking into account that tamoxifen may be acting as an estrogen agonist increasing cell proliferation in gastric cancer cells (170). Then, was hsp27 predicting tamoxifen responsiveness in gastric cancer? Before answering this, we need to know if hsp27 is estrogen receptor associated and an estrogen-regulated marker protein in gastric carcinomas. In any case, the presence of hsp27 in gastric carcinomas has been associated with poor prognosis (78).

Another neoplasm in which hsp27 has been studied is malignant fibrous histiocytoma (90). In this report, the expression of hsp27 was investigated in 13 patients with metastasis who received various salvage chemotherapy protocols including (among others) doxorubicin and vincristine. hsp27 expression did not predict the response to chemotherapy of these patients; in addition, hsp27 expression was associated with a more favorable prognosis. Again, we need clinical studies with groups of patients who are more homogeneous, both in terms of disease stage and chemotherapy treatments, to further evaluate the implications of HSPs in drug resistance.

We also need to mention here another study in which HSPs have been studied, but in relation to disease prognosis. Elevated hsp90 expression was associated with lymph node metastasis and shorter disease-free survival and overall survival in breast cancer patients (73). We have reported that elevated hsp70 levels in breast cancer patients with negative axillary lymph nodes is significantly associated with shorter disease-free survival (72). Overexpression of hsp60 has been associated with poor survival in ovarian cancer patients (82). Although these results are not statistically significant, the authors reported that patients with prior chemotherapy and low hsp60 levels had better survival rates when compared with patients who were high hsp60 expressors, suggesting that hsp60 may be involved in resistance to the platinum-containing drugs.

No significant association of hsp27 content with disease prognosis has been reported for patients with prostate or bladder cancer (65), but increased hsp27 expression in neuroblastomas has been associated with limited-stage disease and more differentiated tumors (69).

We are now studying the expression of hsp27 in breast cancer biopsy samples taken from the same patient before and after chemotherapy in order to have information about the effect of cytotoxic drugs on hsp27 expression. The biopsies have been taken from patients with locally advanced or stage III disease who received neoadjuvant chemotherapy aimed at reducing the primary tumor to allow or facilitate surgical procedures. The biopsies were formalin-fixed and processed for routine histological examination; immunohistochemistry was performed as described previously (171) to

**Table 6**   Changes Induced by Chemotherapy in Breast Cancer Biopsy Samples

| Case (no.) | Chemotherapy | ER[a] | | PR | | hsp27 | | PCNA | |
|---|---|---|---|---|---|---|---|---|---|
| | | Pre | Post | Pre | Post | Pre | Post | Pre | Post |
| 1 | FEC/4c[b] | − | − | − | − | 30% | 66% | 35% | 32% |
| 2 | FAC/3c | + | − | − | − | 60% | 32% | 65% | 44% |
| 3 | FAC/4c | − | − | − | − | 10% | 65% | 80% | 75% |
| 4 | FAC/3c | − | − | − | − | 9% | 68% | 62% | 73% |
| 5 | FEC/8c | + | w+ | w+ | + | 35% | 37% | 67% | 64% |
| 6 | FEC/4c | − | − | − | w+ | 10% | 12% | 85% | 46% |
| 7 | FEC/3c | w+ | − | − | − | 51% | 47% | 44% | 40% |

[a]Abbreviations used: ER, estrogen receptors; PR, progesterone receptors; pre, pre-chemotherapy; post, post-chemotherapy; F, 5-fluorouracil; E, epirubicin; C, cyclophosphamide; A, adriamycin.
[b]3c/4c/8c, number of cycles administered before the second biopsy; w, weak.

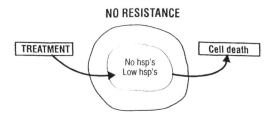

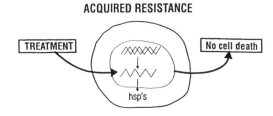

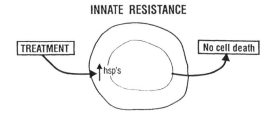

**Figure 4**   Model showing possible situations present in tumor cells where HSPs may be involved in acquired or innate drug resistance.

detect hsp27, estrogen receptors, progesterone receptors, and proliferating cell nuclear antigen (PCNA). At present, seven cases have been analyzed; the results obtained are shown in Table 6.

hsp27 expression was increased two- to sixfold in three of seven (43%) cases; remained without obvious changes in three of seven (43%) cases, and in only one case (14%) was reduced twofold after chemotherapy. Most of the cases studied were estrogen and progesterone receptor negative tumors; however, all of them expressed hsp27 protein. In case number 2, estrogen receptors were positive before chemotherapy and became negative after chemotherapy. hsp27 decreased, but the protein was still expressed in this case. The percentage of proliferating cells evaluated by PCNA staining did not change significantly in the samples where hsp27 increased, but it decreased in case number 2 (case showing decreased hsp27 levels). The presence of PCNA in many tumor cells after chemotherapy suggests that these cells are still cycling and that they were not affected by the cytotoxic drugs. However, we cannot draw conclusions from the response of these tumors to the cytotoxic drugs; this short-term treatment sometimes decreased the tumor size, but we do not know the drug response of the remaining tumor cells. If HSPs are involved in drug resistance, as hypothesized in Figure 4, it is highly probable that large tumors have heterogeneous cell populations, and that the decrease in tumor size following the initial chemotherapy is reflecting the cell killing of the drug-sensitive cell populations only. In any case, it is clear that chemotherapy induced the presence of a larger number of tumor cells expressing hsp27 in certain human breast cancers and that this increase did not correlate with the presence of estrogen and progesterone receptors. We hope that future studies on HSPs and other gene/protein systems will enable us to assess drug resistance with a tangible impact on the selection of the most appropriate therapies for each individual cancer patient.

## REFERENCES

1. Chin K-V, Tanaka S, Darlington G, Pastan I, Gottesman MM. Heat shock and arsenite increase expression of the multidrug resistance (MDR1) gene in human renal carcinoma cells. J Biol Chem 1990; 265:221–226.
2. Matsuo K, Kohno K, Sato S, Uchiumi T, Tanimura H, Yamada Y, Kuwano M. Enhanced expression of the DNA topoisomerase II gene in response to heat shock stress in human epidermoid cancer KB cells. Cancer Res 1993; 53:1085–1090.
3. Chin K-V, Pastan I, Gottesman MM. Function and regulation of the human multidrug resistance gene. Adv Cancer Res 1993; 60:157–180.
4. Matsumoto H, Shimura M, Omatsu T, Okaichi K, Majima H, Ohnishi T. p53 proteins accumulated by heat stress associate with heat shock proteins hsp72/hsc73 in human glioblastoma cell lines. Cancer Lett 1994; 87:39–46.
5. Burdon RH. Heat shock and the heat shock proteins. Biochem J 1986; 240:313–324.
6. Koyasu S, Nishida E, Kadowaki T, Matsuzaki F, Iida K, Harada F, Kasuga M, Sakai H, Yahara I. Two mammalian heat shock proteins hsp90 and hsp100 are actin binding proteins. Proc Natl Acad Sci USA 1986; 83:8054–8058.
7. Subjeck JR, Shyy T, Shen J, Johnson RJ. Association between the mammalian 110,000-dalton heat-shock protein and nucleoli. J Cell Biol 1983; 97:1389–1395.
8. Minami Y, Kawasaki H, Suzuki K, Yahara I. The calmodulin-binding domain of the mouse 90-kDa heat shock protein. J Biol Chem 1993; 268:9604–9610.

9. Sanchez ER, Redmond T, Scherrer LC, Bresnick EH, Welsh MJ, Pratt WB. Evidence that the 90-kDa heat shock protein is associated with tubulin-containing complexes in L cell cytosol and in intact PtK cells. Mol Endocrinol 1988; 2:756–760.

10. Smith DF, Toft DO. Steroid receptors and their associated proteins. Mol Endocrinol 1993; 7:4–11.

11. Rose DW, Wettenhall REH, Kudlicki W, Kramer G, Hardesty B. The 90-kilodalton peptide of the heme-regulated eIF-2a kinase has sequence similarity with the 90-kilodalton heat shock protein. Biochemistry 1987; 26:6583–6587.

12. Oppermann H, Levinson W, Bishop JM. A cellular protein that associates with a transforming protein of Rous sarcoma virus is also a heat shock protein. Proc Natl Acad Sci USA 1981; 78:1067–1071.

13. Jakob U, Buchner J. Assisting spontaneity: the role of hsp90 and small HSPs as molecular chaperones. Trends Biochem Sci 1994; 19:205–211.

14. Perdew GH, Whitelaw ML. Evidence that the 90-kDa heat shock protein (hsp90) exists in cytosol in heteromeric complexes containing hsp70 and three other proteins with Mr of 63,000, 56,000, and 50,000. J Biol Chem 1991; 266:6708–6713.

15. Gething M-J, Sambrook J. Protein folding in the cell. Nature 1992; 355:33–45.

16. Xu Y, Lindquist S. Heat-shock protein hsp90 governs the activity of pp60$^{V-SrC}$ kinase. Proc Natl Acad Sci USA 1993; 90:7074–7078.

17. Kaufman SHE. Heat shock proteins and the immune response. Immunol Today 1990; 11: 129–137.

18. Dahlseid JN, Lill R, Green JM, Xu XX, Qiu Y, Pierce SK. PBP74, a new member of the mammalian 70-kDa heat shock protein family, is a mitochondrial protein. Mol Biol Cell 1994; 5:1265–1275.

19. Sugito K, Yamane M, Hatton H, Hayashi Y, Tohnai I, Veda M, Tsuchida N, Ohtsuka K. Interaction between hsp70 and hsp40, eukaryotic homologues of DnaK and DnaJ, in human cells expressing mutant-type 53. FEBS Lett 1995; 358:161–164.

20. Pinhasi-Kimhi O, Michalovitz D, Ben-Zeev A, Oren M. Specific interactions between the p53 cellular tumour antigen and major heat shock proteins. Nature 1986; 320:182–185.

21. Sánchez C, Padilla R, Paciucci R, Zabala JC, Avila J. Binding of heat-shock protein 70 (hsp70) to tubulin. Arch Biochem Biophys 1994; 310:428–432.

22. Napolitano EW, Pachter JS, Chin SSM, Liem RKH. β-internexin, a ubiquitous intermediate filament-associated protein. J Cell Biol 1985; 101:1323–1331.

23. Margulis BA, Welsh M. Analysis of protein binding to heat shock protein 70 in pancreatic islet cells exposed to elevated temperatures or interleukin 1β. J Biol Chem 1991; 266:9295–9298.

24. Welch WJ, Feramisco JR. Rapid purification of mammalian 70,000-dalton stress proteins: affinity of the proteins for nucleotides. Mol Cell Biol 1985; 5:1229–1237.

25. White E, Spector D, Welch W. Differential distribution of the adenovirus E1A proteins and colocalization of E1A with the 70-kilodalton cellular heat-shock protein in infected cells. J Virol 1988; 62:4153–4166.

26. Sawai ET, Butel JS. Association of a cellular heat-shock protein with simian virus 40 large T antigen in transformed cells. J Virol 1989; 63:3961–3973.

27. Nihei T, Takahashi S, Sagae S, Sato N, Kikuchi K. Protein interaction of retinoblastoma gene product pRb110 with Mr 73,000 heat shock cognate protein. Cancer Res 1993; 53: 1702–1705.

28. Frydman J, Nimmesgern E, Ohtsuka K, Hartl FU. Folding of nascent polypeptide chains in a high molecular mass assembly with molecular chaperones. Nature 1994; 370:111–117.

29. Pelham HRB. Speculations on the functions of the major heat shock and glucose-regulated proteins. Cell 1986; 46:959–961.

30. Chirico WJ, Waters MG, Blobel G. 70k heat shock related proteins stimulate protein translocation into microsomes. Nature 1988; 332:805–810.

31. Chappell TG, Welch WJ, Schlossman DM, Palter KB, Schlesinger MJ, Rothman JE. Uncoating ATPase is a member of the 70 kilodalton family of stress proteins. Cell 1986; 45:3–13.

32. Carper SW, Duffy JJ, Gerner EW. Heat shock proteins in thermotolerance and other cellular processes. Cancer Res 1987; 47:5249–5255.

33. Van Buskirk AM, De Nagel DC, Gugliardi LE, Brodsky FM, Pierce SK. Cellular and sub-cellular distribution of PBP72/74, a peptide-binding protein that plays a role in antigen processing. J Immunol 1991; 146:500–506.

34. Hemmingsen SM, Woolford C, van der Vies SM. Homologous plant and bacterial proteins chaperone oligomeric protein assembly. Nature 1988; 333:330–334.

35. Pratt W, Czar M, Stancato L, Owens J. The hsp56 immunophilin component of steroid receptor heterocomplexes: could this be the elusive nuclear localization signal-binding protein? J Steroid Biochem Mol Biol 1993; 46:269–279.

36. Pratt WB. The role of heat shock proteins in regulating the function, folding, and trafficking of the glucocorticoid receptor. J Biol Chem 1993; 268:21455–21458.

37. Natsume T, Koide T, Yokota S, Hirayoshi K, Nagata K. Interactions between collagen-binding stress protein hsp47 and collagen—analysis of kinetic parameters by surface plasmon resonance biosensor. J Biol Chem 1994; 269:31224–31228.

38. Klemenz R, Fröhli E, Steiger RH, Schäfer R, Aoyama, A. αB-crystallin is a small heat shock protein. Proc Natl Acad Sci USA 1991; 88:3652–3656.

39. Keyse SM, Tyrrell RM. Both near ultraviolet radiation and the oxidizing agent hydrogen peroxide induce a 32-kDa stress protein in normal human skin fibroblasts. J Biochem 1987; 262:14821–14825.

40. Miron T, Vancompernolle K, Vandekerckhove J, Wilchek M, Geiger B. A 25-kD inhibitor of actin polymerization is a low molecular mass heat shock protein. J Cell Biol 1991; 114:255–264.

41. Coffer AI, King RJB. Characterization of p29, an estrogen-receptor associated tumor marker. J Steroid Biochem 1988; 31:745–750.

42. Zhu Y, Tassi L, Lane W, Mendelsohn ME. Specific binding of the transglutaminase, platelet factor XIII to hsp27. J Biol Chem 1994; 269:22379–22384.

43. Jakob U, Gaestel M, Engel K, Buchner J. Small heat shock proteins are molecular chaperones. J Biol Chem 1993; 268:1517–1520.

44. Ciocca DR, Oesterreich S, Chamness GC, McGuire WL, Fuqua SAW. Biological and clinical implications of heat protein 27000 (hsp27): a review. J Natl Cancer Inst 1993; 85:1558–1570.

45. Spector NL, Ryan C, Samson W, Levine H, Nadler LM, Arrigo A-P. Heat shock protein is a unique marker of growth arrest during macrophage differentiation of HL-60 cells. J Cell Physiol 1993; 156:619–625.

46. Kindås-Mügge I, Trautinger F. Increased expression of the Mr 27,000 heat shock protein (hsp27) in in vitro differentiated normal human keratinocytes. Cell Growth Differ 1994; 5:777–781.

47. Cavanagh AC, Morton H. The purification of early-pregnancy factor to homogeneity from human platelets and identification as chaperonin 10. Eur J Biochem 1994; 222:551–560.

48. Hartman DJ, Hoogenraad NJ, Condron R, Hoj PB. Identification of a mammalian 10-kDa heat shock protein, a mitochondrial chaperonin 10 homologue essential for assisted folding of trimeric ornithine transcarbamoylase in vitro. Proc Natl Acad Sci USA 1992; 89:3394–3398.

49. Mager WH, Moradas Ferreira P. Stress response of yeast. Biochem J 1993; 290:1–13.

50. Welch WJ. Mammalian stress response: cell physiology, structure/function of stress proteins, and implications for medicine and disease. Physiol Rev 1992; 72:1063–1081.

51. Ang D, Liberek K, Skowyra D, Zylicz M, Georgopoulos C. Biological role and regulation of the universally conserved heat shock proteins. J Biol Chem 1991; 226:24233–24236.

52. Morimoto RI, Sarge KD, Abravaya K. Transcriptional regulation of heat shock genes. J Biol Chem 1992; 267:21987–21990.

53. Georgopoulos C, Welch WJ. Role of the major heat shock proteins as molecular chaperones. Annu Rev Cell Biol 1993; 9:601–634.

54. Craig EA, Weissman JS, Horwich AL. Heat shock proteins and molecular chaperones: mediators of protein conformation and turnover in the cell. Cell 1994; 78:365–372.

55. Li GC, Werb Z. Correlation between synthesis of heat shock proteins and development of thermotolerance in Chinese hamster fibroblasts. Proc Natl Acad Sci USA 1982; 79:3218–3222.

56. Nover L, Scherf KD. Heat shock proteins. In: Nover L, ed. Heat Shock Response. Boca Raton: CRC Press, 1991:41–127.

57. Riabowol KT, Mizzen LA, Welch WJ. Heat shock is lethal to fibroblasts microinjected with antibodies specific against hsp70. Science 1988; 242:433–436.

58. Landry J. Heat shock proteins and cell thermotolerance. In: Anghileri LJ, Robert J, eds. Hyperthermia in Cancer Treatment. Vol. I. Boca Raton: CRC Press, 1986:37–58.

59. Morimoto RI, Tissieres A, Georgopoulos C, eds. Stress Proteins in Biology and Medicine. Cold Spring Harbor, New York: Cold Spring Harbor Laboratory Press, 1990.

60. Strahler JR, Kuick R, Hanash SM. Diminished phosphorylation of a heat shock protein (hsp27) in infant acute lymphoblastic leukemia. Biochem Biophys Res Commun 1991; 175:134–142.

61. Kimura E, Enns RE, Hohn DK, Arboleda J, Slamon DJ, Howell SB. Expression of the carboxy-terminal portion of P1 mitochondrial chaperonin (CTP1) in normal and cancer tissues (abstr). Proc Am Soc Clin Oncol 1991; 10:101.

62. Mivechi NF, Monson JM, Hahn GM. Expression of HSP-28 and three HSP-70 genes during the development and decay of thermotolerance in leukemic and nonleukemic human tumors. Cancer Res 1991; 51:6608–6614.

63. Mivechi NF, Rossi JJ. Use of polymerase chain reaction to detect the expression of the $M_r$ 70,000 heat shock genes in control or heat shock leukemic cells as correlated to their heat response. Cancer Res 1990; 50:2877–2884.

64. Yufu Y, Nishimura J, Takahira H, Ideguchi H, Nawata H. Down-regulation of a $M_r$ 90,000 heat shock cognate protein during granulocytic differentiation in HL-60 human leukemia cells. Cancer Res 1989; 49:2405–2408.

65. Storm FK, Mahvi DM, Gilchrist KW. HSP-27 has no diagnostic or prognostic significance in prostate or bladder cancers. Urology 1993; 42:379–382.

66. Iwaki T, Iwaki A, Miyazono M, Goldman JE. Preferential expression of B-crystallin in astrocytic elements of neuroectodermal tumors. Cancer 1991; 68:2230–2240.

67. Kato M, Herz F, Kato S, Hirano A. Expression of stress-response (heat-shock) protein 27 in human brain tumors: an immunohistochemical study. Acta Neuropathol 1992; 83:420–422.

68. Yokoyama N, Iwaki T, Goldman JE, Tateishi J, Fukui M. Small heat-shock protein is expressed in meningiomas and granulofilamentous inclusion bodies. Acta Neuropathol 1993; 85:248–255.

69. Ungar DR, Hailat N, Strahler JR, Kuick RD, Brodeur GM, Seeger RC, Reynolds CP, Hanash SM. Hsp27 expression in neuroblastoma—correlation with disease stage. J Natl Cancer Inst 1994; 86:780–784.

70. Ciocca DR, Adams DJ, Edwards DP, Bjercke RJ, McGuire WL. Distribution of an estrogen-induced protein with a molecular weight of 24,000 in normal and malignant human tissues and cells. Cancer Res 1983; 43:1204–1210.

71. Ciocca DR, Stati AO, Amprino de Castro MM. Colocalization of estrogen and progesterone receptors with an estrogen-regulated heat shock protein in paraffin sections of human breast and endometrial cancer tissue. Breast Cancer Res Treat 1990; 16:243–251.

72. Ciocca DR, Clark GM, Tandon AK, Fuqua SAW, Welch WJ, McGuire WL. Heat shock protein hsp70 in patients with axillary lymph node-negative breast cancer: prognostic implications. J Natl Cancer Inst 1993; 85:570–574.

73. Jameel A, Skilton RA, Campbell TA, Chander SK, Coombes RC, Luqmani YA. Clinical and biological significance of HSP89 alpha in human breast cancer. Int J Cancer 1992; 50: 409–415.

74. Ciocca DR, Puy LA, Fasoli LC. Study of estrogen receptor, progesterone receptor, and the estrogen-regulated $M_r$ 24,000 protein in patients with carcinomas of the endometrium and cervix. Cancer Res 1989; 49:4298–4304.

75. Puy LA, Lo Castro G, Olcese JE, Lotfi HO, Brandi HR, Ciocca DR. Analysis of a 24-kilodalton (KD) protein in the human uterine cervix during abnormal growth. Cancer 1989; 64: 1067–1073.

76. Pinder SE, Balsitis M, Ellis IO, Landon M, Mayer RJ, Lowe J. The expression of alpha B-crystallin in epithelial tumours: a useful tumour marker? J Pathol 1994; 174:209–215.

77. Amici C, Sistonen L, Santoro MG, Morimoto RI. Antiproliferative prostaglandins activate heat shock transcription factor. Proc Natl Acad Sci USA 1992; 89:6227–6231.

78. Harrison JD, Jones JA, Ellis IO, Morris DL. Estrogen receptor D5 antibody is an independent negative prognostic factor in gastric cancer. Br J Surg 1991; 78:334–336.

79. Kiyama T, Onda M, Tokunaga A, Oguri T, Teramoto T, Fujita I, Matsukura N, Yamashita K, Todome Y, Ohkuni H. Expression of heat shock protein 70 in cancer and non-cancerous mucosa of the stomach (abstr). Proc AACR 1995; 36:214.

80. Nelson EL, Naftzger C, Welch WJ, Clayberger C, Krensky AM. Involvement of cell surface heat shock 70 protein in autologous, $\gamma/\delta$, cytotoxic T lymphocyte (CTL) recognition of a Burkitt's lymphoma (abstr). Proc AACR 1995; 36:500.

81. Langdon SP, Hirst GL, Rabiasz GJ, King RJB, Miller WR. Expression of HSP27 in human ovarian cancer (abstr). Proc AACR 1995; 36:632.

82. Kimura E, Enns RE, Alcaraz JE, ARboleda J, Slamon DJ, Howell SB. Correlation of the survival of ovarian cancer patients with mRNA expression of the 60-kD heat-shock protein HSP-60. J Clin Oncol 1993; 11:891–898.

83. Terasawa K, Sagae S, Nihei T, Takeda T, Ishioka S, Takashima S, Sato N, Kudo R. Heat shock protein (hsp) 70 family in the carcinogenesis of ovarian cancer (abstr). Proc AACR 1995; 36:197.

84. Mileo AM, Fanuele M, Battaglia F, Scambia G, Benedetti-Panici P, Mancuso S, Ferrini U. Selective over-expression of mRNA coding for 90-KDa stress-protein in human ovarian cancer. Anticancer Res 1990; 10:903–906.

85. Bonay M, Soler P, Riquet M, Battesti J-P, Hance AJ, Tazi A. Expression of heat shock proteins in human lung and lung cancers. Am J Respir Cell Mol Biol 1994; 10:453–461.

86. Ciocca DR, Jorge AD, Jorge O, Milutín C, Hosokawa R, Díaz Lestren M, Muzzio E, Schulkin S, Schirbu R. Estrogen receptors, progesterone receptors and heat-shock 27-kD protein in liver biopsy specimens from patients with hepatitis B virus infection. Hepatology 1991; 13:838–844.

87. Delhaye M, Gulbis B, Galand P, Mairesse N. Expression of 27-kD heat-shock protein isoforms in human neoplastic and nonneoplastic liver tissues. Hepatology 1992; 16:382–389.

88. Protti MP, Heltai S, Bellone M, Ferrarini M, Manfredi AA, Rugarli C. Constitutive expression of the heat shock protein 72kDa in human melanoma cells. Cancer Lett 1994; 85:211–216.

89. Gress TM, Müller-Pillasch F, Weber C, Lerch MM, Friess H, Büchler M, Beger HG, Adler G. Differential expression of heat shock proteins in pancreatic carcinoma. Cancer Res 1994; 54:547–551.

90. Têtu B, Lacasse B, Bouchard H-L, Lagacé R, Huot J, Landry J. Prognostic influence of HSP-27 expression in malignant fibrous histiocytoma: a clinicopathological and immunohistochemical study. Cancer Res 1992; 52:2325–2328.

91. Morimoto RI. Cells in stress: transcriptional activation of heat shock genes. Science 1993; 259:1409–1410.

92. Ciocca DR, Fuqua SAW, Lock-Lim S, Toft DO, Welch WJ, McGuire WL. Response of human breast cancer cells to heat shock and chemotherapeutic drugs. Cancer Res 1992; 52:3648–3654.

93. Bertram J, Palfner K, Hiddemann W, Kneba M. Interrelation between molecular mechanisms of drug resistance and cellular stress response (abstr). Proc AACR 1995; 36:347.

94. Lowe SW, Ruley HE, Jacks T, Housman DE. p53-dependent apoptosis modulates the cytotoxicity of anticancer agents. Cell 1993; 74:957–967.

95. Fan S, El-Deiry WS, Bae I, Freeman J, Jondle D, Bhatia K, Fornace Jr AJ, Magrath I, Kohn KW, O'Connor PM. p53 gene mutations are associate with decreased sensitivity of human lymphoma cells to DNA damaging agents. Cancer Res 1994; 54:5824–5830.

96. Wattel E, Preudhomme C, Hecquet B, Vanrumbeke M, Quesnel B, Dervite E, Morel P, Fenaux P. p53 mutations are associated with resistance to chemotherapy and short survival in hematologic malignancies. Blood 1994; 84:3148–3157.

97. McIlwrath AJ, Vasey PA, Ross GM, Brown R. Cell cycle arrests and radiosensitivity of human tumor cell lines: dependence on wild-type p53 for radiosensitivity. Cancer Res 1994; 54:3718–3722.

98. Sturzbecher H-W, Chumakov P, Welch WJ, Jenkins JR. Mutant p53 proteins bind hsp72/73 cellular heat shock-related proteins in SV 40-transformed monkey cells. Oncogene 1987; 1:201–211.

99. Finlay CA, Hinds PW, Tan T-H, Eliyahu D, Oren M, Levine AJ. Activating mutations for transformation by p53 produce a gene product that forms an hsc70-p53 complex with an altered half-life. Mol Cell Biol 1988; 8:531–539.

100. Sturzbecher H-W, Addison C, Jenkins JR. Characterization of mutant p53-hsp72/73 protein-protein complexes by transient expression in monkey COS cells. Mol Cell Biol 1988; 8:3740–3747.

101. Halevy O, Michalovitz D, Oren M. Different tumor-derived p53 mutants exhibit distinct biological activities. Science 1990; 250:113–116.

102. Tsutsumi-Ishii Y, Tadokoro K, Hanaoka F, Tsuchida N. Response of heat shock element within the human hsp70 promoter to mutated p53 genes. Cell Growth Differ 1995; 6:1–8.

103. Agoff SN, Hou J, Linzer DIH, Wu B. Regulation of the human hsp70 promoter by p53. Science 1993; 259:84–87.

104. Anderson RL, Gabriele T, Strasser A. Bcl-2 and thermotolerance cooperate in cell survival (abstr). J Cell Biochem 1995; suppl 19B:216.

105. Elledge RM, Clark GM, Fuqua SAW, Yu Y-Y, Allred DC. p53 protein accumulation detected by five different antibodies: relationship to prognosis and heat shock protein 70 in breast cancer. Cancer Res 1994; 54:3752–3757.

106. Takahashi S, Mikami T, Watanabe Y, Okazaki M, Okasaki Y, Okasaki A, Sato T, Asaishi K, Hirata K, Narimatsu E, Mori M, Sato N, Kikuchi I. Correlation of heat shock protein 70 expression with estrogen receptor levels in invasive human breast cancer. Am J Clin Pathol 1994; 101:519–525.

107. Wu BJ, Hurst HC, Jones NC, Morimoto RI. The E1A 13S product of adenovirus 5 activates transcription of the cellular human hsp70 gene. Mol Cell Biol 1986; 6:2994–2999.

108. Kaddurah-Daouk R, Greene JM, Baldwin Jr AS, Kingston RE. Activation and repression of mammalian gene expression by c-myc protein. Genes Dev 1987; 1:347–357.

109. Iida H, Yahara I. Durable synthesis of high molecular weight heat shock proteins in $G_0$ cells of the yeast and other eukaryotes. J Cell Biol 1984; 99:199–207.

110. Milarski KL, Morimoto RI. Expression of human hsp70 during the synthetic phase of the cell cycle. Proc Natl Acad Sci USA 1986; 83:9517–9521.

111. Carr BI, Huang TH, Buzin CH, Itakura K. Induction of heat shock gene expression without heat shock by hepatocarcinogens and during hepatic regeneration in rat liver. Cancer Res 1986; 46:5106–5111.
112. Kaczmarek L, Calabretta B, Kao H, Heintz N, Nevins J, Baserga R. Control of hsp70 RNA levels in human lymphocytes. J Cell Biol 1987; 104:183–187.
113. Haire RN, Peterson MS, O'Leary JJ. Mitogen activation induces the enhanced synthesis of two heat-shock proteins in human lymphocytes. J Cell Biol 1988; 106:883–891.
114. Pechan PM. Heat shock proteins and cell proliferation. FEBS Lett 1991; 280:1–4.
115. Amici C, Sistonen L, Santoro MG, Morimoto RI. Antiproliferative prostaglandins activate heat shock transcription factor. Proc Natl Acad Sci USA 1992; 89:6227–6231.
116. Yehiely F, Oren M. The gene for the rat heat-shock cognate, hsc70, can suppress onco-gene-mediated transformation. Cell Growth Differ 1992; 3:803–809.
117. Trieb K, Sztankay A, Amberger A, Lechner H, Grubeckloebenstein B. Hyperthermia in-hibits proliferation and stimulates the expression of differentiation markers in cultured thyroid carcinoma cells. Cancer Lett 1994; 87:65–71.
118. Regazzi R, Eppenberger U, Fabbro D. The 27,000 daltons stress proteins are phosphory-lated by protein kinase C during the tumor promoter-mediated growth inhibition of human mammary carcinoma cells. Biochem Biophys Res Commun 1988; 152:62–68.
119. Spector NL, Samson W, Ryan C, Gribben J, Urba W, Welch WJ, Nadler LM. Growth arrest of human B lymphocytes is accompanied by induction of the low molecular weight mam-malian heat shock protein (hsp28). J Immunol 1992; 148:1668–1673.
120. Knauf U, Bielka H, Gaestel M. Over-expression of the small heat shock protein, hsp25, inhibits growth of Ehrlich ascites tumor cells. FEBS Lett 1992; 309:297–303.
121. Honore B, Rasmussen HH, Celis A, Leffers H, Madsen P, Celis JE. The molecular chap-erones hsp28, grp78, endoplasmin, and calnexin exhibit strikingly different levels in quiescent keratinocytes as compared to their proliferating normal and transformed coun-terparts: cDNA cloning and expression of calnexin. Electrophoresis 1994; 15:3–4.
122. Oesterreich S, Weng C-N, Qiu M, Hilsenbeck SG, Osborne CK, Fuqua SAW. The small heat shock protein hsp27 is correlated with growth and drug resistance in human breast cancer cell lines. Cancer Res 1993; 53:4443–4448.
123. Vargas Roig LM, Fanelli MA, Gago FE, Tello O, Aznar JC, Lucero De Angelis R, Ciocca DR. Heat shock proteins in breast cancer, correlation with cell proliferation (abstr). Proc AACR 1994; 35:227.
124. Hahn GM, Strande DP. Cytotoxic effects of hyperthermia and Adriamycin on Chinese hamster cells. J Natl Cancer Inst 1976; 57:1063–1067.
125. Donaldson SS, Gordon LF, Hahn GM. Protective effect of hyperthermia against the cytotoxicity of actinomycin D on Chinese hamster cells. Cancer Treat Rep 1978; 62: 1489–1495.
126. Li GC, Hahn GM. Ethanol-induced tolerance to heat and to Adriamycin. Nature 1978; 274:699–701.
127. Li GC, Mivechi NF. Thermotolerance in mammalian systems: a review. In: Anghileri LJ, Robert J, eds. Hyperthermia in Cancer Treatment. Vol. I. Boca Raton: CRC Press, 1986:59–77.
128. Burkhardt D, Ghosh P. Synergistic combination of hyperthermia and inhibitors of nucleic acids and protein synthesis. In: Anghileri LJ, Robert J, eds. Hyperthermia in Cancer Treat-ment. Vol. I. Boca Raton: CRC Press, 1986:127–149.
129. Wallner K, Li GC. Adriamycin resistance, heat resistance and radiation response in Chi-nese hamster fibroblasts. Int J Radiat Oncol Biol Phys 1986; 12:829–833.
130. Li GC. Heat shock proteins: role in thermotolerance, drug resistance, and relationship to DNA topoisomerases. NCI Monogr 1987; 4:99–103.
131. Huot J, Roy G, Lambert H, Chretien P, Landry J. Increased survival after treatments with anticancer agents of Chinese hamster cells expressing the human Mr 27,000 heat shock protein. Cancer Res 1991; 51:5245–5252.

132. Chatterjee S, Cheng M-F, Berger SJ, Berger NA. Induction of Mr 78,000 glucose-regulated stress protein in poly(adenosine diphosphate-ribose) polymerase- and nicotinamide adenine dinucleotide-deficient V79 cell lines and its relation to resistance to the topoisomerase II inhibitor etoposide. Cancer Res 1994; 54:4405–4411.

133. Fuqua SAW, Hickey E, Weber L, Lemieux P, Allred C, Ciocca D, Oesterreich S. hsp27 gene expression in human breast tumor cells (abstr). J Cell Biochem 1995; Suppl 19B:191.

134. Rabindraa SK, Brown EB, Greenberger LM. Heat shock proteins are associated with mitoxantrone resistance in human colon carcinoma cells (abstr). Proc AACR 1994; 35:467.

135. Whelan RDH, Hill BT. Differential expression of steroid receptors, hsp27 and ps2 in a series of drug resistant human breast tumor cell lines derived following exposure to antitumor drugs or to fractionated x-irradiation. Breast Cancer Res Treat 1993; 26:23–39.

136. Helburn A, Demolle D, Boeynaems J-M, Fiers W, Dumont JE. Rapid phosphorylation of a 27 Kd protein induced by tumor necrosis factor. FEBS Lett 1988; 227:175–178.

137. Robaye B, Hepburn R, Lecocq R, Fiers W, Boynaems J-M, Dumont JE. Tumor necrosis factor-α induces the phorphorylation of 28-kDa stress proteins in endothelial cells: possible role in protection against cytotoxicity. Biochem Biophys Res Commun 1989; 163:301–308.

138. Nakata B, Barton R, Howell SB, Los G. Association between over-expression of hsp60 and cisplatin resistance in head and neck cancer cells (abstr). Proc AACR 1994; 35:466.

139. Eskenazi AE, Pinkas J, Frantz CN. Induction of heat shock protein 27 (HSP27) and thermotolerance following hydroxyurea (HU) treatment (abstr). Proc AACR 1994; 35:12.

140. Sugita K, Kojika S, Inukai T, Tezuka T, Goi K, Shiraishi K, Del Fierro RS, Kagami K, Nakazawa S. Mechanisms of glucocorticoid resistance in leukemic cells—analysis of ligand-binding receptor and heat shock proteins (abstr). Proc AACR 1994; 35:11.

141. Jaattela M, Wissing D. Hsp70-mediated protection of tumor cells from apoptosis induced by tumor necrosis factor (abstr). J Cell Biol 1995; Suppl 19B:218.

142. Lee W-C, Lin K-Y, Chen K-D, Rai Y-K. Induction of HSP70 is associated with vincristine resistance in heat-shocked 9L rat brain tumour cells. Br J Cancer 1992; 66:653–659.

143. Shen DW, Wang N, Pastan I, Gottesman MM. Identification of a protein overexpressed in cisplatin-resistant cell lines derived from human liver carcinoma and mouse Balb/3T3 cells as the heat shock protein HSP60 (abstr). Proc AACR 1995; 36:401.

144. Wilkes J, Abu-hadid M, Perez R. Relationship between heat shock protein 60 (HSP60) mRNA expression and resistance to platinum analogues in human ovarian and bladder carcinoma cell lines (abstr). Proc AACR 1995; 36:402.

145. Hettinga JVE, Meijer C, Mulder NH, Konings AWT, de Vries EGE, Kampinga HH. Non-correlation between intrinsic cisplatin sensitivity and the levels of a panel of heat shock proteins (27, 60, 72, 73 and 90) in human cell lines (abstr). Proc AACR 1993; 34:24.

146. Kumira E, Hom DK, Isonishi S, Terashima Y, Howell SB. Analysis of the cytotoxic interaction between cis-platin and hyperthermia in a human ovarian carcinoma cell line (abstr). Proc AACR 1993; 34:359.

147. Fisher AM, Ferrario A, Gomer CJ. Adriamycin resistance in Chinese hamster fibroblasts following oxidative stress induced by photodynamic therapy. Photochem Photobiol 1993; 58:581–588.

148. Schardt C, Kasimir-Bauer S, Harstrick A, Hüesker JM, Nettersheim R, Stellberg W, Nowrousian MR, Opalka B, Scheulen ME, Seeber S. Differential mRNA expression of heat shock proteins hsp 27, hsp 60, and hsp 70 in cisplatin and doxorubicin resistant cell lines and regulation by topoisomerase II inhibitors (abstr). Proc AACR 1995; 36:20.

149. Schaefer EL, Morimoto RI, Theodorakis NG, Seidenfeld J. Chemical specificity for induction of stress response genes by DNA-damaging drugs in human adenocarcinoma cells. Carcinogenesis 1988; 9:1733–1738.

150. Kroes RA, Abravaya K, Seidenfeld J, Morimoto RI. Selective activation of human heat shock gene transcription by nitrosourea antitumor drugs mediated by isocyanate-induced

damage and activation of heat shock transcription factor. Proc Natl Acad Sci USA 1991; 88:4825–4829.

151. Murakami Y, Uehara Y, Yamamoto C, Fukazawa H, Mizuno S. Induction of hsp 72/73 by herbimycin A, an inhibitor of transformation by tyrosine kinase oncogenes. Exp Cell Res 1991; 195:338–344.

152. Theodorakis NG, Zand DJ, Kotzbauer PT, Williams GT, Morimoto RI. Hemin-induced transcriptional activation of the hsp70 gene during erythroid maturation in K562 cells is due to a heat shock factor mediated stress response. Mol Cell Biol 1989; 9:3166–3173.

153. Hensold JO, Housman DE. Decreased expression of the stress protein hsp70 is an early event in murine erythroleukemic cell differentiation. Mol Cell Biol 1988; 8:2219–2223.

154. Elia G, Santoro MG. Regulation of heat shock protein synthesis by quercetin in human erythroleukemia cells. Biochem J 1994; 300:201–209.

155. Richards FM, Watson A, Hickman JA. Investigation of the effects of heat shock and agents which induce a heat shock response on the induction of differentiation of HL-60 cells. Cancer Res 1988; 48:6715–6720.

156. Beere HM, Morimoto RI, Hickman JA. Investigations of mechanisms of drug-induced changes in gene expression: N-methylformamide-induced changes in synthesis of the Mr 72,000 constitutive heat shock protein during commitment of HL-60 cells to granulocyte differentiation. Cancer Res 1993; 53:3034–3039.

157. Ferm MT, Soderstrom K, Jindal S, Gronberg A, Ivanyi J, Young R, Kiessling R. Induction of human hsp60 expression in monocytic cell lines. Int Immunol 1992; 4:305–311.

158. Arrigo A-P. Tumor necrosis factor induces the rapid phosphorylation of the mammalian heat shock protein hsp28. Mol Cell Biol 1990; 10:1276–1280.

159. Michishita M, Satoh M, Yamaguchi M, Hirayoshi K, Okuma M, Nagata K. Phosphorylation of the stress protein hsp27 is an early event in murine myelomonocytic leukemic cell differentiation induced by leukemia inhibitory factor/D-factor. Biochem Biophys Res Commun 1991; 176:979–984.

160. Stahl J, Wobus AM, Ihrig S, Lutsch G, Bielka H. The small heat shock protein hsp25 is accumulated in P19 embryonal carcinoma cells and embryonic stem cells of line BLC6 during differentiation. Differentiation 1992; 51:33–37.

161. Bielka H, Hoinkis G, Oesterreich S, Stahl J, Benndorf R. Induction of the small stress protein, hsp25, in Ehrlich ascites carcinoma cells by anticancer drugs. FEBS Lett 1994; 348:165–167.

162. Cano A, Coffer AI, Adatia R, Millis RR, Rubens RD, King RJD. Histochemical studies with an estrogen receptor-related protein in human breast tumors. Cancer Res 1986; 46: 6475–6480.

163. Andersen J, Skovbon H, Poulsen HS. Immunocytochemical determination of the estrogen-regulated protein Mr 24,000 in primary breast cancer and response to endocrine therapy. Eur J Cancer Clin Oncol 1989; 25:641–643.

164. Seymour L, Bezwoda WR, Meyer K. Tumor factors predicting for prognosis in metastatic breast cancer. Cancer 1990; 66:2390–2394.

165. Thor A, Benz C, Moore II D, Goldman E, Edgerton S, Landry J, Schwartz L, Mayall B, Hickey E, Weber LA. Stress response protein (srp-27) determination in primary human breast carcinomas: clinical, histologic, and prognostic correlations. J Natl Cancer Inst 1991; 83:170–178.

166. Damstrup L, Andersen J, Kufe DW, Hayes DF, Skovgaard Poulsen H. Immunocytochemical determination of the estrogen-regulated proteins Mr 24,000, Mr 52,000 and DF3 breast cancer associated antigen: clinical value in advanced breast cancer and correlation with estrogen receptor. Ann Oncol 1992; 3:71–77.

167. Hurlimann J, Gebhard S, Gomez F. Oestrogen receptor, progesterone receptor, pS2, ERD5, hsp27 and cathepsin D in invasive ductal breast carcinomas. Histopathology 1993; 23:239–248.

168. Love S, King RJB. A 27 kDa heat shock protein that has anomalous prognostic powers in early and advanced breast cancer. Br J Cancer 1994; 69:743–748.
169. Harrison JD, Morris DL, Ellis IO, Jones JA, Jackson I. The effect of tamoxifen and estrogen receptor status on survival in gastric carcinoma. Cancer 1989; 64:1007–1010.
170. Harrison JD, Watson S, Morris DL. The effect of sex hormones and tamoxifen on the growth of human gastric and colorectal cancer cell lines. Cancer 1989; 63:2148–2151.
171. Vargas Roig LM, Lotfi H, Olcese JE, Lo Castro G, Ciocca DR. Effects of short-term tamoxifen administration in patients with invasive cervical carcinoma. Anticancer Res 1993; 13:2457–2464.

# 8

## Overcoming Drug Resistance in Ovarian Cancer

**P. H. B. Willemse, G. J. Veldhuis, A. G. J. van der Zee, and E. G. E. de Vries**
*University Hospital Groningen, Groningen, The Netherlands*

### INTRODUCTION

Epithelial carcinoma of the ovary carries a poor prognosis, as most patients are diagnosed at a relatively late stage of development of the disease. Because only a minority of ovarian cancer patients are diagnosed with localized, surgically curable disease, systemic chemotherapy is the treatment modality for the majority of patients suffering from this tumor. Cisplatin-based combination regimens are the basis for most treatment schedules in advanced ovarian cancer, resulting in a median survival of 21–30 months. In these regimens, cisplatin may be combined with cyclophosphamide and doxorubicin. Even patients who achieve a pathological complete remission (pCR) after systemic treatment will have disease recurrence after 5 years in about 70% of cases. These data show that the greater part of patients will ultimately die of their disease as the result of intrinsic or acquired resistance to chemotherapeutic drugs. This phenomenon is the major obstacle in the management of patients with advanced-stage ovarian cancer and is responsible for the poor outlook for these patients (1,2). Therefore, many studies have been directed at the improvement of treatment results. Although our understanding of cell biology and genetic changes involved in drug resistance is developing rapidly, transferral of this knowledge to the clinic is just beginning. In this chapter, we address a number of factors known to be associated with drug resistance in human ovarian cancer, and we describe options used to treat potential drug resistance in the clinic.

### MECHANISMS OF RESISTANCE TO CHEMOTHERAPEUTIC DRUGS IN OVARIAN CANCER

#### Factors Active Within the Cell Membrane

There are a number of factors that act at the level of the cell membrane, P-glycoprotein (Pgp) is a glycoprotein that acts as an efflux pump for certain classes of unrelated drugs, such as doxorubicin, epipodophyllotoxins, and paclitaxel (so-called natural products).

The overexpression of Pgp in tumor cell lines selected for resistance to a single natural product is accompanied by cross-resistance to other natural products, resulting in the so-called multidrug resistance (MDR) phenotype (3). In several human ovarian cancer cell lines, overexpression of Pgp has been found to be (in part) responsible for reduced cytotoxicity of drugs such as doxorubicin and paclitaxel (4). We have shown that there is a significant increase in Pgp-expressing tumors after three cycles of cyclophosphamide, doxorubicin, and cisplatin. Modulation of clinical MDR has been attempted by co-administration of noncytotoxic inhibitors of Pgp, e.g., verapamil (5). The recent introduction of paclitaxel, also an MDR-sensitive drug, in first- and second-line chemotherapy may increase the importance of Pgp-mediated drug resistance in ovarian cancer. Consequently, efforts to modulate Pgp-mediated resistance to paclitaxel may become increasingly relevant to the clinic.

Another member of the ABC-superfamily, the MDR-like protein MRP, has been reported to be actively associated with MDR (6). Cell lines overexpressing MRP often have lower intracellular drug levels than their sensitive counterpart. The putative function of MRP as an ATP-dependent efflux pump for unmodified drugs is as yet undetermined. MRP-overexpressing cell lines are capable of extruding glutathione-drug conjugates (7). Untreated ovarian carcinomas often do express MRP. However, MRP expression did not correlate with response or survival (8). Recently, another protein was described: the lung resistance protein (LRP), which is found in non-Pgp-expressing tumor cell lines with MDR phenotype (6,9). We have found that positive LRP immunostaining in ovarian carcinoma is strongly related to the failure to respond to (mainly platinum) chemotherapy and is also the strongest negative prognostic factor for survival in uni- and multivariate analysis (8,10).

**Intracellular Detoxification**

Increased detoxification of the anticancer drug may also play a role in drug resistance. Glutathione is a tripeptide thiol that has an important role in cellular detoxification of various xenobiotics, such as platinum compounds and alkylating agents (11). In human ovarian cancer cell lines, a strong relation has been found between levels of glutathione and glutathione-synthesizing enzymes and resistance to platinum compounds and alkylating agents. Increased cytosolic glutathione levels have been linked to resistance to platinum compounds and alkylating agents (12,13). In ovarian cancer cell lines that exhibit primary resistance to cisplatin, cross-resistance to drugs such as melphalan and doxorubicin is only correlated with enhanced intracellular glutathione levels (14). This phenomenon reflects the broad cross-resistance patterns encountered in patients with refractory ovarian cancer. Modulation of glutathione metabolism is a way of reversing clinical drug resistance. It has been shown that resistance to these compounds can be reversed by depleting high glutathione levels in ovarian cancer cells—e.g., with buthionine sulfoximine (BSO) (15). In phase I clinical trials, melphalan has been administered in combination with BSO (16). Results on the efficacy of this combination in phase II trials have to be awaited.

Glutathione S-transferases (GSTs) are cytosolic proteins that function as enzymes of detoxification by catalyzing the conjugation of electrophilic agents such as platinum and/or alkylating compounds to glutathione (17). In humans, cytosolic GSTs have been divided into four major classes termed $\alpha$, $\mu$, pi, and theta (18). In several platinum- and alkylating agents–resistant human tumor cell lines, an enhanced content of GST has been described (19). Gene transfection studies showed a role for GSTs in platinum resistance, primarily for GST alpha (for a review, see Ref. 20). In ovarian carcinoma samples, we detected a high level of GST pi. However, overall GST activity as well as GST pi content was lower after chemotherapy in residual and relapsed tumors (21).

## Topoisomerases and DNA Repair

Factors at the DNA level that may also play a role in resistance are the topoisomerases, DNA repair enzymes and suppressor genes. Topoisomerase (Topo) I and II are nuclear enzymes involved in various DNA transactions such as replication, transcription, and recombination. Topo I (topotecan and irinotecan [CPT11]) and Topo II–targeted drugs (etoposide and doxorubicin) produce stabilized drug-Topo-DNA cleavable complexes that result in cell death (22). For the Topo II enzyme, two isozymes—Topo II$\alpha$ and $\beta$—have been described that have different affinities to Topo II–directed drugs. We have shown that Topo II activity is higher in malignant human ovarian tumors than in benign tumors. Topo II activity varies significantly between malignant tumors. After platinum-based chemotherapy, tumors exhibit lower Topo II activity in comparison to untreated tumors, whereas no differences exist for Topo I activity (23). The variation of Topo II levels in ovarian cancer may in part be responsible for the variable response to Topo II–targeted drugs (24,25). In malignant ovarian tumors, topoisomerase II levels were always higher than in benign tumors (23). Based on these studies of ovarian cancer, Topo I may be a potential target for the newly developed camptothecin analogues topotecan, CPT11, and other experimental drugs.

Several platinum-resistant ovarian cancer cell lines show increased levels of DNA repair, as determined by enhanced loss of platinum-DNA adducts and increased synthesis of DNA repair enzymes (19,26). Repair of platinum-DNA adducts occurs primarily by the nucleotide excision repair pathway in which a large number of enzymes are involved (27). A variety of individual DNA repair enzymes have been linked to platinum resistance in (ovarian) tumor cell lines. As DNA damage repair involves many proteins, several opportunities are available to modulate resistance. The drug aphidicolin interferes at different levels in DNA repair and has been found to modulate platinum cytotoxicity in tumor cell lines (28). A phase I clinical trial of aphidicolin showed that prolonged steady-state levels can be achieved at concentrations found to maximally inhibit repair (29). In mice, O'Dwyer et al. found activity of the combination of aphidicolin and platinum compounds to be superior to platinum compounds alone against cisplatin-resistant human ovarian cancer (30). Repair of DNA damage caused by alkylating agents occurs both by DNA base repair and nucleotide excision repair. DNA base repair enzymes such as O6-alkylguanine-DNA-alkyltransferase (ATase) remove alkyl groups from individual nucleotides (31). The jun, fos, and myc oncoproteins act as nuclear transcription factors. Overexpression of these enzymes results in drug resistance by enhanced repair of DNA damage, whereas down-regulation by antifos ribozymes results in restored sensitivity to cisplatin (32,33). Tumors with high expression were found to respond better to platinum based-chemotherapy (34).

## Growth Factors and Tumor Suppressor Genes

There may be a potential role for the tyrosine kinases in drug resistance. Several studies show that c-erbB-2 overexpression may have a role in growth regulation in many ovarian cancers (35). Results from various studies, however, are conflicting. Blocking of c-erbB-2 overexpression with monoclonal antibodies results in increased cisplatin cytotoxicity in cultured ovarian cancer cells, probably because of blocking of DNA repair (36). The same phenomenon has also been reported for anti-epidermal growth factor receptor (EGFR) antibodies (37).

There are now a number of preclinical studies that do suggest a relation between wild-type expression of the tumor suppressor gene p53 and tumor response to chemotherapy. P53 may play an important role in the apoptotic pathway and therefore affect response. Based on the increased protein half-life of mutated p53, immunohistochemistry on tumor samples has become possible and is able to detect mutated p53 expression. Recently, we found p53 immunostaining in 20% of stage I/II and 40% of stage III/IV ovarian cancers (2). In our study, patients with p53-positive ovarian cancer had a shorter progression-free and overall survival. Two other studies also reported a negative prognostic role for mutated p53 immunostaining in ovarian cancer (38,39). This has led to in vitro and clinical studies in which the defective p53 suppressor gene has been replaced by the insertion of the normal tumor suppressor gene. This approach may be especially promising in ovarian cancer (40).

It can be concluded that resistance as a result of decreased intracellular levels of drugs is mediated by presently unknown or poorly defined cell membrane proteins such as MRP. Well-characterized cell membrane glycoproteins such as P-glycoprotein are frequently encountered in resistance to doxorubicin or paclitaxel in cultured tumor cell lines. Studies are currently ongoing to define the role of these factors in patient tumor specimens. Further elucidation of the possible links between frequently observed genetic changes in ovarian cancer such as c-erbB-2 amplification and p53 mutations and other parameters of drug resistance is important because it may offer ways to manipulate drug resistance phenotypes encountered in the clinic.

## CLINICAL STUDIES

### Dose Escalation of Cisplatin

Before the advent of the hematopoietic growth factors (HGF), many studies were undertaken to compare cisplatin alone with combination of cisplatin plus other agents. Combinations of cisplatin with other chemotherapeutic agents will often be limited by their myelotoxicity, and the use of three or four drug schedules has not been shown to improve treatment outcome in the long run (41–43). For a review of the great number of comparative studies, we refer to several excellent papers (41–43). Only studies that have utilized a somewhat more dose-intensive approach will be mentioned here. Many studies have looked at the use of higher doses of single-agent cisplatin in a randomized fashion. In a phase II/feasibility study (only three cycles of cisplatin 200 mg/m$^2$ and cyclophosphamide 1 g/m$^2$), a high (pathological complete response) pCR rate of 32% for patients with stage III disease was found; a median survival was 23 months for all patients and over 47 months for patients who achieved CR. However, the toxicity of this schedule was substantial: 52% of patients develop grade III–IV peripheral neuropathy, and 43% moderate to severe ototoxicity (44). Several randomized studies comparing standard with suprastandard dosing have been published. In a phase III study by Kaye et al., 190 patients with primary ovarian cancer were randomized to receive a fixed dose of cyclophosphamide 750 mg/m$^2$ with cisplatin 50 mg/m$^2$ or 100 mg/m$^2$. All patients received six cycles at 3-weekly intervals, so that both total dose and dose intensity were varied. This study was stopped prematurely because it showed an improved survival in the high-dose arm: 73% for the high-dose arm against 48% for the low-dose arm at 18 months (45). Long-term effects, however, were not affected by the different doses of chemotherapy. These results should be offset against the adverse effects: more neuro- and nephrotoxicity in the high-dose arm. A study by the Gynecologic Oncology Group (GOG) (46) has also looked at dose intensity, but the total dose was kept identical. A group of 460 patients was randomized to receive cisplatin 50 mg/m$^2$ IV and cyclophosphamide 0.5 g/m$^2$ IV every 3 weeks for eight cycles or cisplatin 100 mg/m$^2$ and cyclophosphamide 1 g/m$^2$ every 3 weeks for four cycles. In this study, the two regimens did not differ in terms of response rate, disease-free survival, or overall survival, despite dose intensity being twice as high in the high-dose arm, as the dose actually received was 0.47 versus 0.93 in the low-dose and high-dose arms, respectively. It is unclear why these two studies show different outcomes; the median survival in the lower-dose arm of the Kaye study was inferior to both arms of the GOG study, although the disease volume after operation was actually smaller in that study. These two studies indicate that the total dose of cisplatin may be the critical factor with regard to treatment outcome. In a study from Milan, 254 patients were randomized to either standard therapy (cyclophosphamide 750 mg/m$^2$ and cisplatin 75 mg/m$^2$ IV every 3 weeks for six cycles) or intense therapy (cisplatin 50 mg/m$^2$ IV every week for nine cycles), resulting again in the same total cisplatin dose (47). Response rates were 66% in the dose-intense arm versus 61% in the standard arm. There was a trend toward improvement in progression-free survival in the dose-intense group compared with the conventional group (21 versus 18 months, respectively), and in overall survival (36 versus 33 months, respectively). Ngan et al. reported on a study comparing 50 versus 100 mg/m$^2$ cisplatin in combination with cyclophosphamide 1 g/m$^2$ in patients with stage III or IV ovarian cancer. They found an improved survival with the higher dose, although statistical data were not given (48). In a study by Bella et al., 99 patients were randomly assigned to receive a cumulative dose of 600 mg/m$^2$ cisplatin over a 9- or 20-week period. There was no difference in median survival between the standard group and the high-dose group (25 versus 22 months, respectively), but pCR (9% versus 19%, respectively) and 4-year survival (13% versus 31%, respectively) were different (49). Conte randomized patients to a standard dose of 50 mg/m$^2$ or a high dose of 100 mg/m$^2$ cisplatin in combination with epirubicin and cyclophosphamide 600 mg/m$^2$ every 3 weeks (PEC 50 or PEC 100). The overall response was 43% in the PEC 50 group versus 55% in the PEC 100 group, but median survival has not been reached yet (50).

Overall, most studies using higher dose or dose-intense cisplatin show a slight improvement in treatment results, which often fail to reach statistical significance. The best results (i.e., the most marked differences) are found in those studies that selected patients with small tumor residuals and studies that used different total doses of cisplatin in contrast to studies that compared a similar total amount of cisplatin.

Combinations comprising cisplatin and cyclophosphamide have become the mainstay of primary treatment in advanced ovarian cancer. However, in a meta-analysis, the addition of doxorubicin to standard treatment with cyclophosphamide/cisplatin has been claimed to increase the median survival about 6% (51,52). A retrospective comparison of the schedules that have been used is limited by the fact that the dose intensity of the individual drugs is often different, and that the addition of doxorubicin will compromise the dose of other drugs, mainly cyclophosphamide. Some authors have argued, however, that in first-line treatment, doxorubicin should be the first agent to be combined with platinum compounds, as the addition of cyclophosphamide proved to be of less value than platinum alone in a meta-analysis (53). Others have reported significant activity of higher doses of epirubicin when used in platinum-resistant disease. Depending on the treatment-free interval, varying from 3, 6, 12, or more months, responses were found in respectively 11%, 14%, 20%, and 41% with a suprastandard epirubicin dose of 150–180 mg/m$^2$ once every 3 weeks (54).

### Detoxification of Cisplatin

Several methods have been tried to increase the platinum dose and simultaneously overcome cisplatin nephro- and neurotoxicity. In most instances, this has been done by combining cisplatin with thiol compounds such as sodium thiosulfate, glutathione, or WR 2721 (Ethyol, amifostine), or by direct intraperitoneal instillation of cisplatin IP, in order to achieve high local concentrations without toxic systemic exposure in patients with intra-abdominal disease. Increasing the total amount of platinum has been accomplished by combination with carboplatin. These approaches will be discussed below.

In a recent phase III study, the efficacy of amifostine in preventing cisplatin-induced nephro- and neuropathy was evaluated. Patients received cisplatin 75 mg/m$^2$ and cyclophosphamide 750 mg/m$^2$ for six cycles. Neutropenic infections were reduced by 78%, and 78% less treatment delays due to serum creatinine elevations occurred in the amifostine group; four patients in the control arm left the study because of nephrotoxicity, none in the treatment arm. In a second study, there was 31% less neurotoxicity (76% in the control arm versus 51% in the amifostine arm) and neurotoxicity appeared later, after 600 instead of 500 mg/m$^2$ cumulative cisplatin dose. Overall, neither a difference in tumor response (pCR rates of 15% versus 21% with amifostine), nor progression-free or overall survival (median 33 vs. 34 months) was observed in both studies. In conclusion, amifostine appears to prevent leukopenia and will delay the occurrence of nephro- and neurotoxicity. Side effects of amifostine were nausea, vomiting, sneezing, vasodilatation, rare allergic reactions, and hypotension (55). Smyth et al. have aimed at a higher dose of 100 mg/m$^2$ cisplatin in combination with glutathione to reduce cisplatin toxicity (56). In the group receiving combined treatment, fewer patients had to stop treatment because of toxicity, fewer patients experienced nephro- and neurotoxicity, and more responses were obtained (overall 73% vs. 62%). Subjective tolerance to the combination was higher with glutathione. Overall and progression-free survival are still awaited.

Sodium thiosulfate has mainly been used in combination with the cisplatin IP. Sodium thiosulfate neutralizes the formation of the nephrotoxic aquated species of cisplatin in the renal tubules, thus abrogating renal dysfunction. The most extensive experience with the use of sodium thiosulfate has been reported by Howell, especially after cisplatin IP (57). A dose of 200 mg/m$^2$ cisplatin can be safely administered with sodium thiosulfate without significant renal toxicity, but neurotoxicity is not ameliorated by this approach. This method carries a high rate of CR and long-term remissions, especially in patients with small (i.e., < 5 mm) tumor deposits. An evaluation of IV sodium thiosulfate with IV cisplatin has not been performed. The administration of IP carboplatin has been discouraged because of a slower uptake of carboplatin into tumor tissue and slower formation of platinum-DNA adducts in vitro (58). Recently however, there have been some reports of positive findings with the use of carboplatin IP.

Markman et al. found eight CR among 32 patients after IP carboplatin 200–300 mg/m$^2$ given together with etoposide 100 mg/m$^2$ once every month. All responses were in patients with small tumor deposits (i.e., < 5 mm) (59). With a somewhat higher dose of 500 mg/m$^2$ carboplatin IP every 4 weeks for four times, 10 relapses in 47 patients treated for FIGO stage I–II ovarian cancer were observed; 36 patients were free of tumor at second-look laparotomy (60). The most striking results of the IP route of cisplatin have been recently reported by an Intergroup study comparing a fixed dose of cyclophosphamide IV plus cisplatin 100 mg/m$^2$ IV or IP over six cycles in 539 chemotherapy-naive patients. The IP arm was favored as it had more pCR than the IV arm (40% versus 31%, respectively) and longer survival (51 versus 41 months, respectively) with less hematological and gastrointestinal toxicity (61).

## Dose Escalation by Combining Cisplatin and Carboplatin

Another method of increasing platinum dose intensity is the combination of cisplatin and carboplatin. The rationale for combining these two agents is that both are active and do not share dose-limiting side effects. Two studies have shown that nearly full doses of each drug can be given if carboplatin precedes cisplatin, thus achieving an increased dose intensity of 1.5–2 over that of standard therapy. In this sequence, cisplatin cannot hamper the excretion of carboplatin, which could lead to higher plasma levels and increased myelosuppression. In a phase II trial, carboplatin 300 mg/m$^2$ day 1 was followed by 50 mg/m$^2$ cisplatin days 2 and 3, in 42 previously untreated patients, 80% of whom had bulky tumor residuals. A pathological remission rate of 62% and a pCR rate of 22% were achieved. The dose-limiting toxicity was thrombocytopenia, for which dose reduction was necessary in 22% of cycles and in a further 7% because of neurotoxicity (62).

Although platinum dose intensity is increased by a factor of 1.5–2 by this approach, it is not easily combined with a third alkylating drug. Therefore, a slightly lower dose of carboplatin (200 mg/m$^2$) and cisplatin (50 mg/m$^2$ days 2 and 3), were combined with ifosfamide (1.2 g/m$^2$ days 1–3) in 37 previously untreated patients. This resulted, despite dose modifications, in a 58% overall response rate comprising 42% pCR. Dose-limiting encephalopathy, neurotoxicity, and nephrotoxicity each occurred in 6% of the patients (63). In a phase I–II study in 30 patients with primary ovarian cancer and bulky tumor residuals, carboplatin (300 mg/m$^2$ starting dose day 1) and cisplatin (100 mg/m$^2$ day 2) were combined with vigorous prehydration (64). Toxicity was manageable, although 45% of cycles were delayed, and nephrotoxicity occurred in 12%, neurotoxicity in 21%, and ototoxicity in 39% of patients. Despite the presence of large residual tumors at the start of treatment, the pCR rate in this study also amounted to 22%. Others have used the same approach and have reported similar results (65–69). It has become evident, however, that a substantial increase in dose intensity will not become feasible until myelotoxicity and in particular, thrombocytopenia can be better prevented by the use of specific and active HGF.

## Studies With or Without Hematopoietic Growth Factors

In several large comparative phase III studies, carboplatin has shown clinical activity equivalent to that of cisplatin (70–72). Because of its inherent myelotoxicity, carboplatin is a suitable compound to use in dose-escalation studies, either alone or in combination with an alkylating agent. Some studies have tried to increase the dose of carboplatin by using HGF with varying success, and a number of investigators have tried to increase the dose of carboplatin-based combinations in conjunction with autologous marrow or peripheral stem cell support.

We will first discuss studies that have combined carboplatin with alkylating agents without the support of HGF. Ozols et al. have treated 27 patients with extensive prior cisplatin treatment with a single dose of 800 mg/m$^2$ carboplatin and achieved a response rate of 27% but severe myelosuppression and febrile neutropenia occurred in 40% (73). In another study, carboplatin 400 mg/m$^2$ plus cyclophosphamide 1 g/m$^2$ or ifosfamide 5 g/m$^2$ was given every 3 weeks. The dose intensity reached with the latter combination was markedly higher—carboplatin 124 mg/m$^2$/wk and ifosfamide 2.0 g/m$^2$/wk, versus carboplatin 87 mg/m$^2$/wk and cyclophosphamide 245 mg/m$^2$/wk. No antitumor effects of these combinations were reported (74).

In one of the few randomized studies of dose intensity with carboplatin, Jones et al. have compared either standard or high-dose carboplatin based on a pharmacokinetic model, aiming at an AUC of carboplatin of 7 versus 11, calculated from the creatinine clearance according to the Calvert formula. Responses were higher in the high-dose arm (75).

In combination with an HGF, an increase in dose intensity may be achieved either by administering higher dosages of the cytotoxic compound or by choosing a shorter time interval between cycles. Several groups have investigated this issue, but thus far only feasibility and phase I–II studies have been reported. At present there are no results of phase III studies available that have looked at differences in clinical outcome arising from the addition of an HGF to standard or suprastandard chemotherapy. As myelotoxicity is the dose-limiting factor for carboplatin, it is a suitable drug with which to study increased dose combined with HGF support. At present, there are two HGFs available that stimulate leukocytes. G-CSF mainly stimulates the growth of myeloid precursor cells, especially those of neutrophil lineage (8). GM-CSF induces stimulation of all myeloid progenitors, such as eosinophils, basophils, monocytes, and lymphocytes, in addition to the stimulation of the neutrophil precursors. Most studies with carboplatin have been performed with GM-CSF support; dose-intensity studies with the more recently developed compound paclitaxel have used G-CSF. A number of studies with GM-CSF in ovarian cancer are shown in Table 1. Reed et al. have treated 34 patients with advanced recurrent ovarian cancer with high-dose carboplatin (800 mg/m$^2$, every 35 days) and daily GM-CSF (76). Febrile neutropenia was seen in 33% of the patients, compared to 50% in a historical control group. At 20 $\mu$g/kg GM-CSF, malaise was the dose-limiting toxicity. Thirteen responses were reported (34%). Edmonson et al. (77) tested 17 different regimens with regard to subcutaneous GM-CSF dose and chemotherapy dose in patients with advanced cancer and found that twice-daily 10 $\mu$g/kg/day GM-CSF for 14 days starting the day after chemotherapy resulted in amelioration of both leukopenia and thrombocytopenia and permitted escalation of IV carboplatin dose to 700 mg/m$^2$ in combination with a fixed dose of 1 g/m$^2$ cyclophosphamide. They concluded that 5 $\mu$g/kg GM-CSF twice daily would be optimal. Another group reported that when carboplatin (800 mg/m$^2$) and cyclophosphamide (0.5 g/m$^2$) were administered with GM-CSF (20 $\mu$g/kg/day), no clear benefit was observed with regard to hematological recovery (78). McClay et al. (79) performed a phase I study (n=31) with carboplatin and etoposide, both administered IP with subcutaneous GM-CSF. The authors concluded that with GM-CSF support, the maximal tolerated dose

**Table 1**   Effects of GM-CSF After Chemotherapy for Ovarian Cancer, Feasibility and Phase II Studies

| Ref. | GM-CSF ($\mu$g/kg) | Drug | Dose (mg/m$^2$) | Study type | Int. (weeks) | Comment |
|---|---|---|---|---|---|---|
| 76 | <20 | Carbo | 800 | Phase 1 | 5 | Fever in 30% vs 50% in controls |
| 77 | 10 | Carbo Cyclo | 600 1000 | Phase 1 | 4 | BM dose-limiting |
| 78 | 20 | Carbo Cyclo | 800 500 | Feasibility | 5 | No effect |
| 79 | 500/m$^2$ | Carbo Etop | 500 400 | Phase I | 4 | Myelotoxicity |
| 81 | 10 | Carbo Cyclo | 500 600 | Feasibility | 3 | BM dose-limiting |
| 80 | 5 | Carbo Cyclo | AUC = 7 600 | Feasibility | 2 | Feasible |
| 82 | 5 (7 or 14 days) | Carbo Etop | 500 100 | Feasibility | 3 | GM-CSF given for 7 days gave best results |
| 83 | 1–6 | Carbo Cyclo | 300 750 | Random Placebo | 4 | Reduce or delay in 11% vs 32% |
| 84 | 5 | DDP Cyclo | 75 750 | Repeated × 6 | 2 | 6 of 8 pts had GM-CSF toxicity |
| 85 | 5–10 | Cyclo | 4.5–6 | Phase I | 3 | GM-CSF 5 and 10 $\mu$g were equivalent |

Int. = interval between cycles in weeks; Cyclo = cyclophosphamide; Carbo = carboplatin; Etop = etoposide; BM = bone marrow; DDP = diaminedichloroplatinum; pt = patient.

(MTD) was reached at 600 mg/m$^2$ carboplatin and 400 mg/m$^2$ etoposide. Furthermore, changes of GM-CSF administration to twice daily did not allow for additional carboplatin dose increase. Most nonhematological toxicity concerned allergic skin reactions.

Other studies have aimed at increased dose intensity by shortening the cycle interval. Lind et al. have studied the effect of G-CSF after carboplatin, in an attempt to increase the dose and shorten the interval. The carboplatin dose was based on creatinine clearance, according to the Calvert formula, and carboplatin was administered every 2 weeks for four cycles. A projected carboplatin AUC of 7 mg/L.h every 2 weeks appeared to be feasible (80). GM-CSF allowed carboplatin (500 mg/m$^2$) and cyclophosphamide (600 mg/m$^2$) administration every 3 weeks for four cycles in chemotherapy-naive patients (81). Tafuta et al. (82) compared two GM-CSF schedules of 7 or 14 days after carboplatin 400 mg/m$^2$ and etoposide 100 mg/m$^2$ (days 1–3, IV). They found stimulation of neutrophils, with subsequent increase in nadir levels and accelerated neutrophil recovery after both regimens. When GM-CSF was administered for a brief period (days 12–18), it allowed the chemotherapy to be given every 3 weeks. We have shown in a double-blind placebo-controlled study that GM-CSF after chemotherapy stimulated platelets and leukocytes compared with a non-GM-CSF control group (83). In this study, 15 previously untreated patients with stage III–IV ovarian cancer received carboplatin 300 mg/m$^2$ and cyclophosphamide 750 mg/m$^2$ every 4 weeks for six cycles. Increasing doses of 1.5–6 $\mu$g/kg/day GM-CSF were given subcutaneously on days 6–12. Grade IV neutropenia was more often observed in the control group than the group at the highest dose level. Stimulating effects on platelets were observed for the 6 $\mu$g/ kg/day dose. Chemotherapy dose reduction or delays occurred in nine of 28 cycles for controls versus five of 44 cycles in patients who had received GM-CSF.

Kehoe et al. (84) achieved chemotherapy dose intensification by reducing the treatment interval with GM-CSF support. In this study, eight patients received IV cisplatin (75 mg/m$^2$) and cyclophosphamide (750 mg/m$^2$) on day 1, scheduled every 2 weeks for six cycles with GM-CSF days 3–14 SC. In four patients, all cycles could be given within 3 weeks, and one patient received all the cycles at the scheduled time. This regimen was not without complications, however. Lichtman et al. (85) treated patients (n=51) with four dose levels of IV cyclophosphamide (1.5–6.0 g/m$^2$) and three dose levels of GM-CSF. Each patient was assigned a certain dose of cyclophosphamide and GM-CSF. Cyclophosphamide doses up to 4.5–6.0 g/m$^2$ with GM-CSF support could be given every 15–18 days in most patients. GM-CSF doses of 5.0 and 10.0 $\mu$g/kg/day had comparable efficacy.

The effect of the HGF interleukin-3 (IL-3) has not yet been studied extensively in patients in solid tumors. As IL-3 is a stimulator of the early marrow progenitors, a more pronounced effect on thrombopoiesis could be expected. Biesma et al. (86) gave recombinant (rh) IL-3 as a part of first-line treatment in patients with advanced ovarian carcinoma. The chemotherapy schedule was the same as in the previous study with GM-CSF (83). Compared to control cycles without rhIL-3, IL-3 cycles had enhanced recovery of leukocyte, neutrophil, and platelet counts. Delay of treatment for insufficient bone marrow recovery was necessary in 48% of the control cycles versus 4% of the IL-3 supported cycles. Platelet transfusions were required in 15% of the control cycles versus 6% of the IL-3 cycles. At 15 $\mu$g/kg/day of IL-3, headache was the dose-limiting toxicity. Most patients suffered flu-like symptoms and low-grade fever. Some patients developed a generalized rash, sometimes with facial edema, at doses of 5 $\mu$g/ kg/day and higher, usually during the last days of IL-3 administration after more than three cycles. Thereafter, a study analyzing the feasibility of a shorter treatment interval with the same carboplatin-cyclophosphamide regimen randomly supported by 5 or 10 $\mu$g/kg IL-3 was performed (87). Both IL-3 doses allowed a 3-week interval in 62% and 4 weeks in 81% of cycles without chemotherapy dose reduction. The planned number of six cycles were completed only by 41% of the 17 patients due to untoward allergic side effects of IL-3, such as erythema, fever, urticaria, and facial edema. A dosage regimen of 5 $\mu$g/kg/day of IL-3 proved to be the best tolerated, but cumulative myelotoxicity could not be completely prevented.

In conclusion, the data on the combined use of HGF are still somewhat conflicting, the efficacy being dependent on the cytotoxic dose and its duration and schedule as well as the HGF schedule. The effect in the first two cycles appears to be the most marked; it tends to diminish later on. Another problem is the absence of factors that will stimulate both leukocytes and platelets effectively, but the more recently developed factors (e.g., stem cell factor) may solve this problem. Apart from G-CSF, most HGFs will induce constitutional symptoms, which sometimes resemble an allergic reaction. At present, there are no studies that indicate an improvement in progression-free or overall survival by more dose-intense treatment in conjunction with HGF, and results of phase III studies are eagerly awaited.

## HIGH-DOSE CHEMOTHERAPY

It is questionable whether the increased dose intensity reached by the addition of HGF will be sufficient to reach higher remission rates and a better survival in patients with ovarian cancer. This should be the aim of future phase II–III studies. The two- to threefold increased dose intensity may not be sufficient to change the prognosis in patients with drug-resistant tumors, as five- to 10-fold higher drug concentrations are needed in vitro to overcome drug resistance. These levels can only be reached when drug dosage can be increased adequately and rescue is warranted by the infusion of autologous marrow (ABMT) or peripheral stem cell support (PSCI). However, the application of ablative chemotherapy followed by ABMT or PSCI in conjunction with HGF is hampered by the fact that most schedules cannot be easily repeated, which limits the dose intensity that can be reached by this approach. By the use of repeated rescue with PSCI, this procedure has become feasible, as discussed below. A number of these studies are shown in Table 2.

Mulder et al. (88) have given cyclophosphamide 7 g/m$^2$ and etoposide 1.5 g/m$^2$ followed by ABMT to 11 patients with residual or relapsing ovarian cancer after stan-

**Table 2** Survival and Follow-Up After High-Dose Chemotherapy and Autologous Bone Marrow Support

| Ref. | Combination | Dose (mg/m$^2$) | Med FU (mo) | Number | NED |
|------|-------------|-----------------|-------------|--------|-----|
| 88 | Cyclo | 7000 | 91+,123+ | 11 | 2 |
| | Etop | 1000 | | | |
| 89 | Cyclo + | 7000 | 57+,84+ | 6 | 2 |
| | MX or MX | 30/60 | | | |
| | + Melph | 180 | | | |
| 91 | Carbo | 400–2400 | ns | 11 | ns |
| 90 | Cyclo | 7000 | 3–12+ | 9 | 1 |
| | Etop | 1500 | | | |
| 92 | Melph | 140 | 23 | 35 | 15 |
| 93 | Melph | 140 | 37–58+ | 11 | 5 |
| 95 | Melph | 140 | 52 | 18 | |
| | Cyclo | 6000 | | 13 | |
| | Carbo | 1000–1500 | | | 11 |
| 96 | Cyclo+TBI | 4400 | 37 | 17 | |
| | Melph | 140 | | 3 | |
| | Carbo | 600–1500 | | 14 | |
| | all 3—TBI | | | 3 | 15 |
| 98 | Cyclo | 120 mg/kg | 7–30+ | 6 | 5 |
| | MX | 75 | | | — |
| | Carbo | 1500 | | | |
| 99 | Carbo | 1500 | 4–23 | 9 | — |
| | IFX | 1500–2000 | | | |
| Total | | | | 166 | 56 (33%) |

Comb = cytostatic combination; med FU = median follow-up; NED = no evidence of disease; mo = months; ns = not stated; Cyclo = cyclophosphamide; Etop = etoposide; MX = mitoxantrone; Melph = melphalan; Carbo = carboplatin; TBI = total body irradiation; IFX = ifosfamide.

dard cisplatin-based treatment; two patients are still without evidence of disease (NED) at 91 and 123 months. In a dose-finding study, six patients with ovarian cancer were treated with cyclophosphamide 7 g/m$^2$ and mitoxantrone 30–60 mg/m$^2$ (four patients) or mitoxantrone 60 mg/m$^2$ with melphalan 180 mg/m$^2$ (two patients). Two of these six patients are still NED at 57 and 84 months (89). Shpall et al. combined cyclophosphamide 7 g/m$^2$ with etoposide 1.5 g/m$^2$ and reported that the combination can be given without important extramedullary toxicity (90). Shea et al. treated 11 patients in a phase I study with carboplatin 375–2400 mg/m$^2$ over 4 days. From 1600 mg/m$^2$ carboplatin onwards, ABMT was added and six patients responded; no follow-up data are available (91). In another phase I study, 35 patients were treated after six cycles of a cisplatin-based regimen. Most patients had progressive disease at second-look laparotomy and after extensive surgery received melphalan 120–240 mg/m$^2$ followed by ABMT. Of patients with measurable disease, 75% responded, but response duration generally was short. With a median follow-up of 23 months, 19 patients were alive, 15 without disease progression (92). In a pilot study, high-dose melphalan was combined with bone marrow reinfusion in 11 patients; in five, this was preceded by abdominal radiotherapy (93). Two of the first and three of the second group were disease-free at 37+–58+ months. In five patients with low-volume disease after standard treatment, melphalan 125 mg/m$^2$ was combined with etoposide 600 mg/m$^2$ and carboplatin 2100 mg/m$^2$. Four patients had no evidence of disease at 3–29 months (94). A study was started in 1984 of patients with a positive second-look laparotomy or CR (nine patients) after cisplatin-based regimens. Thirty-one patients were treated with high-dose melphalan 140 mg/m$^2$ (18 patients) or a combination of carboplatin 1000–1500 mg/m$^2$ and cyclophosphamide 6 g/m$^2$ (13 patients). There were no toxic deaths during aplasia, but one patient developed acute leukemia after 60 months. With a median follow up of 60 months, 11 patients were disease-free (95). The group of Marty et al. reported on their experience with high-dose therapy. A total of 37 patients were treated; 17 patients received cyclophosphamide 4.4 g/m$^2$ and abdominal irradiation alone, and this was combined with melphalan 140 mg/m$^2$ (n=3) or with carboplatin 600–1500 mg/m$^2$ (n=14), while three further patients received all three drugs without irradiation. At a median follow-up of 32 months, 15 patients were still without evidence of disease (96).

Also, the increased dose intensity of IP drug administration was combined with bone marrow support (97). In patients with advanced ovarian cancer, one cycle of carboplatin 1600 mg/m$^2$ and etoposide 800 mg/m$^2$ was given IP combined with escalating IV doses of thiotepa and mitoxantrone. Four of seven patients achieved a CR. In a phase I study, patients received carboplatin 1500 mg/m$^2$, escalated bolus mitoxantrone 10–25 mg/m$^2$ × 3, and cyclophosphamide 30–50 mg/kg × 3 combined with ABMT. The maximum tolerated dose was 75 mg/m$^2$ for mitoxantrone and 120 mg/kg for cyclophosphamide. Four patients died, three of sepsis and one of acute respiratory failure. Acute renal failure at the lowest dose level was prevented by hydration in higher dose steps. Five of six ovarian carcinoma patients reached a CR that lasted for 7–30+ months (98). Broun et al. have treated nine patients with refractory ovarian carcinoma with carboplatin 300 mg/m$^2$ × 5 and escalating doses of ifosfamide 1.5–2.0 g/m$^2$ (99). Five patients achieved CR, but all relapsed after respectively 4, 5, 6, 8, and 23 months, with a median duration of 6 months. One death occurred, caused by CNS and renal toxicity.

In an overview of these data, 56 out of 176 patients were disease-free 23–123 months after high-dose treatment. It may well be that this is a highly selected patient group and more definitive data are still needed to substantiate these results, but they suggest that a fraction of patients refractory to treatment with standard-dose therapy may achieve long-term complete remissions with very high dose.

Stiff et al. have reviewed the total experience with ablative chemotherapy for ovarian carcinoma in the United States. Ninety-five percent of 153 patients received transplants during their first remission, with 20 different transplant regimens. There were 43% CR, with an overall response of 71%. The median time to progression was 6 months, and 14% of patients were free of disease after one year (100). The results of high-dose therapy with ABMT in France were reviewed recently. Of a total of 117 patients, 65 patients with macroscopic residuals relapsed over the course of the subsequent years, but 30% of 52 patients with microscopic residuals remained progression free after a 5-year period (109).

The harvesting and subsequent use of PSCI after myelosuppressive chemotherapy followed by a growth factor has been described by several groups (101,102). An interesting new option was described in a study by Tepler et al. (103), in which intensive chemotherapy was used up front. Four courses of dose-intensive chemotherapy (carboplatin 600 mg/m$^2$ and cyclophosphamide 600 mg/m$^2$, day 1) were administered every 4 weeks, with repetitive rescue (except cycle 1) with PSCI. During this dose-intense chemotherapy, GM-CSF was administered. Prior to this regimen, 4 g/m$^2$ cyclophosphamide was administered with subcutaneous GM-CSF to obtain peripheral hematopoietic progenitors. The combination of GM-CSF plus PSCI reduced the duration of thrombocytopenia and neutropenia, compared to GM-CSF alone. These results were comparable with those obtained by Shea et al. (104), who performed a study in which three cycles of 1.2 g/m$^2$ carboplatin were followed by GM-CSF or PSCI plus GM-CSF. No chemotherapy reduction was necessary in the last group, and the total chemotherapy dose was 57% higher than in the group that received GM-CSF alone. A similar approach was used by the group of Fenelly (105), who harvested PSC after a single dose of cyclophosphamide 3.0 g/m$^2$ plus G-CSF, followed by four cycles of carboplatin 1000 mg/m$^2$ and cyclophosphamide 1.5 g/m$^2$ at 16-day intervals. Escalating doses of paclitaxel were given in combination with cyclophosphamide to study its effect on PSC harvest. Nine of 24 paclitaxel/cyclophosphamide courses were followed by febrile neutropenia, and 11 of 12 patients had normalization of CA-125 levels after four cycles of carboplatin/cyclophosphamide, with a median interval of 15 days (range 14–21). There was no dose-limiting mucositis or neurological toxicity (106). Tandem cycles of ifosfamide 1.5 g/m$^2$, carboplatin 200 mg/m$^2$, and etoposide 250 mg/m$^2$, all × 5, were given in a phase I–II setting by Lotz et al. to patients with refractory ovarian carcinoma or germ cell tumors. In five of the 16 patients with germ cell tumors, CRs were achieved and lasted for 2, 6, 8+, 27+, and 37+ months. In the 24 patients with epithelial ovarian cancer, a 78% overall response rate and 14% CR were observed, but none of the responses were durable (107).

## HIGH-DOSE CHEMOTHERAPY IN GERM CELL CARCINOMAS OF THE OVARY

Germ cell tumors (GCT) are prominent in patients who are relatively young; they are among the tumors most responsive to chemotherapy and have proved to be curable by it. It is therefore logical to apply high-dose treatment to this type of tumor. Because these tumors are relatively rare, series of patients treated with intensive chemotherapy and ABMT are even smaller than the series of epithelial carcinoma. Therefore, some studies on high-dose chemotherapy in male or mixed male/female GCT are mentioned here (Table 3). The only study of female GCT was by Culine et al. (108). Broun et al. have studied carboplatin 900–2000 mg/m$^2$ with etoposide 1200 mg/m$^2$ in 40 patients with germ cell tumors in a phase I–II setting. All patients had platinum-refractory disease or failed two cisplatin-based regimens. Twenty-six patients received two cycles. Although most patients received additional G-CSF, all patients suffered from neutropenic fever and seven died during treatment. Eight of 32 evaluable patients achieved a CR and four remained disease-free (109). Eight of 14 responders had progressed while receiving cisplatin. The group at Memorial Sloan-Kettering Cancer Center treated 30 patients with refractory germ cell tumor with carboplatin 1500 mg/m$^2$, etoposide 1200 mg/m$^2$, and cyclophosphamide 60–120 mg/kg, which could be repeated in eight of 17 patients. Two deaths occurred; the main toxicity was hepatic. Thirteen patients achieved a CR (27%) and eight were disease free, one after resection of solitary residual tumor (110). Pico et al. treated 27 patients with solid tumors with a combination of carboplatin 800–1600 mg/m$^2$, cyclophosphamide 6.4 g/m$^2$, and etoposide 1750 mg/m$^2$ followed by ABMT. Eight patients with epithelial ovarian cancer did not achieve CR,

**Table 3**   High-Dose Chemotherapy and ABMT in Germ Cell Tumors

| Ref. | Drug | Support | Pts. | CR | Maint. | Toxic death | Remarks |
|---|---|---|---|---|---|---|---|
| 109 | Carbo 900–2000 Etop 1200 | G-CSF | 40 | 12 | 6 | 7 | [a]6 pts NED at > 2 y, 3 of 28 refractory pts |
| 107 | Carbo 1000 Etop 1250 Ifo 7.5 | PSC × 2 | 16 | 5 | 3 | — | 3 pts NED from 8$^+$–37$^+$ mo |
| 110 | Carbo 1500 Etop 1250 Cyclo 60–120 mg/kg | 8 pts twice 17 – G-CSF 13 + G-CSF | 30 | 13 | 8 | 2 | — |
| 111 | Carbo 800–1600 Etop 1750 Cyclo 6400 | ABM | 15 | 5 | 4 | | 11 refractory pts; 5 pts NED at 5, 22, 27, 40, and 43 mo |
| 108 | DDP 200 Etop 500 Vbl/Bleo | ABM | 3 | 3 | 2 | | ABM as primary treatment; 2 NED at 78$^+$ and 89$^+$ mo |
| 112 | DDP 200 Etop 1750 Cyclo 6400 | ABM | 12 res 6 sens | 3 5 | None 4 | | 4 responders of 6 DDP-sensitive pts are NED at 42$^+$–48$^+$ mo |
| Total | | | 122 | 46 (38%) | 27 (23%) | 9 (8%) | |

Abbreviations: CR = complete remission; res = platinum resistant; sens = platinum sensitive; maint = lasting response; ABMT = autologous bone marrow transfusion; NED = no evidence of disease; DDP = cisplatin; Cyclo = cyclophosphamide; Etop = etoposide; Carbo = carboplatin; Ifo = ifosfamide; Vbl = vinblastine; Bleo = bleomycin.
[a]Ovarian GCT only; pts = patients.

but five of 14 patients with germ cell tumors (11 with platinum-refractory disease) were still disease free at 5, 22, 27, 40, and 43 months after ABMT (111). Culine reported 14 patients with ovarian germ cell tumors who received high-dose cisplatin, vinblastine, bleomycin, and etoposide; four patients had recurrent disease, 10 primary disease. Three also received ABMT. Ten of 13 patients were disease-free (71%) at a median follow-up of 6 years (108). The authors state that treatment with BEP (bleomycin, etoposide, cisplatin) should be preferred, for the undue toxicity of this schedule they have used. The Institut G. Roussy treated 12 cisplatin-refractory patients who had poor prognostic features with an intensive schedule comprising cisplatin 40 mg/m$^2$ for 5 days, etoposide 350 mg/m$^2$ for 5 days, and cyclophosphamide 1.6 g/m$^2$ (PEC) for 4 days. Three achieved CR, but there were no long-term survivors. Four of six patients with "sensitive" (i.e., late) relapse remained long-term NED. There were four treatment-related deaths, three from infection and one from bleeding. The exact value of this approach is difficult to state, as not all patients had cisplatin-refractory disease (112).

In a recent paper, the results of 10 studies with high-dose chemotherapy and ABMT in GCT were reviewed. Of 118 patients with tumors responding to cisplatin, 41 were long-term NED, but only 22 patients in a group of 153 platinum-resistant patients achieved a lasting NED status (113).

In conclusion, female GCT will probably behave in a manner similar to male GCT and react the same way to high-dose therapy. This treatment cannot be recommended for all patients, but patients in late relapse appear to achieve better results than those with progression during cisplatin treatment.

## NEW DRUGS AND THE USE OF HGF

In one study, the dose of paclitaxel could be increased from 175 to 300 mg/m$^2$ as 24-h continuous infusion if combined with G-CSF. The dose-limiting toxicity in this study, however, was neuropathy and not myelotoxicity at 300 mg/m$^2$. Mucositis was rare, and five of the 14 evaluable patients responded to paclitaxel. The recommended dose for further studies was 250 mg/m$^2$ combined with G-CSF (114). With a 3-h infusion, the recommended dose of paclitaxel without G-CSF was 210 mg/m$^2$; with G-CSF, it was 250 mg/m$^2$ in patients with advanced cancer (115). When paclitaxel and cisplatin were combined, neurotoxicity proved also to be dose-limiting at a paclitaxel dose of 250 mg/m$^2$ over 24 h and cisplatin 75 mg/m$^2$, combined with G-CSF starting day 3. Neutropenic fever was not a prominent problem in this two-drug combination (116). In a randomized GOG study of first-line treatment of ovarian carcinoma, the combination of paclitaxel given as a 24-h infusion with cisplatin has shown to be more effective than standard treatment with cisplatin-cyclophosphamide, reaching a pCR rate of 26% versus 19% and a disease-free survival of 13 compared to 18 months; the overall survival was also superior: 24 versus 37 months. Toxicity in the paclitaxel/cisplatin arm proved to be higher, especially myelosuppression and fever (117). The best place for paclitaxel, therefore, seems to be in first-line treatment.

## TOPO I AND II INHIBITORS IN OVARIAN CANCER

Recently, the prolonged oral use of etoposide has regained some interest as a result of studies showing its activity in second-line treatment. A dose of 100 mg/day was given for 14 days every 3 weeks; responses were found in 10 of 47 patients, but because of myelotoxicity the duration of treatment was reduced to 7–10 days and increased if this appeared to be feasible (118). Using a similar dose of etoposide, Hoskins et al. reported eight responses in 31 platinum-resistant patients (119). Other groups found lower activity with an oral dose of 50 mg of etoposide given for 21 days every 4 weeks in second-line treatment (120–122).

The new Topo I inhibitors are currently receiving much interest. Topoisomerase I may function as a repair enzyme in the structural aspects of DNA replication. Topo II may compensate for a loss of topoisomerase I activity. Therefore, synergism is expected from the combined use of topoisomerase I and II inhibitors such as doxorubicin or etoposide.

Depending on its schedule of administration topotecan, the first Topo I inhibitor in clinical use, has shown some activity in phase II studies of ovarian cancer: 14% remissions in 30 patients (123). Its main toxicity is myelosuppression, mostly neutropenia.

Combinations of topotecan with etoposide, doxorubicin, and paclitaxel have been investigated in a phase I setting (124–126). In addition, the combination of topotecan with cisplatin is being tested, as it may possibly retard the development of cisplatin resistance (127,128).

CPT11 or irinotecan is a second-generation Topo I inhibitor, which has shown activity mainly in colon and non–small cell lung cancer. The most commonly employed regimen has been weekly or biweekly infusion. Two Japanese studies have demonstrated activity in advanced ovarian cancer, with this regimen reaching response rates of 24% in 55 patients (128) and 21% in 14 pretreated patients (129). The dose-limiting toxicity is diarrhea, which can usually be managed by the aggressive use of loperamide. Myelosuppression is mostly moderate. CPT11 is a prodrug that is converted into the active compound SN38, which shows a great similarity to its parent drug camptothecin and which has a similar toxicity profile (130). Other Topo I inhibitors, such as G1 147211 (GG 211), have completed phase I investigation and are currently undergoing phase II testing in ovarian cancer (131).

## CONCLUSIONS

Investigators have aimed at improving treatment results in advanced ovarian cancer by many different ways. The most successful method cannot be defined at this moment. The increased dose intensity that is achieved by the use of HGF has not yet been shown to yield a substantial benefit in patients with intrinsic or acquired drug resistance. The use of very high dose chemotherapy with ABMT or PSCI seems to be worthwhile. The newer compounds, such as the taxoids and the Topo I and II inhibitors, have been shown to possess only limited cross-resistance to platinum-resistant cells. Resistance to platinum compounds still is largely ill-defined and appears to be multifactorial. This indicates that it will be difficult to overcome resistance by one sole modality. New ways to circumvent these problems will be found by a better understanding of the underlying mechanism of this phenomenon. New and exciting developments are the possibilities of replacing mutated tumor suppressor genes such as p53 or blocking the expression of growth and metastasis-promoting factors and intracellular signaling pathways. The understanding of the underlying mechanisms of resistance to cytotoxic agents and their transfer to the clinical setting will be one of the major challenges for the next decade.

## REFERENCES

1. Cannistra SA. Cancer of the ovary. N Engl J Med 1993; 329:1550–1559.
2. Van der Zee AGJ, Hollema H, Suurmeyer AH, et al. The value of P-glycoprotein, glutathione S-transferase, c-erbB-2, and p53 as prognostic factors in ovarian carcinomas. J Clin Oncol 1995; 13:70–78.
3. Long V. Charles F. Kettering prize. P-glycoprotein and resistance to anticancer drugs. Cancer 1992; 69:2603–2609.
4. Bradley G, Naik M, Ling V. P-glycoprotein expression in multidrug resistant human ovarian carcinoma cell lines. Cancer Res 1989; 49:2790–2796.
5. Sikic BI. Modulation of multidrug resistance: at the threshold. J Clin Oncol 1993; 11:1629–1635.
6. Cole SP, Bhardwaj G, Gerlach JH, et al. Overexpression of a transporter gene in a multidrug resistant human lung cancer cell line. Science 1992; 258:1650–1654.
7. Müller M, Meijer C, Zaman GJR, et al. Overexpression of the gene encoding the multidrug resistance-associated protein results in increased ATP-dependent glutathione S-conjugate transport. Proc Natl Acad Sci USA 1994; 91:13033–13037.
8. Izquierdo M, Van der Zee AGJ, Vermorken JB, et al. Expression of the new drug resistance-associated marker LRP in ovarian carcinoma predicts poor response to chemotherapy and shorter survival. J Natl Cancer Inst. In press.
9. Scheper RJ, Broxterman HJ, Scheffer GL, et al. Overexpression of a Mr 110,000 vesicular protein in non-P-glycoprotein-mediated multidrug resistance. Cancer Res 1993; 53:1475–1479.
10. Izquierdo MA, Van der Zee AGJ, Vermorken JB, et al. Prognostic significance of the drug resistance associated LRP in advanced ovarian carcinoma. Ann Oncol 1994; 8:98.
11. Arrick BA, Nathan CF. Glutathione metabolism as a determinant of therapeutic efficiency; a review. Cancer Res 1984; 44:4224–4232.
12. Godwin AK, Meister A, O'Dwyer PJ, et al. High resistance to cisplatin in human ovarian cancer cell lines is associated with marked increase of glutathione synthesis. Proc Natl Acad Sci USA 1992; 89:3070–3074.
13. Mistry P, Kelland LR, Abel G, et al. Relationships between glutathione, glutathione S-transferase and cytotoxicity of platinum drugs and melphalan in eight human ovarian carcinoma cell lines. Br J Cancer 1991; 64:215–220.
14. Hamaguchi K, Godwin AK, Yakushiji M, et al. Cross-resistance to diverse drugs is associated with primary cisplatin resistance in ovarian cancer cell lines. Cancer Res 1993; 53:5225–5232.
15. Ozols RF, Loui KG, Plowman J, et al. Enhanced melphalan cytotoxicity in human ovarian cancer in vitro by BSO depletion of GSH. Biochem Pharmacol 1987; 36:147–153.
16. Bailey HH, Mulcahy RT, Ripple GH, et al. Continuous infusion of BSO and melphalan produces depletion of tumor GSH. Proc Am Soc Clin Oncol 1995; 14:181.
17. Boyer TD. The glutathione S-transferases: an update. Hepatology 1989; 9:486–496.
18. Mannervik B. The isoenzymes of glutathione transferase. Adv Enzymol Relat Areas Mol Biol 1985; 57:357–417.
19. Ghu G. Cellular responses to cisplatin. J Biol Chem 1994; 269:787–790.
20. Meijer C, Mulder NH, De Vries EGE. The role of detoxifying systems in resistance of tumor cells to cisplatin and Adriamycin. Cancer Treat Rev 1990; 7:389–407.
21. Van der Zee AGJ, Van Ommen B, Meijer C, et al. Glutathione S-transferase activity and isoenzyme composition in benign ovarian tumours, untreated malignant ovarian tumours, and malignant ovarian tumours after platinum/cyclophosphamide chemotherapy. Br J Cancer 1992; 66:229–234.
22. Liu LF. DNA topoisomerase poisons as antitumor drugs. Annu Rev Biochem 1989; 58:351–375.

23. Van der Zee AGJ, Hollema H, De Jong S, et al. P-glycoprotein and DNA topoisomerase I and II activity in benign tumors of the ovary and in malignant tumors of the ovary, before and after platinum/cyclophosphamide chemotherapy. Cancer Res 1991; 51:5915–5920.

24. Van der Zee AGJ, De Vries EGE, Hollema H, et al. Molecular analysis of the topoisomerase IIα gene and its expression in ovarian cancer. Ann Oncol 1994; 5:75–81.

25. Van der Zee AGJ, De Jong S, Keith WN, et al. Quantitative and qualitative aspects of topoisomerase I and IIα and β in untreated and platinum/cyclophosphamide treated malignant ovarian tumors. Cancer Res 1994; 54:749–755.

26. Johnson SW, Perez RP, Godwin AK, et al. Role of platinum-DNA adduct formation and removal in cisplatin resistance in human ovarian cancer cell lines. Biochem Pharmacol 1994; 47:689–697.

27. Hoeijmakers JHJ. Nucleotide excision repair II: from yeast to mammals. Trends Genet 1993; 9:211–217.

28. Jekunen AP, Homm DK, Alcaraz JE, et al. Cellular pharmacology of dichloro (ethylenediamine)platinum(II) in cisplatin sensitive and resistant human ovarian carcinoma cells. Cancer Res 1994; 54:2680–2687.

29. Sessa C, Zuchetti M, Davoli E, et al. Phase I and clinical pharmacological evaluation of aphidicolin glycinate. J Natl Cancer Inst 1991; 83:1160–1164.

30. O'Dwyer PJ, Moyer JD, Suffness M, et al. Antitumor activity and biochemical effects of aphidicolin glycinate (NSC 303812) alone and in combination with cisplatin in vivo. Cancer Res 1994; 54:724–729.

31. Pegg AE. Mammalian $O^6$-alkylguanine-DNA alkyltransferase: regulation and importance in response to alkylating carcinogenic and therapeutic agents. Cancer Res 1990; 50:6119–6129.

32. Curran T, Franza BR. Fos and jun: The AP-1 connection. Cell 1988; 55:395–397.

33. Kashani-Sabet M, Lu Y, Leong L, et al. Differential oncogene amplification in tumor cells from a patient treated with cisplatin and 5-fluorouracil. Eur J Cancer 1990; 26:383–390.

34. Bauknecht T, Angel P, Kohler M, et al. Gene structure and expression analysis of the epidermal growth factor receptor, transforming growth factor-alpha, myc, jun, and metallothionine in human ovarian carcinomas. Cancer 1993; 71:419–429.

35. Seidman JD, Frisman DM, Norris HJ. Expression of the HER-1/neu proto-oncogene in serous ovarian neoplasms. Cancer 1992; 70:2857–2860.

36. Hancock MC, Langton BC, Chan PT, et al. A monoclonal antibody against the c-erbB-2 protein enhances the cytotoxicity of cis-diamminedichloroplatinum against human breast and ovarian tumor cell lines. Cancer Res 1991; 51:4575–4580.

37. Christen RD, Hom DK, Porter DC, et al. Epidermal growth factor regulates the in vitro sensitivity of human ovarian carcinoma cells to cisplatin. J Clin Invest 1990; 86:1632–1640.

38. Bosari S, Viale G, Radaelli U, et al. P53 accumulation in ovarian carcinomas and its prognostic implications. Hum Pathol 1993; 24:1175–1179.

39. Hartman LC, Podratz KC, Kenney GL, et al. Prognostic significance of p53 immunostaining in epithelial ovarian cancer. J Clin Oncol 1994; 12:64–69.

40. Sikora K. Genes, dreams and cancer. Br Med J 1994; 308:1217–1221.

41. Ozols RF, Young RC. Chemotherapy of ovarian cancer. Semin Oncol 1991; 18:222–232.

42. Ozols RF. Treatment of ovarian cancer: present status. Semin Oncol 1994; 21:1–11.

43. Ozols RF. New developments with carboplatin in the treatment of ovarian cancer. Semin Oncol 1992; 19:85–89.

44. Rothenberg ML, Ozols RF, Glatstein E, et al. Dose-intensive induction chemotherapy for advanced epithelial ovarian cancer. Proc Am Soc Clin Oncol 1990; 9:169.

45. Kaye SB, Lewis CR, Paul J, et al. Randomised study of two doses of cisplatin with cyclophosphamide in epithelial ovarian cancer. Lancet 1992; 340:329–333.

46. McGuire WP, Hoskins WJ, Brady MS, et al. A phase II trial of dose-intensive versus standard dose cisplatin and cytoxan in advanced ovarian cancer. Proc Int Gynecol Cancer Soc 1991; 3:35.

47. Colombo N, Pittelli MR, Parma G, et al. Cisplatin dose-intensity in advanced ovarian cancer. Proc Am Soc Clin Oncol 1993; 12:255.
48. Ngan HYS, Choo YC, Cheung M, et al. A randomized study of high dose versus low-dose cisplatin combined with cyclophosphamide in the treatment of advanced ovarian cancer. Chemotherapy 1989; 35:221.
49. Bella M, Cocconi G, Lotticci R, et al. Conventional versus high-dose intensity regimen of cisplatin in advanced ovarian carcinoma. Proc Am Soc Clin Oncol 1992; 11:223.
50. Conte PF, Bruzzone M, Gaducci A, et al. High-doses versus standard-doses of cisplatin in combination with epirubicin and cyclophosphamide in advanced ovarian cancer patients with bulky residual disease. Proc Am Soc Clin Oncol 1993; 12:273.
51. Williams CJ, Stewart L, Parmar M, et al. Meta-analysis of the role of platinum compounds in advanced ovarian cca. Semin Oncol 1992; 19(suppl 2):120–128.
52. Ovarian cancer meta-analysis project. Cyclophosphamide plus cisplatin versus cyclophosphamide, doxorubicin and cisplatin chemotherapy of ovarian carcinoma: a meta-analysis. J Clin Oncol 1991; 9:1668–1674.
53. A'Hern RP, Gore ME. Impact of doxorubicin on survival in advanced ovarian cancer. J Clin Oncol 1995; 13:726–732.
54. Vermorken JB, Kobierska A, Chevalier B, et al. Phase II study of high-dose epi in ovarian cancer patients previously treated with cisplatin. Proc Am Soc Clin Oncol 1995; 14:176.
55. Roullet B, Bacchini T, Martin C, et al. A phase III study evaluating alfostine cytoprotection in patients with ovarian cancer receiving cisplatin and cyclophosphamide chemotherapy. Proc Eur Soc Med Oncol, Lisbon, 1994.
56. Smyth I, Bowman A, Perren T, et al. Glutathione improves the therapeutic index of cisplatin and quality of life for patients with ovarian cancer (abstr). Proc Am Soc Clin Oncol 1995; 14:273.
57. Howell SB, Zimm S, Markman M, et al. Long-term survival of advanced refractory ovarian carcinoma patients with small volume disease treated with intraperitoneal chemotherapy. J Clin Oncol 1987; 5:1607–1612.
58. Los G, McVie JG. Carboplatin: an alternative for IP cisplatin treatment in cancer restricted to the peritoneal cavity? Proc Am Soc Clin Oncol 1990; 9:157.
59. Markman M, Reichman B, Hakes T, et al. Phase 2 trial of intraperitoneal carboplatin and etoposide as salvage treatment of advanced epithelial ovarian cancer. Gynecol Oncol 1992; 47:353–357.
60. Malmstrom H, Simonsen E, Westberg R. A phase II study of intraperitoneal carboplatin as adjuvant treatment in early-stage ovarian cancer patients. Gynecol Oncol 1994; 52:20–25.
61. Alberts DS, Liu PY, Hannigan EV, et al. Phase III study of IP cisplatin/IV cyclophosphamide vs IV cisplatin/CPA in patients with optimal disease stage III ovarian cancer. Proc Am Soc Clin Oncol 1995; 14:273.
62. Lund B, Hansen M, Hansen OP, et al. High-dose platinum consisting of combined carboplatin and cisplatin in previously untreated ovarian cancer patients with residual disease. J Clin Oncol 1990; 7:1469–1473.
63. Lund B, Hansen M, Hansen OP, et al. Combined high dose carboplatin and cisplatin, and ifosfamide in previously untreated ovarian cancer patients with residual disease. J Clin Oncol 1990; 8:1226–1230.
64. Piccart MJ, Nogaret JM, Marcelis I, et al. Cisplatin combined with carboplatin: a new way of intensification of platinum dose in the treatment of advanced ovarian cancer. J Natl Cancer Inst 1990; 82:703–707.
65. Trump DL, Grem JL, Tutsch KD, et al. Platinum analog combination chemotherapy: Cisplatin and carboplatin: A phase I trial with pharmacokinetic assessment of the effect of cisplatin administration and carboplatin excretion. J Clin Oncol 1987; 5:1281–1289.
66. Gill J, Muggia FM, Terheggen PM, et al. Dose escalation study of carboplatin and cisplatin: tolerance and relation to leucocyte and buccal cell platinum DNA adducts. Ann Oncol 1991; 2:115–121.

67. Hardy JR, Wiltshaw E, Blake PR, et al. Cisplatin and carboplatin in combination for the treatment of stage IV ovarian carcinoma. Ann Oncol 1991; 2:131–136.
68. Dittrich C, Seveld AP, Baur M. In vitro and in vivo evaluation of the combination of cisplatin and its analog carboplatin for platinum dose-intensification in ovarian carcinoma. Cancer 1993; 71:3082–3090.
69. Waterhouse DM, Reynolds RK, Natale RB, et al. Combined carboplatin and cisplatin: limited prospects for dose-intensification. Cancer 1993; 71:4060–4066.
70. Alberts DS, Green S, Hannigan EV, et al. Improved therapeutic index of carboplatin plus cyclophosphamide versus cisplatin plus cyclophosphamide final report. J Clin Oncol 1992; 10:706–717.
71. Swenerton K, Jeffrey J, Stuart G, et al. Carboplatin-cyclophosphamide versus cisplatin-cyclophosphamide in advanced ovarian cancer: a randomized phase III study. J Clin Oncol 1992; 10:718–726.
72. Ten Bokkel Huinink WW, Van den Burg MEL, Van Oosterom AT, et al. Carboplatin combination therapy for ovarian cancer. Cancer Treat Rep 1988; 15:9–15.
73. Ozols RF, Ostchega Y, Curt G, et al. High-dose carboplatin in refractory ovarian cancer patients. J Clin Oncol 1987; 5:197–201.
74. Green JA, Smith K. Dose intensity of carboplatin in combination with Cy or Ifo. Cancer Chemother Pharmacol 1990; 26(suppl):22–25.
75. Jones A, Wiltshaw E, Harper P. A randomized study of high- versus conventional dose carboplatin for previously untreated ovarian cancer. Proc BACR/ACP 1992; 15:C8.
76. Reed E, Janik J, Bookman MA, et al. High-dose carboplatin and recombinant granulocyte-macrophage colony-stimulating factor in advanced-stage recurrent ovarian cancer. J Clin Oncol 1993; 11:2118–2126.
77. Edmonson JH, Hartmann LC, Long HJ, et al. Granulocyte-macrophage colony-stimulating factor. Preliminary observations on the influences of dose, schedule, and route of administration in patients receiving cyclophosphamide and carboplatin. Cancer 1992; 10:2529–2539.
78. Ten Bokkel Huinink WW, Van Warmerdam L, Helmerhorst T. Maximum high-dose chemotherapy for high-risk ovarian cancer. Proc Am Soc Clin Oncol 1992; 11:734.
79. McClay EF, Braly PD, Kirmani S, et al. A phase I trial of intraperitoneal carboplatin and etoposide with granulocyte macrophage colony stimulating factor support in patients with intraabdominal malignancies. Cancer 1994; 2:664–669.
80. Lind MJ, Millward MJ, Chapman F, et al. The use of rhGCSF to increase the delivered dose intensity of carboplatin in women with advanced epithelial ovarian cancer. Proc Am Soc Clin Oncol 1992; 11:A735.
81. Rusthoven J, Levin L, Eisenhauer E, et al. Two phase I studies of carboplatin dose escalation in chemotherapy-naive ovarian cancer patients supported with granulocyte-macrophage colony-stimulating factor. J Natl Cancer Inst 1991; 83:1748–1753.
82. Tafuto S, Abate G, D'Andrea P, et al. A comparison of two GM-CSF schedules to counteract the granulo-monocytopenia of carboplatin-etoposide chemotherapy. Eur J Cancer 1995; 31A:46–49.
83. De Vries EGE, Biesma B, Willemse PHB, et al. A double-blind placebo-controlled study with granulocyte-macrophage colony-stimulating factor during chemotherapy for ovarian carcinoma. Cancer Res 1991; 1:116–122.
84. Kehoe S, Poole CJ, Stanley A, et al. A phase I/II trial of recombinant human granulocyte-macrophage colony-stimulating factor in the intensification of cisplatin and cyclophosphamide chemotherapy for advanced ovarian cancer. Br J Cancer 1994; 3:537–540.
85. Lichtman SM, Ratain MJ, Van Echo DA, et al. Phase I trial of granulocyte-macrophage colony-stimulating factor plus high-dose cyclophosphamide given every 2 weeks: a Cancer and Leukemia Group B study. J Natl Cancer Inst 1993; 85:1319–1326.
86. Biesma B, Willemse PHB, Mulder NH, et al. Effects of interleukin-3 after chemotherapy for advanced ovarian cancer. Blood 1992; 80:1141–1148.

87. Veldhuis GJ, Willemse PHB, Van Gameren MM, et al. Recombinant human interleukin-3 to dose intensify carboplatin and cyclophosphamide chemotherapy in epithelial ovarian cancer: a phase I trial. J Clin Oncol 1995; 13:733–740.

88. Mulder POM, Willemse PHB, Aalders JG, et al. High-dose chemotherapy with autologous bone marrow transplantation in patients with refractory ovarian cancer. Eur J Cancer Clin Oncol 1989; 25:645–649.

89. Mulder POM, Sleijfer DTh, Willemse PHB, et al. HIgh-dose cyclophosphamide or melphalan with escalating doses of mitoxantrone and autologous bone marrow transplantation for refractory solid tumors. Cancer Res 1989; 49:4654–4658.

90. Shpall EJ, Clarke-Pearson D, Soper JT, et al. High-dose alkylating agent chemotherapy with autologous bone marrow support in patients with stage III-IV epithelial ovarian cancer. Gynecol Oncol 1990; 38:294–298.

91. Shea TC, Flaherty M, Elias A, et al. A phase I clinical and pharmacokinetic study of carboplatin and autologous bone marrow support. J Clin Oncol 1989; 7:651–661.

92. Viens P, Maraninchi D, Legros M, et al. High dose melphalan and autologous marrow rescue in advanced epithelial carcinomas: a retrospective analysis of 35 patients treated in France. Bone Marrow Transplant 1990; 5:227–233.

93. Dufour P, Begerat JP, Liu KL, et al. High dose melphalan and ABMT with or without abdominal radiotherapy as consolidation treatment for ovarian carcinoma in complete remission or with microscopic residual disease. Eur J Gynaecol Oncol 1991; 12:457–461.

94. Barnett MJ, Swenerton KD, Hoskins PJ, et al. Intensive therapy with carboplatin, etoposide and melphalan and autologous stem cell transplantation for epithelial ovarian carcinoma. Proc Am Soc Clin Oncol 1990; 9:654.

95. Legros M, Fleury J, Cure H, et al. High-dose chemotherapy and autologous bone marrow transplant in 31 advanced ovarian cancers: long-term results. Proc Am Soc Clin Oncol 1992; 11:A700.

96. Extra JM, Dieras V, Marty M. High-dose chemotherapy with autologous bone marrow reinfusion in patients with advanced ovarian cancer. Proc Am Soc Clin Oncol 1992; 11: A749.

97. Shea TC, Sorniolo AM, Mason JR, et al. High-dose iv and ip combination chemotherapy with autologous stem cell rescue for patients with advanced ovarian cancer. Proc Am Soc Clin Oncol 1992; 11:A756.

98. Stiff PJ, McKenzie RS, Alberts DS, et al. Phase I clinical and pharmacokinetic study of high dose mitoxantrone combined with carboplatin, cyclophosphamide and autologous bone marrow rescue: high response rate for refractory ovarian carcinoma. J Clin Oncol 1994; 12:176–183.

99. Broun ER, Belinson JL, Berek JS, et al. Salvage therapy for recurrent and refractory ovarian cancer with high dose chemotherapy and autologous bone marrow support: a GOG pilot study. Gynecol Oncol 1994; 54:142–146.

100. Stiff P, Antman K, Randolph Broun E, et al. Bone marrow transplantation for ovarian carcinoma in the United States: a survey of active programs. Proc 6th International Autologous Bone Marrow Transplant Symposium 1992:1–9.

101. Gianni AM, Bregni M, Stern AC, et al. Granulocyte-macrophage colony-stimulating factor to harvest circulating haematopoietic stem cells for autotransplantation. Lancet 1989; 2:580–584.

102. Tepler I, Cannistra S, Anderson K, et al. Repetitive dose-intensive chemotherapy made possible by initial collection and repetitive rescue with peripheral blood progenitor cells in previously untreated outpatients with ovarian cancer. Proc Am Soc Oncol 1992; 11:A768.

103. Tepler I, Cannistra SA, Frei E III, et al. Use of peripheral-blood progenitor cells abrogates the myelotoxicity of repetitive outpatient high-dose carboplatin and cyclophosphamide chemotherapy. J Clin Oncol 1993; 8:1583–1591.

104. Shea TC, Mason JR, Storniolo AM, et al. Sequential cycles of high-dose carboplatin administered with recombinant human granulocyte-macrophage colony-stimulating factor

and repeated infusions of autologous peripheral-blood progenitor cells: a novel and effective method for delivering multiple courses of dose-intensive therapy. J Clin Oncol 1992; 10:464–473.

105. Fenelly D, Wasserheit C, Schneider J, et al. Simultaneous dose escalation and schedule intensification of carboplatin-based chemotherapy using peripheral blood progenitor cells and filgrastim: a phase I trial. Cancer Res 1994; 54:1637–1642.

106. Fenelly D, Schneider J, Spriggs D, et al. Dose escalation of paclitaxel with high-dose with analysis of progenitor-cell mobilization and hematologic support of ovarian cancer patients receiving rapidly sequenced high-dose carboplatin/cyclophosphamide courses. J Clin Oncol 1995; 13:1160–1166.

107. Lotz JP, Machover D, Malassagne B, et al. Phase I-II study of two consecutive courses of epipodophyllotoxin, ifosfamide and carboplatin with autologous bone marrow transplantation for treatment of adult patients with solid tumors. J Clin Oncol 1991; 9:1860–1870.

108. Culine S, Kattan J, Lhomme C, et al. A phase II study of high dose cisplatin, vinblastine, bleomycin and etoposide in malignant nondysgerminomatous germ cell tumors of the ovary. Gynecol Oncol 1994; 54:47–53.

109. Broun ER, Nichols CR, Kneebone P, et al. Long-term outcome of patients with relapsed and refractory germ cell tumors treated with high-dose chemotherapy and autologous bone marrow rescue. Ann Intern Med 1992; 117:124–128.

110. Motzer RJ, Gulati SC, Tong WP, et al. Phase I trial with pharmacokinetic analyses of high dose carboplatin, etoposide and cyclophosphamide with ABMT in patients with refractory GCT. Cancer Res 1993; 53:3730–3735.

111. Pico JL, Ibrahim A, Castagna L, et al. Escalating high dose carboplatin and ABMT in solid tumors. Oncology 1993; 50(suppl):47–52.

112. Baume D, Pico JL, Droz JP, et al. Value of high dose chemotherapy followed by bone marrow autograft in NSGT with poor prognosis. Bull Cancer (Paris) 1990; 77:169–180.

113. Droz JP, Kramar A, Pico JL. Prediction of long-term response after high-dose chemotherapy with autologous bone marrow transplantation in the salvage treatment of non-seminomatous germ cell tumors. Eur J Cancer 1993; 29A:818–821.

114. Sarosy G, Kohn E, Stone DA, et al. Phase I study of Taxol and granulocyte colony-stimulating factor in patients with refractory ovarian carcinoma. J Clin Oncol 1992; 10:1165–1170.

115. Schiller JH, Storer B, Tutsch K, et al. Phase I trial of 3-hour infusion of paclitaxel with or without G-CSF in patients with advanced cancer. J Clin Oncol 1994; 12:241–248.

116. Rowinsky EK, Chaudry V, Forastiere AA, et al. Phase I and pharmacologic study of paclitaxel and cisplatin with G-CSF: neuromuscular toxicity is dose-limiting. J Clin Oncol 1993; 11:2010–2020.

117. McGuire WP, Hoskins WJ, Brady MF, et al. Taxol and cisplatin improves outcome in advanced ovarian cancer as compared to cytoxan and cisplatin. Proc Am Soc Clin Oncol 1995; 14:275.

118. Shaffer DW, Smith LS, Burris HA, et al. A randomized phase I trial of chronic oral etoposide with or without granulocyte-macrophage colony-stimulating factor in patients with advanced malignancies. Cancer Res 1993; 24:5929–5933.

119. Hoskins PJ, Swenerton KD. Oral etoposide is active against platinum-resistant epithelial ovarian cancer. J Clin Oncol 1994; 12:60–63.

120. Seymour MT, Mansi JL, Gallagher CJ, et al. Protracted oral etoposide in epithelial ovarian cancer: a phase II study in patients with relapsed or platinum-resistant disease. Br J Cancer 1994; 69:191–195.

121. De Wit R, Van der Burg MEL, Van der Gaast A, et al. Phase II study of prolonged oral etoposide in patients with ovarian cancer refractory to or relapsing within 12 months after platinum-containing chemotherapy. Ann Oncol 1994; 5:656–657.

122. Markman M, Hakes T, Reichman B, et al. Phase 2 trial of chronic low-dose oral etoposide as salvage therapy of platinum-refractory ovarian cancer. J Cancer Res Clin Oncol 1992; 119:55–57.

123. Kudelka A, Edwards C, Freedman R, et al. An open phase II study to evaluate the activity of topotecan. Proc Am Soc Clin Oncol 1993; 12:259.

124. Eckhardt JR, Burris HA, Rodriguez GI, et al. A phase I study of the topoisomerase I and II inhibitors topotecan and etoposide. Proc Am Soc Clin Oncol 1993; 12:137.

125. Tolcher AW, O'Shaunessy JA, Weiss RB, et al. A phase I study of topotecan in combination with doxorubicin. Proc Am Soc Clin Oncol 1994; 13:157.

126. Lilenbaum RC, Rosner GL, Ratain MJ, et al. Phase I study of Taxol and topotecan in patients with advanced solid tumors. Proc Am Soc Clin Oncol 1994; 13:131.

127. Rothenberg ML, Burris HA, Eckardt JR, et al. Phase I/II study of topotecan plus cisplatin in patients with non-small cell lung cancer. Proc Am Soc Clin Oncol 1993; 12:156.

128. Miller AA, Hargis JB, Fields S, et al. Phase I study of topotecan and cisplatin in patients with advanced cancer. Proc Am Soc Clin Oncol 1993; 12:399.

129. Ogawa M, Taguchi T. Clinical studies with CPT 11: the Japanese experience. Ann Oncol 1992; 3(suppl):118–120.

130. Takeuchi S, Takamizawa H, Takeda Y, et al. Clinical study of CPT 11 on gynecological malignancy. Proc Am Soc Clin Oncol 1991; 10:189.

131. Eckardt J, Rodriguez G, Burris H, et al. A phase I and pharmacokinetic study of the topoisomerase I inhibitor GG 211. Proc Am Soc Clin Oncol 1995; 14:476.

# 9

## Protein Kinase C Activation and the Intrinsic Drug Resistance of Human Colon Cancer

**Catherine A. O'Brian, Karen R. Gravitt, Nancy E. Ward, Krishna P. Gupta, Philip J. Bergman, and Constantin G. Ioannides**
*The University of Texas M. D. Anderson Cancer Center, Houston, Texas*

### INTRINSIC DRUG RESISTANCE IN HUMAN COLON CANCER—A CLINICAL PERSPECTIVE

Colorectal cancer is a major cause of cancer-related death in the United States and other industrialized countries (1,2). This unfortunate fact is due in part to the marked resistance of colon cancer cells to available therapeutic agents (Table 1) (2,3). In fact, the sole truly effective therapy available for colorectal cancer at present is surgical intervention. Thus, there is no truly effective therapy available to manage metastatic colorectal cancer. Neither chemotherapeutic drugs nor biological response modifiers (e.g., interferons) have achieved major improvements in the survival of colon cancer patients (2). The inherent resistance of colon cancer to chemotherapeutic agents is termed intrinsic drug resistance. In contrast, acquired drug resistance is commonly observed in cancers that initially respond to chemotherapy (e.g., breast cancer). Acquired drug resistance is defined as resistance that develops as a result of exposure of cancer cells to chemotherapy (4,5).

Because intrinsic drug resistance to cancer chemotherapy is generally observed in cancers that arise from tissues that have detoxifying functions (e.g., the colon, stomach, and kidney), it is thought that tissue-specific detoxification mechanisms are operative in the cancer cells and protect them from chemotherapy (6,7). Evidence has been presented in support of this hypothesis. The drug-efflux pump P-glycoprotein is a contributing factor in drug resistance in cancer, and it is thought to provide a detoxification mechanism in normal cells (6,7). Human colon cancer and other intrinsically drug-resistant cancers have been shown to express the message that encodes P-glycoprotein more abundantly than human cancers that are initially responsive to therapy (5). It should be noted that although this suggests the potential value of P-glycoprotein–targeted drugs in colon cancer therapy, attempts to reverse clinical drug resistance in solid cancers with P-glycoprotein–binding drugs have resulted in unacceptable levels of toxicity, and enthusiasm for this approach in the treatment of solid cancers has declined (8).

**Table 1**  Profile of Intrinsic Drug Resistance in Human Colon
Cancer: Agents That Are Inactive Against the Disease

| | |
|---|---|
| Cisplatin | Vinblastine |
| Carboplatin | Methotrexate |
| Cyclophosphamide | Etoposide |
| Melphalan | Tamoxifen |
| Vincristine | Interferons |
| Mitoxantrone | Interleukin-2 |
| Doxorubicin | Tumor necrosis factor |

5-Fluorouracil is the most effective chemotherapeutic agent available for colon cancer therapy (2). This drug achieves a partial response rate of about 15–20% in advanced colorectal cancers (1,2). Modest improvements in the efficacy of 5-fluorouracil against human colon cancer have been achieved by combination therapy (2,9, 10). Colon cancer therapy has included attempts to combine 5-fluorouracil with other cytotoxic chemotherapeutic agents, with agents that serve as biochemical modulators of 5-fluorouracil, and with biological response modifiers (2). Although the relative merits of these therapies remain controversial, there is a consensus that a combination of 5-fluorouracil and levamisole is indicated as surgical adjuvant chemotherapy in the treatment of advanced colon cancer (10). Levamisole is an anthelminthic agent with immunomodulatory activity (1). The mechanism of action of levamisole in colon cancer therapy remains unclear, and it has yet to be determined whether the combination of 5-fluorouracil and levamisole is actually more effective than 5-fluorouracil alone (9,10).

The lack of a significant breakthrough in the management of advanced colon cancer during the past three decades supports the view that a completely new approach to the treatment of this disease is needed. In this chapter, we will focus on protein kinase C (11) as a potential target for therapeutic intervention in human colorectal cancer. We will review studies on the expression of the protein kinase C isozyme family in the colonic epithelium and in colon carcinomas, and we will also review the evidence that protein kinase C plays a major role in the intrinsic drug resistance of human colon cancer. Finally, we will consider the potential value of inhibiting protein kinase C as a strategy for sensitizing human colon cancer to chemotherapeutic drugs.

## AN OVERVIEW OF THE PROTEIN KINASE C ISOZYME FAMILY

The identification of protein kinase C as the phorbol ester tumor-promoter receptor in 1982 revealed the importance of this enzyme in cell growth and differentiation (12). At approximately the same time, the central importance of protein kinase C in mammalian signal transduction was revealed by the identification of the second messenger diacylglycerol as the endogenous activator of protein kinase C (13). These discoveries set into motion more than a decade of intensive research dedicated to this pivotal signal-transducing enzyme (14,15).

Over the past several years, more than 10 protein kinase C isozymes have been identified (11,16,17). These isozymes can be categorized into three groups, based on structural homology and cofactor requirements (Table 2) (11,14–16). The common protein kinase C isozymes (cPKCs) are activated by diacylglycerol in a $Ca^{2+}$- and

**Table 2** The Protein Kinase C Isozyme Family

| Subfamily | Cofactor dependence | Members |
|---|---|---|
| Common protein kinase C | $Ca^{2+}$, phosphatidylserine, diacylglycerol | cPKC-$\alpha$, cPKC-$\beta_1$, cPKC-$\beta_2$, cPKC-$\gamma$ |
| Novel protein kinase C | Phosphatidylserine, diacylglycerol | nPKC-$\delta$, nPKC-$\varepsilon$, nPKC-$\eta$, nPKC-$\theta$, nPKC-$\mu$ |
| Atypical protein kinase C | Phosphatidylserine, ? | aPKC-$\zeta$, aPKC-$\lambda$ |

phosphatidylserine (PS)-dependent manner. Four cPKCs have been identified: cPKC-$\alpha$, cPKC-$\beta_1$, cPKC-$\beta_2$, and cPKC-$\gamma$. The novel protein kinase C isozymes (nPKCs) are distinguished from the cPKCs by their independence of $Ca^{2+}$. nPKCs are activated by diacylglycerol in a PS-dependent manner. These isozymes are nPKC-$\delta$, nPKC-$\varepsilon$, nPKC-$\eta$, nPKC-$\theta$, and nPKC-$\mu$. The atypical protein kinase C isozymes (aPKCs) are independent of diacylglycerol and phorbol esters (11,16). The messenger molecule(s) responsible for their activation in vivo has not been definitively identified, although evidence has been presented that atypical protein kinase C isozymes can be activated by specific polyphosphoinositides (18). aPKC activity is $Ca^{2+}$-independent and PS-dependent. Two aPKCs have been identified, aPKC-$\zeta$ amd aPKC-$\lambda$ (11,16).

In the cPKC isozymes, the conserved region C2, which is present in the regulatory domain, is responsible for the $Ca^{2+}$-dependence of the kinase activity. The C2 region is not present in $Ca^{2+}$-independent protein kinase C isozymes (11). The shared phorbol ester/diacylglycerol binding site is present in the conserved region C1, which is also within the regulatory domain of protein kinase C. Although the C1 region is present in all protein kinase C isozymes, it is truncated in the diacylglycerol-independent isozymes (i.e., the aPKCs) (11).

In addition to differences in cofactor dependence among protein kinase C isozymes, the isozymes have distinct substrate specificities (16,19,20) and distinct patterns of subcellular localization (21) and tissue expression (11,22). Proteins that anchor particular protein kinase C isozymes appear to play an important role in the subcellular localization of the isozymes (23,24). The isozymes cPKC-$\alpha$, nPKC-$\delta$, and aPKC-$\zeta$ are expressed universally in mammalian tissues; more restricted patterns of expression have been reported for the other isozymes (11). Expression of protein kinase C isozymes is regulated by transcriptional controls and also by protease-mediated down-regulation of activated isozymes (25). Based on distinctions among the catalytic and regulatory properties of the isozymes and their patterns of expression, it has been inferred that the isozymes also have distinct functions in mammalian cells (16). In fact, there is substantial evidence that the contribution of protein kinase C to multidrug resistance in cancer cells, which is the focus of this chapter, is primarily the result of the action of the isozyme cPKC-$\alpha$ (26).

## PROTEIN KINASE C ACTIVITY AND ISOZYME EXPRESSION IN HUMAN COLON CARCINOGENESIS

Protein kinase C activity levels have been determined in normal, premalignant, and transformed human intestinal mucosal tissue specimens. In the normal human intestinal mucosa, the level of protein kinase C activity is highest in the distal ileum, lowest in the rectum, and intermediate in intervening segments (27). Protein kinase C activation is often associated with translocation of cytosolic protein kinase C to the particulate fraction of mammalian cells (25), and approximately the same percentage of protein kinase C activity is membrane-associated in each segment (27). Because cancer is rare in the small intestine, these results indicate that reduced protein kinase C activity levels are associated with increased cancer risk in the intestinal mucosa of healthy individuals (27).

A positive correlation between reduced protein kinase C activity and increased cancer risk is also observed when protein kinase C activity levels are compared in the colonic mucosa of healthy individuals and the uninvolved colonic mucosa of colon cancer patients (28). Both cytosolic and particulate fractions of the uninvolved colonic mucosa have significantly less protein kinase C activity than normal controls, and the uninvolved mucosa has an increased percentage of membrane-associated protein kinase C activity (28). Furthermore, colon adenomas are premalignant lesions, and the level of protein kinase C activity is significantly lower in human colon adenomas (27) and in their particulate fractions (29) than in the adjacent normal-appearing mucosa. Based on these observations, it can be hypothesized that the reduction in the level of colonic mucosal protein kinase C activity may be an early event in human colon carcinogenesis. Furthermore, in human colon carcinomas, the level of protein kinase C activity is significantly reduced with respect to adjacent normal-appearing mucosa in both cytosolic and particulate fractions (27,29,30). This suggests that a progressive down-regulation of protein kinase C may occur during human colon carcinogenesis.

Similarities between 1,2-dimethylhydrazine (DMH)-induced rat colon carcinogenesis and human colon carcinogenesis have been noted in studies of the level of protein kinase C activity and its intracellular distribution in normal, premalignant, and transformed colonic mucosal tissues (31,32). For example, protein kinase C activity in the uninvolved colonic mucosa of tumor-bearing DMH-treated rats is reduced compared with that of control rats, and an even sharper decline in protein kinase C activity is observed in the colon tumors (32). The parallel alterations in colonic mucosal protein kinase C activity in human colon carcinogenesis and DMH-induced rat colon carcinogenesis (27–32) strengthen the evidence that progressive loss of protein kinase C activity is a critical event in human colon carcinogenesis.

Prolonged exposure to phorbol ester tumor promoters results in down-regulation of protein kinase C in mammalian cells (25). Various oncogene-transformed cultured fibroblasts, including ras transformants, express elevated levels of sn-1,2-diacylglycerol and reduced levels of protein kinase C (33–35). Because phorbol ester tumor promoters and sn-1,2-diacylglycerol activate protein kinase C by the same mechanism (25), it is thought that sn-1,2-diacylglycerol may mediate a partial down-regulation of protein kinase C in the transformants (33,35). Because human colon cancers often express activated ras (36), it would seem likely that chronically elevated sn-1,2-diacylglycerol levels in the cancer cells could account for the reduced level of protein kinase C activity. However, this is not the case. In fact, human colon adenomas and carcinomas have less sn-1,2-diacylglycerol than the adjacent normal mucosa (37,38). Thus, cellular sn-1,2-diacylglycerol levels do not offer an explanation for the relative protein kinase C activity levels in these tissues.

Members of the common, novel, and atypical protein kinase C subfamilies have been detected in tissue specimens of normal human colonic mucosa. The isozymes that have been detected in this tissue by Western analysis are cPKC-α, cPKC-β, nPKC-δ, nPKC-ε, nPKC-η, and aPKC-ζ (39–42). There is a lack of agreement among reports from different groups concerning the relative levels of the individual isozymes detected by Western analysis in normal and transformed human colonic mucosal specimens. Three groups report similar levels of cPKC-α in specimens of normal human colonic mucosa and colon carcinoma (39–41), but one group observed decreased cPKC-α expression in human colon carcinomas (42). One report observed decreased cPKC-β and nPKC-ε expression and increased nPKC-δ expression in human colon carcinomas (40); another reported noted increased expression of cPKC-β, nPKC-δ, nPKC-ε, nPKC-η, and aPKC-ζ in the carcinomas (41); and a third report observed decreased expression of nPKC-δ, nPKC-ε, nPKC-η, and aPKC-ζ in human colon carcinomas (42). Further studies will be necessary to address the contradictory conclusions reached by these reports.

In a report that focused on the metastatic potential of human colon carcinomas in nude mice, increased metastatic potential was associated with a loss of the cPKC-β message and increased expression of messages encoding nPKC-δ, nPKC-η, nPKC-θ, and cPKC-α (43). Other investigators have shown that overexpression of rat brain PKC-$\beta_1$ in human colon cancer HT29 cells markedly reduces their tumorigenicity in nude mice (44). These findings suggest that cPKC-$\beta_1$ may be a tumor suppressor in the colonic epithelium (44).

## THE CONTRIBUTION OF PROTEIN KINASE C-α TO THE INTRINSIC DRUG RESISTANCE OF HUMAN COLON CANCER CELLS IN VITRO

Multidrug-resistant (MDR) cancer cells are characterized by broad-spectrum resistance to chemotherapeutic drugs and sharply reduced intracellular accumulation of the drugs (4,6). Typically, MDR tumor cell lines are selected in vitro by exposure to a cytotoxic chemotherapeutic agent, and they express high levels of the drug-efflux pump P-glycoprotein (4,6). The cells are generally resistant to chemotherapeutic drugs that are efficiently transported by P-glycoprotein, and the reduction in the intracellular concentration of the drugs largely accounts for the resistance of the cells to their cytotoxic effects. This type of drug resistance in cancer cells is termed P-glycoprotein–mediated MDR or classical MDR (Table 3) (4,6). A hallmark of classical MDR is potent reversal of the drug resistance by verapamil, which inhibits P-glycoprotein function by directly binding to the drug-efflux pump (4,6,45). The high level of expression of the

Table 3   Anticancer Drugs Affected by P-Glycoprotein–Mediated Multidrug Resistance

| | |
|---|---|
| Adriamycin (doxorubicin) | Daunorubicin |
| Vincristine | Vinblastine |
| Etoposide | Taxol (paclitaxel) |
| Mitoxantrone | Dactinomycin |

P-glycoprotein–encoding message observed in surgical specimens of human colon cancer provides evidence that classical MDR may be a component of the intrinsic drug resistance of clinical colon cancer (5).

A prominent role for protein kinase C in P-glycoprotein–mediated MDR (classical MDR) has been demonstrated (26,46,47). Convincing evidence has been presented that protein kinase C directly stimulates the drug-efflux activity of P-glycoprotein by phosphorylating the pump. Protein kinase C–catalyzed phosphorylation of the linker region of P-glycoprotein in MDR cancer cells is tightly coupled to a sharp reduction in the intracellular accumulation of cytotoxic drugs and a significant enhancement of the drug resistance phenotype (48–52). Although multiple protein kinases have been shown to phosphorylate P-glycoprotein, only protein kinase C has been shown to modulate its function (26).

In human breast cancer drug-sensitive MCF7 cells and doxorubicin selected MCF7-MDR cells, the enhancement of drug resistance and the reduction in intracellular drug accumulation achieved by phorbol ester–mediated activation of protein kinase C is reversed by verapamil. This provides evidence that the phorbol ester effects on MDR are largely the result of protein kinase C–catalyzed P-glycoprotein phosphorylation in the MCF7 cell lines (53,54). Furthermore, transfection of drug-sensitive MCF7 cells with PKC-$\alpha$ does not alter the chemosensitivity of the cells. However, if MCF7 cells are first transfected with P-glycoprotein, transfection with PKC-$\alpha$ significantly enhances the MDR phenotype of the cells, and this is associated with substantial P-glycoprotein phosphorylation (55). Recent studies in a baculovirus expression system have shown that PKC-$\alpha$ directly phosphorylates isolated P-glycoprotein and thereby stimulates the ATPase activity of the pump (56). Thus, PKC-$\alpha$–catalyzed P-glycoprotein phosphorylation may be a contributing factor in the intrinsic drug resistance of human colon cancer.

It is now evident that P-glycoprotein–independent drug resistance mechanisms are of particular importance in the clinical drug resistance of colon and other solid cancers (8). We have developed an in vitro model of the intrinsic drug resistance of human colon cancer (39,57) that shows that protein kinase C activation can play a major role in non–P-glycoprotein–mediated (nonclassical) MDR in colon cancer. In the model, a metastatic human colon cancer cell line that had never been exposed to cytotoxic drugs is rendered transiently multidrug resistant by protein kinase C activation (57). Both phorbol ester and diacylglycerol protein kinase C activators induce resistance to multiple cytotoxic drugs in the cultured human colon cancer KM12L4a cells, and the induction of resistance is antagonized by protein kinase C inhibitors (57). The IC$_{50}$s of the cytotoxic drugs (drug concentrations that cause 50% cell growth inhibition) are increased significantly by two- to threefold as a consequence of phorbol ester exposure, and the phorbol ester–induced resistance correlates with protein kinase C activation (rather than with its down-regulation) (57).

The phorbol ester–induced resistance in human colon cancer KM12L4a cells resembles P-glycoprotein–mediated MDR in three important ways. First, the same spectrum of drugs appears to be affected in the phorbol ester–induced resistance in KM12L4 cells and in the P-glycoprotein–mediated MDR phenotype. Doxorubicin, vincristine, and vinblastine are affected by phorbol esters in KM12L4a cells, and 5-fluorouracil is not (57). Second, the phorbol ester–induced drug resistance in KM12L4a cells and P-glycoprotein–mediated MDR are both associated with a pronounced defect in the intracellular accumulation of affected drugs (39,57). Third, activation of the isozyme PKC-α enhances P-glycoprotein–mediated MDR and triggers the induction of MDR in KM12L4a cells in response to phorbol esters (39).

The phorbol ester–induced MDR phenotype in KM12L4a cells is, however, distinguished from P-glycoprotein–mediated MDR in important ways. P-glycoprotein–mediated MDR is associated with an increased rate of cellular drug efflux (4), whereas phorbol ester–induced MDR in KM12L4a cells is associated with a decreased rate of drug uptake by the cells and with no apparent alteration in the rate of drug efflux (57). Similar phorbol ester effects on cellular drug uptake and efflux rates have been noted in murine leukemia P388 cells (58). Verapamil and cyclosporin A are potent reversal agents of P-glycoprotein–mediated MDR (4), but they have no effect on either phorbol ester–induced resistance or basal chemosensitivity in KM12L4a cells (Gravitt and O'Brian, manuscript in preparation). The apparent P-glycoprotein independence of phorbol ester–induced MDR and basal chemosensitivity in KM12L4a cells is consistent with the lack of detectable P-glycoprotein expression in the cells, as measured by Western analysis (Gravitt and O'Brian, manuscript in preparation). Thus, phorbol ester–induced MDR in KM12L4a cells and P-glycoprotein–mediated MDR are, in fact, distinct phenomena. The mechanism of the phorbol ester–induced MDR phenotype of KM12L4a cells is still unknown.

## THE COLONIC LUMEN AS A REPOSITORY OF ENDOGENOUS PROTEIN KINASE C–STIMULATORY AGENTS—IMPLICATIONS FOR THE PROGRESSION AND INTRINSIC DRUG RESISTANCE OF HUMAN COLON CANCER

Stimulators of protein kinase C activity are included among the major components of the contents of the colonic lumen. These protein kinase C–stimulatory agents include bile acids and dietary fat–derived diacylglycerols and free fatty acids (Table 4) (59–61). Protein kinase C–stimulatory activity appears to be a general feature of bile acids, as it has been observed with primary and secondary bile acids in both conjugated and unconjugated forms (62). Bile acids stimulate protein kinase C by direct effects on the enzyme and by stimulating the production of sn-1,2-diacylglycerol by phospholipase C (62–64). Among diet-derived diglycerides in the colonic lumen, only those with the sn-1,2 configuration have been shown to stimulate protein kinase C activity (65,66). Human fecal bacteria produce sn-1,2-diacylglycerols from dietary lipids in the colon (66). Unsaturated free fatty acids have direct stimulatory effects on protein kinase C and also induce the production of sn-1,2-diacylglycerol in colonic epithelial cells (67).

**Table 4**  Protein Kinase C–Stimulatory Agents Present in the Colonic Lumen

| |
|---|
| Unsaturated free fatty acids |
| sn-1,2-diacylglycerols |
| Unconjugated primary bile acids |
| Tauro- and glyco-conjugated primary bile acids |
| Unconjugated secondary bile acids |
| Tauro- and glyco-conjugated secondary bile acids |

The ability of bile acids such as deoxycholate and free fatty acids to serve as tumor promoters in the colonic lumen has been demonstrated, although the role of protein kinase C modulation in the tumor promotion of the colonic epithelium by these agents has not been defined (61). It has been inferred from the potent tumor-promoting activity of specific protein kinase C activators, such as 12-O-tetradecanoylphorbol-13-acetate (TPA), that chronic activation of colonic epithelial protein kinase C by bile acids and dietary fat metabolites plays an important role in the mediation of tumor promotion by these agents in the colonic epithelium (59–61). Thus, chronic protein kinase C activation has been implicated in the progression of human colorectal cancer. Limiting the activation of colonic epithelial protein kinase C is therefore seen as a potentially valuable strategy for chemoprevention of the malignant disease (60).

Our model of phorbol ester–induced intrinsic drug resistance in cultured human colon cancer cells directly implicates lumenal sn-1,2-diacylglycerols in the intrinsic drug resistance of clinical colon cancer (57), because phorbol esters and sn-1,2-diacylglycerols activate protein kinase C by closely related mechanisms (68). It follows logically that other protein kinase C–stimulatory agents in the colonic lumen (e.g., bile acids and free fatty acids) may also induce multidrug resistance in human colon cancer cells. In fact, we have shown that deoxycholate transiently induces a multidrug resistance phenotype in murine fibrosarcoma cell lines (63). The induction of multidrug resistance in fibrosarcoma cells by deoxycholate appears to be a result of protein kinase C activation, because phorbol ester protein kinase C activators induce a similar response (63). Thus, protein kinase C–stimulatory lumenal contents may induce multidrug resistance in colon cancer cells in vivo and thereby contribute to the intrinsic drug resistance of clinical colon cancer.

## TARGETING PROTEIN KINASE C-α AS A NOVEL STRATEGY FOR REVERSAL OF DRUG RESISTANCE IN COLON CANCER THERAPY

The intrinsic drug resistance of human colon cancer accounts for the limited value of chemotherapy in the management of the disease (1–3). Rational design of strategies to reverse intrinsic drug resistance in human colon cancer will require an understanding of the molecular events underlying the major drug resistance mechanisms operative in the disease. Evidence has been presented that at least three distinct mechanisms of drug resistance may be operative in human colon cancer. These mechanisms are P-glycoprotein–mediated MDR (5), DNA topoisomerase I–mediated MDR (69), and P-glycoprotein–independent, protein kinase C-α–mediated MDR (39,57). The heterogeneous nature of drug resistance mechanisms in human colon cancer suggests that a combination of agents that antagonize drug resistance by distinct mechanisms may be required to reverse clinical drug resistance in colon cancer and improve the ultimate therapeutic outcome for the patient. Conceptually, such an approach to the reversal of drug resistance is analogous to the standard use of combination chemotherapy in cancer treatment to address the heterogeneous nature of tumor cell populations (26).

It is anticipated that P-glycoprotein–binding drugs will be of limited value in colon cancer therapy. This is based on problems of toxicity that have already been encountered in attempts to target P-glycoprotein directly for reversal of clinical drug resistance in solid tumors (8). This underscores the importance of defining the magnitude of the contribution of protein kinase C-α–mediated MDR to the intrinsic drug resistance of clinical colon cancer. Furthermore, definition of the importance of DNA topoisomerase I–mediated resistance in the clinical disease needs to be accomplished. Identification of additional mechanisms of drug resistance in clinical colon cancer is also a worthwhile goal that may lead to effective strategies of chemosensitization of the disease to therapy.

Strategies for the reversal of protein kinase C-$\alpha$–mediated MDR in colon cancer could involve targeting of either protein kinase C-$\alpha$ or molecules that function upstream or downstream of protein kinase C-$\alpha$ in the MDR phenotype. Protein kinase C-$\alpha$ is expressed ubiquitously in mammalian tissues (22,25). If it should turn out that protein kinase C-$\alpha$ inhibition is not well tolerated in cancer patients, effective reversal of intrinsic drug resistance might still be accomplished by blocking downstream events in protein kinase C-$\alpha$–mediated resistance. Elucidation of the mechanism of protein kinase C-$\alpha$–mediated MDR in human colon cancer will be required to identify potential downstream targets for therapeutic intervention.

## ACKNOWLEDGMENTS

This work was supported by grants from the Elsa U. Pardee Foundation, The Physician's Referral Service, National Institutes of Health Award CA52460, and Robert A. Welch Foundation Award G-1141. We thank Patherine Greenwood for expert preparation of the manuscript.

## REFERENCES

1. Hamilton JM. Adjuvant therapy for gastrointestinal cancer. Curr Opin Oncol 1994; 6:435–440.
2. Mayer RJ. Chemotherapy for metastatic colorectal cancer. Cancer 1992; 70(Suppl):1414–1424.
3. Moertel CG. Accomplishments in surgical adjuvant therapy for large bowel cancer. Cancer 1992; 70(Suppl):1364–1371.
4. Gottesman MM, Pastan I. Biochemistry of multidrug resistance mediated by the multidrug transporter. Annu Rev Biochem 1993; 62:385–427.
5. Goldstein LJ, Galski H, Fojo A, Willingham M, Lai SL, Gazdar A, Pirker R, Green A, Crist W, Brodeur G, Lieber M, Cossman J, Gottesman MM, Pastan I. Expression of a multidrug resistance gene in human cancers. J Natl Cancer Inst 1989; 81:116–124.
6. Endicott JA, Ling V. The biochemistry of P-glycoprotein-mediated multidrug resistance. Annu Rev Biochem 1989; 58:137–171.
7. Fojo AT, Ueda K, Slamon DJ, Poplack DG, Gottesman MM, Pastan I. Expression of a multidrug-resistance gene in human tumors and tissues. Proc Natl Acad Sci USA 1987; 84:256–269.
8. Houghton PJ, Kaye SB. Multidrug resistance. J NIH Res 1994; 6:54–61.
9. Moertel CG, Fleming TR, MacDonald JS, Haller DG, Laurie JA, Tangen CM, Ungerleider JS, Emerson WAS, Tormey DC, Glick JH, Veeder MH, Mailliard JA. Fluorouracil plus levamisole as effective adjuvant therapy after resection of stage III colon carcinoma: a final report. Ann Intern Med 1995; 122:321–326.
10. Takimoto CH. Enigma of fluorouracil and levamisole. J Natl Cancer Inst 1995; 87:471–473.
11. Nishizuka Y. Protein kinase C and lipid signaling for sustained cellular responses. FASEB J 1995; 9:484–496.

12. Castagna M, Takai Y, Kaibuchi K, Sano K, Kikkawa U, Nishizuka Y. Direct activation of calcium-activated, phospholipid-dependent protein kinase by tumor-promoting phorbol esters. J Biol Chem 1982; 257:7847–7851.
13. Kishimoto A, Takai Y, Mori T, Kikkawa U, Nishizuka Y. Activation of calcium and phospholipid-dependent protein kinase by diacylglycerol, its possible relation to phosphatidylinositol turnover. J Biol Chem 1980; 255:2273–2276.
14. Lester DS, Epand RM, Eds. Protein Kinase C: Current Concepts and Future Perspectives. New York: Ellis Horwood, 1992.
15. Kuo JF, Ed. Protein Kinase C. New York: Oxford University Press, 1994.
16. Dekker LV, Parker PJ. Protein kinase C—a question of specificity. Trends Biochem Sci 1994; 19:73–77.
17. Grunicke HH, Uberall F. Protein kinase C modulation. Semin Cancer Biol 1992; 3:351–360.
18. Nakanishi H, Brewer KA, Exton JH. Activation of the ζ isozyme of protein kinase c by phosphatidylinositol 3, 4, 5-triphosphate. J Biol Chem 1993; 268:13–16.
19. Kazanietz MG, Areces LB, Bahador A, Mischak H, Goodnight J. Characterization of ligand and substrate specificity for the calcium-dependent and calcium-independent protein kinase C isozymes. Mol Pharmacol 1993; 44:298–307.
20. Fujise A, Mizuno K, Ueda Y, Osada S, Hirai S, Takayanagi A, Shimizu N, Owada MK, Nakajima H, Ohno S. Specificity of the high-affinity interaction of protein kinase C with a physiological substrate, myristoylated alanine-rich protein kinase C substrate. J Biol Chem 1994; 269:31642–31648.
21. Goodnight J, Mischak H, Kolch W, Mushinski JF. Immunocytochemical localization of eight protein kinase C isozymes overexpressed in NIH3T3 fibroblasts. J Biol Chem 1995; 270:9991–10001.
22. Wetsel WC, Khan WA, Merchenthaler I, Rivera H, Halpern AE, Phung HM, Negro-Vilar A, Hannun YA. J Cell Biol 1992; 117:121–133.
23. Mochly Rosen D. Localization of protein kinases by anchoring proteins: a theme in signal transduction. Science 1995; 268:247–251.
24. Ron D, Chen CH, Caldwell J, Jamieson L, Orr E, Mochly-Rosen D. Cloning of an intracellular receptor for protein kinase C: a homolog of the β subunit of G proteins. Proc Natl Acad Sci USA 1994; 91:839–843.
25. Kikkawa U, Kishimoto A, Nishizuka Y. The protein kinase C family: heterogeneity and its implications. Annu Rev Biochem 1989; 58:31–44.
26. O'Brian CA, Ward NE, Gupta KP, Gravitt KR. The contribution of protein kinase C to multiple drug resistance in cancer. In: Kellen JA, ed. Alternative Mechanisms of Multidrug Resistance in Cancer. Boston: Birkhauser, 1995:173–190.
27. Kopp R, Nielke B, Sauter G, Schildberg FW, Paumgartner G, Pfeiffer A. Altered protein kinase C activity in biopsies of human colon adenomas and carcinomas. Cancer Res 1991; 51:205–210.
28. Sakanoue Y, Hatada T, Kusunoki M, Yanagi H, Yamamura T, Utsunomiya J. Protein kinase C activity as a marker for colorectal cancer. Int J Cancer 1991; 48:803–806.
29. Kusunoki M, Sakanoue Y, Hatada T, Yanagi H, Yamamura T, Utsunomiya U. Protein kinase C activity in human colonic adenoma and colorectal carcinoma. Cancer 1992; 69:24–30.
30. Guillem JG, O'Brian CA, Fitzer CJ, Forde KA, LoGerfo P, Treat M, Weinstein IB. Altered levels of protein kinase C and Ca$^{2+}$-dependent protein kinases in human colon carcinomas. Cancer Res 1987; 47:2036–2039.
31. Baum CL, Wali RK, Sitrin MD, Bolt MJG, Brasitus TA. 1,2-dimethyl-hydrazine-induced alterations in protein kinase C activity in the rat preneoplastic colon. Cancer Res 1990; 50:3915–3920.
32. Wali RK, Baum CL, Bolt MJG, Dudeja PK, Sitrin MD, Brasitus TA. Downregulation of protein kinase C activity in 1,2-dimethylhydrazine-induced rat colonic tumors. Biochim Biophys Acta 1991; 1092:119–123.

33. Wolfman A, Wingrove TG, Blackshear PJ, Macara IG. Downregulation of protein kinase C and of an endogenous 80-kDa substrate in transformed fibroblasts. J Biol Chem 1987; 262:16546–16552.

34. Fleischman LF, Chahwala SB, Cantley L. Ras-transformed cells: altered levels of phosphatidylinositol-4,5-bissphosphate and catabolites. Science 1986; 231:407–410.

35. Weyman CM, Taparowsky EJ, Wolfson M, Ashendel CL. Partial downregulation of protein kinase C in C3H10T½ mouse fibroblasts transfected with the human Ha-ras oncogene. Cancer Res 1988; 48:6535–6541.

36. Vogelstein B, Fearon ER, Hamilton SR, Kern SE, Preisinger AC, Leppert M, Nakamura Y, White R, Smits AMM, Bos JL. Genetic alterations during colorectal-tumor development. N Engl J Med 1988; 319:525–532.

37. Phan SC, Morotomi M, Guillen JG, LoGerfo P, Weinstein IB. Decreased levels of 1,2-sn-diacylglycerol in human colon tumors. Cancer Res 1991; 51:1571–1573.

38. Sauter G, Nerlich A, Spengler U, Kopp R, Pfeiffer A. Low diacylglycerol values in colonic adenomas and colorectal cancer. Gut 1990; 31:1041–1045.

39. Gravitt KR, Ward NE, Fan D, Skibber JM, Levin B, O'Brian CA. Evidence that protein kinase C-α activation is a critical event in phorbol ester-induced multiple drug resistance in human colon cancer cells. Biochem Pharmacol 1994; 48:375–381.

40. Pongracz J, Clark P, Neoptolemos JP, Lord JM. Expression of protein kinase C isoenzymes in colorectal cancer tissue and their differential activation by different bile acids. Int J Cancer 1995; 61:35–39.

41. Davidson LA, Jiang YH, Derr JN, Aukema HM, Lupton JR, Chapkin RS. Protein kinase C isoforms in human and rat colonic mucosa. Arch Biochem Biophys 1994; 312:547–553.

42. Kahl-Rainer P, Karner-Hanusch J, Weiss W, Marian B. Five of six protein kinase C isoenzymes present in normal mucosa show reduced protein levels during tumor development in the human colon. Carcinogenesis 1994; 15:779–782.

43. Kuranami M, Cohen AM, Guillem JG. Analysis of protein kinase C isoform expression in a colorectal cancer liver metastasis model. Am J Surg 1995; 169:57–64.

44. Choi PM, Tchou-Wong KM, Weinstein IB. Overexpression of protein kinase C in HT29 colon cancer cells causes growth inhibition and tumor suppression. Mol Cell Biol 1990; 10:4650–4657.

45. Fan D, Beltran PJ, O'Brian CA. Reversal of multidrug resistance. In: Kellen JA, ed. Reversal of Multidrug Resistance in Cancer. Boca Raton: CRC Press, 1994:93–125.

46. O'Brian CA, Ward NE, Gravitt KR, Fan D. The role of protein kinase C in multidrug resistance. In: Goldstein LJ, Ozols RF, eds. Anticancer Drug Resistance: Advances in Molecular and Clinical Research. Boston: Kluwer Academic Publishers, 1994:41–55.

47. Glazer RI. Protein kinase C in multidrug resistance, neoplastic transformation, and differentiation. In: Kuo JF, ed. Protein Kinase C. New York: Oxford University Press, 1994:171–198.

48. Chambers TC, McAvoy EM, Jacobs JW, Eilon G. Protein kinase C phosphorylates P-glycoprotein in multidrug resistant human KB carcinoma cells. J Biol Chem 1990; 265:7679–7686.

49. Chambers TC, Pohl J, Raynor RL, Kuo JF. Identification of specific sites in human P-glycoprotein phosphorylated by protein kinase C. J Biol Chem 1993; 268:4592–4595.

50. Chambers TC, Zheng B, Kuo JF. Regulation by phorbol ester and protein kinase C inhibitors, and by a protein phosphatase inhibitor (okadaic acid) of P-glycoprotein phosphorylation and relationship to drug accumulation in multidrug resistant human KB cells. Mol Pharmacol 1992; 41:1008–1015.

51. Bates SE, Currier SJ, Alvarez M, Fojo AT. Modulation of P-glycoprotein phosphorylation and drug transport by sodium butyrate. Biochemistry 1992; 31:6366–6372.

52. Bates SE, Lee JS, Dickstein B, Spolyar M, Fojo AT. Differential modulation of P-glycoprotein transport by protein kinase inhibition. Biochemistry 1993; 32:9156–9164.

53. Blobe GC, Sachs CW, Khan WA, Fabbro D, Stabel S, Wetsel WC, Obeid LM, Fine RL, Hannun YA. Selective regulation of expression of protein kinase C (PKC) isoenzymes in multidrug-resistant MCF7 cells. J Biol Chem 1993; 268:658–664.

54. Fine RL, Patel J, Chabner BA. Phorbol esters induce multidrug resistance in human breast cancer cells. Proc Natl Acad Sci USA 1988; 85:582–586.

55. Yu G, Ahmad S, Aquino A, Fairchild CR, Trepel JB, Ohno S, Suzuki K, Tsuruo T, Cowan KH, Glazer RI. Transfection with protein kinase C-α confers increased multidrug resistance to MCF7 cells expressing P-glycoprotein. Cancer Commun 1991; 3:181–189.

56. Ahmad S, Safa AR, Glazer RI. Modulation of P-glycoprotein by protein kinase C-α in a baculovirus expression system. Biochemistry 1994; 33:10313–10318.

57. Dong Z, Ward NE, Fan D, Gupta KP, O'Brian CA. An in vitro model for intrinsic drug resistance: effects of protein kinase C activators on the chemosensitivity of cultured human colon cancer cells. Mol Pharmacol 1991; 39:563–569.

58. Kessel D. Effects of phorbol esters on doxorubicin transport systems. Biochem Pharmacol 1988; 37:2297–2299.

59. O'Brian CA, Ward NE. Relevance of the tumor promoter receptor protein kinase C in colon carcinogenesis. In: Riddell RH, ed. Dysplasia and Cancer in Colitis. New York: Elsevier Press, 1991:135–139.

60. O'Brian CA, Ward NE, Ioannides CG, Dong Z. Potential strategies of chemoprevention through modulation of protein kinase C activity. In: Steele VE, Stoner GD, Boone CW, Kelloff GJ, eds. Cellular and Molecular Targets for Chemoprevention. Boca Raton, FL: CRC Press, 1992:161–170.

61. O'Brian CA, Ward NE, Ioannides CG. Altered signal transduction in carcinogenesis. Adv Mol Cell Biol 1993; 7:61–88.

62. Fitzer CJ, O'Brian CA, Guillem JG, Weinstein IB. The regulation of protein kinase C by chenodeoxycholate, deoxycholate, and several structurally related bile acids. Carcinogenesis 1987; 8:217–220.

63. O'Brian CA, Fan D, Ward NE, Dong Z, Iwamoto L, Gupta KP, Earnest LE, Fidler IJ. Transient enhancement of multidrug resistance by the bile acid deoxycholate in murine fibrosarcoma cells in vitro. Biochem Pharmacol 1991; 41:797–806.

64. Craven PA, Pfanstiel J, DeRubertis FR. Role of activation of protein kinase C in the stimulation of colonic epithelial proliferation and reactive oxygen formation by bile acids. J Clin Invest 1987; 79:532–541.

65. Friedman E, Isaksson P, Rafter J, Marian B, Winawer S, Newmark H. Fecal diglycerides as selective endogenous mitogens for premalignant and malignant human colonic epithelial cells. Cancer Res 1989; 49:544–548.

66. Morotomi M, Guillem JG, LoGerfo P, Weinstein IB. Production of diacyglycerol, an activator of protein kinase C, by human intestinal microflora. Cancer Res 1990; 50:3595–3599.

67. Craven PA, DeRubertis FR. Role of activation of protein kinase C in the stimulation of colonic epithelial proliferation by unsaturated fatty acids. Gastroenterology 1988; 95:676–685.

68. Bell RM, Burns DJ. Lipid activation of protein kinase C. J Biol Chem 1991; 266:4661–4664.

69. Giovanella BC, Stehlin JS, Wall ME, Wani MC, Nichols AW, Liu LF, Silber R, Potmesil M. DNA topoisomerase I-targeted chemotherapy of human colon cancer in xenografts. Science 1989; 246:1046–1048.

# 10

## Clinical Relevance of P-glycoprotein-Related Multidrug Resistance in Hematological Malignancies

Petra C. Pasman and Harry C. Schouten
*University Hospital Maastricht, Maastricht, The Netherlands*

### INTRODUCTION

Hematological malignancies tend to respond reasonably well to chemotherapy. However, a number of patients do not achieve a complete remission or have relapsing disease. This poor response to chemotherapy has given rise to the question whether the tumor cells have the intrinsic (or acquired) property to detoxify these cytotoxic drugs. Clinically, there are patients who are refractory to a whole range of chemotherapeutic agents, even without prior exposure—this is called multidrug resistance (MDR). Some cellular mechanisms have been identified that are able to explain the clinical MDR phenotype. For instance, the detoxifying glutathione system is related to resistance for alkylating agents (1,2). Alteration of topoisomerase II leads to resistance to anthracyclines, epopodophylotoxins, mitoxantrone, and amsacrine (3).

P-glycoprotein (Pgp) is an energy-dependent protein located in the cell membrane that is able to extrude drugs such as vinca alkaloids, anthracyclines, and epopodophylotoxins. Recently another protein, the multidrug resistance–associated protein (MRP), has been discovered (4). MRP mediates resistance to drugs such as doxorubicin, vincristine, and etoposide (5).

This chapter gives an overview of the role of Pgp and (if known) MRP in specific hematological malignancies. Studies aimed at detecting *MDR1*/mRNA are reviewed separately from those studies that analyzed Pgp expression, as these methods of detection differ in sensitivity (6–8).

### ACUTE MYELOID LEUKEMIA

#### Frequency of Expression

Initially, patients with acute myeloid leukemia (AML) respond well to chemotherapy: 60–80% of patients may achieve a complete remission. However, most patients relapse early. Five-year disease-free survival is 10–30%. Secondary AML has a very poor prognosis; few patients survive for more than 1 year.

Only larger studies that were able to perform statistical analyses are reviewed here. Amplification of *MDR1*/DNA was not observed (9,10). Generally, *MDR1*/mRNA detection in untreated patients is 40%, ranging from 18 to 54% (Table 1). Although the polymerase chain reaction (PCR) is regarded as the most sensitive technique at present, the studies that used PCR have detected the lowest incidence (14,16). This incidence seems comparable to the presence of *MDR1*/mRNA in the treated group (overall 51%).

Table 2 shows an overview of those studies that detected Pgp with the use of monoclonal antibodies such as C219, JSB1, and MRK16. The range of Pgp expression in the untreated group was comparable to the detection of *MDR1*/mRNA: 18–58%, with an overall incidence of 44%. Generally, it can be concluded that Pgp is expressed in about 40% of the patients with de novo AML.

Most studies (11,13,17,19,29) have not been able to detect a difference in Pgp expression for the individual FAB subtypes. However, some have described a higher frequency of positivity in cases with M0 (25), M1 (14,15), and M4 (12) and a lower frequency in M3 (21,26). However, because of small population sizes, no definite conclusions can yet be drawn.

MRP/mRNA was detected in 9 of 51 (18%) untreated patients and in 13 of 30 (43%) treated patients (16). Schneider et al. found significantly higher levels of MRP/mRNA at relapse than at diagnosis (27).

Patients with secondary AML have a significantly higher level of *MDR1*/mRNA than do those with de novo AML (28). *MDR1*/mRNA was detected by Gruber et al. in eight of 13 (62) and by Holmes et al. in four of five (80%) patients (9,13). Pgp expression was seen in 30 of 45 (67%) patients (21,29,30).

## Clinical Relevance

All studies that we found, except two (17,23), detected a significant negative correlation between Pgp expression and complete remission (CR) rates (12,13,15,18–22,24). Presence of Pgp correlated especially with primary resistant disease (and not relapse rate). Probably as a consequence, survival was also adversely influenced by the presence of Pgp (11,12,15,19,21,23,24). Meta-analysis including 859 patients has been performed

**Table 1** The Presence of *MDR1*/mRNA in Previously Untreated and Treated Patients with Acute Myeloid Leukemia

| Untreated number positive/total patients (%) | Treated number positive/total patients (%) | Ref. |
|---|---|---|
| 18/36  (50%) | 13/18 (72%) | 11 |
| 22/51  (42%) | 21/35 (60%) | 12 |
| 20/44  (46%) | | 13 |
| 15/50  (30%) | | 14 |
| 34/63[a]  (54%) | | 15 |
| 9/51  (18%) | 13/40 (33%) | 16 |
| 118/295 (40%) | 47/93 (51%) | Overall |

[a]Low mRNA level not taken into account.

by Holmes et al., and a relative risk of 0.7 for Pgp expression to achieve CR was estimated (31).

In three studies (14,21,32), correlation was found between CD34 positivity and
Pgp expression, but in three other studies (18,20,24) there was no such correlation.
However, the outcome of patients whose sample was CD34+/Pgp+ was significantly
poorer than that of CD34–/Pgp– patients (18,20,21). The combination of an abnormal
karyotype and Pgp expression was also correlated with a poor outcome (18,20).

Zhou et al. found MRP/mRNA correlated with lower complete remission rates
(16). MRP and Pgp were usually both expressed in the same patient sample.

In five studies, a multivariate analysis was done: Lamy et al. and Wood et al. did
not find Pgp to be an independent prognostic factor (18,20). In contrast, Campos et
al., Musto et al., and Leith et al. found Pgp to be such a factor (21,23,33).

### Therapy with MDR-Reversing Agents

*In Vitro/Ex Vivo*

Agents such as verapamil, nifedipine, quinidine (a quinoline derivative), colchicine,
tamoxifen, RU 486 (an experimental antiprogestin), and cyclosporin A have been
shown to modulate daunorubicin and vincristine accumulation and retention in AML-
resistant cell lines (K562 and HL60) (34–41). Verapamil and cyclosporin A were shown
to act synergistically (42). Muller et al. did a very interesting study showing that verapamil down-regulates the transcription of the *MDR1* gene (43,44). Ross et al. proved
that the vehicle for intravenous administration of cyclosporin A, Cremophor EL, also
has MDR-reversing capacity in fresh AML samples (not in an AML cell line) (36).
Elgie et al. showed that both activators and an inhibitor of protein kinase C enhances
cytotoxicity (45). Mechetner et al. effectively used a monoclonal antibody to inhibit the
efflux of Pgp substrates and to significantly increase the cytotoxicity of Pgp-transported
drugs (46). Marie et al. and Nooter et al. used samples from AML patients for functional assays with daunorubicin (47,48). They found a significant increase in uptake of
daunorubicin with cyclosporin A in untreated patients; in treated patients, however,
cyclosporin A did not have such an effect.

**Table 2**  The Expression of Pgp in Previously Untreated and Treated Patients with Acute
Myeloid Leukemia

| Untreated number positive/total patients (%) | Treated number positive/total patients (%) | Ref. |
|---|---|---|
| 18/67  (18%) | 19/46 (41%) | 12 |
| 14/52  (27%) |  | 17 |
| 27/51  (53%) |  | 18 |
| 19/52  (37%) |  | 19 |
| 30/52  (58%) |  | 20 |
| 52/122 (43%) |  | 21 |
| 15/26  (58%) |  | 22 |
| 70/145 (48%) |  | 23 |
| 30/54  (55%) |  | 24 |
| 275/621 (44%) | 19/46 (41%) | Overall |

*Clinical Trials*

Although only a small number of AML patients have undergone treatment with an MDR-reverser, the first results are promising. Several of these poor-prognosis patients achieved CR, although it was short lasting (Table 3).

Pgp expression was investigated in four of these studies (50–52,54). A patient described by Sonneveld et al. was Pgp negative at diagnosis, positive at relapse, and negative when a second CR was achieved after the use of the original remission-induction chemotherapy in addition with cyclosporin A (50). However, as the myeloid blasts returned, so did Pgp expression. In the study by Marie et al., five of nine patients were Pgp positive at original diagnosis (54). After treatment with mitoxantrone, etoposide, and cyclosporin A, one of seven patients tested had Pgp expression. This one patient had been negative at diagnosis. Of the patients who were Pgp positive before treatment, two achieved CR. Solary et al. mention two of four tested patients being positive for Pgp; however, they did not correlate this finding with clinical outcome (52). List et al. could not detect a significant correlation between Pgp expression and response (51). They followed up five patients for Pgp expression and saw either a decrease or disappearance of Pgp expression.

Side effects varied from none (50) to severe myelosuppression (51,52,54) and cardiac toxicity (49,52). A transient conjugated hyperbilirubinemia was seen when cyclosporin A was used (51,54). List et al. found a rise in serum bilirubin correlating with a better response (51). However, side effects were usually well tolerated and did not lead to discontinuation of the applied drugs.

## Myelodysplastic Syndromes

High-risk myelodysplastic syndromes (MDS), including refractory anemia with excess blasts (in transformation) and chronic myelomonocytic leukemia, were associated with a higher incidence of Pgp expression than low-risk MDS, including refractory anemia and sideroblastic anemia (9,29,30,55): 50% (n=95) and 19% (n=54), respectively. CD34 was correlated with Pgp expression (29,30,55).

Interestingly, Pgp expression was correlated with poor response to intensive anthracycline/cytarabine (ara-C) treatment. As may be expected, treatment with low-dose ara-C leads to responses regardless of Pgp expression (29). In some patients, ara-C

**Table 3** Overview of Patients with Acute Myeloid Leukemia in Clinical Trials with Pgp-Reversing Agents

| Chemotherapy | MDR-reverser | Total number of patients | Response | Ref. |
|---|---|---|---|---|
| DNR, ara-C | Dexverapamil | 6 | 2 CR, 2 PR, 2 NR | 49 |
| DNR, ara-C | CsA | 1 | 1 CR | 50 |
| DNR, ara-C | CsA | 31 | 11 CR, 1 PR, 17 NR | 51 |
| ara-C, mitoxantrone | Quinine | 5 | 3 CR, 1 PR, 1 NR | 52 |
| Vinblastine, VP-16 | Verapamil | 2 | 2 PR | 53 |
| Mitoxantrone, etoposide | CsA | 9 | 2 CR, 4 PR, 3 NR | 54 |

DNR = daunorubicin, CR = complete remission, PR = partial remission, NR = no response, CsA = cyclosporin A, ara-C = cytarabine, VP-16 = etoposide.

combined with granulocyte-macrophage colony-stimulating factor (GM-CSF) or inter-
leukin-3 (IL-3) induced Pgp (56).

## Conclusion

With the limited data available, the presence of Pgp seems to predict resistant disease
and poor survival in patients with AML, which is supported by the meta-analysis by
Holmes et al. (31). When Pgp is present in combination with CD34 positivity, MRP,
and an abnormal karyotype, the predictive value for a poor prognosis may be enhanced.
Secondary AML and high-risk MDS seem to have a higher incidence of Pgp expression,
which may be related to the poor prognosis.

Large clinical trials are necessary to assess the final role of MDR-reversing
agents.

## CHRONIC MYELOID LEUKEMIA

For patients with chronic myeloid leukemia (CML), treatment with cytostatic drugs is
not a curative option: currently, CML can be cured only by high-dose therapy followed
by allogeneic bone marrow transplantation.

Only limited data are available on large groups of patients with CML. In (untreated and treated) patients with CML in chronic phase, *MDR1*/mRNA was not detected (n=18) (57–59). However, Pgp expression was found in 42% (n=88) (60–66).
In blastic phase, *MDR1*/mRNA was detected in 37% (n=35) (47,57–59,67), and Pgp
expression was found in 60% (n=52) (60–62,65–67). Michelutti et al. found the proportion of Pgp positive cells to be significantly higher in blastic phase (65). Weide et
al. found the more mature granulocytes bearing Pgp, whereas the blast cells were negative (62). In contrast, Sato et al. found a trace of *MDR1*/mRNA in the immature subpopulation; the whole population of chronic phase cells was negative (58). Not one
study was able to implement a statistical analysis because of small group sizes.

Several studies (58,64,68) describe patients that had no Pgp expression in the first
blast crisis but had acquired Pgp during the second blast crisis. Weide et al. found Pgp
presence in CML not to be correlated with Pgp expression in blast crisis (62).

List et al. treated 10 CML patients in blastic phase with daunorubicin and cyclosporin A (51). The type of blastic crisis was not given. Six patients achieved CR; five
patients were restored to the chronic phase, with a median duration of 4 months. One
patient achieved a cytogenetic CR that lasted 7 months. Pgp expression was not correlated with response. Side effects of nausea, vomiting, dysesthesias, hypomagnesemia,
transient hyperbilirubinemia, and prolonged myelosuppression were reported.

Although there is a tendency for higher expression of Pgp in blastic crisis, larger
studies are necessary to elucidate the expression of Pgp and its clinical relevance in
CML.

## ACUTE LYMPHOCYTIC LEUKEMIA

### Frequency of Expression

Acute lymphocytic leukemia (ALL) is a disease that generally responds well to chemotherapy, resulting in a remission rate of 90% in standard-risk children and 50–70% in
poor-risk children and adults. Although these results are promising, relapses frequently

occur, with finally 20–30% of standard-risk patients and 50–70% of poor-risk patients dying of leukemia.

Two studies (10,69) investigated the cell samples from patients with ALL for *MDR1* gene expression. Both studies found no amplification of the gene.

The results of those studies directed to detect *MDR1*/mRNA are shown in Table 4. At diagnosis, *MDR1*/mRNA was detected in 33% (26/79) of all studied cases, with larger studies (13,14,57) having results ranging from 13% to 36%. Miwa, using PCR, found *MDR1*/mRNA in 30% of the samples studied (14). In previously treated patients, *MDR1*/mRNA was detected in 14 of 41 (34%) samples.

The overall rate of Pgp positivity in untreated patients was 25% (70/321); however, the interstudy variation ranged from 0% to 36% (Table 5). Limiting the analysis to those studies with 10 patients or more, four of six studies found an equal result (Pgp positivity 36%). Pieters et al., however, found no presence of Pgp in 28 cases, Fennetau et al. saw only two of 51 cases positive for Pgp (79,80). All studies used similar staining techniques; therefore, lack of uniform techniques is unlikely to explain the observed discrepancy.

The range of Pgp positivity was large in the group of treated patients, varying from 0% to 100%; this may be explained by small numbers of patients studied and variation in histocytochemical techniques used. Overall, 43% (22/51) of treated patients were positive for Pgp.

Musto et al. and Gruber et al. described a number of patients evaluated both at time of diagnosis and at relapse (13,81). In nine patients, Pgp was detected only at relapse, indicating a form of acquired resistance. In five patients, the amount of Pgp at relapse had increased compared to the level of Pgp at diagnosis. This may be the result of the selection of Pgp-positive cells when using MDR-related agents.

When studies that analyzed children were compared to investigations analyzing adults, no difference in incidence of Pgp positivity for untreated patients was seen: children 26% (n=178) and adults 26% (n=26). However, treated children are more often Pgp positive than are adults, 72% (n=32) and 27% (n=26), respectively. It must be taken into account that the group sizes are very small. Goasguen et al. evaluated children and adults separately (78). In children, Pgp positivity was significantly corre-

**Table 4**  The Presence of *MDR1*/mRNA in Previously Untreated and Treated Patients with Acute Lymphocytic Leukemia

| Untreated number positive/total patients (%) | Treated number positive/total patients (%) | Ref. |
|---|---|---|
| 2/15 (13%) | 1/1 (100%) | 57 |
| 1/9 (11%) | 3/20 (15%) | 69 |
| 1/2 (50%) | 1/3 (33%) | 70 |
| 5/8 (63%) | 1/1 (100%) | 71 |
| 0/2 (0%) | 0/2 (0%) | 10 |
| 4/4 (100%) | 6/6 (100%) | 72 |
| 8/25 (32%) | | 14 |
| 5/14 (36%) | 2/8 (25%) | 13 |
| 26/79 (33%) | 14/41 (34%) | Overall |

**Table 5** The Expression of Pgp in Previously Untreated and Treated Patients with Acute Lymphocytic Leukemia

| Untreated number positive/total patients (%) | Treated number positive/total patients (%) | Ref. |
|---|---|---|
| 0/6 (0%) | 10/11 (91%) | 73 |
| | 1/3 (33%) | 63 |
| 0/3 (0%) | 1/1 (100%) | 60 |
| | 1/1 (100%) | 74 |
| 4/11 (36%) | 6/9 (67%) | 75 |
| 4/11 (36%) | 3/6 (50%) | 76 |
| 0/3 (0%) | 0/5 (0%) | 10 |
| | 0/1 (0%) | 68 |
| 36/104 (35%) | | 77 |
| 16/45 (36%) | | 23 |
| 17/59 (29%) | | 78 |
| | 3/5 (60%) | 61 |
| 2/51 (4%) | | 79 |
| 0/28 (0%) | 0/14 (0%) | 80 |
| 79/321 (25%) | 25/56 (45%) | Overall |

lated with the achievement of second remission. In adults, the achievement of first and second remission was significantly correlated.

## Clinical Relevance

A number of studies have correlated the presence of Pgp with clinical outcome. Sauerbrey et al., Goasguen et al., and Musto et al. found Pgp to be an independent prognostic unfavorable factor in a multivariate analysis (23,77,78). Goasguen et al. showed a significant correlation between Pgp presence, relapsing disease, and survival rate. Musto et al. could not detect a correlation between the presence of Pgp and the achievement of complete remission, yet the number of Pgp-positive cells was significantly correlated with disease-free and overall survival (23). Gekeler et al. observed a tendency for high expression in second and third relapses (81).

Pgp in correlation with other markers such as glutathione-$\pi$ (77) or the proliferation marker Ki67 (23) indicated more significantly a poor clinical outcome than did Pgp alone. T-cell ALL is more frequently Pgp-positive than B-cell ALL (14).

## Therapy with MDR-Reversing Agents

In vitro studies with the MDR-resistant lymphoblastic leukemia cell line CEM/VLB (ADM) have shown that a large range of agents such as verapamil (82–84), cyclosporin A (82,85), SDZ-PSC 833 (analogue of cyclosporin A) (85), chlorpromazine, chloroquine, quinacrine, quinine (86), reserpine, and (trimethox)yombine (87) are able to reverse sensitivity to a variable extent. Verapamil and cyclosporin A showed significant synergism when used in combination (88). Lemoli et al. showed that a dye-mediated photolysis was capable of specifically eliminating MDR+ cells (89).

Four clinical trials with MDR-reversing agents included also ALL patients. Bessho et al. treated five refractory patients with diltiazem and vincristine (90). All patients showed a dramatic drop in leukocyte count; however, Pgp expression was not evaluated. Cardiac toxicity was seen. Cairo et al. described two ALL patients who were treated with verapamil in combination with etoposide and mitoxantrone (53). Both achieved a partial response. Cardiac toxicity was observed, but well tolerated. Again, Pgp was not analyzed. Three patients were treated with quinine, mitoxantrone, and ara-C by Solary et al. (91). One patient did not respond; two patients achieved CR (however, both died within a year). The patients who achieved CR were positive for Pgp; the other patient was Pgp-negative. Side effects were severe myelosuppression, cardiac toxicity, tinnitus, and vertigo. Miller et al. treated two patients who had refractory disease with trifluoperazine and doxorubicin (92); no responses were seen. Pgp expression was not evaluated. Extrapyramidal side effects were observed.

## Conclusion

Comparing the results of Pgp expression at the protein and the mRNA level, no significant difference can be seen. Although the range is large in the treated group (especially when the protein is detected), there seems no difference in presence of Pgp in untreated and treated patients, this being present in about one third of the patients. Pgp expression may explain drug resistance in some cases. However, different mechanisms are likely involved. Further studies investigating other mechanisms of drug resistance are needed. Preliminary results from clinical trials also indicate that reversing only Pgp is not sufficient to cure patients.

## CHRONIC LYMPHOCYTIC LEUKEMIA

### Frequency of Expression

First of all, it must be mentioned that the treatment of chronic lymphocytic leukemia (CLL) often does not include MDR-related drugs. Also, with a median survival depending on the stage of the disease—varying from 2.5 years to more than 10 years—it is a relatively indolent disease.

Rochlitz et al. detected amplification of the *MDR1* gene in nine of nine untreated cases and in 20 of 21 treated cases (93). Holmes et al. did not detect any amplification of the *MDR1* gene in 18 patients (94). When regarding both *MDR1*/mRNA and *MDR3*/mRNA transcription, several studies (95–97) reported 91–100% positive cases (Table 6); others (98–100) reported an incidence of 14–46%, despite the use of very sensitive techniques such as PCR. Table 7 shows that both untreated and treated patients have a high incidence of Pgp expression: 83% (n=48) and 88% (n=80), respectively.

Shustik et al. described the follow-up of a few patients (98): six mdr1/mRNA-negative patients remained negative; five of six mdr1/mRNA-positive patients lost *MDR1*/mRNA transcription. They did not see any patient that acquired mdr1/mRNA positivity.

MRP/mRNA was detected in 10 of 13 untreated patients and five of eight treated patients (104). High levels of MRP/mRNA were found in 33 samples (100). Beck et al.

**Table 6** The Presence of *MDR1*/mRNA and *MDR3*/mRNA in Previously Untreated and Treated Patients with Chronic Lymphocytic Leukemia

| Untreated mdr1 number positive/ total patients (%) | Untreated mdr3 number positive/ total patients (%) | Treated mdr1 number positive/ total patients (%) | Treated mdr3 number positive/ total patients (%) | Ref. |
|---|---|---|---|---|
| 10/10 (100%) | 10/10 (100%) | 15/16 (94%) | 16/16 (100%) | 97 |
| 4/28 (14%) | 5/19 (26%) | | | 98 |
| 4/7 (57%) | | 14/27 (67%) | | 94 |
| 3/3 (100%) | 2/3 (67%) | 3/13 (23%) | 6/13 (46%) | 99 |
| 11/12 (92%) | | 8/8 (100%) | | 95 |
| 19/21 (91%) | 19/21 (91%) | 10/10 (100%) | 10/10 (100%) | 96 |
| 62/90 (69%) | 36/53 (68%) | 70/95 (74%) | 32/39 (82%) | |

found a significant positive correlation of the *MDR1* gene with the *MRP* gene in samples from treated patients (105).

## Clinical Relevance

None of the studies were able to correlation Pgp with response or survival. However, several studies tried to correlate Pgp expression with different parameters: Sonneveld et al. found a significant correlation between a high level of *MDR3*/mRNA and advanced CLL (Rai classification 3 and 4) (96). Michieli et al. observed a higher level of positive cells in patients treated with interferon-$\alpha$ (101). Ludescher et al. reported that patients treated with MDR-related drugs had a higher level of cells capable of drug efflux in the functional assay indicating Pgp induction (97).

## Conclusion

Because of present-day treatment strategies, MDR is not very important in CLL, and Pgp does not seem to influence clinical outcome, despite its frequent expression. The expression and role of MRP has to be further defined.

**Table 7** The Expression of Pgp in Previously Untreated and Treated Patients with Chronic Lymphocytic Leukemia

| Untreated number positive/total patients (%) | Treated number positive/total patients (%) | Ref. |
|---|---|---|
| 22/22 (100%) | 41/41 (100%) | 101 |
| | 0/2 (0%) | 63 |
| 11/11 (100%) | 9/9 (100%) | 102 |
| 4/8 (50%) | 4/9 (44%) | 95 |
| 0/1 (0%) | | 60 |
| 3/6 (50%) | 10/19 (53%) | 103 |
| 40/48 (83%) | 64/80 (80%) | Overall |

## NON-HODGKIN'S LYMPHOMA

### Frequency of Expression

Response rates and survival vary greatly, depending on histology and stage. Therefore, the studies are reviewed according to histology.

   If studies are paired according to histology, high-grade lymphoma may have a tendency toward higher Pgp expression. For untreated patients with low-grade lymphoma, the incidence of Pgp expression is 19% (n=36); in intermediate grade, 29% (n=21); and in high-grade lymphoma, 45% (n=102). The incidence of Pgp positivity in already treated patients was more or less comparable: low grade 36% (n=14), intermediate grade 30% (n=32), and high grade 42% (n=12). Pileri et al. found no difference in Pgp expression and histology (106). In contrast, Moscow et al. reported lymphomas with an indolent histology being more likely *MDR1*/mRNA positive than cases with aggressive histologies (109).

   Schlaifer et al. did detect Pgp-positive cells; however, they did not belong to the neoplastic population (108).

**Table 8**  The Presence of *MDR1*/mRNA and Pgp in Previously Untreated and Treated Patients with Non-Hodgkin's Lymphoma Grouped According to Histology

| Histology | Untreated number positive/total patients | Treated number positive/total patients | Ref. |
|---|---|---|---|
| Low grade | 9/16 | | 106 |
| | 0/3 | 0/1 | 107 |
| | 0/1 | 0/3 | 108 |
| | 3/7 | 3/4 | 109 |
| | 4/9 | 2/6 | 110 |
| | | 1/1 | 111 |
| | 0/16 | 0/2 | 112 |
| Overall (%) | 16/52 (31%) | 6/17 (35%) | |
| Intermediate grade | 0/3 | 4/11 | 107 |
| | 0/3 | 0/4 | 108 |
| | 1/3 | 1/6 | 109 |
| | 5/12 | 4/10 | 110 |
| | 1/2 | 0/1 | 111 |
| | 1/19 | 5/7 | 112 |
| | | 1/1 | 113 |
| Overall (%) | 8/42 (19%) | 15/40 (38%) | |
| High grade | 28/57 | | 114 |
| | 15/34 | | 106 |
| | 1/4 | 5/9 | 107 |
| | 0/2 | 0/2 | 108 |
| | 0/1 | 0/1 | 109 |
| | 2/4 | | 110 |
| | 0/3 | 1/3 | 111 |
| | 0/4 | | 112 |
| Overall (%) | 46/109 (42%) | 6/15 (40%) | |

## Clinical Relevance

Several studies did not detect any significant correlation between Pgp expression and response or survival rates (109,110,114). Gascoyne et al. found that only in B-cell lymphomas was Pgp presence negatively correlated with outcome (115). However, Pileri et al. and Cheng et al. reported a significant correlation with response (106,107). Cheng et al. also found survival after recurrence to be significantly better in Pgp-negative cases (107). Rodriguez et al. saw a high treatment failure rate when *MDR1*/mRNA was present together with glutathione-S-transferase π/mRNA (110). Patient numbers were too small to apply statistical analyses. Although small numbers were tested in vitro, doxorubicin resistance was correlated with Pgp expression (116). However, Pgp was not correlated with clinical drug resistance.

## Therapy with MDR-Reversing Agents

Three studies have investigated the effect of verapamil in refractory/relapsed NHL. Wilson treated 30 patients with verapamil and EPOCH (etoposide, doxorubicin, vincristine, cyclophosphamide, prednisone) (117). One patient achieved CR, five had partial response (PR), and 24 patients had no response. Four responders had intermediate levels of *MDR1*/mRNA, 11 nonresponders had low (n=9) or high (n=2) levels. Fourteen patients were treated with CVAD (cyclophosphamide, vincristine, doxorubicin, dexamethasone) and verapamil by Miller et al. (112). Four patients achieved CR, seven PR, and three had no response. Response was not correlated with histology. Eleven samples were analyzed for Pgp expression (including cases of Hodgkin's disease). Five of seven Pgp-positive patients responded to treatment and two of four Pgp-negative patients (difference not significant). Dalton et al. treated one Pgp-positive patient with verapamil in addition to VAD (113). This patient achieved a CR for 6 months. These studies reported cardiac toxicity, which was dose-related but reversible.

Miller et al. treated three patients with doxorubicin and trifluoperazine. Two patients had a partial response, and one patient did not respond. Pgp expression was not analyzed (92).

## Conclusion

In 20–30% of lymphoma patients, Pgp is expressed. Whether Pgp is correlated with histology needs further investigation. Large studies are necessary to determine the clinical relevance of Pgp. Results from first clinical trials are promising and warrant future studies.

## HODGKIN'S DISEASE

Hodgkin's disease responds very well to chemotherapy, and more than 70% of patients can be cured.

Few patients with Hodgkin's disease have undergone tissue sampling for Pgp analysis. At diagnosis, samples from 19 patients were analyzed and four were positive (61,107,108,111,112,118). Six of 23 patients tested Pgp-positive at relapse. These numbers are too small to evaluate clinical relevance.

Seven patients have been described in clinical MDR-reversing trials. Miller et al. (112) treated four patients with CVAD and verapamil. One patient achieved CR, one patient PR. Pgp was not mentioned specifically. Another patient was treated with lomustine, etoposide, prednimustine, and verapamil (119). Disappearance of pruritus was seen after the first course. This patient was positive for Pgp. A partial remission was achieved when a drug-refractory patient was treated with 4'-epidoxorubicin and verapamil (120). Yahanda et al. (121) described one patient treated with etoposide and cyclosporin A. This patient achieved a PR after 12 cycles. Pgp was present at relapse, and its level increased in the course of the disease.

In conclusion, for Hodgkin's disease insufficient data are available to evaluate the presence of Pgp. Larger studies, correlated with clinical outcome, are necessary to establish the role of Pgp.

## MULTIPLE MYELOMA

### Frequency of Expression

Chemotherapy is able to postpone multiple myeloma (MM) related deaths; however, truly curative treatment is not available.

Only one study has looked at $MDR1$/mRNA (122) in MM. The investigators found $MDR1$/mRNA expression in all patients. However, cutoff values for positivity were not defined.

Table 9 gives an overview of Pgp positivity in multiple myeloma. Overall positivity in untreated patients is 22% (74/336). Only four studies have evaluated more than 10 untreated patients; in these series, Pgp positivity ranged from 6% to 31%. The percentage of positive cases among treated patients is higher: overall 47% (85/182). The three largest studies (127–129) agree remarkably on the number of positive patients: 41%, 43%, and 45%.

**Table 9**  The Expression of Pgp in Previously Untreated and Treated Patients with Multiple Myeloma

| Untreated number positive/total patients (%) | Treated number positive/total patients (%) | Ref. |
|---|---|---|
| 0/5   (0%) | 1/5   (20%) | 75 |
|  | 5/7   (71%) | 113 |
|  | 12/15  (80%) | 123 |
| 33/105 (31%) |  | 124 |
|  | 5/10  (50%) | 125 |
| 3/47   (6%) | 21/49  (43%) | 126 |
|  | 26/63  (41%) | 127 |
| 9/29  (31%) | 15/33  (45%) | 128 |
| 29/150 (19%) |  | 129 |
| 74/336 (22%) | 85/182 (47%) | Overall |

## Clinical Relevance

Several studies have dealt with the issue of Pgp expression in multiple myeloma (Table 10). Resistance to therapy was correlated with a higher level of *MDR1*/mRNA (122) and a higher number of cells positive for Pgp (130). Interestingly, Grogan et al. (126) found a correlation between the presence of Pgp and total dose of doxorubicin and/or vincristine previously administered. This could imply the agents used induce Pgp. Raaij-makers et al. confirm this observation (128). They report that Pgp positivity found at remission has disappeared at relapse in six of seven cases, suggesting either drug-mediated Pgp induction or suppression of Pgp-positive cells. In contrast to these studies, Cornelissen et al. and Musto et al. detected no relation between Pgp and clinical response (127,129). Several authors could not detect any relation with survival (122,126, 127). However, Musto et al. found Pgp to be an independent prognostic factor in a multivariate analysis (129).

MDR-related drugs (such as vincristine, daunorubicin, doxorubicin) have been shown to induce Pgp expression (131). Therefore, the applied drugs may be the cause of higher Pgp levels in treated myeloma patients.

## Therapy with MDR-Reversing Agents

### In Vitro/Ex Vivo

Interesting work has been done with the human myeloma cell line 8226. Synergistic effects of verapamil and quinine were observed (132). Kulkarni et al. was able to selectively kill resistant cells by treating them with the MRK16 monoclonal antibody in combination with rabbit complement (133). This may become a useful technique for bone marrow purging.

### Clinical Trials

Seven studies included 83 MM patients in clinical MDR-reversing trials (Table 10). Only two patients achieved CR, and 35 patients achieved PR.

Several patients were evaluated for expression of Pgp. In the investigation by Salmon et al. (134), four of 10 Pgp-positive patients achieved PR; none of three Pgp-negative patients had a response. Eleven of 14 evaluable patients were Pgp positive in

**Table 10** Overview of Patients with Multiple Myeloma in Clinical Trials with Pgp-Reversing Agents

| Chemotherapy | MDR-reverser | Total patients | Response | Ref. |
|---|---|---|---|---|
| VAD | Verapamil | 22 | 5 PR, 17 NR | 134 |
| VAD | Verapamil | 9 | 1 PR, 8 NR | 135 |
| VAD | Verapamil | 1 | 1 PR | 136 |
| VAMP | Verapamil | 7 | 1 CR, 3 PR, 3 NR | 137 |
| VAD | CsA | 20 | 1 CR, 9 PR, 10 NR | 123 |
| VAD | SCD PSC833 | 23 | 10 PR, 10 NR, 3 D | 138 |
| Doxorubicin | Trifluoperazine | 1 | 1 NR | 92 |

VAD = vincristine/doxorubicin/dexamethasone, CR = complete remission, PR = partial remission, NR = no response, D = death.

the study by Sonneveld et al. (123). Patients were treated with VAD (vincristine, doxorubicin, and dexamethasone) in combination with cyclosporin A. A response was seen in six of 11 Pgp-positive patients and in none of three Pgp-negative patients. Sonneveld et al. could no longer detect Pgp in six of eight patients after treatment. The response rate of patients refractory to melphalan did not differ from that of VAD-refractory patients (138).

Reversible cardiac toxicity was observed when verapamil was used; one patient had to discontinue further treatment (135). Besides a transient hyperbilirubinemia when cyclosporin A was used, mostly mild, reversible side effects were seen (123). Seven patients, however, experienced musculoskeletal pain, which was dose dependent. Three toxic deaths occurred with PSC833. And in 10 patients, the dose of vincristine and doxorubicin had to be reduced by 75% (138).

## Conclusion

The level of Pgp positivity is about 40% in previously treated patients and seems to be lower in untreated patients. Treatment may induce Pgp expression. MDR-reversing agents may be important but are not the only answer for drug-refractory MM patients.

## GENERAL CONCLUSIONS

The frequencies of multidrug resistance and Pgp expression and the role they play in the clinical setting still remain unclear for most hematological malignancies. This may be the result of the different laboratory techniques used to assess MDR/mRNA and Pgp presence and also the small numbers of patients analyzed in each study. Importantly, there may also be a publication bias; those studies that found negative results are less likely to be published.

In the future, however, MDR/Pgp expression may prove to be a prognostic factor in some diseases. But whether this implies that additional treatment with MDR-reversing drugs improves the prognosis still has to be assessed. Early clinical results indicate MDR reversers have some impact, but still many cases appear to be refractory—suggesting the importance of different mechanisms for resistance.

## REFERENCES

1. Robson CN, Alexander J, Harris AL, Hichson ID. Isolation and characterization of a Chinese hamster ovary cell line resistant to bifunctional nitrogen mustards. Cancer Res 1986; 46:6290–6294.
2. Dulik D, Fenselau C, Hilton J. Characterization of melphalan-glutathione adducts whose formation is catalyzed by glutathione transferases. Biochem Pharmacol 1986; 35:3405–3409.
3. Alton PA, Harris AL. The role of DNA topoisomerases II in drug resistance. Br J Haematol 1993; 85:241–245.
4. Cole SPC, Bhardwaj G, Gerlach JH, et al. Overexpression of a transporter gene in a multidrug-resistant human lung cancer cell line. Science 1992; 258:1650–1654.
5. Grant CE, Valdimarsson G, Hipfner DR, Almquist KC, Cole SPC, Deeley R. Overexpression of multidrug resistance-associated protein (MRP) increases resistance to natural product drugs. Cancer Res 1994; 54:357–361.

6. Brophy NA, Marie JP, Rojas VA, et al. Mdr1 gene expression in childhood acute lympho-blastic leukemias and lymphomas: a critical evaluation by four techniques. Leukemia 1994; 8:327–335.

7. Herzog CE, Trepel JB, Mickley JA, Bates SE, Fojo AT. Various methods of analysis of mdr-1/P-glycoprotein in human colon cancer cell lines. J Natl Cancer Inst 1992; 84:711–716.

8. Gala JL, McLachlan JM, Bell DR, Michaux JL, Ma DDF. Specificity and sensitivity of im-munocytohistochemistry for detecting P-glycoprotein in haematological malignancies. J Clin Pathol 1994; 47:619–624.

9. Holmes J, Jacobs A, Carter G, Janowska-Wieczorek A, Padua RA. Multidrug resistance in haemopoietic cell lines, myelodysplastic syndromes and acute myeloblastic leukemia. Br J Haematol 1989; 72:40–44.

10. Ito Y, Tanimoto M, Kumazawa T, et al. Increased P-glycoprotein expression and multidrug-resistant gene (mdr1) amplification are frequently found in fresh acute leukemia cells. Can-cer 1989; 63:1534–1538.

11. Sato H, Preisler H, Day R, et al. MDR1 transcript levels as an indication of resistant disease in acute myelogenous leukemia. Br J Haematol 1990; 75:340–345.

12. Zhou DC, Marie JP, Suberville AM, Zittoun R. Relevance of mdr1 gene expression in acute myeloid leukemia and comparison of different diagnostic methods. Leukemia 1992; 6:879–885.

13. Gruber A, Vitols S, Norgren S, et al. Quantitative determination of mdr1 gene expression in leukaemic cells from patients with acute leukemia. Br J Cancer 1992; 66:266–272.

14. Miwa H, Kita K, Nishii K, et al. Expression of MDR1 gene in acute leukemia cells: associa-tion with CD7+ acute myeloblastic leukemia/acute lymphoblastic leukemia. Blood 1993; 82:3445–3451.

15. Pirker R, Wallner J, Geissler K, et al. MDR1 gene expression and treatment outcome in acute myeloid leukemia. J Natl Cancer Inst 1991; 83:708–712.

16. Zhou DC, Zittoun R, Marie JP. Expression of multidrug resistance-associated protein (MRP) gene in acute myeloid leukemia and correlation with expression of multidrug resis-tance (mdr1) gene (abstr). Leukemia 1995; 9:535.

17. Ino T, Miyazaki H, Isogai M, et al. Expression of P-glycoprotein in de novo acute myelo-genous leukemia at initial diagnosis: results of molecular and functional assays, and corre-lation with treatment outcome. Leukemia 1994; 8:1492–1497.

18. Lamy T, Goesguen JE, Mordelet E, et al. P-glycoprotein (P-170) and CD34 expression in adult acute myeloid leukemia (AML). Leukemia 1994; 8:1879–1883.

19. Zöchbauer S, Gsur A, Brunner R, Kyrle PA, Lechner K, Pirker R. P-glycoprotein expression as unfavourable prognostic factor in acute myeloid leukemia. Leukemia 1994; 8:974–977.

20. Te Boekhorst PW, Leeuw K, Schoester M, et al. Predominance of functional multidrug resistance (MDR-1) phenotype in CD34+ acute myeloid leukemia cells. Blood 1993; 82:3157–3162.

21. Campos L, Guyotat D, Archimbaud E, et al. Clinical significance of multidrug resistance P-glycoprotein expression on acute nonlymphoblastic leukemia cells at diagnosis. Blood 1992; 79:473–476.

22. Chitnis M, Hegde U, Chavan S, Juvekar A, Advani S. Expression of the multidrug trans-porter P-glycoprotein and in vitro chemosensitivity: correlation with in vivo response to chemotherapy in acute myeloid leukemia. Sel Cancer Ther 1991; 7:165–173.

23. Musto P, Matera R, Carotenutto M. Multidrug resistance (mdr) in phenotype in acute leu-kemia: prognostic aspects and relationship to proliferative activity (abstr). Leukemia 1995; 9:547.

24. Wood P, Burgess R, MacGregor A, Liu Yin JA. P-glycoprotein expression on acute myeloid leukaemia blast cells at diagnosis predicts response to chemotherapy and survival. Br J Haematol 1994; 87:509–514.

25. Stasi R, Poeta G, Venditti A, et al. Analysis of treatment failure in patients with minimally differentiated acute myeloid leukemia (AML-M0). Blood 1994; 83:1619–1625.

26. Paietta E, Andersen J, Racevskis J, et al. Significantly lower P-glycoprotein expression in acute promyelocytic leukemia than in other types of acute myeloid leukemia: immunological, molecular and functional analyses. Leukemia 1994; 8:968–973.

27. Schneider E, Cowan K, Bader H, et al. Increased expression of the multidrug resistance-associated protein gene in relapsed acute leukemia. Blood 1995; 85:186–193.

28. Hart SM, Ganeshaguru K, Hoffbrand AV, Prentice HG, Mehta AB. Expression of the multidrug resistance-associated protein (MRP) in acute leukemia. Leukemia 1994; 8:2163–2168.

29. Lepelley P, Soenen V, Preudhomme C, Lai JL, Cosson A, Fenaux P. Expression of multidrug resistance P-glycoprotein and its relationship to haematological characteristics and response in treatment in myelodysplastic syndromes. Leukemia 1994; 8:998–1004.

30. List AF, Spier CM, Cline A, et al. Expression of the multidrug resistance gene product (P-glycoprotein) in myelodysplasia is associated with a stem cell phenotype. Br J Haematol 1991; 78:28–34.

31. Holmes JA, West RR. The effect of MDR-1 gene expression on outcome in acute myeloblastic leukaemia. Br J Cancer 1994; 69:382–384.

32. Tiirikainen MI, Syrjälä MT, Jansson SE, Krusius T. Flow cytometric analysis of P-glycoprotein in normal and leukemic cells. Ann Hematol 1992; 65:124–130.

33. Leith PC, Kopecky KJ, Chen IM, et al. Multidrug resistance (mdr1) expression and function in acute myeloid leukemia (AML) in the elderly: mdr1 and secondary AML status are dependent predictors of complete remission (CR) (abstr). Leukemia 1995; 9:535.

34. Tsuruo T, Iida H, Nojiri M, Tsukagoshi S, Sakurai Y. Circumvention of vincristine and doxorubicin resistance in vitro and in vivo by calcium influx blockers. Cancer Res 1983; 43: 2905–2910.

35. Tsuruo T, Iida H, Kitatani Y, Yokota K, Tsukagoshi S, Sakurai Y. Effects of quinidine and related compounds on cytotoxicity and cellular accumulation of vincristine and doxorubicin in drug-resistant tumor cells. Cancer Res 1984; 44:4303–4307.

36. Ross DD, Wooten PJ, Tong Y, et al. Synergistic reversal of multidrug-resistance phenotype in acute myeloid leukemia cells by cyclosporin A and Cremophor EL. Blood 1994; 83:1337–1347.

37. Berman E, Adams M, Duigou-Osterndorf R, Godfrey L, Clarkson B, Andreeff M. Effect of tamoxifen on cell lines displaying the multidrug-resistant phenotype. Blood 1991; 77:818–825.

38. Berman E, McBride M, Tong W. Comparative activity of tamoxifen and N-desmethyltamoxifen in human multidrug resistant leukemia cell lines. Leukemia 1994; 8:1191–1196.

39. Jiang XR, Macey MG, Collins PW, Newland AC. Characterization and modulation of drug transport kinetics in K562 cl.6 daunorubicin-resistant cell line. Br J Haematol 1994; 86:547–554.

40. Lecureur V, Fardel O, Guillouzo A. The antiprogestatin drug RU 486 potentiates doxorubicin cytotoxicity in multidrug resistant cells through inhibition of P-glycoprotein function. FEBS Lett 1994; 355:187–191.

41. Sato W, Fukazawa N, Nakanishi O. Reversal of multidrug resistance by a novel quinoline derivative, MS-209. Cancer Chemother Pharmacol 1995; 35:271–277.

42. Ishida Y, Shimada Y, Shimoyama M. Synergistic effect of cyclosporin A and verapamil in overcoming vincristine resistance of multidrug-resistant cultured human leukemia cells. Jpn J Cancer Res 1990; 81:834–841.

43. Muller C, Bailly JD, Goubin F, et al. Verapamil decreases P-glycoprotein expression in multidrug-resistant human leukemic cells. Int J Cancer 1994; 56:749–754.

44. Muller C, Goubin F, Ferrandis E, et al. Evidence for transcriptional control of human mdr1 gene expression by verapamil in multidrug-resistant leukemic cells. Mol Pharmacol 1995; 47:51–56.

45. Elgie A, Sargent J, Taylor C. In vitro study of PKC modulators in acute myeloid leukemia (abstr). Leukemia 1995; 9:538.
46. Mechetner EB, Roninson IB. Efficient inhibition of P-glycoprotein-mediated multidrug resistance with a monoclonal antibody. Proc Natl Acad Sci USA 1992; 89:5824–5828.
47. Marie JP, Faussat-Suberville AM, Zhou D, Zittoun R. Daunorubicin uptake by leukemic cells: correlations with treatment outcome and mdr1 expression. Leukemia 1993; 7:825–831.
48. Nooter K, Sonneveld P, Oostrum R, Herweijer H, Hagenbeek T, Valerio D. Overexpression of the mdr1 gene in blast cells from patients with acute myelocytic leukemia is associated with decreased anthracycline accumulation that can be restored by cyclosporin-A. Int J Cancer 1990; 45:263–268.
49. Pirker R, Zöchbauer S, Kupper H, et al. Dexverapamil as resistance modifier in acute myeloid leukemia (abstr). Leukemia 1995; 9:539.
50. Sonneveld P, Nooter K. Reversal of drug-resistance by cyclosporin-A in a patient with acute myelocytic leukaemia. Br J Haematol 1990; 75:208–211.
51. List AF, Spier C, Greer J, et al. Phase I/II trial of cyclosporine as a chemotherapy-resistance modifier in acute leukemia. J Clin Oncol 1993; 11:1652–1660.
52. Solary E, Caillot D, Chauffert B, Dumas M, Casanovas RO, Guy H. Phase I/II study of quinine associated with mitoxantrone and aracytine in refractory and relapsed acute leukemias (abstr). Proc Am Assoc Cancer Res 1992; 33:236.
53. Cairo MS, Siegel S, Anas N, Sender L. Clinical trial of continuous infusion of verapamil, bolus vinblastine, and continuous infusion VP-16 in drug-resistant pediatric tumors. Cancer Res 1989; 49:11063–11066.
54. Marie JP, Bastie JN, Coloma F, et al. Cyclosporin A as a modifier agent in the salvage treatment of acute leukemia (AL). Leukemia 1993; 7:824–824.
55. Sonneveld P, Dongen Van J, Hagemeijer A, et al. High expression of multidrug resistance P-glycoprotein in high risk myelodysplasia is associated with immature phenotype. Leukemia 1993; 7:963–969.
56. Nüssler V, Pelka-Fleischer R, Zwierzina H, et al. Clinical importance of P-glycoprotein-related resistance in leukemia and myelodysplastic syndromes—first experience with their reversal. Ann Hematol 1994; 69:S25–S29.
57. Goldstein LJ, Galski H, Fojo A, et al. Expression of a multidrug resistance gene in human cancers. Cancer Inst 1989; 81:116–124.
58. Sato H, Gottesman MM, Goldstein LJ, et al. Expression of the multidrug resistance gene in myeloid leukemias. Leukemia Res 1990; 14:11–22.
59. Gekeler V, Beck J, Noller A, et al. Drug-induced changes in the expression of MDR-associated genes: investigations on cultured cell lines and chemotherapeutically treated leukemias. Ann Hematol 1994; 69:S19–S24.
60. Sugawara I, Kodo H, Ohkochi E, Hamada H, Tsuruo T, Mori S. High-level expression of MRK 16 and MRK 20 murine monoclonal antibody-defined proteins (170,000-180,000 P-glycoprotein and 85,000 protein) in leukaemias and malignant lymphomas. Br J Cancer 1989; 60:538–541.
61. Umeda Y, Tsuruo T, Mori S, Arimori S, Sugawara I. High-level expression of P-glycoprotein and 85 kD protein as assessed by flow cytometry and immunohistochemistry in leukemias and malignant lymphomas. Tokai J Exp Clin Med 1990; 15:179–187.
62. Weide R, Dowding C, Paulsen W, Goldman J. The role of the MDR-1/P-170 mechanism in the development of multidrug resistance in chronic myeloid leukemia. Leukemia 1990; 4:695–699.
63. Mattern J, Efferth T, Bak M, Ho AD, Volm M. Detection of P-glycoprotein in human leukemias using monoclonal antibodies. Blut 1989; 58:215–217.
64. Kuwazura Y, Yoshimura A, Hanada S, et al. Expression of the multidrug transporter, P-glycoprotein, in chronic myelogenous leukaemia cells in blast crisis. Br J Haematol 1990; 74:24–29.

65. Michelutti A, Michieli M, Damiani D, et al. Overexpression of mdr-related p170 glycopro-
    tein expression in chronic myeloid leukemia. Haematologica 1994; 79:200–204.
66. Joncourt F, Oberli A, Redmond SMS, et al. Cytostatic drug resistance: parallel assessment
    of glutathione-based detoxifying enzymes, O6-alkylguanine-DNA-alkyltransferase and P-
    glycoprotein in adult patients with leukaemia. Br J Haematol 1993; 85:103–111.
67. Tsuruo T, Sugimoto Y, Hamada H, et al. Detection of multidrug resistance markers,
    p-glycoprotein and mdr1 mRNA in human leukemia cells. Jpn J Cancer Res 1987; 78:
    1415–1419.
68. Carulli G, Petrini M, Marini A, Vaglini F, Cracciolo F, Grassi B. P-glycoprotein and drug
    resistance in acute leukemias and in the blastic crisis of chronic myeloid leukemia. Haema-
    tologica 1990; 75:516–521.
69. Rothenberg ML, Mickley LA, Cole DE, et al. Expression of the mdr-1/P-170 gene in patients
    with acute lymphoblastic leukemia. Blood 1989; 74:1388–1395.
70. Marie JP, Zittoun R, Sikic BI. Multidrug resistance (mdr1) gene expression in adult acute
    leukemias: correlations with treatment outcome and in vitro drug sensitivity. Blood 1991;
    78:586–592.
71. Herweijer H, Sonneveld P, Baas F, Nooter K. Expression of mdr1 and mdr3 multidrug-re-
    sistance genes in human acute and chronic leukemias and association with stimulation of
    drug accumulation by cyclosporine. J Natl Cancer Inst 1990; 82:1133–1140.
72. Fojo AT, Ueda K, Salmon DJ, Poplack DG, Gottesman MM, Pastan I. Expression of a
    multidrug-resistance gene in human tumors and tissues. Proc Natl Acad Sci USA 1987;
    84:265–269.
73. Haddad G, Thorner PS, Bradley G, Dalton WS, Ling V, Chan HSC. A sensitive multilayer
    immunoalkaline phosphatase method for detection of P-glycoprotein in leukemic and tumor
    cells in the bone marrow. Lab Invest 1994; 71:595–603.
74. Redner A, Hegewisch S, Haimi J, Steinherz P, Jhanwar S, Andreeff M. A study of multidrug
    resistance and cell kinetics in a child with near-haploid acute lymphoblastic leukemia. Leu-
    kemia Res 1990; 14:771–777.
75. Musto P, Cascavilla N, Di Renzo N, et al. Clinical relevance of immunocytochemical detec-
    tion of multidrug-resistance-associated P-glycoprotein in haematological malignancies. Tu-
    mori 1990; 76:353–359.
76. Kawazuru Y, Yoshimura A, Hanada S, et al. Expression of the multidrug transporter, P-gly-
    coprotein, in acute leukemia cells and correlation to clinical drug resistance. Cancer 1990;
    66:868–873.
77. Sauerbrey A, Zintl F, Volm M. P-glycoprotein and glutathione S-transferase π in childhood
    acute lymphoblastic leukemia. Br J Cancer 1994; 70:1144–1149.
78. Goasguen JE, Dossot JM, Fradel O, et al. Expression of the multidrug resistance-associated
    P-glycoprotein (P-170) in 59 cases of de novo acute lymphoblastic leukemia: prognostic
    implications. Blood 1993; 81:2394–2398.
79. Fennetau O, Marie JP, Lescoeur B, Vilmer E, Schlegel N. Expression of the multidrug
    resistance associated P-glycoprotein (P-170) in acute lymphoblastic leukemia. Blood 1993;
    82:3787–3788.
80. Pieters R, Hongo T, Loonen AH, et al. Different types of non-P-glycoprotein mediated
    multiple drug resistance in children with relapsed acute lymphoblastic leukaemia. Br J Can-
    cer 1992; 65:691–697.
81. Gekeler V, Frese G, Noller A, et al. MDR1/P-glycoprotein, topoisomerase, and glutathione-
    s-transferase π gene expression in primary and relapsed state adult and childhood leukae-
    mias. Br J Cancer 1992; 66:507–517.
82. Hill BT, Hosking LK. Differential effectiveness of a range of novel drug-resistance modu-
    lators, relative to verapamil, in influencing vinblastine or teniposide cytotoxicity in human
    lymphoblastoid CCRF-CEM sublines expressing classic or atypical multidrug resistance.
    Cancer Chemother Pharmacol 1994; 33:317–324.

83. Tsuruo T, Iida-Saito H, Kawabata H, Oh-Hara T, Hmada H, Utakoji T. Characteristics of resistance to doxorubicin in human myelogenous leukemia K562 resistant to doxorubicin and in isolated clones. Jpn J Cancer Res 1986; 77:682–692.

84. Beck TW, Cirtain MC, Glover CJ, Felsted RL, Safa AR. Effects of indole alkaloids on multidrug resistance and labelling of P-glycoprotein by a photoaffinity analog of vinblastine. Biochem Biophys Res Commun 1988; 153:959–966.

85. Michieli M, Damiani D, Michelutti A, et al. p170-dependent multidrug resistance. Restoring full sensitivity to idarubicin with verapamil and cyclosporin A derivatives. Haematologica 1994; 79:119–126.

86. Zamora JM, Pearce HL, Beck WT. Physical-chemical properties shared by compounds that modulate multidrug resistance in human leukemia cells. Mol Pharmacol 1987; 33:454–462.

87. Pearce HL, Safa AR, Bach NJ, Winter MA, Cirtains MC, Beck WT. Essential features of the P-glycoprotein pharmacophore as defined by a series of reserpine analogs that modulate multidrug resistance. Proc Natl Acad Sci USA 1989; 86:5128–5132.

88. Hu XF, Martin TJ, Bell DR, Luise M, Zalcberg JR. Combined use of cyclosporin A and verapamil in modulating multidrug resistance in human leukemia cell lines. Cancer Res 1990; 50:2953–2957.

89. Lemoli RM, Igarashi T, Knizewski M, et al. Dye-mediated photolysis is capable of eliminating drug-resistant (MDR+) tumor cells. Blood 1993; 81:793–800.

90. Bessho F, Kinumaki H, Kobayashi M, et al. Treatment of children with refractory acute lymphocytic leukemia with vincristine and diltiazem. Med Pediatr Oncol 1985; 13:199–202.

91. Solary E, Caillot D, Chauffert B, et al. Feasibility of using quinine, a potential multidrug resistance-reversing agent, in combination with mitoxantrone and cytarabine for the treatment of acute leukemia. J Clin Oncol 1992; 10:1730–1736.

92. Miller RL, Bukowski RM, Budd GT, et al. Clinical modulation of doxorubicin resistance by the calmodulin-inhibitor, trifluoperazine: a phase I/II trial. J Clin Oncol 1988; 6:880–888.

93. Rochlitz CF, De Kant E, Neubauer A, et al. PCR-determinated expression of the MDR1 gene in chronic lymphocytic leukemia. Ann Hematol 1992; 65:241–246.

94. Holmes JA, Jacobs A, Carter G, Whittaker JA, Bentley DP, Padua RA. Is the mdr1 gene relevant in chronic lymphocytic leukemia? Leukemia 1990; 4:216–218.

95. Perri RT, Louie SW, Espar WG. Expression of the multidrug resistance (mdr) gene mdr1 in chronic lymphocytic leukemia (CLL) B cells (abstr). Blood 1989; 74(suppl 1):198a.

96. Sonneveld P, Nooter K, Burghouts JThM, Herweijer H, Adriaansen HJ, Van Dongen JJM. High expression of the mdr3 multidrug-resistance gene in advanced-stage chronic lymphocytic leukemia. Blood 1992; 79:1496–1500.

97. Ludescher C, Hilbe W, Eistererr W, et al. Activity of p-glycoprotein in B-cell chronic lymphocytic leukemia determined by a flow cytometric assay. J Natl Cancer Inst 1993; 85:1751–1758.

98. Shustik C, Groulx N, Gros P. Analysis of multidrug resistance (MDR-1) gene expression in chronic lymphocytic leukaemia (CLL). Br J Haematol 1991; 79:50–56.

99. El Rouby S, Thomas A, Costin D, et al. p53 Gene mutation in B-cell chronic lymphocytic leukemia is associated with drug resistance and is independent of MDR1/MDR3 gene expression. Blood 1993; 82:3452–3459.

100. Hart SM, Ganeshaguru, Robinson L, Hoffbrand AV, Mehta AB. Expression of the multidrug resistance (mdr1) and multidrug resistance-associated protein (MRP) genes in chronic lymphocytic leukaemia (CLL) (abstr). Leukemia 1995; 9:535.

101. Michieli M, Raspadori D, Damiani D, et al. The expression of the multidrug resistance-associated glycoprotein in B-cell chronic lymphocytic leukemia. Br J Haematol 1991; 77:460–465.

102. Sparrow RL, Hall FJ, Siregar H, Van der Weyden MB. Common expression of the multidrug resistance marker P-glycoprotein in B-cell chronic lymphocytic leukemia and correlation with in vitro drug resistance. Leuk Res 1993; 17:941–947.

103. Cumber PM, Jacobs A, Hoy T, et al. Expression of the multiple drug resistance gene (mdr-1) and epitope masking in chronic lymphatic leukaemia. Br J Haematol 1990; 76:226–230.
104. Burger H, Nooter K, Zaman GJR, et al. Expression of the multidrug resistance-associated protein (MRP) in acute and chronic leukemias. Leukemia 1994; 8:990–997.
105. Beck J, Niethammer D, Gekeler V. High mdr1- and mrp-, but low topoisomerase II alpha-gene expression in B-cell chronic lymphocytic leukaemias. Cancer Lett 1994; 86:135–142.
106. Pileri SA, Sabattini E, Falini B, et al. Immunohistochemical detection of the multidrug transport protein P170 in human normal tissues and malignant lymphomas. Histopathology 1991; 19:131–140.
107. Cheng AL, Su IJ, Chen YC, Lee TC, Wang CH. Expression of P-glycoprotein and glutathione-S-transferase in recurrent lymphomas: the possible role of Epstein-Barr virus, immunophenotypes, and other predisposing factors. J Clin Oncol 1993; 11:109–115.
108. Schlaifer D, Laurent G, Chittal S, et al. Immunohistochemical detection of multidrug resistance associated P-glycoprotein in tumour and stromal cells of human cancers. Br J Cancer 1990; 62:177–182.
109. Moscow JA, Fairchild CR, Madden MJ, et al. Expression of anionic glutathione-S-transferase and P-glycoprotein genes in human tissues and tumors. Cancer Res 1989; 49:1422–1428.
110. Rodriguez C, Commes T, Robert J, Rossi JF. Expression of P-glycoprotein and anionic glutathione S-transferase genes in non-Hodgkin's lymphoma. Leuk Res 1993; 17:149–156.
111. Dan S, Esumi M, Sawada U, et al. Expression of a multidrug-resistance gene in human malignant lymphoma and related disorders. Leuk Res 1991; 15:1139–1143.
112. Miller TP, Grogan TM, Dalton WS, Spier CM, Scheper RJ, Salmon SE. P-glycoprotein expression in malignant lymphoma and reversal of clinical drug resistance with chemotherapy plus high-dose verapamil. J Clin Oncol 1991; 9:17–24.
113. Dalton WS, Grogan TM, Meltzer PS, et al. Drug-resistance in multiple myeloma and non-Hodgkin's lymphoma; detection of P-glycoprotein and potential circumvention by addition of verapamil to chemotherapy. J Clin Oncol 1989; 7:415–424.
114. Niehans G, Jaszcz W, Brunetto V, et al. Immunohistochemical identification of P-glycoprotein in previously untreated, diffuse large cell and immunoblastic lymphomas. Cancer Res 1992; 52:3768–3775.
115. Gascoyne R, Hoskins P, Connors J, Coldman A, Klasa R, O'Reilly S. A study of clinical and pathological variables affecting disease specific survival (DSS) of patients with diffuse large cell lymphoma treated with MACOP-B or VACOP-B: univariate and multivariate analyses (abstr). Proc ASCO 1994; 13:374.
116. Salmon SE, Grogan TM, Miller T, Scheper R, Dalton WS. Prediction of doxorubicin resistance in vitro in myeloma, lymphoma, and breast cancer by P-glycoprotein staining. J Natl Cancer Inst 1989; 81:696–701.
117. Wilson WH, Bates S, Kang YK, et al. Reversal of multidrug resistance (mdr-1) with R-verapamil and analysis of mdr-1 expression in patients with lymphoma refractory to EP-OCH chemotherapy (abstr). Proc Am Assoc Cancer Res 1993; 34:212.
118. Pasman PC, Erdkamp FLG, Vrints L, Breed WP, Arends JW, Schouten HC. P-glycoprotein expression in Hodgkin's disease. Fifth International Conference on Malignant Lymphoma. Lugano, Switzerland, June 9–12, 1993.
119. Gisslinger H, Pirker R, Wallner J, Watzke H, Ludwig H. Effect of combination therapy with verapamil. Lancet 1990; 336:1078.
120. Demichelli R, Jirillo A, Bonciarelli G, Lonardi F, Balli M, Bandello A. 4*epidoxorubicin plus verapamil in anthracycline-refractory cancer patients. Tumori 1989; 75:245–247.
121. Yahanda AM, Adler KM, Fisher GA, et al. Phase I trial of etoposide with cyclosporine as a modulator of multidrug resistance. J Clin Oncol 1992; 10:1624–1634.
122. Linsenmeyer ME, Jefferson S, Wolf M, Matthews JP, Board PG, Woodcock DM. Levels of expression of the mdr1 gene and glutathione S-transferase genes 2 and 3 and response to chemotherapy in multiple myeloma. Br J Cancer 1992; 65:471–475.

123. Sonneveld P, Durie BG, Lokhorst HM, et al. Modulation of multidrug-resistant multiple myeloma by cyclosporin. Lancet 1992; 340:255–259.

124. Sonneveld P, Durie BGM, Lokhorst HM, Frutiger Y, Schoester M, Vela EE. Analysis of multidrug-resistance (MDR-1) glycoprotein and CD56 expression to separate monoclonal gammopathy from multiple myeloma. Br J Haematol 1993; 83:63–67.

125. Carulli G, Petrini M, Marini A, et al. P-glycoprotein expression in multiple myeloma. Haematologica 1990; 75:288–290.

126. Grogan TM, Spier CM, Salmon SE, et al. P-glycoprotein expression in human plasma cell myeloma: correlation with prior chemotherapy. Blood 1993; 81:490–495.

127. Cornelissen JJ, Sonneveld P, Schoester M, et al. MDR-1 expression and response to vincristine, doxorubicin, and dexamethasone chemotherapy in multiple myeloma refractory to alkylating agents. J Clin Oncol 1994; 12:115–119.

128. Raaijmakers HGP, Izquierdo MA, Beliën J, Scheper RJ, Lokhorst HM. Induction of ndr1 expression after successful alkylating chemotherapy in multiple myeloma (abstr). Leukemia 1995; 9:547.

129. Musto P, Matera R, Carotenutto M. Multidrug resistance (mdr) in phenotype in multiple myeloma: prognostic aspects and relationship to proliferative activity (abstr). Leukemia 1995; 9:547.

130. Epstein J, Xiao H, Oba BK. P-glycoprotein expression in plasma-cell myeloma is associated with resistance to VAD. Blood 1989; 74:913–917.

131. Kohno K, Sato S, Takano H, Matsuo K, Kuwano M. The direct activation of human multidrug resistance gene (MDR1) by anticancer agents. Biochem Biophys Res Commun 1989; 165:1415–1421.

132. Lehnert M, Dalton WS, Roe D, Emerson S, Salmon SE. Synergistic inhibition by verapamil and quinine of P-glycoprotein-mediated multidrug resistance in a human myeloma cell line. Blood 1991; 77:348–354.

133. Kulkarni SS, Wang Z, Spitzer G, et al. Elimination of drug-resistant myeloma tumor cell lines by monoclonal anti-P-glycoprotein antibody and rabbit complement. Blood 1989; 74:2244–2251.

134. Salmon SE, Dalton WS, Grogan TM, et al. Multidrug-resistant myeloma: laboratory and clinical effects of verapamil as a chemosensitizer. Blood 1991; 78:44–50.

135. Trümper LH, Ho AD, Wulf G, Hunstein W. Addition of verapamil to overcome drug resistance in multiple myeloma: preliminary clinical observations in 10 patients. J Clin Oncol 1989; 7:1578.

136. Durie BNGM, Dalton WS. Reversal of drug-resistance in multiple myeloma with verapamil. Br J Haematol 1988; 68:203–206.

137. Gore ME, Selby PJ, Millar B, et al. The use of verapamil to overcome drug resistance in myeloma. Proc ASCO 1988; 7:882.

138. Sonneveld P, Marie JP, Schoester M, Groenewegen A. Phase 1 study of SDZ PSC833 combined with VAD in patients with refractory multiple myeloma (abstr). Leukemia 1995; 9:539.

# 11

## Prediction of Cytotoxic Drug Resistance in Acute Leukemia

**Rolf Larsson**
*Uppsala University Hospital, Uppsala, Sweden*

### INTRODUCTION

#### Acute Leukemia

Acute leukemia (AL) is a clonal disorder characterized by aberrant hematopoietic cellular proliferation and maturation. Acute leukemia is generally divided into two subgroups, acute myelocytic leukemia (AML) and acute lymphoblastic leukemia (ALL). Acute leukemia presents itself either as a de novo disease or secondary as a result of exposure to marrow toxins (1,2) or following myeloproliferative disorders (3). Untreated AL is rapidly fatal, with a median survival of less than 2 months (4).

From the mid-1960s, AL has been treated with induction therapy using combinations of cytotoxic drugs. Chemotherapy is generally divided into two phases, remission induction therapy and consolidation or maintenance therapy. Today, complete remissions are obtained in most patients under the age of 60 (5). Despite increasing remission rates, however, only a small fraction—approximately 15% of patients with AML—will experience continued complete remission (6). The prognosis for adults with ALL is better than that of AML, but still only 35–45% of patients will become long-term survivors. For childhood ALL, the prognosis is excellent, with a cure rate above 80% (7).

Conventional chemotherapy for acute leukemia is cyclic, and sensitivity to a given treatment is clinically determined at the point of remission evaluation (usually > 21 days after beginning of therapy after a defined number of courses, generally 1 to 3). Complete and in some cases partial remissions (CR and PR, respectively) are the common indicators of drug sensitivity. A patient with a residual leukemic cell mass in the bone marrow at remission evaluation in excess of the definitions for CR (or PR) is consequently judged as resistant or refractory, depending on previous response to chemotherapeutic drug regimens.

#### Causes of Treatment Failures

Treatment failure in AL may be caused by several different factors. A simple way of classifying these factors into three major groups has been described previously (8). The principal determinants of drug resistance in AL according to this model include (1) low cellular sensitivity to cytotoxic drugs—*cellular drug resistance*; (2) increased proliferative potential of the leukemic cells between courses of chemotherapy—*regrowth resistance*; and (3) low systemic exposure of antileukemic drugs—*pharmacokinetic resistance*.

Treatment failure caused by drug-induced nontolerable toxicity is not considered in the above classification but may be a major problem for certain groups of patients, especially elderly patients and patients with vital organ dysfunction (9).

Figure 1 illustrates the concept of apparent clinical drug resistance associated with induction or reinduction chemotherapy. For the sake of simplicity, the graph considers only one course of chemotherapy, and the achievement of CR is the criterion for drug sensitivity. It is assumed that the biological characteristics and drug sensitivity of the leukemic cells are constant over time. Curve A represents the cytolytic response of a CR patient during and shortly after a course of chemotherapy, whereas curve B illustrates the comparably poorer response of a patient with resistant disease (RD). Curve C represents the regrowth phase of leukemic cells typical of CR patients, whereas curve D illustrates an increased regrowth rate typical of a RD patient. Although the shapes of these curves are illustrated conceptually, the principal features are based on published data from serial studies (day 0, 6, 17 > weekly) of the effect of chemotherapy on bone marrow content of leukemic cells from patients with AML (10,11).

According to this model, only curve A–C will lead to CR at day 28 (final remission evaluation). Substituting the regrowth rate of the CR patient (C) with that of the RD patient (D) will offset the benefits of high initial cell kill and lead to RD outcome. Similarly, changing the initial cell kill rate of CR with that of RD patients will obviously

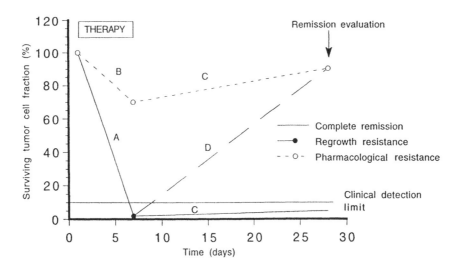

**Figure 1**  Basis for principal classification of treatment failures in acute leukemia in response to a 7-day induction or reinduction course of chemotherapy. *Curve A* illustrates the initial killing of leukemic cells in a patient showing drug sensitivity, and *curve B* the poor cell kill typical of a patient with resistance due to cellular drug resistance and/or too low systemic exposure. *Curve C* represents the regrowth phase of leukemic cells typical of a CR patient and *curve D* represents the increased leukemic cell growth defining regrowth resistance.

lead to RD. Thus, the presence of any component of a RD curve B or D will result in RD outcome.

The factors that determine which of the curves will apply to the individual patient are depicted in Figure 2. Whether the initial cell killing of leukemic cells will follow the steep A curve or the more shallow B curve depends on intrinsic leukemic *cellular drug sensitivity* and/or the level of *systemic exposure* of the chemotherapeutic drug, the latter often quantified by the area under the plasma-concentration-time curve (AUC). The factors that determine which of the two curves C and D will apply is related to the *regrowth potential* of the remaining leukemic cells, which in turn may be determined by several biological and cell kinetic factors (see below).

I will now briefly discuss these principal determinants separately and discuss possible ways of obtaining laboratory estimates of these parameters for clinical use. Special focus will be placed on measurement of cellular drug resistance because this area has attracted much interest in recent years and is also the primary research area of the author.

## CELLULAR DRUG RESISTANCE

The development of mechanisms for detoxification of foreign, potentially toxic chemicals was probably a requirement for survival early in the course of evolution (12). In

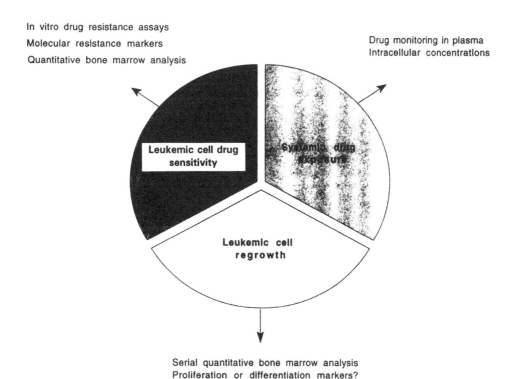

**Figure 2**  Schematic illustration of the principal determinants of clinical tumor response and their possible principles of measurement.

simple eukaryotes, the protective mechanisms were developed in the single cell, whereas in multicellular organisms, many detoxification processes were localized to specialized organs, such as the kidney or liver. Most antileukemic agents are recognized by these detoxification systems, which are present in both normal and neoplastic cells (13). Development of an increased capacity of these systems in the neoplastic cell is thus believed to be the cause of drug resistance.

## Mechanisms of Leukemic Cell Resistance

Most of the various mechanisms of leukemic cell resistance can be classified into four major groups: (1) altered plasma membrane transport; (2) decreased cellular drug activation; (3) increased drug inactivation; and (4) alteration of cellular drug targets. It should be noted that most of these mechanisms have been defined using established cell lines selected for resistance to a particular chemotherapeutic agent. Resistance to any particular drug can occur through one or more of these mechanisms, acting either alone or in combination. The principal mechanisms are illustrated in Figure 3.

### Plasma Membrane Transport

Many drugs used for treatment of leukemia show structural similarity to natural metabolites with which they share common carrier systems for cellular uptake (13). Such drugs can be taken up across cell membranes by cells by energy-dependent processes, and alterations of the number or structure of the carrier proteins may lead to decreased uptake and increased resistance. Cell lines selected for methotrexate resistance have

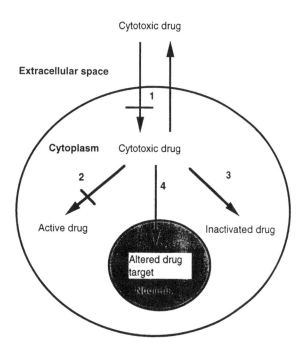

**Figure 3**   Mechanisms of cytotoxic drug resistance at the level of the leukemic cell. See text for explanation.

thus been reported to display a significantly reduced uptake compared to the parental cell line, possibly due to a reduction of both the affinity to, and number of, carrier molecules (14). Melphalan has been reported to be accumulated inside cells by active membrane transport systems normally used by amino acids and alterations of the affinity of these carriers for melphalan have been found to cause decreased uptake of the drug, leading to resistance (15).

Perhaps the most well-studied mechanism of resistance involving altered membrane transport is "classical" multidrug resistance (MDR). MDR defines a cellular phenotype in which the development of resistance in vitro to one "natural product" derived cytotoxic drug, such as the vinca alkaloids, anthracyclines, and podophyllotoxins, also confers cross-resistance to the other MDR-related drugs (16,17). Classical MDR is believed to be mediated by a transmembrane 170-kd permeability glycoprotein (Pgp), a product of the *MDR1* gene (16–19). Pgp is a transmembrane protein and probably functions as an energy-dependent drug efflux channel for the MDR-associated drugs but not for alkylating agents or antimetabolites (17). Many cell lines selected for doxorubicin (Dox), vincristine (Vcr), or etoposide (VP-16) resistance show increased expression of both MDR1 RNA and Pgp (20). Other forms of cytotoxic drug efflux mechanisms dissimilar from Pgp have recently been described for Vcr and Dox selected cell lines (21–23). Perhaps the most well characterized of these is the non–Pgp-mediated MDR variant that expresses the multidrug resistance associated protein (MRP), which has a cross-resistance pattern similar to that of Pgp (22). MRP expression appears to be preferentially induced by vinca alkaloids and often precedes the expression of Pgp (23).

*Decreased Drug Activation*

To be effective, some important antileukemic agents require activation after entering the cell. A decrease of enzyme activity responsible for this conversion may thus lead to resistance. This has been described for cytarabine (ara-C)-resistant cells (24,25), for example. Ara-C is phosphorylated by deoxycytidine kinase to its phosphorylated congeners, of which the triphosphate is believed to be active (24,25). A significantly lower level of deoxycytidin kinase has been reported for ara-C resistant cells (26). A similar process of decreased drug activation may account for resistance to the purine analogue 6-thioguanine (6-TG). This compound requires conversion to the active nucleotide 6-thioguanylate to cause damage to DNA, and in vitro studies have indicated that resistance may be caused by reduction of the conversion ability (13,25).

*Increased Drug Inactivation*

Cellular mechanisms for inactivation of xenobiotics, including cytotoxic drugs, involve increased activity of glutathione S-transferase (GST) and/or increased levels of glutathione (GSH) (13,27). GSH-utilizing enzymes play important roles in detoxification by scavenging free radicals and by conjugating toxins and xenobiotics with GSH, rendering them inactive (28). The GSTs are highly conserved enzymes (29), of which the pi and alpha forms have been implicated in cytotoxic drug resistance (28). Alteration of the GSH/GST system has been correlated with development of resistance to a variety of drugs, including bifunctional alkylating agents, Dox and cisplatin (27,30,31). However, a direct causal association with drug resistance has not been completely established; for instance, transfection of the GST pi gene has failed to confer the drug-resistant phenotype to human recipient cells (32). Furthermore, increased glutathione peroxidase activity in Dox-resistant cells has been linked to an increased rate at which free radicals generated by Dox exposure are converted to inactive forms (33).

Alterations occurring in the subcellular distribution of cytotoxic drugs by incorporation and trapping of the cytotoxic drug in intracellular organelles is another way for cells to "inactivate" drugs. This mechanism will prevent the drug from interaction with its target molecule and has been described for the anthracyclines (34,35). This cellular alteration appears to be part of the classical and the non-Pgp-mediated MDR phenotypes (36,37).

Limiting drug-induced damage by compensatory changes in other cellular functions also falls into this category of resistance mechanisms. The ability of drug-resistant cells to repair DNA damage induced by alkylating agents has received increasing attention. A range of repair enzymes may be responsible for resistance through excision repair of damaged sections of DNA. However, the relationship between changes in DNA repair activity and drug resistance is incompletely understood, possibly because of difficulties in detecting the low levels of alkylation required for inducing lethal effects (13).

*Altered Target Molecules*

Resistance to a given cytotoxic drug may result from changes in the level of expression or the biochemical properties of a target molecule. A classic example of this type of mechanism is acquired resistance to methotrexate: increased levels of the target enzyme, dihydrofolate reductase, allow the metabolic pathway for tetrahydrofolate formation to proceed at a normal rate despite presence of the drug (38). The increased enzyme expression may be the result of an increased translation or transcription or may be secondary to gene amplification (13). In addition to these quantitative changes in dihydrofolate reductase levels, there may also be qualitative changes that reduce the susceptibility of the enzyme to methotrexate inhibition (39).

A recently discovered cellular target for many important antileukemic drugs is topoisomerase II (Topo II). Topoisomerases are nuclear enzymes that modulate the topological structure of DNA by making transient DNA breaks (40). Topo II inhibitors are thought to act by stabilization of enzyme-DNA binding. Drugs that inhibit Topo II belong to diverse chemical classes of importance for the treatment of leukemia, including the anthracyclines, epipodophyllotoxins, anthracenediones, and acridines. Both quantitative reduction of enzyme activity and qualitative changes in Topo II function have been associated with development of resistance to these drugs in cell lines (16,41). The resulting cellular phenotype is denoted atypical MDR to distinguish it from classical MDR. It is characterized by cross-resistance between Topo II inhibitors but retained sensitivity to vinca alkaloids (13,41).

Recently, several molecules have been discovered that may be of prime importance in the regulation of the sensitivity of the cell to apoptosis. Many, if not all, currently used cytotoxic drugs kill cells by inducing apoptosis (42,43); therefore, regulatory mechanisms for this process may be highly relevant as determinants for drug sensitivity in leukemia. Indeed, increased expression of the *bcl-2* gene has been found to protect many cell types from apoptosis (42). Expression of the p53 protein, on the other hand, may facilitate apoptosis, and mutant cell lines lacking normal p53 survive even high concentrations of cytotoxic drugs (44). Increased knowledge of these and other molecules involved in regulation of cell death is probably important for the understanding of cellular cytotoxic drug resistance.

## Resistance Markers in Leukemic Cells from Patients

Compared to cell line models, much less is known about cellular resistance mechanisms operative in the leukemic cells from patients. However, many of the preclinically defined mechanisms have been implicated in clinical drug resistance based on correlative studies using mechanism-specific assays on patient cells. During recent years, much effort has been directed toward the evaluation of cellular markers for the various forms of MDR, including atypical and non-Pgp-mediated MDR forms as well as MDR associated with resistance to alkylating agents. The methods used have been based primarily on measurements of gene expression at the level of mRNA or the detection of resistance-associated molecules by immunocytochemical techniques.

Pgp is the most studied molecule in this context. In AML, several studies have shown increased *MDR1* gene and Pgp expression to be associated both with poor treatment outcome and decreased survival (45–48), although there are contradictory results (49). In contrast, ALL samples have been reported to express Pgp in only a small fraction of cases, and Pgp is believed to be of less importance for the development of drug resistance in this disease (50). However, contradictory results also exist for ALL, and the role of Pgp still appears controversial in this disease (51).

Alteration in the GSH/GST system has repeatedly been associated with clinical outcome in AL. Low GST levels have been associated with a favorable prognosis in AL whereas high levels, especially of GST pi, were related to poor clinical outcome in terms of both response and disease-free survival (52,53). A significant correlation also has been observed between GST and Pgp expression (54). Little is known about the role of other more recently discovered MDR-associated molecules (e.g., MRP and Topo II) in clinical drug resistance in AL, although some preliminary studies indicate the feasibility of performing future correlative studies in a larger number of patients (55–57).

There are few data on samples from the same patient before and after chemotherapy. However, preliminary results suggest that Pgp and GST appear to be raised more often in leukemic cells from resistant and relapsed patients; but it is quite clear that such mechanisms can be active in de novo malignancy and not necessarily emerge as a consequence of prior chemotherapy.

Many of the postulated mechanisms of resistance described for the antimetabolite drugs in cell lines also have been observed in clinical samples from patients with AL. Thus, for AL samples obtained in conjunction with methotrexate therapy, both quantitative and qualitative changes in dihydrofolate reductase have been reported in addition to altered membrane transport (38). For ara-C, reported mechanisms of resistance encompass changes in transport, activation, and inactivation as well as interaction with target molecules (24,25). Because many of the transport-related mechanisms may be overcome by high-dose regimens, focus has been put on the activation step where ara-C is phosphorylated to the active triphosphate. The ability of AML blast cells to form the triphosphate has also been shown to be correlated to clinical outcome (24,25). However, as for the markers of MDR, the actual and relative contributions of all the reported cellular changes for observed clinical resistance to antimetabolites in different forms of AL have not yet been firmly established.

Clinical evaluation of mechanism-specific assays is only just beginning and some of the data are clearly contradictory. To some extent, this may reflect the complex way in which the various resistance mechanisms may interact in vivo. Resistance to one drug may also be caused by a variety of potential mechanisms yet to be discovered.

## Cell Culture Drug Resistance Assays

Development of laboratory tests for measurement of resistance to cytotoxic drugs in tumor cells dates from the beginning of the twentieth century. The first report was made by Pappenheimer in 1917 (58). He added trypan blue to fresh thymic lymphocytes that had been exposed to different toxic agents. Trypan blue stained the dead cells blue, while the living cells remained unstained and clear. In 1954, Black and Speer (59) reported a variation in drug responsiveness among tumor biopsy specimens using a tetrazolium reduction assay (MTT-assay), based on the reduction of a tetrazolium salt to a colored product by living cells. During the 1960s, Schrek published several papers on the effect on lymphocytes exposed to heat and the in vitro cytotoxicity of L-asparaginase using a modified trypan blue assay (60,61).

The most commonly used in vitro assay for chemosensitivity testing during the past decade has been the clonogenic assay, assays based on measurement of proliferation, and assays based on the concept of total tumor cell kill. The various end points are discussed below and summarized in Figure 4.

### Clonogenic Assay

In the late 1970s, Salmon and Hamburger reported clinical correlations using a clonogenic assay for patient tumor cells (62,63) and the interest in drug resistance assays increased dramatically. The technique is based on single cell culture in soft agar and the subsequent counting of formed colonies, 2–3 weeks after exposure to cytotoxic drugs. The assay relies on the proliferative capacity of a small fraction of the cells, presumed to be the stem cells (64). The clonogenic assay has been used successfully to predict response to chemotherapy in AML (65–67). However, the method has several limitations, including generally low evaluability rates, clumping artifacts, and a lengthy performance time (68–70). Drug effects are measured only in a small fraction of cells, and drug effects in resting $G_0$ cells, which may well be proliferative in vivo, are not measured (69). Some clones may also be derived from contaminating normal cells (71). Clonogenic assays are also of limited value for lymphatic neoplasms because of their low colony formation (72). This makes clonogenic assays unsuitable for large-scale testing of clinical samples from patients with leukemia. A modification of the assay with higher success rates measuring DNA precursor incorporation has been developed but has mainly been applied to solid tumors (73,74). The overall reported sensitivities and specificities are in the range of 0.8 (75).

### Cell Proliferation Assays

Cell proliferation assays are short-term assays (1–7 days) based on measurement of DNA precursor incorporation in the proliferative fraction of cells. In vitro response to antileukemic drugs using these assays has been shown to correlate with clinical response to therapy in hematological malignancies (72,76–79). Agreement between in vitro results and survival has also been observed (79). The ability of AML blasts unexposed to cytotoxic drugs to incorporate DNA precursors during in vitro culture has also been found to be associated with treatment outcome (80). These assays have higher reported technical success rates than clonogenic assays. The major drawbacks with this assay type are that drug effects are dependent on the degree of DNA synthesis and—just as with the clonogenic assay—$G_0$ cell effects may not be adequately measured. Artifactual alterations of nucleoside pools and in purine and pyrimidine pathways are potential

| Endpoint | Technique | Assay type | Measured cell population |
|---|---|---|---|
| **Reproductive capacity** | Clonogenic assay | Colony formation | CC |
| **DNA synthesis** | DNA precursor uptake assays | 3H-thymidine incorporation 3H-uridine incorporation | CC+TC |
| **Membrane function** | DiSC assay | Vital dye exclusion | CC+TC+EC |
| | FMCA | Fluorescein production from FDA | CC+TC+EC |
| **Cell metabolism** | MTT assay | Colorimetric measurement of formazan production | CC+TC+EC |
| | ATP assay | Measurement of ATP luminiscence | CC+TC+EC |

## CELL POPULATIONS ACCORDING TO THE STEM CELL CONCEPT

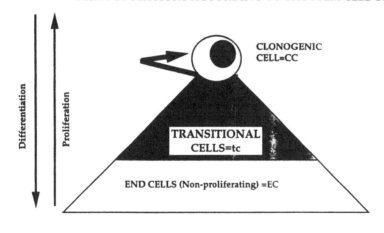

**Figure 4** *Top*. Some currently used methods for predicting drug resistance in leukemia and the cell populations estimated. *Bottom*. Tumor cell populations according to the stem cell concept (see Ref. 64). Abbreviations: DiSC, differential staining cytotoxicity; FMCA, fluorometric microculture cytotoxicity assay; MTT, dimethylthiazole tetrazolium.

technical pitfalls. The calculated sensitivities and specificities for this test are roughly in the range of 0.8–0.9 and 0.6–0.7, respectively (75).

*Total Cell Kill Assays*

Although a dye-exclusion test had already been used in 1917 by Pappenheimer, it was not until the late 1970s that Weisenthal further developed this principle and introduced the differential staining cytotoxicity (DiSC) assay (81,82) by which the interest in these nonclonogenic assays was regained. The DiSC assay is a short-term dye-exclusion test based on the concept of total tumor cell kill in the whole, largely nondividing tumor-cell population (81,83). After 96 h of continuous exposure to the cytotoxic drug, the cells are incubated with the vital dyes fast green and nigrosin, spun onto slides, and counterstained, followed by quantification of the proportion of living cells in relation to an internal standard of a fixed number of added duck erythrocytes (81,83). The assay has a high technical success rate, and because individual cells are examined under the microscope, it can also be used in cases of high contamination of nontumor cells. Furthermore, it can distinguish between resistant and sensitive cell populations; and assay results correlate well with clinical response and survival (75,84–87), with an overall sensitivity and specificity of about 0.95 and 0.70, respectively (75). However, the DiSC assay is labor-intensive and time-consuming, and the evaluation is quite subjective and requires a highly skilled observer for the slide counting.

An alternative method that has been used for chemosensitivity testing of both solid tumors (88) and leukemias (89–93) is the semiautomated 96-well MTT assay, originally described in 1954 by Black and Speer (59). It is based on measurement of drug-induced changes in cellular reduction of a tetrazolium salt to a colored product generated by the mitochondrial dehydrogenase activity of living cells (89,94). After the salt crystals are dissolved, the color change can be measured spectrophotometrically in 96-well plates. Compared to the DiSC assay, the MTT assay is more objective and less labor-intensive. However, the MTT assay requires a fairly pure tumor cell population because it cannot distinguish between drug effect in normal and tumor cells. The MTT and DiSC assays are comparable when using pure tumor cell populations (89,90,95) and the MTT assay has also shown good clinical correlations (91,92,95,96) and may be predictive of patient survival (93). The sensitivity and specificity from more than 300 correlations from different studies have been reported to be around 0.8 and 0.7, respectively (75).

The fluorometric microculture cytotoxicity assay (FMCA) also belongs to this category of tests. The FMCA is based on the measurement of fluorescence generated from nonfluorescent fluorescein diacetate (FDA), which rapidly enters cells with intact plasma membranes and is hydrolyzed to its fluorescent derivative, fluorescein (96). The FMCA has been successfully applied for drug-sensitivity testing using cell lines (97). The intra- and inter-assay variations have been estimated to be less than 5% and less than 10–15%, respectively (98,99). The FDA fluorescence was linearly related to the number of living cells and showed good correlation with the MTT (99) and DiSC assay (99,100). Good correlations with clinical response has been obtained for both ALL and AML, with sensitivities and specificities of 0.8–0.9 and 0.6–0.7, respectively (100–102).

Another assay based on metabolic activity within the cell is the ATP assay (103, 104), which measures cellular ATP content. Comparatively little experience has yet been gained with this assay in leukemia but the initial results appear promising (105, 106). The advantages and disadvantages of the FMCA and ATP assays are similar to those of the MTT assay.

## Methodological Considerations of Cell Culture Assays

### Drug Exposure

Selection of concentrations for in vitro cytotoxic drug resistance assays is an important issue. Although some investigators obtain full concentration-response curves and use

$IC_{50}$ or $IC_{10}$ as a measure of drug activity (84,93), the majority employ one or a few fixed concentrations and measure a variable effect at those concentrations (74,85,107).

Clonogenic assays have traditionally used a short (1-h) drug exposure, and early studies with other assay types often used a similar drug exposure strategy, although longer incubations were often needed for the time-dependent antimetabolites (85). Subsequently, for short-term assays it was shown that continuous exposure could be used for all drugs with retained predictive ability (83). Many investigators, especially those using clonogenic assays, have attempted to mimic the in vivo situation by using cutoff concentrations similar to clinically achievable peak plasma concentrations or some fraction thereof (63,74,108). A major concern with this approach is the lack of information on stability under assay conditions for many important drugs (109), making in vivo–like exposure difficult to achieve. Differences in serum protein concentrations between culture medium and patient plasma may also distort in vivo modeling. The design of in vitro drug exposure procedures resulting in intracellular exposure similar to that of in vivo has been described for some antileukemic drugs and is an interesting approach that may partly circumvent these problems (87).

An alternative approach for selecting cutoff concentrations for prediction of tumor response has been developed for nonclonogenic total cell kill assays (83,85). For each drug, concentration-response curves spanning a large range of concentrations are generated for a number of samples. The cutoff concentration is then defined as the concentration producing the largest scatter of test results. This approach does not require drug concentrations or the mechanisms for drug induced cell kill in vitro to be the same as in vivo, provided that the mechanisms determining drug resistance are the same (110).

It has been suggested that the predictive performance of cell culture assays at least in part may be influenced by the drug exposure strategy chosen (75). The relative high accuracy of the classical clonogenic assays in predicting drug sensitivity may be the result of the lower drug exposure (usually 1/10 of peak plasma levels), whereas the suprapharmacological exposure employed in the Kern assay is suggested to contribute to its excellent ability for prediction of drug resistance (74).

*Selection of Cutoff Lines*

In most of the described assay types, the measured in vitro drug response is categorized using one or more cutoff values (75). In the early studies, a cutoff limit was often empirically chosen to maximize assay performance. A 70% or 50% inhibition of the assay-specific parameter measured was used in many of these studies to distinguish sensitive from resistant samples (74,76,84,110). An underlying assumption for this approach is that all drugs with similar clinical activity will produce a similar distribution of cell survival measured in vitro. The validity of this assumption is not well established and may be seriously undermined depending on the uncertainties related to the selection of drug-exposure strategy.

In recent years, relative, rather than absolute, cutoff lines have been increasingly employed. Drug response in vitro for samples from each individual patient is compared and related to that of other patients' samples analyzed for the same drug. The main advantage of this approach is that test results are normalized for differences in cell survival between different drugs at the chosen cutoff concentration. In the much-cited calibration procedure, described by Kern and Weisenthal, for the clonogenic and DNA precursor uptake "Kern" assay, the drug-specific median cell survival index value for a large number of samples was used to classify samples into low and intermediate drug resistance categories for any particular drug (74). A second cutoff limit was set to 1 standard deviation above the median derived from a large number of samples. The category of samples above the second cutoff line was termed extreme drug resistance (EDR), and comparison with clinical outcome showed that patients with samples in this category receiving only EDR drugs had an extremely low probability of response (74,111). The EDR phenotype appears to be detected also by nonclonogenic assays based on total tumor cell kill by using a similar calibration procedure (84). The relationship between assay results calibrated this way and clinical outcome for patients with AL using the FMCA is shown in Figure 5.

*Statistical Considerations*

An appreciation of the usefulness of any laboratory test requires some quantitative knowledge of the performance characteristics of the test, often described in terms of sensitivity and specificity (112). The sensitivity of a test is defined as the number of true positive test results/true positive plus false negative test results whereas specificity is

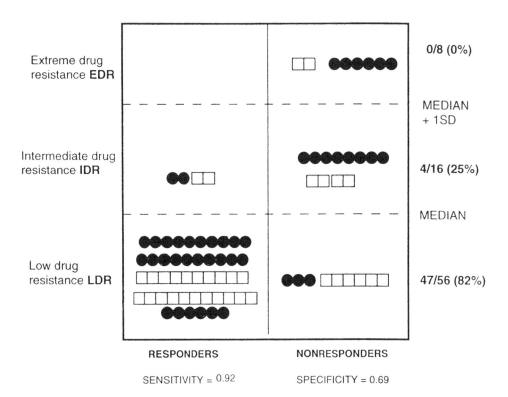

**Figure 5** Single drug activity as the basis for correlation with clinical outcome (n=80) using drug specific cutoff lines. The median survival index spearates low drug resistance (LDR) from intermediate drug resistance (IDR), and median + 1 SD separates IDR from extreme drug resistance (EDR). The sensitivity and specificity using the median as cutoff are indicated. Unfilled symbols = acute lymphoblastic leukemia (ALL); filled symbols = acute myelocytic leukemia (AML) samples. Overall response rate (CR) for the included patients was 64%.

the number of true negative test results/true negative plus false positive test results. In the case of in vitro prediction of clinical response to chemotherapy, a high level of sensitivity means that the ability of the test to predict drug resistance generally is good, whereas a high specificity implies a test with good ability to predict drug sensitivity.

However, the predictive value or accuracy of a test is not only dependent on the sensitivity and specificity but also highly influenced by the prevalence of the event to be predicted, sometimes referred to as pretest probability. In the case of in vitro predictions of clinical response to cytotoxic agents, pretest probability may be estimated from known response rates for the particular drug in the patient population under investigation. Thus, for a given sensitivity and specificity, increasing the pretest probability will increase the predictive accuracy for drug sensitivity, whereas decreasing pretest probability will increase the predictive accuracy of drug resistance (111,112).

The continuous relationship between pretest and post-test probability can be described by Bayes' theorem and, provided that the sensitivities and specificities of the test are constant over the range of pretest probabilities of interest, a simple nomogram can be constructed to translate an individual pretest probability to post-test probability of response given either a positive or negative test (111). Such a nomogram is shown in Figure 6 based on the data in Figure 5. Indeed, meta-analyses of many studies of different diagnoses, from different laboratories and assay types, have shown that the predictive values obtained appear to vary in accordance with Bayesian expectations over a wide range of pretest probabilities (113). The principal steps involved in the calibration of a cell culture drug-resistance assay are listed in Table 1.

Because many antileukemic drugs have a relatively high pretest probability of response, the predictive accuracy of drug resistance may be less than for drug sensitivity

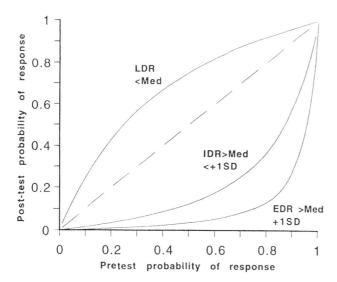

**Figure 6** Calculated relationship between pre- and post-test probability of response for the fluorometric microculture cytotoxicity assay (FMCA) based on Bayes' theorem. The specific categories (LDR, IDR, and EDR) and cutoff limits are indicated (filled lines). Broken line is the line of unity. Sensitivity and specificity values from Figure 5 are used. The sensitivity value for EDR was set to 0.99 (75).

**Table 1**  Uniform Calibration Procedure for Cell Culture Drug Resistance Assays

Step 1.  Test drugs at several logs of concentrations in pilot series of drug-sensitive tumor types.

Step 2.  Select concentrations at which a significant scatter of test results is obtained (generally 1–10 × clinically achievable drug exposure) as cutoff concentrations.

Step 3.  For each drug, calculate median value (Med) and standard deviation (SD) based on at least 30–50 samples from tumors, including those with documented response rate for the particular drug.

Step 4.  Use these values to define the uniform statistical cutoff lines by dividing test results into LDR, low drug resistance (< Med); IDR, intermediate drug resistance (> MED < + 1 SD); EDR, extreme drug resistance > (Med + 1 SD).

Step 5.  Evaluate and verify the validity and reliability of the assay by prospective clinical correlations and calculate assay sensitivity and specificity.

Step 6.  Describe the relationship between pretest information and post-test probability of tumor response using the test characteristics and Bayes' theorem.

Step 7.  Feedback adjustments of drug-specific calibration procedure (cutoff levels and concentrations 1–4).

unless the test sensitivity is high. For many of the assay systems discussed previously, the sensitivity was higher than the specificity, partly compensating for this. For the EDR category, sensitivity appears to be very high (>0.99) irrespective of assay type (74,84). However, even in the case of moderate sensitivities and specificities (0.70–0.80), for drugs that have equal pretest probability of response and that are equally acceptable clinically, an assay-positive drug will, on average, be more likely to produce a clinical response than an assay-negative drug. In leukemic patients with pretest probabilities of response of 30–80%, the difference in the likelihood of clinical response will be approximately two- to sevenfold.

### Clinical Implications of Cell Culture Assays

There are several possible clinical applications of laboratory tests for predicting resistance to cytotoxic drugs in tumor cells from individual patients:

1. To avoid the use of drugs with a predicted low probability of response.
2. To select the best alternative among drugs that are considered equally active.
3. To identify possible treatment alternatives.
4. To direct patients with a high degree of cellular drug resistance to investigational treatment alternatives.
5. To identify drug candidates for adjuvant therapy or dose intensification treatments.
6. To direct investigational drugs in the phase II setting to patients with in vitro sensitive tumors.

Retrospective comparisons of test results with treatment outcome is the common method for evaluating the accuracy of a laboratory test. Over the past decade, the numerous studies from many different laboratories using different types of in vitro assays has demonstrated a remarkably consistent ability to predict clinical drug resistance, with predictive values in the range of 0.8–0.95 (for reviews, see Refs. 75,111).

This level of performance compares well with antibiotic sensitivity testing, estrogen receptor determinations in breast cancer, fecal blood testing for colon cancer, and digoxin toxicity (112), to name a few laboratory tests that are felt to be of clinical use. In addition, there have been several studies demonstrating a correlation with patient survival (75). Thus, from the standpoint of clinical utility, in vitro drug resistance assays appear to meet the criteria for clinical application. To exclude drugs showing extreme drug resistance (EDR) and to aid in the selection of the best alternative among otherwise equally clinically acceptable treatment options may be the most appropriate and uncontroversial applications. However, as for most other laboratory or radiological tests, prospective clinical studies of the impact of this technology on patient care have been sparse. Nevertheless, at least four prospective studies, three of which were randomized, have shown advantages in clinical outcome for assay-positive drugs (110,114–116). These encouraging reports should promote larger prospective studies evaluating the optimal role of drug-resistance assays in various clinical settings.

Based on the overall published data on cell culture assay performance characteristics, no one assay has an apparent advantage over the other. For AL, however, total cell kill assays provide a practical, robust, and theoretically sound alternative to proliferation-based assays. Regarding the total cell kill assays, the use of 96-well microtiter plate technology in parallel with morphological evaluation for determination of drug effects may be required for optimal performance and measurement quality.

## PHARMACOKINETIC RESISTANCE

Dose intensity in chemotherapy has been shown to be of great importance for the clinical outcome in many drug-sensitive tumors, including the leukemias (117,118). These observations imply that reducing the dose to lower toxicity may seriously undermine the therapeutic responses in drug-sensitive patients. The correlation obtained between dose and tumor response clearly suggests a relationship also between plasma concentration (systemic exposure) and dose (118).

### Pharmacokinetic Variability

For the individual patient, not only dose but also interindividual variations in pharmacokinetic parameters such as absorption, distribution, and elimination of drugs play an important role in determining treatment intensity. The cytotoxic effect of many cytotoxic drugs, especially the non-cell cycle phase-specific drugs, is most closely related to the product of a drug concentration (C) and exposure time (T). Clinically, $C \times T$ is represented by systemic exposure, defined as the area under the plasma concentration-time curve where plasma concentration is related to time (AUC; 119). For some antileukemic drugs, notably the antimetabolites, the cytotoxic effect is more a function of the duration of exposure over a threshold concentration or of the dosing administration schedule (e.g., total dose given as a prolonged infusion rather than as a bolus; 119).

Most antileukemic drugs display a large interindividual variation in systemic exposure (two- to 10-fold) in patients with normal liver and renal function (118). For certain drugs, there is also an intraindividual variability between courses (120). These facts make the systemic exposure for different patients receiving the same dose very unpredictable. This is illustrated in Figure 7, where two hypothetical patients receive

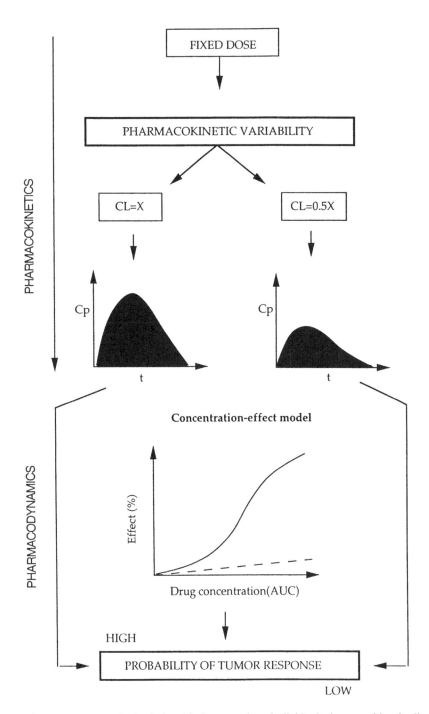

**Figure 7** Theoretical relationship between interindividual pharmacokinetic disposition, systemic exposure, and clinical response. CL = systemic clearance, T = time, Cp = plasma concentration, AUC = area under the plasma concentration-time curve. See text for explanation.

the same dose but have a plasma clearance (CL) varying with a factor 2. This will lead to different plasma concentrations (Cp) over time (t) and consequently different AUCs. These AUCs will translate into different clinical outcome probabilities depending on a the steep concentration-response curve (solid line). The classic sigmoidal concentration-response curve is the one expected to result from application of non-phase-specific drugs to drug-sensitive tumors. Note that for a patient with leukemic cells resistant to clinically achievable AUCs (broken line), no difference in effect will be observed. An increase in AUC in this case will only add to toxicity. The great heterogeneity among tumors with respect to cellular drug sensitivity makes measurements of AUC alone difficult to interpret and is undoubtedly a major reason for the lack of success of therapeutic drug monitoring in clinical oncology. This lack of enthusiasm is somewhat surprising, considering that for drug-sensitive patients with steep concentration-effect relationships, small changes in AUC may be of major importance for the final oncolytic activity achieved.

## Concentration-Effect Relationships

Several studies in drug-sensitive tumors have demonstrated positive relationships between plasma concentration (in most cases, its time integral, the AUC) and therapeutic effect (118). Such a relationship has been shown for several important antileukemic drugs, including anthracyclines, vinca alkaloids, teniposide, methotrexate, and 6-mercaptopurine (121–126). Correlations between plasma concentration and toxicity have also been increasingly reported, especially frequently for new agents undergoing pharmacokinetically monitored phase I trials. The end point generally considered is the acute decrease in blood cell counts compared to the pretreatment status. In general, the correlation coefficient between the pharmacokinetic parameter and efficacy or toxicity does not exceed 0.7, meaning that no more than 50% of the variability in tumor response may be explained by pharmacokinetic factors (121). Nevertheless, the absolute frequency of cases with suboptimal systemic exposures (pharmacokinetic resistance) for most tumor types is currently unknown. The often-held argument that dose escalation based on dose-limiting toxicity (to maximally tolerated dose, MTD) should prevent undertreatment may not always hold, because the dose-toxicity relationship seldom is known and dose escalation based on graded toxicity is in fact a rare clinical event. Even if dose adjustment to MTD is performed stepwise, there is still an appreciable time between courses for drug-resistant subclones to emerge under suboptimal systemic exposure. The situation becomes even more complex because combination therapy is often given and the component drugs often have similar dose-limiting toxicities, making judgment on which drug to escalate very difficult, not to say impossible. Surprisingly, there is virtually no information on the variability and pharmacokinetic behavior of drugs given in chemotherapeutic combinations. One recent study of the combination fluorouracil, cyclophosphamide, and epirubicin, determined in parallel in patients with breast cancer, showed a lack of correlation between the systemic exposures for the different components (127).

For some drugs, the intracellular concentration of the active metabolite appears to correlate better with clinical tumor response than the plasma concentration. Ara-C and 6MP exemplify drugs for which the clinical effects are more closely linked to the intracellular accumulation (in tumor or red blood cell) of their active metabolites, ara-CTP and 6TG, respectively (128–130). However, from a practical clinical perspective, the repeated sampling of representative material is difficult to obtain on a routine basis. Also, because most methods require an overall extraction and analysis, tumor cell heterogeneity and normal cell contamination clearly limits the interpretation of results.

## Measurement of Systemic Exposure

Monitoring drug levels in plasma for dose adjustment—with the aim of maximizing the therapeutic effect and minimizing toxicity (therapeutic drug monitoring, TDM)—is widely used clinically for many types of drugs, including heart glycosides and the anti-epileptics. Although anticancer drugs fulfill many criteria for drugs suitable for TDM (steep dose-response curves, narrow therapeutic window, large interindividual variability in drug disposition), only methotrexate is routinely monitored with this technology (119). The reasons for this are many, including lack of adequate analytical techniques, the frequent use of bolus administration, the requirement for multiple sampling, the use of combination therapy, and the occurrence of cellular drug resistance. However, recent developments in analytical and statistical pharmacokinetics have made TDM easier to perform in the clinical setting (119,131).

Prolonged infusion of drugs with sufficiently short half-life to allow rapid establishment of the steady-state concentration (Css) (which requires 4–5 half-lives to pass) offers the most simple situation. In this case, a single measurement at steady state can be used as an estimate of systemic exposure, and it is then possible to modify the rate of infusion for the remainder of the course to reach a preset target Css. This situation is rare, and more often one has to deal with non-steady-state situations resulting from bolus injections or short-term infusions. However, the recent development of robust "limiting sampling" techniques for anticancer drugs can allow the investigator to estimate AUC from 1–2 timed blood samples, even in the case of bolus administration (119,131). If previous estimates on pharmacokinetic parameters (and their intra- and interindividual variation) have been established using population-based pharmacokinetic methods (131), safe dose adjustment can be accomplished for the next course by revising the individual pharmacokinetic parameters using Bayesian feedback (131). In this procedure, the initial mean parameter value (prior estimates) for the population is revised by taking the measured individual estimates into account. The subsequent dose required to reach the desired target AUC can then easily be calculated for the next course. One important requirement is that the course-course variability is small. Population models and limited sampling strategies have been developed for many anticancer drugs (119). There are also several easy-to-operate computer programs available for these types of analysis (132).

With the strategy described above, the dosing of first course will be similar for all patients, a priori based on the mean population parameters and the desired target concentration. However, the population approach may also provide correlations with clinical descriptors (for example, age, gender, creatinine, bilirubin levels, etc.), which may explain at least part of the pharmacokinetic variability (131). Such information can then be used to individualize the dose and limit variability without measurement of plasma concentration. Such an approach may give plasma levels closer to those desired compared to the conventional normalization to body surface area for which the rationale is weak (119). Another way of adjusting the dose for the first course would be to administer a small test dose before the course, measuring plasma concentrations and subsequently calculating the individual parameters as described above. Such test dose procedures have been developed for high-dose methotrexate therapy (119,133). Finally, several enzymes involved in drug detoxification may be subjected to genetic variability testing. For example, acetylation of the drug amonafide inactivates this agent, and patients with genetically determined deficiency in enzyme activity (slow acetylators) will thus require higher doses than those with a normal acetylation ability (134). Measurement of the individual pheno- or genotype with respect to drug-metabolizing enzyme activity may thus help in individualizing the dose. Improvements in these areas will hopefully lead to a more systematic investigation of the potential role of "pharmacokinetic" resistance in the clinical setting.

## REGROWTH RESISTANCE

The importance of regrowth resistance as an explanation for treatment failure was recognized some years ago by detailed studies of determinants of response in AML by Dr. H. D. Preisler and coworkers (10,11,135). Regrowth resistance has been estimated to be a major cause of treatment failure in about 50% of patients with poor-prognosis AML (10) and is probably the most recently described clinical phenomenon that has been directly linked to drug resistance in AML. Although investigated primarily in AML, regrowth resistance may be relevant for other forms of leukemia as well (136).

### Causes of Regrowth Resistance

The extent of leukemic cell regrowth between courses of therapy is probably determined by several factors: (1) the number of cells surviving chemotherapy; (2) percentage of cells in cycle; (3) proliferative potential (number of cell divisions each cell is capable of); (4) cell cycle time; (5) the ability to differentiate; and (6) yet-undefined factors. High levels of the oncogene *c-myc* and low levels of *c-fms* have repeatedly been associated with short remission durations (137) and ascribed a role in determining regrowth. Also, the expression of IL-1B—a stimulator of growth factor release from stromal cells, T cells, and monocytes, leading to leukemic cell proliferation—has been associated with short remissions (138). (For a more detailed review of the biology of proliferation in leukemia, see Ref. 135.)

### Treatment of Regrowth Resistance

Even if the leukemic cells are pharmacodynamically sensitive to the drug and high systemic exposure is achieved, treatment will fail if the surviving leukemic cells regrow as fast as or faster than they can be killed. Conversely, for leukemic cells inherently resistant to the chemotherapeutic drug attempted, the proliferative rate of leukemic cells is of no consequence for the clinical response. The primary treatment strategy would then be to maximize leukemic cell kill by increasing systemic exposure, frequency of therapy (fractionation), or circumventing cellular drug resistance mechanisms (by adding resistance-modifying agents). However, a 50% reduction in the extent of regrowth can have as much effect on the remaining leukemic cell mass as would a doubling of the number of cells actually killed by the chemotherapy given. Hence, an appealing alternative approach would be to reduce leukemic regrowth between courses of therapy. Several maneuvers appear possible to accomplish this. For example, agents such as 1,25-dihydroxy vitamin $D_3$ and retinoic acid have been shown to inhibit prolif-eration and induce terminal myeloid differentiation of leukemic blasts (139). Recently, it was also demonstrated that a combination of interferon alpha and 13-cis-retinoic acid was able to slow leukemia proliferation in patients (140). Recombinant GM-CSF was also shown to slow proliferation of leukemia cells in vivo (140). Moreover, IL-1B-re-ceptor antagonists were able to reduce the clonogenic capacity of AML cells and inhibit DNA synthesis (141). The clinical testing of these and other protocols aiming at block-ing regrowth between courses of therapy will determine the utility of the approach.

Hitherto, only the leukemic cell progeny has been considered, for reasons of simplification. However, the cellular drug sensitivity and the extent and rate of normal hematopoietic cell repopulation also may be important factors for clinical outcome and the acceptable timepoint for subsequent courses of chemotherapy. Indeed, some pa-tients with AML, especially AML associated with myelodysplastic syndrome, fail to enter CR despite the disappearance of leukemic cells from the bone marrow. Some of these marrows remain empty while others are repopulated by myelodysplastic cells. In this situation, recombinant growth factors such as rhGM-CSF would theoretically be beneficial.

## Measurement of Regrowth Potential

Because this is a newly discovered clinical phenomenon, little information has yet been gained with respect to potential laboratory parameters that may be reflective of cellular regrowth. In describing regrowth resistance in AML, Preisler et al. used serial quanti-tative bone marrow examinations to measure both the level of cell kill and leukemic cell regrowth after termination of therapy (142). This technique is labor-intensive, and results cannot be obtained before therapy is terminated. Using the expression of the proliferation-associated oncogene *c-myc* as a predictor of clinical outcome, Preisler et al. (135,137) suggested this marker is reflective of proliferative potential in AML. High *c-myc* expression was associated with short remission durations, and CRs could be obtained only in patients in whom a high degree of leukemic cell kill had taken place, as judged by marrow examination immediately after termination of therapy and on day 6 (137). Northern blotting of mRNA appears impracticable for clinical use; it requires a large number of cells per sample, and results may easily be distorted by contamination with normal cell elements. Detection of the protein by immunohistochemistry may be more feasible, but, unfortunately, there appear to be some technical difficulties with measurement of *c-myc* with this technique (143). The spontaneous proliferation of AML blasts in vitro measured by simple thymidine labeling has also been shown to predict clinical outcome of chemotherapy (80). Measurement of IL-1B expression may be another alternative (138). These and other potentially useful markers, including cell cycle kinetics, spontaneous clonal growth, and differentiation ability of the leukemic cells, should be reinvestigated with respect to regrowth after chemotherapy and pref-erably in combination with measurement of cellular drug sensitivity.

## FUTURE DIRECTIONS

According to the present classification, clinically resistant disease can be the result of "classical" cellular drug resistance, low systemic exposure, the ability of the surviving

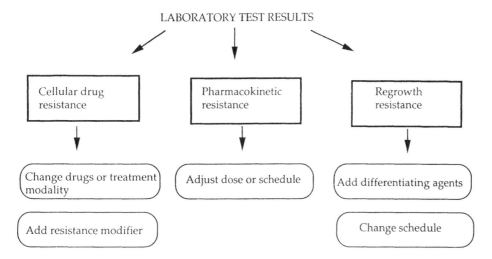

**Figure 8** Hypothetical illustration of laboratory diagnosis of drug resistance and some suggested potential clinical actions to counteract the mechanisms of resistance.

cell to regrow rapidly after chemotherapy, or a combination of these factors. If it were possible to accurately predict cellular drug sensitivity, regrowth potential of leukemic cells, and (as early as possible after the start of chemotherapy) the expected systemic exposure for individual patients, patient-specific treatment regimens could be designed and hopefully result in improved therapeutic outcome. This is illustrated in Figure 8 where a patient with a test result showing cellular drug resistance will require a change of drugs or addition or resistance modifiers to increase the probability of response. The patient with a test result showing high regrowth potential will require maneuvers designed to limit leukemic cell growth between courses, whereas low systemic exposure will be corrected by increasing the dose.

What then are the current possibilities for measuring these parameters (Fig. 2)? As discussed above, cellular drug sensitivity can be measured before start of therapy in vitro with nonclonogenic fresh tumor assays with relatively high accuracy. Alternatively, these measurements can be performed by serial bone marrow examinations (135, 142). Measurement of regrowth potential may require direct quantification of leukemic cells in the bone marrow samples while other pretherapeutic measures, such as *c-myc* expression and/or other proliferative characteristic features of the leukemic cell, are evaluated. Measurement of systemic exposure for all important antileukemic drugs can currently be performed with existing analytical and pharmacokinetic technologies.

## CONCLUDING REMARKS

In this chapter, an attempt to describe the principal determinants for clinical drug resistance in acute leukemia was made. Although the focus was placed on cellular causes and cell culture assays, it is my personal belief that taking pharmacokinetic and regrowth resistance into consideration will provide an even better understanding and prediction of clinical drug resistance. Research in this area will require collaboration between specialists from different fields, including clinical oncology and hematology, tumor biology, and clinical pharmacology. Such concentrated interdisciplinary efforts may be required to expand our knowledge of determinants of clinical drug resistance in acute leukemia and other forms of human cancer.

## ACKNOWLEDGMENTS

The author wants to specifically thank Dr. Peter Nygren, department of oncology, Uppsala University, for many helpful discussions and advice during the writing of this chapter. Drs. Jorgen Kristensen and Bertil Jonsson are also acknowledged for fruitful discussions.

## LIST OF ABBREVIATIONS

| | |
|---|---|
| AL | acute leukemia |
| ALL | acute lymphocytic leukemia |
| AML | acute myelocytic leukemia |
| AUC | area under the plasma concentration-time curve |
| Amsa | amsacrine |
| Ara-C | cytarabine |
| Ara-CTP | cytarabine triphosphate |
| CR | complete remission |
| Css | steady-state concentration |
| CV | coefficient of variation |
| $C \times T$ | concentration $\times$ time product |
| DiSC | differential staining cytotoxicity |
| Dox | doxorubicin |
| EDR | extreme drug resistance |
| FDA | fluorescein diacetate |
| FMCA | fluorometric microculture cytotoxicity assay |
| GSH | glutathione |
| CST | glutathione S-transferase |
| $IC_{50}$ | concentration inhibiting tumor cell survival to 50% |
| $IC_{10}$ | concentration inhibiting tumor cell survival to 10% |
| IL-1B | interleukin-1 beta |
| IDR | intermediate drug resistance |
| LDR | low drug resistance |
| MTT | dimethylthiazole tetrazolium |
| MDR | multidrug resistance |
| MRP | multidrug resistance associated protein |
| Mitox | mitoxantrone |
| PBS | phosphate buffered saline |
| Pgp | permeability-glycoprotein |
| RD | resistant disease |
| 6-TG | 6-thioguanine |

Topo II    topoisomerase II
Vcr        vincristine
VP-16      etoposide

## REFERENCES

1. Kyle R. Second malignancies associated with chemotherapeutic agents. Semin Oncol 1982; 9:133–139.
2. Kantarjian HM, Keating MJ. Therapy-related leukemia and myelodysplastic syndrome. Semin Oncol 1987; 14:435–443.
3. Bloomfield CD, Brunnig RD. Acute leukemia as a terminal event in leukemic hematopoietic disorders. Semin Oncol 1976; 3:297–303.
4. Tivey H. The natural history of untreated acute leukemia. Ann NY Acad Sci 1995; 60:322.
5. Poplack DG, Kun LE, Cassady JR, Pizzo PA. Leukemias and lymphomas of childhood. In: deVita VT Jr, Hellman S, Rosenberg SA, eds. Cancer: Principles and Practice of Oncology. Philadelphia: Lippincott, 1989:1671–1683.
6. Preisler HD, Anderson K, Rai K, et al. The frequency of long-term remission in patients with acute myelogenous leukaemia treated with conventional maintenance chemotherapy. A study of 760 patients with a minimal follow-up time of 6 years. Br J Haematol 1989; 71:189–195.
7. Wiernik PH. Acute leukemias. In: DeVita VT Jr, Hellman S, Rosenberg SA, eds. Cancer: Principles and Practice of Oncology. Philadelphia: Lippincott, 1989:1809–1835.
8. Larsson R, Nygren P. Laboratory prediction of clinical chemotherapeutic drug resistance: a working model exemplified by acute leukemia. Eur J Cancer 1993; 29A:1208–1212.
9. Larson RA, Sandler DP, Le Beau M. Acute leukemia: biology and treatment. Educ Prog Am Soc Hematol 1994; 2:34–42.
10. Preisler H, Raza A, Larson R, Goldbergh J, Tricot J, Carey M, Kukla C. Some reasons for the lack of progress in the treatment of acute myelogenous leukemia: a review of three consecutive trials of the treatment of poor prognosis patients. Leuk Res 1991; 15:773–780.
11. Preisler HD. Poor prognosis acute myelogenous leukemia. Leuk Lymphoma 1993; 9:273–283.
12. Jacoby WB. The natural substrates of the enzymes of detoxification are foreign compounds: a comment. Rev Biochem Toxicol 1982; 4:1–4.
13. Hall AG, Cattan AR. Drug resistance mechanisms in leukemia. Baillieres Clin Haematol 1991; 4:655–681.
14. Hill BT, Bailey BD, White JC, Goldman ID. Characteristics of transport 4-amino antifolates and folate compounds by two lines of L5178Y lymphoblasts, one with impaired transport of methotrexate. Cancer Res 1979; 39:2440–2446.
15. Redwood WR, Colvin M. Transport of melphalan by sensitive and resistant L1210 cells. Cancer Res 1980; 40:1144–1149.
16. Beck WT. The cell biology of multiple drug resistance. Biochem Pharmacol 1987; 36:2879–2887.
17. Lum BL, Gosland MP, Kaubisch S, Sikic BI. Molecular targets in oncology: implications of the multidrug resistance gene. Pharmacotherapy 1993; 13:88–109.
18. Kartner N, Riordan JP, Ling V. Cell surface P-glycoprotein associated with multidrug resistance in mammalian cell lines. Science 1983; 221:1285.
19. Chen CJ, Chin JE, Ueda K, Clark D, Pastan I, Gottesman MM, Roninson I. Internal duplication and homology with bacterial transport proteins in the MDR-1 gene from multidrug-resistant human cells. Cell 1986; 47:381.
20. Hill BT. Differing patterns of cross resistance resulting from exposures to specific antitumor drugs or to radiation in vitro. Cytotechnology 1993; 12:265–288.

21. McClean SM, Hill BT. An overview of membrane, cytosolic and nuclear proteins. Biochim Biophys Acta 1992; 114:107–127.

22. Cole SPC, Bhardwaj G, Gerlach JH, Mackie JE, Grant CE, Almqvist KC, Stewart AJ, Kurz EU, Duncan AMV, Deeley RG. Overexpression of a transporter gene in a multidrug-resistant human lung cancer cell line. Science 1992; 258:1650–1654.

23. Sugawra I. Multidrug resistance: role of multidrug resistance-associated protein (MRP). Cancer J 1995; 8:59–61.

24. Ross D. Cellular and pharmacologic aspects of drug resistance in acute myeloid leukemia. Curr Opin Oncol 1991; 3:21–29.

25. Capizzi RL, White JC, Fernandes DJ. Antimetabolites. Baillieres Clin Haematol 1991; 4:15–39.

26. Drahovsky D, Kreis W. Studies on drug resistance-II. Kinase patterns in P815 neoplasms sensitive and resistant to 1-beta-D-arabinofuranosylcytosine. Biochem Pharmacol 1970; 19:940–944.

27. Kramer RA, Zakher J, Kim G. Role of the glutathione redox cycle in acquired and de novo multidrug resistance. Science 1988; 24:694–697.

28. Moscow AM, Cowan KH. Glutathione S-transferase and drug resistance. Cancer Cells 1990; 2:15–22.

29. Mannervik B, Lin P, Guthenberg C, Jensson H, Tahir KM, Warholm M, Jörnval H. Identification of three classes of cytosolic glutathione transferases common to several mammalian species: correlation between structural data and enzymatic properties. Proc Natl Acad Sci USA 1985; 82:7202–7206.

30. Batist G, Tulpule A, Sinha BK, Katki AG, Myers CE, Cowan KH. Overexpression of a novel anionic glutathione transferase in multidrug-resistant human breast cancer cells. J Biol Chem 1986; 261:15544–15549.

31. Gupta V, Singh SV, Ahmad H, Medh RD, Awasthi YC. Glutathione and glutathione S-transferase in a human plasma cell line resistant to melphalan. Biochem Pharmacol 1989; 38:1993–2000.

32. Moscow AM, Townsend AJ, Cowan KH. Elevation of pi-class glutathione S-transferase activity in human breast cancer cells by transfection of the GST-pi gene and its effect on sensitivity to toxins. Mol Pharmacol 1989; 36:22–28.

33. Sinha BK, Mimnaugh EG, Rajagopalan S, Myers CE. Adriamycin activation and oxygen free radical formation in human breast tumor cells: Protective role of glutathione peroxidase in Adriamycin resistance. Cancer Res 1989; 49:3844–3848.

34. Coley HM, Amos WB, Twentyman PR, Workman P. Examination by laser scanning confocal fluorescence imaging microscopy of the subcellular localisation of anthracyclines in pare nt and multidrug resistant cell lines. Br J Cancer 1993; 67:1316–1323.

35. Schuurhuis GJ, van Heijningen THM, Cervantes A, Pinedo HM, De Lange JH, Keizer HG, Broxterman HJ, Baak JPA, Lankelma J. Changes in subcellular doxorubicin distribution and cellular accumulation alone can largely account for doxorubicin resistance in SW-1573 lung cancer and MCF-7 breast cancer multidrug resistant tumour cells. Br J Cancer 1993; 68:898–908.

36. Barrand MA, Rhodes T, Center MS, Twentyman PR. Chemosensitisation and drug accumulation effects of cyclosporin A, PSC-833 and verapamil in human MDR large cell lung cancer cells expressing a 190k membrane protein distinct from P-glycoprotein. Eur J Cancer 1993; 29A:408–415.

37. Simon SM, Schindler M. Cell biological mechanisms of multidrug resistance in tumors. Proc Natl Acad Sci USA 1994; 91:3497–3504.

38. Jolivet J. Methotrexate and leucovorin in malignant blood diseases. Baillieres Clin Haematol 1991; 4:1–11.

39. Jackson RC, Niethammer D. Acquired methotrexate resistance in lymphoblasts resulting from altered kinetic properties of dihydrofolate reductase. Eur J Cancer 1977; 13:567–575.

40. Liu LF. DNA topoisomerase poisons as antitumor drugs. Annu Rev Biochem 1989; 58:351–375.

41. Beck WT, Cirtain MC, Danks MK, Felsted RL, Safa AR, Wolverton JS, Suttle DP, Trent JM. Pharmacological, molecular and cytogenetic analysis of "atypical" multidrug-resistant human leukemic cells. Cancer Res 1987; 47:5455–5460.

42. Green DR, Bissonnette RP, Cotter TG. Apoptosis and cancer. Princ Prac Oncol 1994; 8:1.

43. Dive C, Hickman JA. Drug-target interactions: only the first step in the commitment to a programmed cell death? Br J Cancer 1991; 64:192–196.

44. Scott WL, Ruley HE, Jacks T, Housman DE. p53-dependent apoptosis modulates the cyto-toxicity of anticancer agents. Cell 1993; 74:957–967.

45. Sato H, Preisler H, Day R, Raza A, Larson R, Browman G, Goldberg J, Vogler R, Grunwald H, Gottlieb A, Bennett J, Gottesman M, Pastan I. MDR1 transcript levels as an indication of resistant disease in acute myelogenous leukemia. Br J Haematol 1990; 75:340–345.

46. Marie JP, Zittoun R, Sikic BI. Multidrug resistance (mdr1) gene expression in adult acute leukemias: correlation with treatment outcome and in vitro drug sensitivity. Blood 1991; 78: 586–592.

47. Pirker R, Götzl M, Gsur A, Havelec L, Wallner J, Michl I, Zöchbauer S, Knapp W, Haas O, Linkesch W, Lechner K. MDR-1 gene expression: an independent prognostic factor in acute myeloid leukemia. In: Kaspers GJL, Pieters R, Twentyman PR, Weisenthal LM, Veer-man AJP, eds. Drug Resistance in Leukemia and Lymphoma: The Clinical Value of Labo-ratory Studies. Chur: Harwood, 1993:41–47.

48. Campos L, Guyotat D, Archimbaud E, Calmard-Oriol P, Tsuruo T, Troncy J, Treille D, Fiere D. Clinical significance of multidrug resistance P-glycoprotein expression on acute nonlymphoblastic leukemia cells at diagnosis. Blood 1992; 79:473–476.

49. Ball ED, Lawrence D, Malnar M, Ciminelli N, Mayer D, Wurster-Hill A, Davey FR, Bloom-field CD. Correlation of CD34 and multidrug resistance P170 with FAB and cytogenetics but not prognosis in acute myeloid leukemia (AML). Blood 1990; 76:252.

50. Pieters R, Hongo T, Loonen A, Huismans D, Broxterman H, Hählen K, Veerman A. Dif-ferent types of non-P-glycoprotein mediated multi drug resistance in children with relapsed acute lymphoblastic leukemia. Br J Cancer 1992; 65:691–697.

51. Gosaguen J, Dossot J, Fardel O, Le Mee F, Le Gall E, Leblay R, Leprise P, Chaperon J, Fauchet R. Expression of the multidrug resistance associated P-glycoprotein (P-170) in 59 cases of de novo acute lymphoblastic leukemia: prognostic implications. Blood 1993; 81: 2394–2398.

52. Tidefelt U, Elmhorn-Resenborg A, Paul C, Hao XY, Mannervik B, Eriksson LC. Expression of glutathione transferase pi as a predictor for treatment results at different stages of acute nonlymphoblastic leukemia. Cancer Res 1992; 52:3281–3285.

53. Koberda J, Hellmann A. Glutathione S-transferase activity of leukemic cells as a prognostic factor for response to chemotherapy in acute leukemias. Med Oncol Tumor Pharmacother 1991; 8:35–38.

54. Zhou DC, Hoang-Ngoc L, Delmer A, Faussat AM, Russo D, Zittoun R, Marie JP. Expres-sion of resistance genes in acute leukemia. Leuk Lymphoma 1994; 13(suppl 1):27–30.

55. Burger H, Nooter K, Zaman GJ, Sonneveld P, van Wingerden KE, Oostrum RG, Stoter G. Expression of the multidrug resistance-associated protein (MRP) in acute and chronic leu-kemias. Leukemia 1994; 8:990–997.

56. McKenna SL, West RR, Whittaker JA, Padua RA, Holmes JA. Topoisomerase II alpha expression in acute myeloid leukemia and its relationship to clinical outcome. Leukemia 1994; 8:1498–1502.

57. Kaufmann SH, Karp JE, Jones RJ, Miller CB, Schneider E, Zwelling LA, Cowan K, Wendel K, Burke PJ. Topoisomerase II levels and drug sensitivity in adult acute myelogenous leu-kemia. Blood 1994; 15:83, 517–530.

58. Pappenheimer AM. Experimental studies upon lymphocytes. I. The reactions of lympho-cytes under various experimental conditions. J Exp Med 1917; 25:633.

59. Black MM, Speer FD. Further observations on the effects of cancer chemotherapeutic agents on the in vitro dehydrogenase activity of cancer tissue. J Natl Cancer Inst 1954; 14:1147–1158.
60. Schrek R. In vitro methods for measuring viability and vitality of lymphocytes exposed to 45 degree, 47 degree, and 50 degree C. Cryobiology 1965; 2:122–128.
61. Schrek R, Dolowy WC. In vitro cytotoxicity of L-asparaginase on rodent and human neoplastic cells. Lancet 1970; 2:722.
62. Hamburger AW, Salmon SE. Primary bioassay of human tumor cells. Science 1977; 54: 2475–2479.
63. Salmon SE, Hamburger SW, Soehlen B, Durie BGM, Alberts DS, Moon TE. Quantitation of differential sensitivity of human-tumor stem cells to anticancer drugs. N Engl J Med 1978; 298:1321–1327.
64. Buick RN, Pollak MN. Perspectives on clonogenic tumor cells, stem cells, and oncogenes. Cancer Res 1984; 44:4909–4918.
65. Preisler HD, Azarnia N. Assessment of the drug sensitivity of acute nonlymphocytic leukemia using the in vitro clonogenic assay. Br J Haematol 1984; 58:361–367.
66. Smith PJ, Lihou MG. Prediction of remission induction in childhood acute myeloid leukemia. Aust N Z J Med 1986; 16:39–42.
67. Dow LW, Dahl GV, Kalwinsky DK, Mirro J, Nash MB, Roberson PK. Correlation of drug sensitivity in vitro with clinical response in childhood acute myeloid leukemia. Blood 1986; 68:400–405.
68. Selby P, Buick RN, Tannock I. A critical appraisal of the "human tumor stem cell assay." N Engl J Med 1983; 308:129–134.
69. Weisenthal LM, Lippman ME. Clonogenic and nonclonogenic in vitro chemosensitivity assays. Cancer Treat Rep 1985; 69:615–632.
70. Weisenthal LM, Su YZ, Duarte TE, Nagourney RA. Non-clonogenic, in vitro assays for predicting sensitivity to cancer chemotherapy. Prog Clin Biol Res 1988; 276:75–92.
71. Drexler HG. Which cells do respond during in vitro stimulation of B-CLL and HCL cultures? Leukemia 1989; 3:240–241.
72. Veerman AJP, Pieters R. Annotation. Drug sensitivity assays in leukemia and lymphoma. Br J Haematol 1990; 74:381–384.
73. Kern DH, Sondak VK, Morgan CR, Hildebrandt-Zanki SU. Clinical application of the thymidine incorporation assay. Ann Clin Lab Sci 1987; 17:383–388.
74. Kern D, Weisenthal L. Highly specific prediction of antineoplastic drug resistance with an in vitro assay using suprapharmacologic drug exposures. J Natl Cancer Inst 1990; 82:582–586.
75. Fruehauf JP, Bosanquet AG. In vitro determination of drug response: a discussion of clinical applications. Princ Prac Oncol 1993; 7:1–16.
76. Mattern J, Volm M. Clinical relevance of predictive tests for cancer chemotherapy. Cancer Treat Rev 1982; 9:267–298.
77. Lepri E, Liberati M, Menconi E, Santucci A, Piselli F, Barzi A. In vitro chemosensitivity testing in acute leukemia. Results of a retrospective study. Anticancer Res 1990; 10:1735–1738.
78. Schwarzmeier JD, Paietta E, Mittermayer K, Pirker R. Prediction of the response to chemotherapy in acute leukemia by a short-term test in vitro. Cancer 1984; 53:390–395.
79. Silvestrini R, Sanfilippo O, Daidoni MG, Zaffaroni N. Predictive relevance for clinical outcome of in vitro sensitivity evaluated through antimetabolic assay. Recent Results Cancer Res 1984; 94:140–150.
80. Löwenberg B, van Putten WLJ, Touw IP, Delwel R, Santini V. Autonomous proliferation of leukemic cells in vitro as a determinant of prognosis in adult acute myeloid leukemia. N Engl J Med 1993; 328:614–619.
81. Weisenthal LM, Marsden JA, Dill PL, Macaluso CK. A novel dye exclusion method for testing in vitro chemosensitivity of human tumors. Cancer Res 1983; 43:749–757.

82. Weisenthal LM, Dill PL, Kurnick NB, Lippman ME. Comparison of dye exclusion assays with a clonogenic assay in the determination of drug-induced cytotoxicity. Cancer Res 1993; 43:258–264.

83. Bird MC, Bosanquet AG, Gillby ED. In vitro determination of tumor sensitivity in haematological malignancies. Hematol Oncol 1985; 3:1–9.

84. Bosanquet AG. Correlations between therapeutic response of leukemias and in vitro drug-sensitivity assay. Lancet 1991; 1:711–714.

85. Weisenthal LM, Dill PL, Finklestein JZ, Duarte TE, Baker JA, Moran EM. Laboratory detection of primary and acquired drug resistance in human lymphatic neoplasms. Cancer Treat Rep 1986; 70:1283–1295.

86. Bird MC, Bosanquet AG, Forskitt S, Gillby ED. Longterm comparison of results of a drug-sensitivity assay in vitro with patient response in lymphatic neoplasms. Cancer 1988; 61: 1104–1109.

87. Tidefelt U, Sundman-Engberg B, Rhedin A-S, Paul C. In vitro drug testing in patients with acute leukemia with incubations mimicking in vivo intracellular drug concentrations. Eur J Haematol 1989; 43:374–384.

88. Suto A, Kubota T, Yutaka S, Ishibiki K, Abe O. MTT assay with reference to the clinical effect of chemotherapy. J Surg Oncol 1989; 42:28–32.

89. Pieters R, Huismans DR, Leyva A, Veerman AJP. Comparison of a rapid automated MTT assay with a dye-exclusion assay for chemosensitivity testing of childhood leukemia. Br J Cancer 1989; 59:217–220.

90. Twentyman PR, Fox NE, Rees JKH. Chemosensitivity testing of fresh leukemia cells using the MTT colorimetric assay. Br J Haematol 1989; 71:19–24.

91. Sargent JM, Taylor CG. Appraisal of the MTT-assay as a rapid test of chemosensitivity in acute myeloid leukemia. Br J Cancer 1989; 60:206–210.

92. Hongo T, Fujii Y, Igarashi Y. An in vitro chemosensitivity test for the screening of anti-cancer drugs in childhood leukemia. Cancer 1990; 15:1263–1272.

93. Pieters R, Huisman DR, Loonen A, Hählan K, Van der Does-van den Berg A, Van Wering ER, Veerman AJP. Relation of cellular drug resistance to long-term clinical outcome in childhood acute lymphoblastic leukemia. Lancet 1991; 338:399–403.

94. Mosmann T. Rapid colorimetric assay for cellular growth and survival. Application to proliferation and cytotoxicity assays. J Immunol Meth 1983; 65:55–63.

95. Kirkpatrick DL, Duke M, Goh TS. Chemosensitivity testing of fresh human leukemia cells using both a dye exclusion assay and a tetrazolium dye (MTT) assay. Leuk Res 1990; 14: 459–466.

96. Rotman B, Papermaster BW. Membrane properties of living mammalian cells studied by enzymatic hydrolysis of fluorogenic esters. Proc Natl Acad Sci USA 1966; 55:134–141.

97. Larsson R, Nygren P. Pharmacological modification of multi-drug resistance (MDR) in vitro detected by a novel fluorometric microculture cytotoxicity assay. Reversal of resistance and selective cytotoxic actions of cyclosporin A and verapamil on MDR leukemia T-cells. Int J Cancer 1990; 46:67–72.

98. Larsson R, Nygren P, Ekberg M, Slater L. Chemotherapeutic drug sensitivity testing of human leukemia cells in vitro using a semiautomated fluorometric assay. Leukemia 1990; 4:567–571.

99. Larsson R, Kristensen J, Sandberg C, Nygren P. Laboratory determination of chemotherapeutic drug resistance in tumor cells from patients with leukemia, using a fluorometric microculture cytotoxicity assay (FMCA). Int J Cancer 1992; 51:177–185.

100. Nygren P, Kristensen J, Jonsson B, Sundström C, Lönnerholm G, Kreuger A, Larsson R. Feasibility of the Fluorometric Microculture Cytotoxicity Assay (FMCA) for cytotoxic drug sensitivity testing of tumor cells from patients with acute lymphoblastic leukemia. Leukemia 1992; 6:1121–1128.

101. Kristensen J, Jonsson B, Sundström C, Nygren P, Larsson R. In vitro analysis of drug resistance in tumor cells from patients with acute myelocytic leukemia. Med Oncol Tumor Pharmacother 1992; 9:65–74.

102. Larsson R, Jonsson B, Kristensen J, Öberg G, Simonsson B, Sundström C, Lönnerholm G, Kreuger A, Glimelius B, Hagberg H, Nygren P. Drug sensitivity testing of tumor cells from patients with acute leukemia and non-Hodgkin's lymphoma using a fluorometric microculture cytotoxicity assay. In: Kaspers GJL, Pieters R, Twentyman PR, Weisenthal LM, Veerman AJP, eds. Drug Resistance in Leukemia and Lymphoma. The Clinical Value of Laboratory Studies. Chur: Harwood, 1993:399–407.

103. Kangas L, Gronroos M, Nieminen AL. Bioluminescence of cellular ATP: a new method for evaluating cytotoxic agents in vitro. Med Biol 1984; 62:338–343.

104. Nishiyama M, Takagami S, Kirihara Y, Saeki T, Niimi K, Nosoh Y, Hirabayashi N, Niimoto M, Hattori T. The indications of chemosensitivity tests against various anticancer agents. Jpn J Surg 1988; 18:647–652.

105. Kumits R, Rumbold H, Muller MM, et al. The use of bioluminescence to evaluate the influence of chemotherapeutic drugs on ATP levels of malignant cell lines. J Clin Chem Biochem 1986; 24:293–296.

106. Rhedin AS, Tidefelt U, Jonsson K, Lundin A, Paul C. Comparison of a bioluminescence assay with differential staining cytotoxicity for cytostatic drug testing in vitro in human leukemic cells. Leuk Res 1993; 17:271–276.

107. Von Hoff DD, Casper J, Bradley E, Sandbach J, Jones D, Makuch R. Association between human tumor colony-forming assay results and response of an individual patient's tumor to chemotherapy. Am J Med 1981; 70:1027–1032.

108. Von Hoff DD. Send this patient's tumor for culture and sensitivity. N Engl J Med 1983; 308:154–155.

109. Bosanquet AG, Bell PB. Handling requirements to achieve active drugs in in vitro drug sensitivity and resistance assays. In: Kaspers GJL, Pieters R, Twentyman PR, Weisenthal LM, Veerman AJP, eds. Drug Resistance in Leukemia and Lymphoma. The Clinical Value of Laboratory Studies. Chur: Harwood, 1993:227–255.

110. Wilbur DW, Camacho ES, Hilliard DA, Dill PL, Weisenthal LM. Chemotherapy of non-small cell lung carcinoma guided by an in vitro drug resistance assay measuring total tumour cell kill. Br J Cancer 1992; 65:27–32.

111. Weisenthal LM. Predictive assays for drug and radiation resistance. In: Masters JRW, ed. Human Cancer in Primary Culture, A Handbook. Boston: Kluwer Academic Publishers, 1991:103–147.

112. Sox HC, Blatt MA, Higgins MC, Marton KI. Medical Decision-Making. Stoneham: Butterworths, 1990:67–111.

113. Weisenthal LM. Clinical correlations for cell culture assays based on the concept of total tumor cell kill. In: Köchli OR, Sevin B-U, Haller ?, eds. Chemosensitivity Testing in Gynecologic Malignancies and Breast Cancer. Contrib. Gynecol. Obstet. Basel: Karger, 1994: 82–90.

114. Von Hoff DD, Clark GM, Stogdill BJ, Sarosdy MF, O'Brien MT, Casper JT, Mattox DE, Cruz AB, Sandbach JF. Prospective clinical trial of a human tumor cloning system. Cancer Res 1983; 43:1926–1931.

115. Yamaue H, Tanimura H, Tsunoda T, Tani M, Iwahashi M, Noguchi K, Tamai M, Hotta T, Arii K. Chemosensitivity testing with highly purified fresh human tumour cells with the MTT colorimetric assay. Eur J Cancer 1991; 27:1258–1263.

116. Gazdar AF, Steinberg SM, Russell EK, et al. Correlation of in vitro drug sensitivity testing results with response to chemotherapy and survival in extensive-stage small cell lung cancer: a prospective clinical trial. J Natl Cancer Inst 1990; 82:117–123.

117. Hryniuk W. Average relative dose intensity and the impact on design of clinical trials. Semin Oncol 1987; 14:65–74.

118. Evans R, Relling M. Clinical pharmacokinetics-pharmacodynamics of anticancer drugs. Clin Pharmacokinet 1989; 16:327–336.

119. Galpin AJ, Evans WE. Therapeutic drug monitoring in cancer management. Clin Chem 1993; 39:2419–2430.

120. Morris R, Kotasek D, Paltridge G. Disposition of epirubicin and metabolites with repeated courses to cancer patients. Eur J Clin Pharmacol 1991; 40:481–487.

121. Desoize B, Robert P. Individual dose adaptation of anticancer drugs. Eur J Cancer 1994; 30A:844–851.

122. Borsi J, Moe P. Systemic clearance of methotrexate in the prognosis of acute leukemia in children. Cancer Treat Rep 1987; 20:3020–3024.

123. Koren G, Ferrazini G, Sulh H, Langevin AM, Kapulushnik J, Klein Geisbrecht E, Soldin S, Greenberg M. Systemic exposure to mercaptopurine as a prognostic factor in acute lymphocytic leukemia in children. N Engl J Med 1990; 323:17–21.

124. Rodman J, Abromowitch M, Sinkule J, Rivera GK, Evans WE. Clinical pharmacodynamics of continuous infusion teniposide: systemic exposure as a determinant of response in a phase I trial. J Clin Oncol 1987; 5:1007–1014.

125. Lu K, Yap HY, Loo TL. Clinical pharmacodynamics of vinblastine by continuous intravenous infusion. Cancer Res 1983; 43:1405–1408.

126. Preisler HD, Gessner T, Azarnia N, Bolanowska W, Epstein J, Early J, D'Arrigo P, Vogler R, Winton L, Chervenik P. Relationship between plasma Adriamycin levels and the outcome of remission induction therapy for acute nonlymphocytic leukemia. Cancer Chemother Pharmacol 1984; 12:125–130.

127. Sandström M, Freijs A, Larsson R, Nygren P, Fjällskog M-L, Bergh J, Karlsson MO. Lack of relationship between systemic exposure for the component drugs of the FEC regimen in breast cancer patients. J Clin Oncol (submitted).

128. Liliemark J, Dixon DO, Plunkett W. The relationship between 1-B-D-arabino-furanosylcytosine in plasma to 1-B-D-arabino-furanosylcytosine 5-triphosphate in leukemic cells during treatment with high dose 1-B-D-arabino-furanosylcytosine. Cancer Res 1985; 5: 5952–5960.

129. Plunkett W, Iancoboni S, Estey E, Danhauser L, Liliemark JO, Keating M. Pharmacologically directed ara-C therapy for refractory leukemia. Semin Oncol 1985; 12(suppl 3):20–30.

130. Lennard L, Lilleyman JS. Variable mercaptopurine metabolism and treatment outcome in childhood lymphoblastic leukemia. J Clin Oncol 1989; 7:1816–1823.

131. Paalzow L. Therapeutic monitoring of anticancer drugs. In: Domelöf L, ed. Drug Delivery in Cancer Treatment. Berlin: Springer-Verlag, 1990:85–96.

132. Buffington DE, Lampasona V, Chandler HH. Computers in pharmacokinetics. Clin Pharmacokinet 1993; 25:205–216.

133. Stoller RG, Hande KR, Jacobs SA, Rosenberg SA, Chabner BA. Use of plasma pharmacokinetics to predict and prevent methotrexate toxicity. N Engl J Med 1977; 297:630–634.

134. Ratain MJ, Mick R, Berezin F, Janisch L, Schilsky RL, Williams SF, Smiddy J. Paradoxical relationship between acetylator phenotype and amonafide toxicity. Clin Pharmacol Ther 1991; 50:573–579.

135. Preisler HD. Determinants of response and prediction of response to chemotherapy in acute myelogenous leukemia. Baillieres Clin Haematol 1991; 4:68–82.

136. Preisler HD, Raza A, Baccarani M. Proliferative advantage rather than classical drug resistance as the cause of treatment failure in chronic myelogenous leukemia. Leuk Lymphoma 1993; 11(suppl 1):303–306.

137. Preisler HD, Raza A, Larson R, LeBeau M, Browman G, Goldberg J, Grunwald H, Volger R, Verkh L, Singh P, Block AM, Sandberg A. Protooncogene expression and the clinical characteristics of acute nonlymphocytic leukemia: a leukemia intergroup pilot study. Blood 1989; 73:255–266.

138. Preisler HD, Raza A, Kukla C, Larson R, Goldberg J. Browman G. IL-1B expression and treatment outcome in acute myelogenous leukemia (AML). Blood 1991; 78:849–850.
139. Koeffler HP, Amatruda T, Ikekawa N, Kobayashi Y, DeLucca HF. Induction of macrophage differentiation of human normal and leukemic myeloid stem cells by dihydroxyvitamin D3 and its fluorinated analogues. Cancer Res 1984; 44:5664–5628.
140. Preisler HD, Raza A. Alteration of the proliferative rate of acute myelogenous leukemia cells in vivo in patients. Blood 1992; 80:1–4.
141. Yin M, Gopal V, Banavali SD, Preisler HD. Effects of an IL-1B receptor antagonist on acute myelogenous leukemia cells. Leukemia 1992; 6:898–901.
142. Preisler HD, Larson RA, Raza A, Browman G, Goldberg J, Volger R, Day R, Gotlieb A, Vardiman JW, Bennett J, Kukla C, Grunwald H. The treatment of patients with newly diagnosed poor prognosis acute myelogenous leukemia: response to treatment and treatment failure. Br J Haematol 1991; 79:390–397.
143. Preisler HD, Sati H, Yang P, Wilson M, Kaufman C, Watt R. Assessment of c-myc expression in individual leukemic cells. Leuk Res 1988; 12:507–516.

# 12

## Determinants of Estramustine Resistance

**Lisa A. Speicher**
*Wyeth-Ayerst Research, Philadelphia, Pennsylvania*

**Kenneth D. Tew**
*Fox Chase Cancer Center, Philadelphia, Pennsylvania*

### DRUG STRUCTURE/FUNCTION ANALYSIS

Over the past three decades, a number of steroid–alkylating agent conjugates have been synthesized and tested for antitumor potential. Estramustine is a conjugate of estradiol and nor-nitrogen mustard linked by a carbamate ester. The feature that distinguishes estramustine from other similar conjugates is the N–C=O motif (Fig. 1). The carbamate is especially resistant to enzymatic cleavage. An agent such as prednimustine (a prednisolone ester of chlorambucil) has an ester linkage, which is readily hydrolyzed by serum esterases. The presence of the carbamate group in estramustine creates a substrate with a biological half-life in humans that is greater than 16 h (1). This stabilization by the carbamate group has produced a drug with an unpredicted and unexpected mechanism of action.

Conceptually, the estradiol portion of this molecule was designed to facilitate uptake by steroid receptors in malignant cells. The nitrogen mustard alkylating moiety would be released intracellularly to exert cytotoxicity, following cleavage of both the carbamate and ester bonds shown in Figure 1. In its proprietary form, Estracyt has a phosphate group at the 17$\beta$ position of the steroid D ring. This substituent makes the molecule more water soluble and thus more suitable for clinical administration. The drug is readily absorbed following oral administration, with relatively rapid dephosphorylation by serum and intracellular phosphatases. A complication, noted in early clinical studies, involves the formation of an insoluble calcium phosphate salt of estramustine. This occurs when the drug is administered with antacids or with a diet high in calcium (such as dairy products). The calcium phosphate salt formed is not amenable to intestinal absorption, resulting in a significant reduction in bioavailability and a substantial reduction from the presumed administered dose of the drug (2). Such issues have served to complicate the interpretation of early clinical trials with estramustine.

With the generalities of these structure-activity relationships in mind, hydrated and anhydrous crystals of estramustine were grown and the crystal and molecular structures of the drug determined by x-ray crystallographic techniques (3). The mustard

279

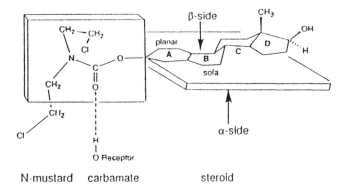

**Figure 1** Diagram of features of the molecular structure of estramustine, showing intermolecular interactions that may be significant in its binding in vivo. (From Ref. 3.)

substituents had little effect on the overall conformation of the steroid nucleus, so that it resembled that found in estradiol. One chlorine atom of the mustard group was found to make a close contact (3.13 Å) with the nitrogen atom. This favorable Cl–N interaction may be important for the inherent stability of estramustine. It is also possible that the chlorine atoms hinder accessibility to the carbamate group by hydrolytic enzymes.

Figure 1 shows that the carbamate group, the three carbon atoms bonded directly to the nitrogen of the mustard group, and the C(3) of the steroid all line in a plane. The steroid ring system is, in each case, approximately perpendicular to this carbamate plane. The carbonyl of the carbamate group points to the α side of the steroid. The nitrogen atom of the carbamate group is not involved in hydrogen bonding, but the oxygen of the carbonyl is capable of hydrogen bonding to target proteins. The x-ray diffraction analysis has shown that the carbamate group, with a short C–N bond (Fig. 1) analogous to that found in peptides, has considerable double-bond character, thereby precluding formation of an aziridine ring. In effect, the carbamate has converted the mustard nitrogen atom from an amine to an amide, thereby obviating the drug's alkylating potential.

An overview of the structures of many antimitotic drugs shows that an aminocarboxyalkyl group occurs in many of them. By a series of chemical substitution studies, Gupta (4) was able to show that the antimicrotubule properties of nocodazole and other benzimidazole carbamates were diminished or abolished if the aminocarboxylalkyl group was replaced by another group. Many other antimicrotubule agents have this motif in their structure, including the simplest, isopropyl-*N*-phenylcarbamate. Furthermore, virtually all antimicrotubule drugs have aliphatic or aromatic ring substituents of varying degrees of complexity (5), indicating that binding must involve not only hydrogen bonding but also hydrophobic interactions. This would explain the noncovalent reversible effects of estramustine on the cytoskeletons of cells in culture (6). Substituents that alter the planarity and/or hydrophobicity of the ring structures can influence the binding of the drug to its target protein. The steroid ring of estramustine provides a hydrophobicity that contributes to overall binding. The antimitotic properties of diethylstilbestrol (7,8), although certainly not its primary pharmacological property, also indicate the possible role of the planar hydrophobic aromatic groups of this agent in binding to microtubule structures.

In fact, structural explanations of noncovalent binding to protein targets were secondary to the early observations that questioned the alkylating agent classification (9,10). The intervening decade has provided evidence for a fascinating dualistic antitumor activity. Antimicrotubule activity is accompanied by testosterone lowering potential (in vivo) and the drug has recently gone through a renaissance period, gaining widespread usage in the clinical management of hormone-refractory prostate carcinoma.

## PRECLINICAL PHARMACOLOGY—MECHANISM OF ACTION

An appreciation of the complexity of the cytoskeleton of cells is important in defining the mechanisms of action of chemotherapeutic agents that target microtubule components. Neoplastic cell growth is less sensitive to changes in cell shape than that of normal cells, which exhibit a growth control tightly coupled to morphology. Tumor progression is hypothesized to be correlated to altered cellular morphology through a failure of the cytoskeleton to transduce cell shape and surface signals (11). In addition, the metastatic ability of malignant cells is greatly increased when they are grown on nonadhesive surfaces and lose their "well-spread" morphology (12). Thus, it is likely that the morphology of a cell is somehow involved in expression of the malignant phenotype.

The cell's internal architecture or cytoskeleton consists of a complex network of filamentous proteins that are involved in a plurality of functions, including (1) regulation of cell shape, adhesion, and cell-cell interactions; (2) cell division; (3) cell motility; and (4) intracellular organelle movement and protein synthesis. The three principal components of the cytoskeleton are actin microfilaments, intermediate filaments, and microtubules. A number of accessory proteins link these components together as well as to other cellular structures. In addition, accessory proteins play an important role in the regulation of actin and microtubule polymerization and depolymerization.

Most of the anticancer agents currently employed that target the cytoskeleton do so through interactions with the microtubules. Although a great number of both natural and synthetic compounds are effective microtubule poisons, the number of agents affecting either actin or intermediate filaments are quite sparse. This could indicate a more important role of functioning microtubules with respect to cell viability and proliferation as compared to the microfilaments/intermediate filaments. However, this does raise an interesting question as to why a protein as abundant as actin is such a poor target for anticancer agents. Because actin is so well conserved throughout the various phyla, it is unlikely that a significant therapeutic advantage could be gained through tumor–normal cell differences in actin expression. Although similar arguments could be applied to microtubules and by extension tubulin and microtubule-associated proteins (MAPs), heterogeneity of expression and the presence of multiple tubulin isoforms serves to broaden the "target base" for these drugs. In addition, the reduced role of actin in mitotic spindle formation presumably serves to make it a less critical target in dividing cells.

Microtubules are polymers formed by the energy-dependent assembly of heterodimer subunits, $\alpha$ and $\beta$ tubulins (13). Microtubules are present in all eukaryotic cells. A group of proteins, collectively referred to as microtubule-associated proteins (MAPs), has been described on the basis of their ability to associate physically with microtubules, stimulate microtubule assembly, and/or stabilize microtubules under conditions that would normally lead to disassembly (14,15). The best-characterized MAPs are found in brain tissue and include a group of high-molecular-weight (MW) proteins, MAP1, MAP2, and a group of proteins of intermediate MW, collectively referred to as tau. The MAPs in tumor tissue and cell lines have been less well characterized, but appear to include MAP1 and a group of proteins with MW between 120 kd and 210 kd, including MAP4. The expression of these MAPs varies according to cell and tissue type (15,16).

Estramustine-induced destabilization of the structural and functional aspects of microtubules has been fairly extensively covered in the literature in the past 5–10 years. In vitro experiments showed that estramustine (EM) and estramustine phosphate inhibit microtubule assembly (17,18), bind MAP2 and tau (19,20), and cause the dissociation of MAP1 and MAP2 from paclitaxel-stabilized isolated microtubules (20). Based on such results, it was suggested that estramustine exerted its cytotoxic properties by interaction with the MAP component of microtubules. More recently, direct EM effects upon tubulin polymerization have been reported (21), and these authors have suggested that the antimicrotubule properties of the drug are mediated by tubulin binding. Demonstration of specific binding to both tubulin and MAPs was achieved by design and synthesis of a photoaffinity analogue of estramustine (Fig. 2) (22). This analogue, 17-O-[[2-[3-(4[azido-3-[$^{125}$I]]iodophenyl)-propionamido]ethyl]carbamyl]estradiol-3-N-bis(2-chloroethyl)carbamate ([$^{125}$I]AIPP-EM), was reacted in competition assays with cytoskeletal protein preparations from a number of sources. By attaching the photoaffinity ligand to the 17β-position of the steroid D-ring, the basic pharmacological and cytotoxic properties of the drug were maintained. In cytoskeletal protein preparations from human prostate carcinoma cells (DU 145) or a clonally selected, estramustine-resistant cell line (E4), the major MAP present was MAP4. In both cytoskeletal fractions and reconstituted microtubules, [$^{125}$I]AIPP-EM bound to both MAP4 and tubulin. From competition assays, the apparent binding constant for MAP4 from DU 145 cells was 15 μM. Similar calculations for tubulin gave values of 13 μM (E4 cells). The identification of these cytoskeletal proteins as specific drug targets provides a direct explanation for the antimicrotubule and antimitotic effects of estramustine. It does not, however, distinguish between the contribution of each interaction in delineating such effects. It is apparent from Figures 3 and 4 that tubulin is the most prevalent of the drug targets, and it is also the most common protein in these preparations. Also of note is the fact that the binding constants of other antimicrotubule drugs for tubulin are generally 1–3 log units lower than those we report for estramustine. Indeed, although many of the antimicrotubule effects that are produced by estramustine are

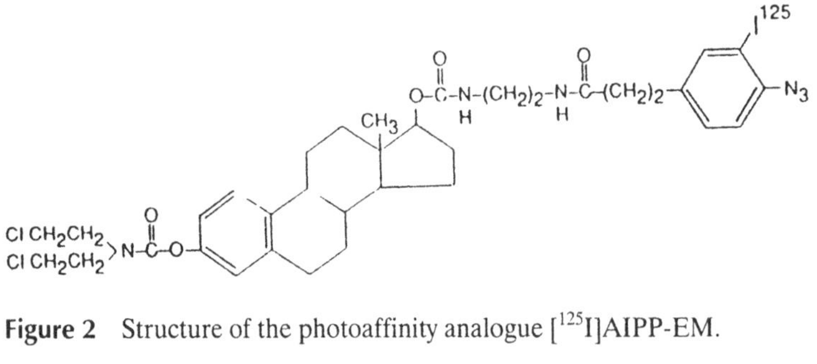

**Figure 2**   Structure of the photoaffinity analogue [$^{125}$I]AIPP-EM.

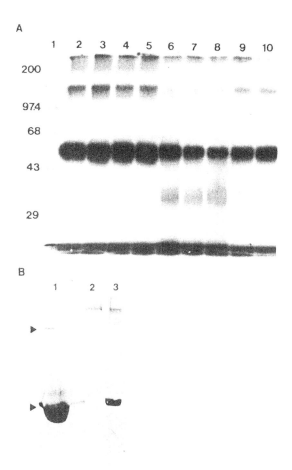

**Figure 3** (A) Photolabeling of reconstituted microtubules separated by 8% SDS-PAGE. Bovine tubulin was used to purify MAP4 from wild-type DU 145 cells. Large molar excesses of bovine tubulin were used to facilitate purification of MAP4. Competitive concentrations of unlabeled estramustine were as follows: lane 1, molecular mass markers; lane 2, $0\ \mu$M; lane 3, 0.1 $\mu$M; lane 4, $1.0\ \mu$M; lane 5, $10\ \mu$M; lane 6, $20\ \mu$M; lane 7, $30\ \mu$M; lane 8, $50\ \mu$M; lane 9, $75\ \mu$M; lane 10, $100\ \mu$M. (B) Lane 1, Western blot of purified bovine brain tubulin probed with a monoclonal antibody to $\beta$-tubulin. Monomeric and dimeric bovine tubulin bands are apparent (*arrowheads*). Lane 2, Western blot of the MAP4-enriched extract from DU 145 cells probed with anti-MAP4 polyclonal antibody. Lane 3, Western blot of the microtubule pellet from the polymerization of bovine tubulin with the MAP4 extract, probed with both anti-$\beta$-tubulin and anti-MAP4 antibodies. *A* and *B* represent different gels run for different lengths of time, and therefore the tubulin bands exhibited different migration rates. (From Ref. 22.)

consistent with those of standard tubulin-binding agents, the cytotoxicity profiles are distinct (23). In addition, the synergistic antimitotic and cytotoxic effects of estramustine in combination with vinblastine (24) or paclitaxel (25) argue against duplicate or overlapping effects, because purely additive antimicrotubule and cytotoxic effects would then be predicted. Thus, the antimicrotubule and antimitotic properties of estramustine could conceivably be the product of the combined MAP and tubulin binding.

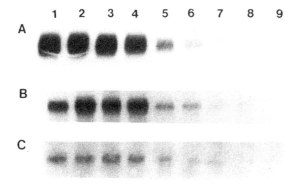

**Figure 4** Photolabeling of tubulin purified from bovine brain (A), DU 145 wild-type cells (B), and E4 cells (C). Increasing concentrations of unlabeled estramustine were used with 1 nm [$^{125}$I]AIPP-EM and 0.03–0.1 $\mu$M tubulin. (A) Drug concentrations were as follows: lane 1, 0 $\mu$M; lane 2, 0.1 $\mu$M; lane 3, 1 $\mu$M; lane 4, 10 $\mu$M; lane 5, 20 $\mu$M; lane 6, 30 $\mu$M; lane 7, 50 $\mu$M; lane 8, 75 $\mu$M; lane 9, 100 $\mu$M. (B) and (C). Drug concentrations were as follows: lane 1, 0 $\mu$M; lane 2, 0.1 $\mu$M; lane 3, 1 $\mu$M; lane 4, 10 $\mu$M; lane 5, 25 $\mu$M; lane 6, 35 $\mu$M; lane 7, 50 $\mu$M; lane 8, 75 $\mu$M; lane 9, 100 $\mu$M. Data are representative blots from at least three experiments. (From Ref. 22.)

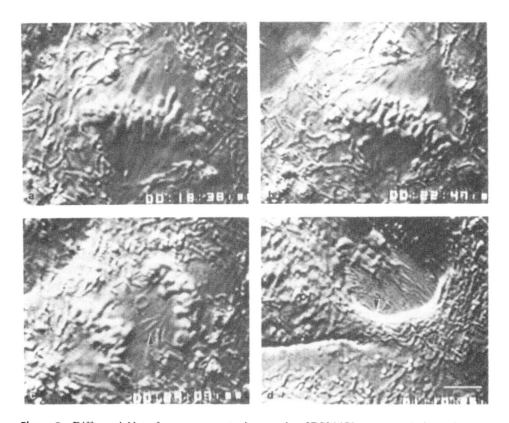

**Figure 5** Differential interference contrast micrographs of DU 145 human prostatic carcinoma cells treated with 60 $\mu$M estramustine after the onset of anaphase (between a and b). -a-: meta-phase, -b-, -c-: anaphase; mitochondria in the spindle zone are indicated by the arrowhead in (c). -d-: cytokinesis, cleavage furrow represented by arrowhead. Bar equals 10 $\mu$m. (From Ref. 26.)

**Table 1** Estramustine Treatment During Anaphase

|  | Mean metaphase pole-to-pole distance ($\mu$M) prior to addition of drug[a] | Mean anaphase spindle pole separation ($\mu$M)[b,c] | Individual high/low values for anaphase chromosome separation ($\mu$M) |
|---|---|---|---|
| Control | 19.5 ± 2.19 (N=7) | 28.7 ± 2.39 (N=8) | 32.5/25.3 |
| 2.5 $\mu$M | 19.1 ± 1.97 (N=5) | 25.0 ± 2.20 (N=8) | 27.7/21.7 |
| 10 $\mu$M | 19.1 ± 1.09 (N=8) | 22.0 ± 21.0 (N=8) | 24.1/17.6 |
| 30 $\mu$M | 18.6 ± 0.94 (N=7) | 20.1 ± 2.27 (N=8) | 24.1/17.6 |
| 60 $\mu$M | 18.9 ± 1.43 (N=8) | 18.7 ± 3.08 (N=8) | 22.9/14.5 |

[a]The means of controls vs. each treated population are not significantly different ($p > .05$).
[b]The means of controls vs. each treated population are significantly different ($p < .05$).
[c]Anaphase spindle pole separation was measured as the distance from the centrosomal side of each separated chromosome set prior to the onset of cytokinesis.
*Source*: Reprinted from Ref. 26.

Video-enhanced differential interference contrast (DIC) microscopy (Fig. 5) has been used to examine the effects of estramustine on dividing human prostate cancer cell lines (26,27). The mitotic progression of a number of individual cells was followed: estramustine was found to delay the onset of anaphase, to reduce the anaphase spindle-pole elongation (anaphase B, Table 1), and to delay cytokinesis. The integrity of the spindle apparatus was also disrupted. Infiltration of the spindle area by mitochondria was apparent in drug-treated cells.

## IN VITRO RESISTANCE

A number of drug-resistant cell lines have been developed by exposing cultures to incrementally increased concentrations of estramustine and selecting for an acquired resistant phenotype (27). These resistant cell lines, cultured in the continued presence of estramustine, have acquired a number of morphological adaptations. The cells are smaller, have slightly slower doubling times, and traverse mitosis more quickly. Concomitantly, their mitotic spindles are smaller and they have reduced nodal chromosome numbers (the parent cells are aneuploid), compared with the wild-type cell line (26,27). This in vitro reduction in chromosome complement provides an interesting analogy with a clinical trial that was carried out in the 1970s (28). These investigators found that the DNA contents of tumor cells of poorly differentiated prostate malignancies decreased more after estramustine than after conventional estrogen therapy. The precise cause(s) of this reduction were not investigated; however, their flow cytometry data would certainly be consistent with a loss of chromosomes. Whether this is linked with the development of the acquired resistant phenotype is impossible to predict. Indeed, while it is apparent that estramustine causes chromosome shedding during mitosis (26) and estramustine-resistant cells maintain a lower aneuploid state, whether this is a cause or effect of the resistant phenotype is not yet clear. Although there is a difference in the apparent binding constants of estramustine for tubulin (as determined from the ability of estramustine to prevent labeling by [$^{125}$I]AIPP-EM) from the wild-type

(19.5 $\mu$M) and resistant E4 (24.6 $\mu$M) cells, at present it is not clear whether this is a major factor contributing to the resistant phenotype. There are subsequent changes in the total transcript levels of cytoskeletal elements in resistant cells. Aberrant expression of mRNA for tubulin and MAP4 is found in E4 cells, compared with wild-type cells (29). This may indicate that multiple differences in microtubule regulation and organization may contribute to the resistant phenotype.

Most cell lines resistant to antimicrotubule drugs fall into two categories: (1) efflux mutants (i.e., cells expressing the multidrug-resistant phenotype [MDR]) (30,31) and (2) mutants exhibiting tubulin subunit alterations (32). Frequently, the degree of resistance for the MDR phenotype is many thousandfold. For estramustine, however, resistance levels did not exceed four- to fivefold, and such levels were attained only after multiple rounds of selection in increasing drug concentrations. A series of collateral resistance and biological characterization assays indicated that estramustine resistance is distinct from the MDR phenotype. Estramustine-resistant clones exhibit no cross-resistance to other antimitotic/MDR agents, including doxorubicin, cytochalasin B, paclitaxel, and vinblastine (Table 2). In addition, two cell lines known to be part of the MDR phenotype—SKVLB (human ovarian cells) and ARN (mouse leukemia cells)—do not exhibit increased resistance to estramustine. Finally, estramustine-resistant clones do not express increased mRNA or protein levels of P-glycoprotein. These results led to the conclusion that the estramustine resistance is distinct from the MDR phenotype.

Despite this negative correlate with the MDR phenotype, the photoaffinity analogue of estramustine was shown to be a substrate for the P-glycoprotein of MDR cell lines (33). For example, membrane fractions from a human ovarian carcinoma cell line, SKOV3 and SKVLB1 cells, were analyzed for proteins that could be photoaffinity-labeled with [$^{125}$I]AIPP-EM (Fig. 6). The primary difference between membranes from the multidrug-resistant SKVLB 1 cells and the wild-type SKOV3 cells was the presence of an intensely labeled band at approximately 170 kd. This protein was consistently the heaviest labeled in membranes from SKVLB1 cells and was shown to migrate with P-glycoprotein by Western blot analysis (Fig. 6, panel B). Competition assays with 100 $\mu$M of each agent (equivalent to approximately 100,000 times the concentration of [$^{125}$I]AIPP-EM) demonstrated that binding was substantially reduced by estramustine, vinblastine, progesterone, verapamil, and, to a lesser degree, by paclitaxel. In contrast,

**Table 2** Cross-Resistance of Estramustine-Resistant DU 145 Cells Toward Antimitotic/MDR Drugs

| | IC$_{50}$ values (relative degree of resistance) | | | |
|---|---|---|---|---|
| | Wild type | EMR 4 | EMR 9 | EMR 12 |
| Estramustine ($\mu$g/mL) | 2.8 (1) | 9.2 (3.3) | 8.1 (2.9) | 8.8 (3.2) |
| Doxorubicin (ng/mL) | 6.9 (1) | 8.7 (1.3) | 6.1 (0.9) | 3.0 (0.4) |
| Cytochalasin B ($\mu$g/mL) | 14.0 (1) | 5.0 (0.4) | 5.5 (0.4) | 4.8 (0.3) |
| Paclitaxel (ng/mL) | 2.5 (1) | 1.7 (0.7) | 2.7 (1.1) | 3.1 (1.2) |
| Vinblastine (ng/mL) | 1.8 (1) | 1.6 (0.9) | 1.8 (1.0) | 1.6 (0.9) |

Colony-forming assays were performed in continuous exposure to drug. IC$_{50}$ values were calculated by linear regression analysis of results of at least three experiments performed in triplicate. EMR clones do not exhibit increased resistance to any of the drugs tested; however, an increased sensitivity to cytochalasin B is noted. Source: Reprinted from Ref. 27.

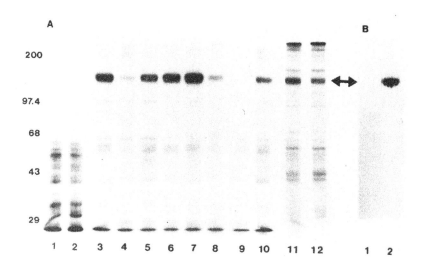

**Figure 6** (A) Photolabeling of membrane proteins from SKOV3 and SKVLB1 cell lines. Fifty micrograms of membrane proteins were incubated with [$^{125}$I]AIPP-estramustine in the presence or absence of 100 $\mu$M unlabeled competitors. Lane(s) 1 and 2: SKOV3 cells; 3–12: SKVLB cells. Lanes 1, 3, and 11: [$^{125}$I]AIPP-estramustine only; 2 and 4: +100 $\mu$M estramustine; 5: +100 $\mu$M estramustine phosphate; 6: +100 $\mu$M estradiol; 7: +100 $\mu$M estriol; 8: +100 $\mu$M progesterone; 9: +100 $\mu$M vinblastine; 10: +100 $\mu$M verapamil; 12: +100 $\mu$M paclitaxel. Numbers on the side indicate molecular weights in kilodaltons. Photolabeling of the ~170 kd P-glycoprotein (*arrow*) is prevalent and competitively inhibited by some of the agents in SKVLB membranes. (B) Western blot analysis for P-glycoprotein detection. Arrow shows ~170 kd protein present in the SKVLB1 (lane 2), but not in SKOV3 (lane 1), which cross-reacts with the P-glycoprotein–specific polyclonal antibody. (From Ref. 33.)

labeling of lower-molecular-weight proteins by [$^{125}$I]AIPP-EM was not significantly reduced by these agents, suggesting high specificity of ligand binding to P-glycoprotein. Essentially no competition of labeling of P-glycoprotein was seen with estramustine phosphate, estradiol, and estriol. These data suggested that the hormonal moiety of estramustine was not a determinant factor in the noncovalent binding of estramustine to the P-glycoprotein.

It is also apparent that the polarity of the competing agents has an influence on the binding assays. Estramustine phosphate is a water-soluble agent that behaves very differently from estramustine under in vitro conditions. Under in vivo conditions, dephosphorylation must occur before the drug can cross the cell membrane. Thus, intracellular drug effects are attributable to the dephosphorylated molecule.

As would be predicted from the high-avidity binding of estramustine to the P-glycoprotein, the drug significantly increased the accumulation of either vinblastine or paclitaxel in the MDR cell line (Fig. 7). Estramustine caused a concentration-dependent enhancement of drug accumulation in the SKVLB1 cells to a maximum of approximately 12-fold. No effect of estramustine was apparent for the wild-type SKOV3 cells. Estramustine was more effective than verapamil in enhancing drug accumulation in SKVLB1 cells (histogram; Fig. 7), allowing [$^3$H]paclitaxel to accumulate to levels at

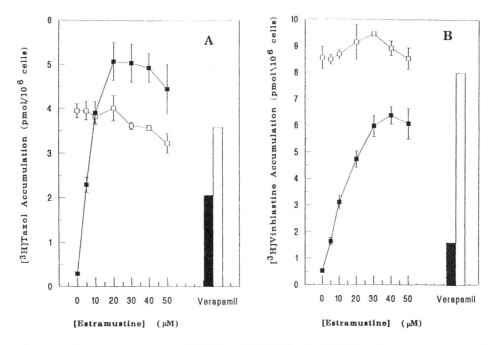

**Figure 7**  Drug accumulation by SKOV3 and SKVLB1 cells. SKOV3 cells (*open symbols*) and SKVLB1 cells (*closed symbols*) were incubated with the indicated concentrations of estramustine for 60 min or with 20 $\mu$M verapamil (histograms) before the addition of 6 nM [$^3$H]paclitaxel (A) or 14 nM [$^3$H]vinblastine (B). In all cases, the cultures were further incubated for 60 min before the levels of intracellular [$^3$H]-drug were determined. Values represent the mean $\pm$ SD for triplicate cultures. (From Ref. 33.)

least as high as those in SKOV3 cells and [$^3$H]vinblastine to 70% of the level in SKOV3 cells. Given such data, it is surprising that estramustine in combination with other MDR drugs did not achieve the same degree of cytotoxicity enhancement as verapamil (33). This was true for dactinomycin, vinblastine, paclitaxel, and daunomycin, although in the case of the first three drugs, some enhancement was observed. The reasons for this difference became apparent when the affinity of estramustine for serum proteins was considered (34). Without serum, the sensitivities of a human breast carcinoma MDR cell line (MCF-7/ADR) to several P-glycoprotein–transported drugs were increased by estramustine and verapamil. Conversely, when the cells were treated with a 10% serum, the cytotoxicities of these drugs were increased by verapamil, but not by estramustine. Without serum, intracellular accumulation of [$^3$H]vinblastine and [$^3$H]paclitaxel by MCF-7/ADR cells was increased markedly by verapamil and estramustine; however, serum suppressed the effects of estramustine much more strongly than those of verapamil. Equilibrium dialysis experiments demonstrated that [$^3$H]paclitaxel binds to albumin and alpha$_1$-acid-glycoprotein, and [$^3$H]vinblastine binds predominantly to alpha$_1$-acid-glycoprotein (Fig. 8).

The attenuation of estramustine activity by serum proteins reduces the propensity of the drug to act as an MDR modulator in vivo. By the same principles, such interactions may serve to limit the circulating levels of available drug for tissue uptake.

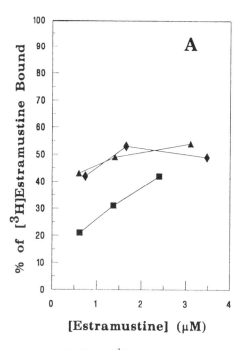
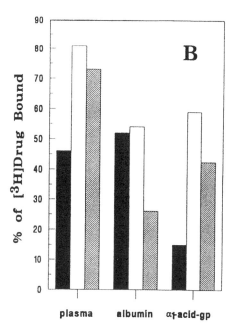

**Figure 8** Binding of [$^3$H]estramustine to plasma proteins. (A) Several concentrations of [$^3$H]estramustine were dialyzed against plasma for 24 (■), 48 (◆), or 96 (▲) h. The indicated concentrations of estramustine (abscissa) are calculated from the total counts per minute (cpm) on the side of the chamber containing protein, whereas bound [$^3$H]estramustine is calculated from the difference in cpm between the two sides of the chamber. Values represent the mean of duplicate samples in a representative experiment. (B) [$^3$H]estramustine (2 $\mu$M; filled bars), [$^3$H]paclitaxel (0.1 $\mu$M; open bars), or [$^3$H]vinblastine (0.1 $\mu$M; cross-hatched bars) was dialyzed against plasma, 40 mg human albumin/mL, or 1 mg $\alpha_1$-acid-glycoprotein/mL for 48 h. The percentage of [$^3$H]drug bound was calculated as indicated. Values represent the mean of duplicate samples in a representative experiment. (From Ref. 34.)

These factors will all play a role in determining pharmacokinetic and pharmacodynamic aspects of drug delivery in the clinical situation.

## CLINICAL STUDIES

In the absence of dietary calcium, approximately 75% of an oral dose of EM phosphate (usual dose range 140–1400 mg/day in up to three divided doses) is absorbed into the systemic circulation. Plasma half-lives of the active constituents estramustine and estromustine range between 9 and 23 h. Both species are excreted primarily via the bile. Uptake and retention in the prostate tissue is facilitated by a protein called prostatin, or estramustine-binding protein (EMBP), which concentrates the drug in the prostate. This serves to enhance the therapeutic index of the drug in a prostate-specific fashion.

In noncomparative trials, objective response rates in hormone-refractory patients ranged from 19–69% with estramustine as a single agent (35). These rates have been

**Table 3** Summary of Phase II Noncomparative Studies of Oral Estramustine Phosphate (E) in Combination with Vinblastine (VB), Paclitaxel (PT), or Etoposide (ET) in Patients with Histologically Confirmed Advanced Hormone-Refractory Prostate Cancer

| Reference | Dosage (mg) [no. of evaluated patients] | Age range (years) | Reduction in PSA levels [no. of patients (%)] | Other evaluation criteria | CR | PR | PD | Duration of response (months) |
|---|---|---|---|---|---|---|---|---|
| (41) | E 420/d PO + VB 6/m²/w IV for 6w [28] | 45–73 | 13/28 (46)[a] | PAP,BS,NMM | | 3/11 (27)[b] | | |
| (42) | E 600/m²/d PO d1–42 + VB 4/m²/w IV for 6w q8w [36] | 59–85 | 22/36 (61)[c] 8/36 (22)[c] | STLM | | 11/36 (30.5)[d] (ORR), 1/7 (14)[f] | | |
| (43) | E 600/m²/d PO + PT 120–140/m²/96h IV q3w [17] | 45–79 | 10/17 (58.8)[g] 6/17 (35.2)[h] | NMM, STLM | | 3/6[f] | | 7 (median) |
| (44) | E 15/kg/d PO + ET 50/m²/d PO for 21d q4w [52] | 58–83 | 28/52 (54)[c] | 13/52 (25)[e] | STLM, BMD | 3/20 (15)[f] | 6/20 (30)[f] [OR], 17/52 (33) [ORR] | 12 |
| (45) | E 10/kg/d PO + VB 4/m²/w IV for 6w q8w [24] | 69 (median) | 13/24 (54)[a,i] | | | 2/5 (40)[f] | 4/24 (16) | 7 (median) |

[a]PSA levels decreased >50% from baseline on three consecutive occasions.
[b]Improvements in nodal metastases.
[c]Maximum number of patients with a decrease in PSA levels >50% from baseline.
[d]Patients with ≥50% decrease in PSA levels on three consecutive 2-week measurements plus an improved/stable pain score, performance status, and measurable tissue disease.
[e]Maximum number of patients with a decrease in PSA levels ≥75% from baseline.
[f]Patients with measurable soft tissue disease.
[g]Patients with sustained declines in PSA levels ≥50% below baseline.
[h]Patients with >80% decreases in PSA levels.
[i]The median decrease in PSA was 64%.

*Abbreviations:* BMD = bidimensionally measurable measurable soft tissue disease; BS = bone scan; CR = complete response; d = day(s); IV = intravenous nodal metastases measurements; OR = objective response; ORR = overall response rate; P = progressive disease; PAP = prostatic acid phosphatase; PO = orally; PR = partial response; PSA = prostate-specific antigen; qxw = every x weeks (x = number of weeks); STLM = soft tissue lesion measurements; w = week(s).
Source: Modified from Ref. 46.

found to be equivalent to or better than other standard antineoplastic drug treatments. As a first-line therapy in advanced metastatic disease patients, estramustine has been reported to have objective response rates of up to 96% (36–38).

More recently, effective combinations of estramustine with other antimicrotubule drugs have been utilized. The rationale for such combinations was based on a number of factors: (1) in vitro survival data suggested greater than additive cytotoxicity; (2) the molecular targets, although affecting microtubule dynamics, do not appear to be identical; (3) mechanisms of resistance to estramustine are primarily distinct from those of either vinblastine or paclitaxel; (4) host and dose-limiting toxicities of these agents are distinct; and (5) any tumor cells expressing the P-glycoprotein may be sensitized, if the extracellular serum concentration of estramustine is high enough. Such encouraging factors have had an impact on the apparent success of a number of completed phase II noncomparative combination studies, the results of which are summarized in Table 3.

Continuing efforts to improve the response rates are ongoing. Initial results of a phase II combination regimen involving estramustine and paclitaxel in hormone-refractory prostate cancer are encouraging (39). A phase II/III trial with the same drug treatment (estramustine/paclitaxel) given to patients as an adjuvant therapy with standard irradiation is also currently under way (Hudes et al., personal communication). This approach in early-stage prostate cancer is supported by data from preclinical studies that show estramustine to be an effective radiation sensitizer (40).

Although each of the antimitotic drug combination regimens has provided an incremental but meaningful advance in the management of hormone-refractory cancer, more experimentation should lead to better multiple-drug regimens. The continued premise of these combinations should be based on those preclinical factors that avoid collateral resistance. Fortunately, estramustine appears to have pharmacological properties unique among antimitotic drugs. These features, together with the mainly tolerable host toxicities, suggest that the use of estramustine in the management of prostate cancer will continue for the foreseeable future.

## REFERENCES

1. Gunnarsson PO, Forshall GP. Clinical pharmacokinetics of estramustine phosphate. Urology 1984; 23:22–27.
2. Gunnarsson PO, Davidsson T, Andersson SB, Backman C, Johansson SA. Impairment of estramustine phosphate absorption by concurrent milk and food. Eur J Clin Pharmacol 1990; 38:189–193.
3. Punzi JS, Duax WL, Strong P, Griffin JF, Flocco MM, Zacharias DE, Carrell HL, Tew KD, Glusker JP. Molecular conformation of estramustine and two analogs. Mol Pharmacol 1992; 41:569–576.
4. Gupta RS. Cross-resistance of nocodazole-resistant mutants of CHO cells toward other microtubule inhibitors: similar mode of action of benzimidazole carbamate derivatives and NSC 181928 and TN-16. Mol Pharmacol 1986; 30:142–148.
5. Speicher LA, Tew KD. Fluorescent probes in antimicrotubule drug activity. J Cell Pharmacol 1992; 3:86–93.
6. Tew KD, Hartley-Asp B. Cytotoxic properties of estramustine unrelated to alkylating and steroid constituents. Urology 1984; 23:28–33.
7. Parry EM, Danford N, Parry JM. Differential staining of chromosomes and spindle and its use as an assay for determining the effect of diethylstilbestrol on cultured mammalian cells. Mutat Res 1982; 105:243–252.

8. Hartley-Asp B, Deinum J, Wallin M. Diethylstilbestrol induces metaphase arrest and inhibits microtubule assembly. Mutat Res 1985; 143:231–235.

9. Tew KD. The mechanism of action of estramustine. Semin Oncol 1983; 10:21–26.

10. Tew KD, Erickson LC, White G, Wang AL, Schein PS, Asp B. Cytotoxicity of estramustine, a steroid nitrogen mustard derivative, through non-DNA targets. Mol Pharmacol 1983; 24: 324–328.

11. Wittelsberger SC, Kleene K, Penman S. Progressive loss of shape-responsive metabolic controls in cells with increasing transformed phenotype. Cell 1981; 24:859–866.

12. Raz A, Ben-Ze'ev A. Modulation of the metastatic capability in B16 melanoma by cell shape. Science 1983; 221:1307–1310.

13. Darnell JE, Lodish H, Baltimore D. Molecular Cell Biology, Part III. New York: Scientific American Books, Inc., 1986.

14. Kim H, Binder LI, Rosenbaum JL. The periodic association of MAP2 with brain microtubules in vitro. J Cell Biol 1979; 80:266–276.

15. Olmsted JB. Microtubule-associated proteins. Annu Rev Cell Biol 1986; 2:421–457.

16. Wiche G, Herrman H, Dalton JM, Roisner R, Leichtfired FE, Lassman H, Koszka C, Briones E. Molecular aspects of MAP-1 and MAP-2: microheterogeneity, in vitro localization and distribution in neuronal and non-neuronal cells. Ann N Y Acad Sci 1986; 466:180–198.

17. Stearns ME, Jenkins DP, Tew KD. Dansylated estramustine, a fluorescent probe for studies of uptake and identification of intracellular targets. Proc Natl Acad Sci USA 1985; 82:8483–8487.

18. Wallin M, Deinum J, Friden B. Interaction of estramustine phosphate with microtubule-associated proteins. Fed Eur Biochem Soc Lett 1985; 179:289–293.

19. Friden B, Wallin M, Deinum J, Prasade V, Luduena R. Effect of estramustine phosphate on the assembly of trypsin-treated microtubules and microtubules reconstituted from purified tubulin with either tau, MAP-2 or the tubulin binding fragment of MAP-2. Arch Biochem Biophys 1987; 257:123–130.

20. Stearns ME, Tew KD. Estramustine binds MAP-2 to inhibit microtubule assembly in vitro. J Cell Sci 1988; 89:331–342.

21. Dahllof B, Billstrom A, Carbral F, Hartley-Asp B. Estramustine depolymerized microtubules by binding to tubulin. Cancer Res 1993; 53:4573–4581.

22. Speicher LA, Laing N, Barone L, Robbins JD, Seamon KB, Tew KD. Interaction of estramustine photoaffinity analog with cytoskeletal proteins in prostate carcinoma cells. Mol Pharmacol 1994; 46:866–872.

23. Tew KD, Glusker JP, Hartley-Asp B, Hudes G, Speicher LA. Preclinical and clinical perspectives on the use of estramustine as an antimitotic drug. Pharmacol Ther 1992; 56:323–339.

24. Mareel MM, Storme GA, Dragonetti CH, De Bruyne GK, Hartley-Asp B, Segers JL, Rabaey ML. Antiinvasive activity of estramustine on malignant MO4 mouse cells and on DU-145 human prostate carcinoma cells in vitro. Cancer Res 1988; 48:1842–1849.

25. Speicher LA, Barone L, Tew KD. Combined antimicrotubule activity of estramustine and Taxol in human prostatic carcinoma cell lines. Cancer Res 1992; 52:4433–4440.

26. Sheridan VR, Speicher LA, Tew KD. The effects of estramustine on mitotic progression in DU 145 human prostatic carcinoma cells. Eur J Cell Biol 1991; 54:268–276.

27. Speicher LA, Sheridan VR, Godwin A, Tew KD. Resistance to the antimitotic drug estramustine is distinct from the multidrug resistant phenotype. Br J Cancer 1991; 64:267–273.

28. Leistenschneider W, Nagel R. Control of response to estramustine phosphate therapy through cytology and DNA analysis of cell nuclei in prospective study. Urology 1984; 23: 81–88.

29. Speicher LA, Barone L, Tew KD. Altered regulation of cytoskeletal elements in estramustine resistant cell lines. Cell Pharmacol 1995; 2:91–96.

30. Ling V. Drug resistance and membrane alteration in mutants of mammalian cells. Can J Genet Cytol 1975; 17:503–508.

31. Schibler MJ, Cabral F. Microtubule mutants. In: Gottesman M, ed. Molecular Cell Genetics. New York: John Wiley, 1985:669–710.

32. Cabral F, Barlow S. Mechanisms by which mammalian cells acquire resistance to drugs that affect microtubule assembly. FASEB J 1989; 3:1593–1598.

33. Speicher LA, Barone LR, Chapman AE, Hudes GR, Laing N, Smith CD, Tew KD. P-glycoprotein binding and modulation of the MDR phenotype by estramustine. J Natl Cancer Inst 1994; 86:688–694.

34. Smith CD, Zilfou JT, Zhang X, Hudes GR, Tew KD. Modulation of P-glycoprotein activity by estramustine is limited by binding to plasma proteins. Cancer 1995; 75:2597–2604.

35. Dexeus F, Logothetics CJ, Samuels ML, Hossan E, von Eschenbach AC. Continuous infusion of vinblastine for advanced hormone-refractory prostate cancer. Cancer Treat Rep 1985; 69:885–886.

36. Nilsson T, Jonsson G. Estramustine phosphate (Estracyt) as a primary treatment of prostatic carcinoma. Curr Chemother 1978; 1282–1283.

37. Asakawa M, Wada S, Yayumoto R, et al. Clinical study of estramustine phosphate disodium (Estracyt) on prostatic cancer. Results of long-term therapy for 38 patients with prostatic cancer [in Japanese]. Hinyokika Kiyo 1990; 36:1361–11369.

38. Brausi M, Reich A, Micali F, et al. Estramustine phosphate in escalating dose in previously untreated metastatic prostate cancer. A multicenter study. Urol Res 1992; 20:453.

39. Hudes GR, Obasaju C, Chapman A, Gallo J, McAleer C, Greenberg R. Phase I study of paclitaxel and estramustine: preliminary activity in hormone refractory prostate cancer. Semin Oncol 1995; 22:6–11.

40. Kim JH, Khil MS, Kim SH, Ryu S, Gabel M. Clinical and biological studies of estramustine phosphate as a novel radiation sensitizer. Int J Radiat Oncol Biol Phys 1994; 29:555–557.

41. Amato RJ, Ellerhorst J, Sella A, et al. Estramustine and vinblastine for patients with progressive androgen-independent adenocarcinoma of the prostate. Pharmacia (Milan). Data on file.

42. Hudes GR, Greenberg R, Krigel RL, Fox S, Scher R, Litwin S, Watts P, Speicher L, Tew K, Comis R. Phase II study of estramustine and vinblastine, two microtubule inhibitors, in hormone-refractory prostate cancer. J Clin Oncol 1992; 10:1754–1761.

43. Hudes G, Nathan R, Chapman A, et al. Combined antimicrotubule therapy of metastatic prostate cancer with 96-hr paclitaxel (P) and estramustine (EM): activity in hormone-refractory disease (HRPC). Proc ASCO, March, 1995.

44. Pienta KJ, Redman BG, Hussain M, et al. Inhibition of prostate cancer growth by estramustine and etoposide. Cancer 1995;75:1920–1926.

45. Seidman AD, Scher HI, Petrylak D, et al. Estramustine and vinblastine: use of prostate specific antigen as a clinical trial end point for hormone refractory prostatic cancer. J Urol 1992; 147:931–934.

46. Perry CM, McTavish D. Estramustine phosphate sodium: a review of its pharmacodynamic and pharmacokinetic properties, and therapeutic efficacy in prostate cancer. Drugs Aging 1995; 7:49–74.

# 13

## Strategies for Overcoming Anthracycline Resistance

**Daniel J. Booser**
*The University of Texas M.D. Anderson Cancer Center, Houston, Texas*

Drugs of the anthracycline class have been used to treat human malignancies since 1965. Several thousand analogues have been developed in the laboratory and hundreds studied in animal tumor systems. The first two anthracyclines reported in clinical studies, daunorubicin and doxorubicin (Adriamycin), remain in widespread use, although the newer analogues idarubicin and epirubicin are perceived by many to have a slightly improved therapeutic index (decreased mucosal and cardiac toxicity). Daunorubicin and idarubicin are regarded as drugs for the treatment of acute leukemias, although they are also active against solid tumors. Doxorubicin and epirubicin are used clinically against a broader spectrum of tumor types.

Despite their ability to shrink tumors of many histological origins, anthracycline regimens only rarely prove to be curative in the treatment of disseminated malignancy. After an initial response, tumors generally develop secondary resistance to the anthracycline. Occasionally tumors of potentially responsive cell types show de novo resistance to anthracyclines, and many other tumor types are completely refractory to this class of drugs.

Overcoming resistance has proved difficult. Anthracyclines have many mechanisms of interaction with cells, and little is known about the differences of interaction with neoplastic compared with normal cells. Entry of drug and its retention in the cell is a current focus of therapeutic research, but pharmacological attempts to modify this have been limited by a lack of selectivity for malignant cells. Much has been learned in the laboratory about the interaction of anthracyclines with cellular functions, but here too the precise mechanisms of cytotoxicity remain poorly understood.

Most recent efforts to overcome clinical resistance have focused on drug dosage and delivery and on agents that reverse the multidrug resistance associated with P-glycoprotein (Pgp). Anthracycline analogues less affected by Pgp have been developed. Additional resistance mechanisms have been identified and are coming into clinical study. The identification of cellular oncogenes and proteins involved in growth regulation, including programmed cell death (apoptosis), offers potential targets to increase the selectivity of drug action. However, these mechanisms show a daunting heterogeneity. Cellular differentiation induced by anthracyclines may become an area of expanded interest.

This chapter reviews significant findings from recent work. Although these efforts have failed to produce a major improvement in the therapeutic index of this class of drugs, some of the most recent results may guide clinical investigators in designing new treatment protocols. Some interesting preclinical discoveries may lead to entirely new approaches for anthracycline use in clinical medicine. A recent review provides background on many aspects of anthracycline biology and chemistry that are not covered here (1).

## DOSE AND DOSE INTENSITY

The traditional approach to cancer chemotherapy has been to kill cells by interfering with the structure and function of nuclear DNA, although protein or lipid interactions independent of DNA damage may also be critical (2). Drug dosage is important in direct cell killing. The original concept of increased effectiveness with higher drug dose (dose response) has been refined by the concept of dose intensity as expressed by the measurement of milligrams per meter squared per week ($mg/m^2/wk$) (3). Increased dose intensity may be gained by increasing the doses given at a fixed interval or by shortening the interval between fixed doses.

Chemotherapy doses are limited by the effects of drugs on normal cells, most commonly the bone marrow. To overcome this limitation, techniques of hematopoietic progenitor storage and transplantation were developed, originally with bone marrow and now with peripheral stem cells. Growth factor support using granulocyte colony-stimulating factor (G-CSF) (filgrastim, lenograstim) and granulocyte-macrophage colony-stimulating factor (GM-CSF) (sargramostim) to accelerate granulocyte recovery, as well as platelet-stimulating factors (now undergoing promising clinical studies) may also permit much higher drug doses to be given with acceptable acute hematological toxicity.

Unfortunately, anthracycline dosage is also limited by cardiac and mucosal toxicity. Cardiac damage can be reduced by infusion of anthracycline over several days, but this increases mucosal toxicity. Dexrazoxane (formerly known as ICRF-187, then ADR-529; now commercially available) can be given with quick infusions of anthracycline to protect the heart, although it may reduce its effect against the tumor target (4) (see below). Swainsonine, an alkaloid that inhibits Golgi α-mannosidase II in cellular carbohydrate processing, facilitated recovery of mice from doxorubicin-induced neutropenia and protected against cardiac toxicity (5). This new class of anticancer agents may prove to be of particular interest for clinical trials in combination with anthracyclines.

There is limited evidence in support of dose intensity as a determinant of response to anthracyclines within the standard dose range. The standard combination of 5-fluorouracil, doxorubicin, and cyclophosphamide (FAC) in adjuvant treatment of node-positive breast cancer produced poorer disease-free and overall survival at the lowest dose intensity (including doxorubicin 7.5 $mg/m^2/wk$) than a 33% higher intensity (including doxorubicin 10 $mg/m^2/wk$). However, there was no additional benefit in a group treated at a still higher intensity that included doxorubicin at 15 $mg/m^2/wk$. This is most consistent with a threshold level of the dose rather than a dose-response effect or dose intensity (6). It confirms earlier studies that failed to show an advantage to higher dose intensity for regimens that include doxorubicin (7,8) or epirubicin (9) at or near the maximum tolerated dose (MTD) in the adjuvant setting.

The inferiority of doxorubicin at 35 mg/m$^2$ compared with 70 mg/m$^2$ every 3 weeks (10) and the equivalence of epirubicin at 50 mg/m$^2$ and 75 mg/m$^2$ (11) or 100 mg/m$^2$ (12) suggests a threshold rather than dose-response effect in the treatment of metastatic breast cancer, although an earlier small study of 26 women treated with high doses of doxorubicin alone (75 to 135 mg/m$^2$) did suggest a close relationship between dose and response (13). In a series of 287 patients, epirubicin at 40, 60, and 90 mg/m$^2$ produced 20%, 20%, and 38% response rates, respectively. However, a further dose increase to 135 mg/m$^2$ gave only a 36% response rate (14). Of 197 patients randomized to treatment with epirubicin at 60 mg/m$^2$ or 120 mg/m$^2$ in combination with a fixed dose of cyclophosphamide, those in the higher dose arm showed a higher rate of response (including complete response). Unfortunately, even though the goal of relative dose intensity was nearly achieved, there was no difference in time to progression or survival (15).

In other diseases, intensification of only the doxorubicin dose in combination chemotherapy for non-Hodgkin's lymphomas (13.5 vs. 10.4 mg/m$^2$/wk, $P<0.01$) did not improve the rate of response or rate of survival (16). Unfortunately, dose escalation was limited by the decision to avoid a granulocyte nadir of <1000/mm$^3$. Even higher doses (doxorubicin 34.4 mg/m$^2$/wk or epirubicin 54.9 mg/m$^2$/wk) have been given in combination regimens for lymphomas with acceptable toxicity, but these were not compared directly with a standard-dose arm for response or survival (17). In a retrospective review of osteogenic sarcoma and Ewing's sarcoma, doxorubicin dose intensity seemed to be an important determinant of favorable outcome (18).

Unfortunately, efforts to increase dose intensity by protecting the marrow or improving its ability to recover have so far had little effect on survival. Elderly patients with acute myelogenous leukemia treated with daunorubicin at 135 mg/m$^2$ (19) or 180 mg/m$^2$ (20) combined with cytarabine had no improvement in survival if randomized to receive growth factor support. Lenograstim reduced morbidity but did not change the response rate in a randomized study of patients with inflammatory breast cancer who were receiving epirubicin 105 mg/m$^2$ as part of a standard combination regimen given every 3 weeks (21).

In a preliminary report (22) of patients with locally advanced breast cancer, those randomized to FAC treatment at a 30% increase in dose intensity (including doxorubicin 60 mg/m$^2$ every 18 days rather than 50 mg/m$^2$ every 21 days) with filgrastim support had a higher incidence of neutropenic fever and required more red blood cell and platelet transfusions. A similar combination, with *Escherichia coli*–derived GM-CSF, produced cumulative dose-limiting myelosuppression and significant clinical toxicity in patients with advanced breast cancer. The doxorubicin was delivered at a dose intensity of 14.8 mg/m$^2$/wk (23). It remains to be seen whether the modest 60% increase in dose intensity made possible by using growth factors and achieved primarily by using a 2-week rather than 3-week treatment interval (24) will increase the cure rate.

In preliminary reports, doxorubicin can be given in a dose of 165 mg/m$^2$ in a combination single-dose regimen for metastatic breast cancer if marrow or peripheral stem cell support is given; mucositis is the dose-limiting toxicity (25). Epirubicin can be given safely in a dose of 225 mg/m$^2$ over 96 h in repeated cycles of combination chemotherapy if dexrazoxane cardioprotection and G-CSF with peripheral blood stem cell support are added (26).

High-dose regimens are difficult to sustain in combination with high dose intensity because of cumulative toxicities, and often the two concepts are, at least to some extent, mutually exclusive. The highest doses of anthracyclines reported to have acceptable toxicity are at most two to three times the standard doses even if steps are taken to protect the bone marrow. When one considers the much higher in vitro resistance factors seen in many cell cultures, it should not be too surprising that neither high-dose nor high-dose-intensity anthracycline regimens as given in clinical chemotherapy to date have had a major impact on cancer cure rates.

It should be noted that occasional patients will have a much better response to anthracyclines given at a higher dose and/or dose intensity well above the threshold level, although this is hard to show for populations of patients. Also, it is important to note that for some diseases not treated with anthracyclines, such as metastatic germ cell carcinomas treated with platinum, the relationship between dose and cure is unequivocal.

## TARGETED CHEMOTHERAPY

### Arterial Infusion

Arterial infusion has been used to deliver high local doses of anthracycline chemotherapy to tumors, primarily extremity sarcomas and hepatocellular carcinomas. This approach avoids venous dilution and hepatic metabolism of the drug before it reaches the tumor.

Although intra-arterial doxorubicin is very effective in permitting limb-conserving treatment of extremity sarcomas, its superiority over standard intravenous chemotherapy has not been established for local failure rate or overall survival (27). A relatively conservative dose (50–60 mg/m$^2$) is required because of poor tissue tolerance, especially with concomitant radiotherapy. A recent refinement of this technique uses extracorporeal carbon chemofilters to extract remaining drug from the venous effluent before return of the blood to the systemic circulation, thus reducing systemic toxicity. The maximum tolerated dose (MTD) in a phase I study of patients with hepatocellular carcinoma was 120 mg/m$^2$ for doxorubicin given over 20 min into the hepatic artery, with grade 3 liver toxicity the dose-limiting factor (28).

### Liposomes

Another way to increase intensity to the target while limiting damage to normal tissues is to encapsulate the drug. Anthracyclines given in lipid vesicles with a diameter of 0.05 to 0.5 $\mu$m are not significantly taken up by the heart, probably because of the structure of cardiac vascular basement membrane. Thus, the potential for heart damage as a dose-limiting toxicity is reduced. Although liposomes are targeted to certain tumors because of the microvascular structure, they are also concentrated in the liver, spleen, and bone marrow.

At least eight formulations of anthracyclines in liposomes have been tested in humans. These are generally classified as small unilamellar vesicles (SUVs). Although investigational lipophilic anthracyclines may be better trapped in multilamellar liposomes, which have a smaller (about 10%) hydrophilic compartment (29), SUVs measuring 0.03 to 0.15 $\mu$m in diameter appear to have superior targeting and thus improved drug delivery to the tumor. Clinical trials were started in the late 1980s, after animal studies suggested some improvement in the therapeutic index of liposomal anthracyclines. The results of phase I and phase II studies remain preliminary.

AIDS-related Kaposi's sarcoma is a disease of particular interest. A liposomal daunorubicin preparation with significant antitumor activity can be given safely at doses of up to 60 mg/m$^2$ every 2 weeks (30). Doxorubicin in polyethyleneglycol (PEG)-coated liposomes is highly active at a dose of 20 mg/m$^2$ every 3 weeks, but cumulative neutropenia develops after several courses of chemotherapy (31). Skin toxicity was reported as the dose-limiting toxicity if doxorubicin was given at 50 mg/m$^2$ every 3 weeks or 60 mg/m$^2$ every 4 weeks in PEG liposomes (32). Both formulations were recently approved for the treatment of Kaposi's sarcoma.

Muramyltripeptide-phosphatidylethanolamine (MTP-PE) is a lipophilic synthetic molecule that resembles the minimal structural unit of the cell wall of mycobacterium and other bacteria and is a potent activator in vitro of tumor cell killing by monocytes and macrophages. A liposomal formulation (L-MTP-PE) plus doxorubicin may have enhanced monocyte activation in children with osteosarcoma (33). Subsequent studies in dogs showed a sustained enhancement of serum tumor necrosis factor activity and monocyte activation following L-MTP-PE with doxorubicin compared with either drug alone (34). Dogs randomized to receive L-MTP-PE in combination with adjuvant doxorubicin and cyclophosphamide for splenic hemangiosarcoma had significantly prolonged survival compared with those receiving the chemotherapy alone (35).

Iodized poppy-seed oil deposits selectively in the cells of hepatocellular carcinoma. A water-in-oil-in-water emulsion of this containing epirubicin is undergoing clinical study in Japan (36).

Receptors for folic acid are frequently overexpressed on epithelial cancer cells. To take advantage of this, folate liposomes (PEG-DSPE) were loaded with doxorubicin. They showed 1.6-fold increased uptake and 2.7-fold the cytotoxicity compared with free doxorubicin in KB cell culture (37).

## Antibodies

Preclinical studies since the early 1980s have shown the ability of antibodies to target anthracyclines to tumors in animals. BR96-Dox, a conjugate of doxorubicin with a chimeric monoclonal antibody that binds an antigen related to Lewis Y, produced complete regressions and cures of subcutaneously xenografted human lung, breast, and colon carcinomas in athymic mice (38). Unfortunately, a phase I study using this conjugate for patients with Lewis Y–positive tumors at doxorubicin doses of up to 19 mg/m$^2$ every 3 weeks produced diffuse hemorrhagic gastritis of the body of the stomach. Steroid premedication allowed for further dose escalations (39).

Increasingly specific antibody development may enhance the selective targeting of anthracycline delivery. Daunorubicin coupled with monoclonal antibody 19-24, which recognizes the sarcoma-associated antigen p102, appeared more efficient and less cytotoxic than free drug to normal tissues in athymic mice with human fibrosarcoma xenografts (40). Doxorubicin-containing PEG liposomes whose surface was tagged with antibodies to KLN-205 squamous lung carcinoma eradicated tumor in about half of DBA/2 mice bearing KLN-205 transplants (41).

A cephalosporin derivative of doxorubicin (C-Dox) was evaluated as a prodrug for activation by lung adenocarcinoma or melanoma-directed monoclonal antibody conjugates of β-lactamase. Immunospecific activation took place when cells were pretreated with β-lactamase conjugate that could bind to antigens on the tumor cells. In athymic mice, C-Dox was at least 7-fold less toxic than Dox on a molar basis, despite a ≥320-fold greater area under the curve (AUC) of C-Dox in the first 2 h after administration. Intratumoral levels of Dox were higher after treatment with C-Dox following delivery of adenocarcinoma antibody–β-lactamase conjugate, which suggested that the conversion of C-Dox to Dox was tumor-specific and dependent on the presence of the targeted antigen (42).

## Albumin Conjugates

A conjugate of daunomycin with maleylated bovine serum albumin was efficiently internalized by transformed macrophage cells. When 0.8 μg of conjugated daunorubicin was injected into BALB/c mice bearing the macrophage tumor cell line J774A.1, a 50% reduction of tumor mass was elicited; 28 μg of free drug was required to achieve a similar reduction (43). This relatively simple preparation may merit clinical study in the treatment of histiocytic malignancies bearing the scavenger receptors.

In a combined targeting approach, albumin microspheres loaded with only 9 mg doxorubicin injected through an internal mammary arterial catheter produced a dramatic local tumor response in a patient with locally advanced breast cancer. This was probably caused by embolization of the capillary bed and release of anthracycline into the target organ. However, this response was complicated by necrosis of subcutaneous fat over adjacent areas of the abdomen (44).

## MOLECULAR MECHANISMS OF ANTHRACYCLINE RESISTANCE

Drug entry and retention in the cell is a basic premise of effective chemotherapy. The demonstration of a 170-kd cell-surface glycoprotein in a multidrug-resistant (MDR) Chinese hamster ovary cell line (45) and its subsequent identification in patients with clinically MDR ovarian cancer (46) opened the door to the rapidly expanding study of molecular mechanisms accounting for tumor resistance to a variety of chemically unrelated natural product drugs, including anthracyclines.

The 170-kd permeability glycoprotein (Pgp), acting as a channel regulator (47) and pumping drug out of the cell, remains the most widely studied mechanism of MDR. Many clinical studies have attempted to reverse its function, and most clinicians regard MDR and Pgp as synonymous. However, a number of other MDR mechanisms have been described in the laboratory (Table 1) and are beginning to be studied in clinical materials. Some cell lines have more than one mechanism of MDR, and so improving drug retention in the cell by blocking Pgp may still be insufficient to reverse an MDR phenotype.

## MDR1 (P-Glycoprotein)

Pgp-mediated resistance is known as MDR1. In addition to some tumors, a variety of normal tissues with diverse physiologic functions express Pgp. Pharmacological attempts to regulate tumor Pgp expression or function thus have the risk of interfering with many normal physiological processes, including hepatic and renal excretion. The timing of the dosages and specific interactions of the drug and its modulator probably will prove to be important in developing a strategy to inhibit tumor Pgp specifically.

**Table 1** Anthracycline Resistance Mechanisms[a]: Reported Spectra of Associated Drug Resistance (reference numbers in parentheses)

| Drug | MDR1 | MRP (100,101) | AT-MDR | LRP (107) | Apoptosis | | HER-2 (191) | Unknown (111) | GSH? (112) | Unknown (113) | Unknown (222) |
|---|---|---|---|---|---|---|---|---|---|---|---|
| | | | | | BCL-2 Pos (157) | BCL-2 Neg (149,164) | | | | | |
| Anthracycline[b] | Yes | Yes | Yes | Yes | Yes | Yes | Yes | Yes | Yes | Yes | No |
| Actinomycin | Yes | No | | | | | | | | | |
| Amsacrine | Yes[c] | | Yes | | | | | | | | |
| AD-198[d] | No | | | | | | | | | | |
| Cisplatin | No | No[e] | | | No | No | Yes | No | Yes | Yes | |
| Epipodophyllotoxin | Yes | Yes | Yes | Yes | No | Yes | Yes | Yes | Yes | Yes | |
| 5-FU | No[f] | | | | | Yes | | | | No | |
| Melphalan | No | | | | | No | Yes | | | | |
| Methotrexate | No | | | | No | Yes[c] | | | | Yes | |
| Mitomycin | Yes | | | | Yes | | Yes | | | | |
| Mitoxantrone | Yes | Yes | Yes | Yes | | | | Yes | | | |
| Morpholinyl anthracycline | Rarely | | | | | | | | | | Yes |
| Nitrosoureas | No | | | | No | No | Yes | | | | |
| Taxanes | Yes | Yes[c] | No | | No | Yes | | | Yes | No | |
| 6-Thioguanine | No | | | | | | | No | | | |
| Vinca alkaloids | Yes | Yes | No | Yes | | | | | | No | |

[a]More than one mechanism may coexist.
[b]May not include some analogues.
[c]Low-level resistance.
[d]Non-MRP p190 resistance protein (see text).
[e]May depend on glutathione-S conjugation (see text).
[f]High thymidylate synthase may be coexpressed (see text).

In vitro colon carcinoma cells grown in high culture density and large tumor volume down-regulated the expression of the MDR1 gene (48). The half-life of Pgp was four- to sixfold longer when cultures were maintained at a high cell density (49).

MDR1 SW-1573 lung cancer and MCF-7 breast cancer cells in vitro may show alterations in intracellular drug localization, characterized by decreased nuclear/cytoplasmic doxorubicin fluorescence ratios (50). Pgp was found in the Golgi apparatus of resistant MCF cells, with doxorubicin accumulating in the perinuclear region (51). Modifiers of Pgp may have cellular effects in addition to those on the cell membrane. Verapamil induced redistribution of doxorubicin from the cytoplasm to the nucleus (52). It also caused down-regulation of MDR1 gene transcription in two resistant leukemic cell lines at concentrations between 15 and 50 $\mu$M, probably by decreasing MDR1 proximal promoter activity (53).

Some in vitro studies of MDR1 cells have shown a striking range of resistance factors for the drugs involved in the MDR1 phenotype, suggesting a heterogeneity in the interaction of drug with the Pgp pump. This heterogeneity may be related to transmembrane topology of the transporter or to the extent of phosphorylation of the protein. Both the initial association of Pgp with a drug and the subsequent dissociation necessary to release the drug from the cell appear to be important in this dynamic process (54), but other factors are also involved. The modulator may interact with separate or overlapping domains of Pgp (55). In addition, substances such as progesterone that efficiently bind to Pgp are not necessarily transported by Pgp (56). Prolonged drug exposure may also have differing effects on resistance to various cytotoxic agents (57). In the small cell lung cancer cell line H69/LX4, the MDR1-phenotype drugs paclitaxel and vinblastine did not share the same binding site on Pgp, and paclitaxel acted as an allosteric regulator by slowing association of vinblastine with Pgp (58). The high affinity of Pgp for paclitaxel suggests that it may have a role in overcoming the MDR1 phenotype in combination chemotherapy (59) and may contribute to the increased clinical toxicity when doxorubicin follows rather than precedes it in the treatment of breast cancer (60).

Interferon-$\alpha$ (IFN-$\alpha$) is not a substrate of Pgp, but in MDR cell line ChRC5 it enhanced the ability of verapamil to modulate doxorubicin accumulation and cytotoxicity, probably by altering the accessibility of Pgp binding sites to verapamil (61). It also enhanced the reversal of doxorubicin and vincristine resistance in retrovirus-infected HT-29 colon carcinoma cells by MRK-16 monoclonal antibody (62). IFN-$\alpha$ with all-trans retinoic acid increased doxorubicin cytotoxicity in resistant K562 cells despite an increase in MDR1 gene expression (63).

Although the frequency of mutations in Pgp structure is not known and is probably quite low, studies with NIH3T3 cells containing a transfected MDR1 vector mutant at residue 185 showed interesting differences from transfected wild-type in degree of resistance (the mutant had increased resistance to colchicine, less resistance to daunorubicin, paclitaxel, and vinblastine). MDR1-reversing agents had different potencies if the transporter was a mutant instead of wild-type, and the extent of the difference depended on the cytotoxic drug whose resistance was being reversed (64). A mutant human leukemic cell line K562/RDC selected in cyclosporine and doxorubicin was resistant to modulation with the cyclosporine analogue PSC 833 and with verapamil (65).

Though treatment with doxorubicin (or other MDR1 drugs) may result in a mutational selection of resistant cells (66), it is also true that fractionated X irradiation in vitro (67) and short-term exposure to a number of non-Pgp substrate drugs including antimetabolites (68) induce Pgp overexpression. Estrogen activated the MDR promoter in a human hepatoblastoma cell line (69). Doxorubicin in the leukemic cell line K562/ADR$_{500}$ appeared to modulate both the expression and function of Pgp (70).

Liposomal encapsulation of doxorubicin increased the in vitro cytotoxicity at least tenfold against MDR1 Chinese hamster lung fibroblast LZ cells, probably by increasing cellular drug accumulation and by changing intracellular drug distribution (71). This suggests the increased effectiveness of the liposomal drug in MDR1 transgenic mice (72) is the result of a more specific mechanism than just an increased plasma AUC for doxorubicin.

Other, more exotic mechanisms have been used to overcome the MDR1 phenotype. A hammerhead ribozyme recognized the GUC sequence in codon 196 of MDR1 mRNA was transfected into a resistant MOLT-3 human leukemia cell line. The level of resistance and the amount of MDR1 mRNA appeared to correlate inversely with the amount of ribozyme expression. For some reason, a ribozyme directed to codon 179 was less active in this system (73). Leukoregulin, a 50-kD cytokine from human lymphocytes, caused a simultaneous increase in plasma membrane permeability and a decrease in Pgp expression with enhanced doxorubicin uptake in resistant 8226/Dox$_{40}$ myeloma cells. A number of other cytokines, however, had no effect on Pgp expression (74).

A mixture of three oligonucleotides targeted to adjacent binding sites of the MDR1 mRNA reduced the level of both MDR1 mRNA and Pgp and doubled the sensitivity of a resistant LoVo/Dx human colorectal cell line to doxorubicin (75).

Cyclosporine analogue PSC 833 suppressed the emergence of MDR1-mutant MES-SA sarcoma cells treated with 40 nmol/L doxorubicin, apparently suppressing MDR1 gene activation. This suggests that the routine use of PSC 833 (and perhaps other resistance modulators) would suppress the activation of MDR1 and prevent the emergence of cells with this phenotype. Of concern, doxorubicin-resistant cells that did emerge had a significant decrease in topoisomerase II$\alpha$ mRNA and protein (76).

In addition to effects on drugs in the MDR1 resistance spectrum, cyclosporine also modulates platinum resistance in vitro. This appears to be related to its suppression of the expression of genes related to the repair of platinum-mediated DNA damage, including *c-fos*, *c-myc*, and *c-H-ras* (77).

Because of the nonhematological toxicity of anthracyclines, protection of bone marrow by the introduction of a MDR1 gene (78) is unlikely to provide a significant advantage for this class of drugs. A retrovirus carrying both MDR1 and glutathione S-transferase $\pi$ to normal cells offers an example of an additional conceptual strategy for protection against toxic side effects (79).

*Clinical Studies with Pgp Modifiers*

Considering the cardiotoxic potential of anthracyclines, the use of MDR1-reversing agents has only a limited window of opportunity. Even if a highly effective and selective modifier were identified, concerns about the effects of cumulative anthracycline dose on cardiac function would soon require a change to another chemotherapeutic class except for patients receiving brief, potentially curative treatment courses.

Clinical studies with MDR1-reversing agents in solid tumors have been flawed by methodological problems. These include the failure to strictly define anthracycline resistance, to check whether potentially significant drug levels were reached, and to look for any potential resistance factors in tumor cells. Many resistant tumors do not express either Pgp or MDR1 mRNA, and so Pgp modifiers should have no effect. Even when these assays are done, there are many methodological pitfalls. Although the correlation is usually good, Pgp level is not always proportional to MDR1 mRNA. Furthermore, expressed Pgp may be nonfunctional, perhaps related to low phosphorylation by protein kinase C and other factors. Limited information suggests a resistance factor less than 5 in most tumors overexpressing MDR1 mRNA (80), much lower than that seen in many cell cultures and potentially within a therapeutic range for clinical modulation.

Several clinical studies have found that the toxicity of doxorubicin as well as several other drugs in the MDR1 spectrum was increased when they were given with cyclosporine as a modulator of Pgp, with altered pharmacology (81–83). Lack of enhanced toxicity in another study (84) may be attributed to the use of a relatively low dose (36 mg/m$^2$) of doxorubicin.

Verapamil is one of the most extensively studied Pgp modulators, but it has been toxic and only marginally active in clinical trials. Dexverapamil (R-verapamil), with less cardiovascular toxicity, is being studied as a second-generation modifier of MDR1 function but with limited success to date. Conversion of a bolus chemotherapy treatment schedule including doxorubicin to a 96-h infusion produced responses in patients with relapsed or refractory non-Hodgkin's lymphoma (NHL). Unfortunately, neither MDR1 nor pharmacology was studied. Both groups received two MDR1 drugs (doxorubicin and etoposide) (85), and one group a third (vincristine), by continuous infusion (86). Perhaps these drugs served as modulators of Pgp for one another during the infusion. When dexverapamil was added to the latter regimen (EPOCH), there were additional responses but hematopoietic toxicity increased. It was concluded that although Pgp inhibition may be necessary, it is probably insufficient to significantly improve the control of refractory lymphomas (87). It has been suggested that the presence of Pgp may be not simply a marker of chemosensitivity but also a sign of tumor aggressiveness (88).

Clinical studies have been conducted in plasma cell myeloma. Unfortunately, the great majority of peripheral B cells in myeloma express Pgp independent of treatment status, which may make them a potential reservoir of MDR1 disease (89). The development of Pgp expression by tumor cells correlated with a cumulative dose of vincristine >20 mg and doxorubicin 340 mg (90). When these drugs and dexamethasone (VAD) were given by 96-h infusion with cyclosporine as a Pgp modulator, six patients had at least a 50% reduction in the Pgp-positive tumor cell population. When two of these relapsed, the only tumor cells remaining were Pgp negative. One patient's Pgp-positive cells increased markedly despite infusion of the two MDR1 chemotherapeutic agents and a modifier (91). In another study of 63 myeloma patients with tumor cells refractory to alkylating agents, 59% of the samples were Pgp positive according to monoclonal antibody C219 technique. No association could be demonstrated between response to VAD chemotherapy and Pgp. Dexamethasone may have induced some of the responses in Pgp-positive tumors (92), or perhaps there was modulation of Pgp by the simultaneous doxorubicin and vincristine infusion. Obviously, Pgp alone is not sufficient to explain these heterogeneous results.

It is counterproductive to reduce the dose of a chemotherapeutic agent because of enhanced toxicity unless a schedule or modulator can be found with significant selectivity for tumor compared with normal tissue Pgp. Recent potentially selective candidate modulator drugs include progesterone, which enhanced the hematological toxicity of doxorubicin without altering its pharmacokinetics. This suggested that progesterone affected Pgp at the level of the pluripotent hematopoietic stem cell (93), hence making toxicity potentially amenable to growth factor support. Tamoxifen combined with doxorubicin may also enhance toxic effects on normal bone marrow progenitors (94). Its action is probably unrelated to estrogen receptor. In MDR1 MCF-7 cells, tamoxifen is synergistic with doxorubicin at lower concentrations (1–2.5 $\mu$M), but the synergism is lost at higher concentrations (5 $\mu$mol/L). Although another study (95) did not show this loss of synergy at 5 or 8 $\mu$mol/L, pharmacological monitoring may be needed to avoid either excessive or inadequate doses of the modifier (96). The antiprogestin RU 486 inhibited rhodamine 127 efflux more effectively than progesterone did, and so it too deserves careful study as a modulator of drug efflux (97). Although GF-120918, an acridine carboxamide derivative, is a potent Pgp inhibitor, it did not significantly modify the distribution or elimination of doxorubicin in mice (98). In a phase I clinical study, the triazinoaminopiperidone derivative S9788 did not alter the pharmacokinetics of doxorubicin (99). Many other drugs are undergoing preclinical study as potential modulators of Pgp.

## MRP and Other Resistance Proteins

Identification of the 190-kd multidrug resistance–associated protein (MRP) in the small cell lung cancer line H69AR (100) was greeted with some concern that its spectrum of drug resistance and response to resistance modulators would be somewhat different from that of Pgp. However, their potential clinical spectra appear to be quite similar (including resistance to doxorubicin, daunorubicin, and epirubicin) (Table 1), with differences probably no greater than those seen among various MDR1 cell lines (although the modulators may involve mechanisms independent of MRP expression) (101,102). MRP appears to be ubiquitously expressed at low levels in all normal tissues, and increased expression has been found in many human tumors (103). Its distribution of expression in normal tissues is different from that of MDR1, with low levels in liver, kidney, and bowel (104). Functionally, MRP mediates the ATP-dependent transport of glutathione-S conjugates (105), with cisplatin as well as doxorubicin serving as a substrate of the MRP/GS-X pump (106).

The 110-kd lung resistance protein (LRP) was found originally in the cytoplasm of the non–small cell lung cancer line SW-1573/2R120 and several other doxorubicin-resistant cell lines. It is found also in a number of normal and malignant human tissues (107). Its gene maps in close proximity to MRP on the short arm of chromosome 16, but the two are rarely coamplified and are not normally located within the same amplicon. The LRP gene encodes a major vault protein associated with drug resistance (108). What effect resistance modulators have on LRP is not yet known. In clinical materials it appears to be an indicator of poor response to platinum or to alkylating agents (109), but there are no reports of anthracycline resistance.

Several other resistance proteins have been reported, including a second 190-kd protein associated with resistance to the Pgp-independent investigational anthracycline AD198 (110). Profiles of some other drug-resistant cell lines have been described but no definite resistance protein was identified (111–113) (see Table 1). It remains to be determined whether any of these will be found commonly in clinical material, and if they are, whether there are any differences in the spectra of drug resistance or resistance modulators compared with Pgp.

## Topoisomerase II

The MDR associated with altered topoisomerase II (at-MDR) is a well-defined system of drug resistance in tissue culture for which a clinical correlate has not yet been found. The spectrum of drug resistance is similar but not identical to that of Pgp. at-MDR cells are resistant to amsacrine but sensitive to vinca alkaloids and taxanes. Both Pgp and at-MDR systems are resistant to epipodophyllotoxins and most anthracycline analogues and are sensitive to cisplatin and alkylating agents (Table 1).

Resistant human lymphoblastic leukemia cell lines showed quantitative changes in the $\alpha$ (170-kd) and $\beta$ (180-kd) forms of topoisomerase II that correlated with the cytocidal activity of doxorubicin. Specifically, increased $\alpha$ levels or decreased $\beta$ levels were associated with increased doxorubicin resistance (114). Another leukemic cell line showed normal topoisomerase II mRNA levels ($\alpha$ and $\beta$ not measured separately) and function, but there was overexpression of the topoisomerase I gene in these doxorubicin-resistant cells (115). The failure of doxorubicin to arrest T47D breast cancer cells at the $G_1$/S checkpoint of the cell cycle correlated with a reduction in topoisomerase II (116).

Several mutations of this enzyme were described in cell culture. One of these, in HL60/AMSA leukemic cells, resulted in resistance to idarubicin but not doxorubicin (117). An interesting mutation in doxorubicin-resistant P388 leukemia cells appeared to be a gene fusion between the loci encoding topoisomerase II and retinoic acid receptor $\alpha$ (118). The small cell lung cancer line H209/V6 with fourfold doxorubicin resistance had a mutant 160-kd topoisomerase II$\alpha$ form located in the cytoplasm rather than the nucleus; it lacked three putative bipartite nuclear localization signals (119).

Phosphorylation may be a key to topoisomerase modulation. Trifluoroperazine, a calmodulin inhibitor that also interacts with Pgp, produced an increase in DNA strand breaks at lower doxorubicin levels in resistant L1210 leukemia cells, probably because of an increase in the basal level of topoisomerase II phosphorylation (120). The $\beta_{II}$ protein kinase C activator byrostatin I also up-regulated topoisomerase II phosphorylation (121).

Interference with the topoisomerase II catalytic cycle at four distinct steps has been described. The anthracycline aclarubicin inhibited binding of topoisomerase II to its DNA substrate. Etoposide caused reversible and clerocidin caused irreversible inhibition of DNA religation. Of potential clinical concern, the cardioprotector dexrazoxane (ICRF-187) partakes in an energy-dependent inappropriate binding of the enzyme to DNA after the religation step (122). Nontoxic concentrations of aclarubicin can increase intracellular daunorubicin accumulation in an MDR cell line (presumably MDR1), but it inhibits daunorubicin cytotoxicity by interacting with topoisomerase II (123). The topoisomerase I inhibitors camptothecin and topotecan also inhibited the cytotoxicity of daunorubicin. This probably was not related to any alteration in the drug-induced function of topoisomerase II–DNA cross-links but instead to the inhibition of nucleic acid (especially RNA) synthesis by the topoisomerase I inhibitor (124).

The topoisomerase II–mediated cleavage sequence of DNA is different for some anthracycline analogues. 3'-Epidaunorubicin cleaves preferentially when there is a guanine at position -2, whereas daunorubicin and doxorubicin prefer thymine and exclude guanine. Interestingly, an analogue with no substitutes at the 3' C of the sugar stimulated DNA-cleavage at sites stimulated by the parent drugs as well as those stimulated by 3'-epidaunorubicin (125). Further study of the critical role of the 3' position for optimal anthracycline interactions in the ternary complex would be of interest.

Genetic suppressor elements (GSEs) were isolated from a retroviral library containing random fragments complementary to human topoisomerase IIα cDNA. These were used to encode either dominant-negative mutant proteins (which were likely to interfere with protein processing or function rather than expression) or antisense RNA (which was postulated to inhibit topoisomerase II through a decrease in protein synthesis). In fact, both sense- and antisense-oriented GSEs inhibited topoisomerase II with a 2.5- to 3-fold increase in relative resistance to doxorubicin (126). Down-regulation of kinesin (a microtubular transport protein) may be a natural mechanism of becoming resistant, especially to etoposide and amsacrine but also to doxorubicin and cisplatin (127).

*Clinical Studies with Topoisomerase II*

Clinical information about topoisomerase II remains quite limited. A study of 140 newly diagnosed and 57 relapsed or refractory patients with acute myelogenous leukemia failed to demonstrate topoisomerase II gene mutations that could account for the resistance in 20 patients examined for a G-A mutation at position 1493. Content of the α and β isoenzymes varied over a 20-fold range, but did not correlate with drug sensitivity in vitro or in vivo. There was marked cell-to-cell heterogeneity. Levels of topoisomerase IIα and β in 46 of 47 clinical samples were lower than in human AML cell lines (128).

One of 13 patients with small cell lung cancer had two mutations in topoisomerase II DNA after treatment with etoposide (129). In ovarian cancer, topoisomerase IIα expression was detected in 65% of 54 tumors, with a 16-fold range in level. The frequency of heterozygosity at the topoisomerase IIα locus was not significantly different from that of the normal population (130). Median topoisomerase II catalytic activity was significantly lower ($p < 0.05$) in nine tumors after platinum/cyclophosphamide therapy than in eight untreated patients, whereas expression of the enzyme was not significantly different (131).

## Multiple Resistance Mechanisms

More than one resistance mechanism may be found in tumor cells. Small cell lung cancer H69/VP overexpressed first MRP mRNA and then MDR1, and immunocytochemical staining demonstrated both MRP and Pgp in the same cells (132). Increased MDR1 and MRP and decreased topoisomerase II were described in relapsed acute lymphoblastic leukemia treated with a combination including doxorubicin and daunorubicin (133). Human colon carcinoma LoVo cells had decreased topoisomerase II and also expressed MDR1. The cells were more resistant to daunorubicin than to idarubicin because of differences in intracellular distribution, probably related to the high lipophilicity of idarubicin (134). MDR P388 mouse leukemia cells overexpressed Pgp and had a decreased amount and DNA cleavage activity of topoisomerase II, although the decatenation (unwinding) activity was unchanged (135).

MRP overexpression and reduced sensitivity of topoisomerase II were found in the breast carcinoma MCF-7 cell line (136). Small cell lung cancer line H69AR overexpressing MRP had reduced levels of topoisomerase IIα and β with decreased cleavable complex formation but normal strand-passing activity (137). A third doxorubicin-resistant line, small cell carcinoma $GLC_4/ADR_{150x}$, also overexpressed MRP mRNA and had decreased topoisomerase IIα and β mRNA levels (138).

Another member of the ABC transporter family (which includes Pgp and MRP), the transporter associated with antigen presentation (TAP) was overexpressed in three of three MRP+ and two of five Pgp+ cell lines. TAP genes modestly contributed to MDR, perhaps by transporting drugs into the endoplasmic reticulum (139). A panel of 61 cell lines examined for Pgp, MRP, and LRP showed coexpression of more than one in 64% of the lines. Coexpression was, in general, associated with high levels of drug resistance (140).

The induction of MDR1-mediated doxorubicin resistance in MCF-7 cells has resulted in the development of resistance to tumor necrosis factor (TNF). TNF resistance may have involved an overexpression of endogenous TNF and manganese superoxide dismutase genes; it did not require MDR1 gene expression (141).

MDR1 human breast and colon carcinoma cells overexpressed thymidylate synthase and were cross-resistant to 5-fluorouracil (5-FU) (142). The MDR1 ovarian carcinoma line OAW42-A was not resistant to the MDR1 drug colchicine (nor to 5-FU) but was resistant to cisplatin, suggesting there were additional mechanisms of resistance (143).

In 94 fresh paraffin-embedded non–small cell lung carcinomas, 44 overexpressed Pgp, 67 were positive for thymidylate synthase, and 43 stained negatively for topoisomerase II. Although the report did not give details, two or three of these potential resistance mechanisms must have coexisted in at least some of the tumors (144).

## ONCOGENES: REGULATION OF APOPTOSIS AND OTHER FUNCTIONS

Recently, the scope of interest in mechanisms of cell killing by chemotherapeutic agents has expanded to include the function of oncogenes and tumor suppressor genes. These genetic elements, activated in many types of human cancers, encode proteins implicated in cellular signal transduction and regulation of gene expression. Thus, growth-regulatory messages are transmitted from outside the cell to the nucleus, controlling cellular function, replication, and death. Point-mutated oncogenes such as *p53* and *ras* offer specific targets for therapeutic intervention, whereas overexpressed oncogenes such as *Her-2/neu* offer a nonspecific but quantitatively useful target. The interactions of anthracyclines and other chemotherapeutic agents with oncogenes and other regulators of cell function are of interest as potential mechanisms to regulate neoplastic cells.

In addition to the traditional direct cell killing (by irreversible damage to cellular function leading to degeneration and necrosis), mechanisms of apoptosis (programmed cell death by activation of metabolic pathways involving gene expression, protein synthesis, and activation of endogenous nucleases) are being studied (145). Many cell types with mutant (overexpressed) *p53* suppressor genes are resistant to the induction of apoptosis. The *Bcl-2* proto-oncogene inhibits apoptosis, whereas *c-myc* and *ras* can enhance it.

Inhibition of protein synthesis with cycloheximide or 2-deoxy-D-glucose abrogated doxorubicin toxicity and inhibited apoptosis even when the inhibitor was given 30–45 min after the doxorubicin (146,147). Growth inhibition of HeLa $S_3$ cells treated with doxorubicin and daunorubicin was observed at concentrations about 10 times lower than those inhibiting DNA synthesis. At lower concentrations of anthracyclines, apoptosis was inhibited by post-incubation with cycloheximide, whereas higher

($\times 10$) concentrations potentiated cell death. This suggested that apoptosis may be directly responsible for cell killing that follows the cytostatic effect of these anthracyclines (148).

Acquired MDR in a MOLT-4 (T-lymphoblastic leukemia) cell line appeared to be the result of diminished apoptotic response. The resistance factors were relatively low (two- to fourfold). The drug spectrum included antimetabolites (6-thioguanine, methotrexate, and cytarabine) and two drugs involved in both MDR1 and at-MDR (doxorubicin and etoposide), but the cells remained sensitive to cisplatin and melphalan (149).

Aclarubicin reduced the extent of apoptosis induced by etoposide in most intestinal crypt cells, which may explain how nontoxic doses of aclarubicin interfere with the effectiveness of etoposide against Ehrlich ascites tumors (150). G-CSF and interleukin-6 inhibited apoptosis induced by several classes of drugs including doxorubicin in two cell lines of myeloid leukemia (151).

The dose of anthracycline appears very important in apoptosis. Murine thymocytes were cultured in dexamethasone at 0.1 $\mu$mol/L, a concentration that induces apoptosis. Doxorubicin in low concentrations (0.001–1.0 $\mu$mol/L) produced additive induction, whereas high concentrations (2–10 $\mu$mol/L) completely inhibited apoptosis (152). This dose effect may explain why idarubicin at 1 $\mu$mol/L produced apoptosis in HL-60 human leukemic cells but doxorubicin at 5 $\mu$mol/L did not (117), rather than reflecting an intrinsic difference between the two drugs.

When cellular energy was depressed, a lower dose of doxorubicin (approximately 50%) produced a better response against autochthonous breast tumors in CD8F1 mice. Histological examination (a relatively crude technique) suggested the mechanism was enhanced apoptosis (153). Studies of MCF7 cell nuclear matrix showed differences in the staining pattern of cells killed by doxorubicin compared with those killed by serum growth factor deprivation (154).

## Bcl-2

Bcl-2 is a protein located on the inner mitochondrial membrane that blocks programmed cell death (155). Originally described in malignant lymphomas, it was recently identified in 70% of breast cancers (156). Evidence for the role of Bcl-2 in drug resistance is emerging.

For example, doxorubicin-induced apoptosis was inhibited by *Bcl-2* transfected into human cell lung cancer line SBC-3; however sensitivity to cisplatin, etoposide, methotrexate, and paclitaxel were unchanged (157). Transfection of human pre-B-cell leukemia 697 cell lines with *Bcl-2* vectors produced markedly elevated resistance to apoptotic changes induced by doxorubicin and daunorubicin. This correlated with elevations of Bcl-2 protein levels. Conversely, antisense-mediated reductions in Bcl-2 protein levels in t(14:18)-containing NHL cell lines resulted in enhanced sensitivity. Similar results were seen for other drugs, including methotrexate, vincristine, and 2-chlorodeoxyadenosine (158).

High expression of Bcl-2 was associated with a low complete remission rate and significantly shortened survival in patients treated intensively for acute myeloid leukemia with chemotherapy combinations including anthracyclines (159). However, Bcl-2 abnormalities were sometimes reversed with treatment. Nineteen patients with stage IV low-grade lymphomas had pretreatment *Bcl-2* rearrangements demonstrated by polymerase chain reaction (PCR). Following intensive chemotherapy with conventional doses including doxorubicin, 13 (68%) achieved negative PCR status, including 11 of 14 with complete response as defined by conventional criteria (160).

Bax is a homologue of Bcl-2 that promotes apoptosis. In a group of 199 patients with metastatic breast cancer, reduced Bax correlated with failure to respond and shorter overall survival in those randomized to receive weekly injections of an epirubicin-based chemotherapy regimen. This difference was not significant in those given monthly standard doses, although the epirubicin dose intensity was the same as in the weekly schedule. The authors speculated that administration of chemotherapy as a single monthly dose allowed drugs to surpass a critical threshold concentration tolerated by Bax-negative tumor cells, but decreased the finding as highly preliminary (161).

Antisense oligodeoxynucleotides can reduce Bcl-2 expression in small cell lung cancer lines, increasing the sensitivity to doxorubicin (162). Retinoic acid (RA) treatment of neuroblastoma cell lines abolished the cytotoxic effect of doxorubicin (as well as cisplatin) with a loss of the apoptotic response. There was a marked induction of Bcl-2 expression in cells undergoing differentiation after RA treatment, suggesting a mechanism for the clinical observation that tumor cell differentiation parallels the emergence of drug resistance (163).

## p53

The *p53* gene is located on the short arm of chromosome 17. It encodes a 53-kd nuclear phosphoprotein that acts as a transcription factor. It regulates apoptosis triggered by radiation and many chemotherapeutic agents including doxorubicin (164), but not that induced by glucocorticoids (165). It also blocks cell entry into S phase if DNA damage has been inflicted (166). Most mutant *p53* proteins have a much longer half-life than the wild-type protein—hours rather than minutes. The relatively low levels of *p53* protein in normal cells are generally undetectable when examined by immunohistochemical techniques, whereas in neoplastic cells carrying a mis-sense mutation it is easily demonstrated (overexpressed) because of its prolonged half-life. It is mutated in about half of almost all types of cancer (167). Although most *p53* mutations involve loss of function, gain-of-function mutations have also been described (168).

In a fibrosarcoma model, tumors expressing the normal *p53* gene contained a high proportion of apoptotic cells and regressed after treatment with doxorubicin, but deficient tumors lacking the *p53* gene continued to enlarge and contained few apoptotic cells. Acquired mutations in *p53* were associated with treatment resistance and relapse in *p53*-expressing tumors (169).

A mutant *p53* specifically stimulated the human MDR1 promoter gene and wild-type *p53* specifically repressed it. This implies that the MDR1 gene could be activated during tumor progression, with mutant cells expressing it permitted to pass into S phase during tumor progression by the lack of normal *p53* checkpoint regulation. The *C-Ha-ras*-1 oncogene also had a stimulatory effect on the MDR1 gene promoter (170). In addition, the transcriptional regulatory effects of *p53* are mediated through interactions with MDR1 core promoter sequences (171). Several different *p53* mutants trans-activated MDR1 promoter in several different cell types (172). Transfection of a hammerhead ribosome into A2780AD cells resulted in decreased expression of mutant *p53* and the MDR1 gene, as well as *c-jun* and *c-fos* (173).

In two reports of untreated breast cancer specimens, one found a significant ($P < .001$) correlation of Pgp expression with *p53* expression (mutation) among 213 tumors tested (174), whereas the other found coexpression only in three of 71 tumors. The latter report, however, described higher levels of thymidylate synthase in Pgp-positive tumors ($P=.05$) (175).

Reports of chemoresistance and of shortened survival in patients with mutant (overexpressed) *p53* cannot be evaluated with regard to any specific chemotherapeutic agent or regimen because of the heterogeneity of treatments given to small numbers of patients included in clinical reports.

## Ras

The *ras* oncogene has a central role in the control of cellular growth, regulating a number of genes (176). Transformation of rat liver epithelial cells with retroviral *H-ras* or *raf* oncogenes resulted in increased doxorubicin resistance accompanied by increasing expression of Pgp and glutathione-S transferase P (177). Transformed NIH-3T3 mouse fibroblasts were also less sensitive to cisplatin, but not the MDR1 drugs vincristine or etoposide, and Pgp expression was unchanged although doxorubicin accumulation was decreased. The activity of thymidylate synthase was decreased (178).

The rat cell line R2T24, which was produced by stable *ras* transfection of the R2NEO line, showed significantly less apoptosis and three- to fivefold less cytotoxicity when it was treated with doxorubicin, although no difference was observed in intracellular doxorubicin concentration (179). However, total topoisomerase II activity was higher after *ras*-transformation of NIH-3T3 cells, the higher proportion being the 170-kd α form. The *ras*-transformed cells were more sensitive to the cytotoxic effect of several topoisomerase II inhibitors (180), but anthracyclines were not tested. This was related to increased expression of the RIα isoform of protein kinase type I. It was suggested that events downstream of the topoisomerase II–DNA cleavable complex were modulated by the kinase (181).

## FOS

The *c-fos* oncogene, which is regulated by *ras*, may be important in the function of MDR1 cells. The MDR phenotype of A2780S human ovarian carcinoma cells was reversed four times more rapidly by an anti-*fos* hammerhead ribozyme than by a separate anti-MDR1 ribozyme (173). *Fos* RNA can be induced by a wide variety of DNA-damaging agents, including doxorubicin (182).

## HER-2/neu

*Her-2/neu* (otherwise known as *erbB-2*) encodes a growth factor receptor with extensive homology to the epidermal growth factor receptor (EGFR) and is overexpressed in many human malignancies including breast, ovarian, and non–small cell lung cancers. There is conflicting information about the significance of *Her-2/neu* and its gene product p185 (a growth factor receptor tyrosine kinase) in drug resistance, perhaps related in part to variations in drug dosage.

A retrospective clinical study suggested *Her-2/neu* overexpression may be associated with a significant dose-response effect of FAC adjuvant chemotherapy for breast cancer (183). This effect may be due to an up-regulation of topoisomerase II in cells with activated *Her-2* receptor (184,185), although topoisomerase II deletion was also described in breast cancer cells amplifying *Her-2/neu* (186). MCF-7 subclones selected for MDR by exposure to doxorubicin showed lower amounts of protein encoded by *Her-2/neu* (187). In contrast, coexpression of Pgp and *Her-2/neu* was described in a subgroup of clinically inoperable breast cancer specimens but not in operable tumors (188). Anthracycline-based chemotherapy modified the expression of *Her-2/neu* (and also *p53*) in a minority of cases of breast cancer, usually resulting in the acquisition of oncoprotein (189).

H460 large cell lung cancer cells expressing Pgp showed enhanced chemoresistance to doxorubicin (also etoposide and mitomycin) when transfected with *Her-2/neu*. Interestingly, cisplatin resistance also increased in this cell line (190). In a panel of 20 non–small cell lung cancer cell lines, there was a correlation between *Her-2/neu* expression and the $IC_{50}$ of these drugs as well as for carmustine and melphalan, neither of which is part of the MDR1 spectrum (191). All of this would suggest a deleterious effect of *Her-2/neu* expression on drug response. Interestingly, estrogen stimulated growth of breast cancer cell lines T470 and MCF7 in vitro while inhibiting *Her-2/neu* expression at both the mRNA and protein levels (192). This effect may be potentially beneficial if high levels of *Her-2/neu* are causally related to decreased chemosensitivity.

Emodin, an anthraquinone that inhibits tyrosine kinase, synergistically inhibited the proliferation of non–small cell lung cancer cells overexpressing *Her-2/neu* when given with doxorubicin (and also with cisplatin or etoposide). This synergy did not occur for cells with low expression of *Her-2/neu* (193). The adenovirus type 5 early region 1A (E1A) gene product, transduced by a replication-deficient adenovirus into *Her-2/neu*-overexpressing human cancer cell line Sk-OV3.ip1 in mice, suppressed expression of the p185 tyrosine kinase (194). It would be interesting to study whether the E1A gene product is similarly synergistic with anthracyclines and other chemotherapeutic agents.

Immunoliposomes targeted to the p185 gene product are markedly and specifically cytotoxic in vitro when loaded with doxorubicin and can deliver the drug in vivo in Scid mice bearing human breast tumor BT-474 (195). A disulfide-linked Fvβ-lactamase fusion protein is being developed for activation of a cephalosporin-doxorubicin prodrug against p185[HER2]-overexpressing tumors (196).

## Epidermal Growth Factor Receptor (EGFR)

Doxorubicin causes up-regulation of EGFR in actively growing cells (197). In addition, epidermal growth factor (EGF) increased the sensitivity of two doxorubicin-resistant squamous carcinoma A431 cell lines to doxorubicin (198). In these cells, EGFR was inactivated at 5 min, but then increased and reached its maximum 4–8 h after doxorubicin treatment. The mutated form of *p53* carried by these cells increased, coincident with the doxorubicin-induced $G_2M$ block (199). Because EGF can mediate apoptosis in EGFR-overexpressing MDA-MB-468 human breast cancer cells, this may prove to have important clinical implications (200).

MDR1 Chinese hamster and mouse tumor cells were found to have increased EGFR (201). The function of Pgp in MCF-7/AdrR cells is regulated by EGF through phospholipase C, increasing phosphorylation of Pgp and thus its activity (202).

Antibodies against the extracellular domain of EGFR delivered doxorubicin specifically and efficiently to tumor sites that expressed high receptor levels (203). This resulted in a dose-dependent enhanced antitumor activity capable of complete tumor eradication in some mice bearing A431 xenografts (204). Doxorubicin conjugated to the EGFR monoclonal antibody mAb425 showed striking antitumor activity in a pre-clinical model of spontaneous metastatic human melanoma that was insensitive to free doxorubicin (205).

## Myc

The *myc* oncogene has a role in mitogenesis and also is a potent inducer of apoptosis. Bcl-2 protein abrogates this apoptosis but does not affect the mitogenic function (206). Acute exposure of MCF-7 cells in vitro to a clinically relevant concentration of doxorubicin (1 $\mu$mol/L) or idarubicin (0.01 $\mu$mol/L) resulted in an early reduction in *myc* RNA levels, corresponding closely with growth arrest. This may represent a component of a nonapoptotic mode of cell death (207,208).

The level of regulated *myc* expressed in myeloid leukemias was not associated with susceptibility to induction of apoptosis by doxorubicin, although transfection with deregulated *myc* increased susceptibility. The addition of mutant *p53* transfection to deregulated *myc* suppressed the increased susceptibility to apoptosis (209).

Childhood neuroblastoma cell lines and primary tumors with amplification of *n-myc* oncogene were found to have significantly higher MRP expression than those with no amplification. Decreased expression of *n-myc* in two cell lines following treatment with retinoic acid was paralleled by down-regulation of MRP gene expression, contrasting with increased expression of the MDR1 gene (210).

## INDUCTION OF CELLULAR DIFFERENTIATION

There is some limited information about the ability of anthracyclines and other chemotherapeutic agents (especially cytarabine and dactinomycin) to induce differentiation of malignant cells. The evaluation of increased differentiation is based on morphological changes and on the development of normal cellular functions by neoplastic cells.

Among such agents is the oligosaccharide anthracycline marcellomycin. It was a potent maturation inducer in vitro of the human promyelocytic cell line HL-60 (doxorubicin was inactive) but did not induce differentiation of Friend murine erythroleukemia cells (211). A low concentration of doxorubicin (40 nmol/L) stimulated the synthesis of both hemoglobin and nonhemoglobin proteins in human erythroleukemia K562 (212). Daunorubicin inhibited DNA synthesis, after which differentiation markers accrued in the myeloblastic cell line ML-1 (unlike the mechanism by which retinoic acid stimulates differentiation) (213), and enhanced the ability of lipopolysaccharide to induce differentiation of rat myelomonocytic leukemia c-WRT-7 cells (214).

Epirubicin induced morphological and biochemical differentiation of several human neuroblastoma cell lines in vitro, coincident with growth of neurites and increased acetylcholinesterase activity (215). Cytostatic drug concentrations of doxorubicin in vitro appeared to induce morphological signs of differentiation, including increased melanin content and tyrosinase activity in murine B16 melanoma cells. However, the overgrowth of a few partially differentiated drug-resistant cells from the parental population could not be excluded (216).

Normal cell phenotypes of NIH-3T3 cells transformed by *ras* oncogenes were induced in vitro by doxorubicin. The effect was less prominent on cell lines transformed by other oncogenes and was also seen with pirarubicin but not with the oligosaccharide aclarubicin (217).

Ultrastructural examination of MCF-7 breast carcinoma cells exposed for 24 h to a therapeutic concentration of doxorubicin (50 nmol/L) in vitro showed morphological changes consistent with differentiation induction, with a sustained decline in *c-myc* mRNA levels. This may be the result of damage of nascent DNA, leading to down-regulation of *c-myc* expression and the induction of differentiation (218). In a Friend leukemia cell line, doxorubicin had no effect on *c-myc* (or on *c-myb*) expression or on differentiation, although aclarubicin produced erythroid differentiation and a rapid decrease in oncogene levels (219).

Noncytotoxic concentrations of anthracyclines inhibited angiogenesis in two in vitro systems (220). This may be important for the growth and metastatic potential of tumors.

Future research directions and the potential clinical significance of these interesting observations are not clear.

## ANTHRACYCLINE ANALOGUES

More than 2000 anthracycline analogues have been developed in the search for better drugs than the original daunorubicin and doxorubicin, now in use since the 1960s. Although this number may at first appear absurd, increased understanding about drug-target interactions and the ability to use lipid carriers to deliver water-insoluble drugs clearly justify the continued search for safer and more effective anthracycline drugs. Although modifications of the 4-ring aglycone structure also change the biological interactions with cells, recent interest has been focused primarily on the daunosamine (sugar) molecule of the anthracycline structure.

### Morpholinyl Anthracyclines

Morpholinyl anthracyclines, with a morpholino ring at the 3'-position of the sugar molecule, have been in phase I and II clinical studies since about 1990. These lipophilic molecules are effective against most MDR1 and at-MDR cells, and are active against topoisomerase I rather than topoisomerase II. The methoxymorpholino anthracyclines have a DNA-alkylating activity as a result of metabolic activation in vivo (221). A line of L1210 cells resistant to methoxymorpholino doxorubicin by an unidentified mechanism is sensitive to the parent doxorubicin (222). Similarly, L5178Y murine lymphoblasts were resistant to cyanomorpholinyl doxorubicin but not to doxorubicin itself (223). Detoxifying systems such as GSH and GST may have a role, because a morpholino-resistant small cell line GLC4 was also resistant to cisplatin (224).

A phase I study of 53 patients treated with IV bolus methoxymorpholinyl doxorubicin defined a maximum tolerated dose of 1.5 mg/m$^2$ every 3 weeks. Plasma data suggested linear kinetics, although there was considerable interpatient variability. One patient with a pelvic recurrence of cervical cancer had a complete response. No patient received more than six courses, and no cardiotoxicity was observed (225).

### Annamycin

Reduction of basicity by substitution of hydroxyl for the 3'-amino on the daunosamine sugar molecule increases drug accumulation in MDR1 cells. The introduction of a halogen molecule into the daunosamine increases lipophilicity of the anthracycline. When iodide was added to the 2′ position of the 3′-hydroxyepirubicin derivative, the resultant compound was less water soluble but could be entrapped in liposomes. Removal of the methoxy group at C4 of the aglycone D ring improved the efficiency of liposomal entrapment.

The resulting anthracycline drug, annamycin (3′-deamino-4′-epi-3′-hydroxy-2′-iodo-4-demethoxydoxorubicin), has the potential double advantages of circumventing the MDR1 resistance pump and also relatively selective targeting of drug to tumors by the liposomal carrier (226).

In preclinical studies, annamycin was more effective than doxorubicin against several tumor models, and MDR1 tumors were only partially cross-resistant to annamycin both in vitro and in vivo. Small liposomes (0.03 $\mu$m) enhanced the in vivo antitumor properties of annamycin (227). A clinical phase I trial using 0.15 $\mu$m liposomes under the direction of the author is in progress at the M. D. Anderson Cancer Center.

### Interesting Preclinical Analogues

An interesting nitrosourea-anthracycline hybrid AD312 (2-chlorethylnitrosoureido-daunorubicin) is undergoing preclinical evaluation. It is highly effective against doxorubicin-resistant ovarian, lung, and bladder carcinoma xenografts as well as P388/DOX leukemia. Surprisingly, this compound lacks signs of toxicity, except for weight loss, but dose escalations to date have been limited by the toxicity of its surfactant formulation (228,229).

Conjugates of anthracyclines with DNA minor groove-binding oligopeptides may prove interesting as sequence-specific DNA-binding agents (230).

Two doxorubicin derivatives (DNC$_4$ and DNC$_5$) with pronounced selectivity against doxorubicin-resistant MDR1 human melanoma xenografts have been described (231). Previous anthracyclines are generally inactive in the treatment of melanoma.

### SUMMARY

Anthracycline resistance in cancer patients remains poorly understood despite rapidly emerging information about resistance factors in laboratory systems. It is unlikely that a single approach directed to any one of these currently known factors will have a major impact in overcoming clinical drug resistance. An improved understanding of cellular signaling mechanisms may eventually provide unifying approaches with wide applications for patient care.

### ACKNOWLEDGMENTS

The author is grateful to many colleagues for advice and critical review; to Walter Pagel for both substantive and stylistic editorial suggestions; and to Bonnie Schoenbein for superb secretarial assistance.

## REFERENCES

1. Booser DJ, Hortobagyi GN. Anthracycline antibiotics in cancer therapy: focus on drug resistance. Drugs 1994; 47(2):223–258.
2. Vichi PJ, Tritton TR. Protection from Adriamycin cytotoxicity in L1210 cells by brefeldin A. Cancer Res 1993; 53:5237–5243.
3. Hryniuk W, Bush H. The importance of dose intensity in chemotherapy of metastatic breast cancer. J Clin Oncol 1984; 11:1281–1288.
4. Sehested M, Jensen PB, Sorensen BS, Holm B, Friche E, Demant EJF. Antagonistic effect of the cardioprotector (+)-1,2-bis(3,5-dioxopiperazinyl-1-yl) propane (ICRF-187) on DNA breaks and cytotoxicity induced by the topoisomerase II directed drugs daunorubicin and etoposide (VP-16). Biochem Pharmacol 1993; 46:389–393.
5. Oredipe OA, F-Harris P, Griffin W. Potential importance of swainsonine in doxorubicin therapy (abstr). Proc Am Assoc Cancer Res 1995; 36:355 (2116).
6. Wood WC, Budman DR, Korzun AH, Cooper MR, Younger J, Hart RD, Moore A, Ellerton JA, Norton L, Ferree CR, Ballow AC, Frei E, Henderson IC. Dose and dose intensity of adjuvant chemotherapy for stage II, node-positive breast carcinoma. N Engl J Med 1994; 330:1253–1259.
7. Ang P-T, Buzdar AU, Smith TL, Kau S, Hortobagyi GN. Analysis of dose intensity in doxorubicin-containing adjuvant chemotherapy in stage II and III breast carcinoma. J Clin Oncol 1989; 7:1677–1684.
8. Buzdar AU, Hortobagyi GN, Kau S-WC, Smith TL, Fraschini G, Holmes FA, Gutterman JU, Hug VM, Singletary SE, Ames FC, McNeese MD. Adjuvant therapy with escalating doses of doxorubicin and cyclophosphamide with or without leukocyte-interferon for stage II or III breast cancer. J Clin Oncol 1992; 10:1540–1546.
9. Fumolaeu P, Devaux Y, Vo Van ML, Kerbrat P, Fargeot P, Schraub S, Mihura J, Namer M, Mercier M. Premenopausal patients with node-positive resectable breast cancer. Drugs 1993; 45(suppl 2):38–45.
10. Carmo-Pereira J, Costa FO, Henriques E, Godinho F, Cantinho-Lopes MG, Sales-Luis A, Rubens RD. A comparison of two doses of Adriamycin in the primary chemotherapy of disseminated breast carcinoma. Br J Cancer 1987; 56:471–473.
11. French Epirubicin Study Group. A prospective randomized trial comparing epirubicin monochemotherapy to two fluorouracil, cyclophosphamide, and epirubicin regimens differing in epirubicin dose in advanced breast cancer patients. J Clin Oncol 1991; 9:305–312.
12. Habeshaw T, Paul J, Jones R, Stallard S, Stewart M, Kaye SB, Soukop M, Symonds RP, Reed NS, Rankin EM. Epirubicin at two dose levels with prednisolone as treatment for advanced breast cancer: the results of a randomized trial. J Clin Oncol 1991; 9:295–304.
13. Jones RB, Holland JF, Bhardwaj S, Norton L, Wilfinger C, Strashun A. A phase I-II study of intensive-dose Adriamycin for advanced breast cancer. J Clin Oncol 1987; 5:172–177.
14. Bastholt L, Dalmark M, Gjedde S, Pfeiffer P, Petersen D, Sandberg E, Kjaer M, Mouridsen HT, Rose C, Nielsen OS, Jakobsen P, Bentzen SM. Dose-response relationship of epirubicin in the treatment of postmenopausal patients with metastatic breast cancer: a randomized study of epirubicin at four different dose levels performed by the Danish Breast Cancer Cooperative Group. J Clin Oncol 1996; 141:1146–1155.
15. Marschner N, Krelenberg R, Souchon R, Räth U, Eggeling B, Voigtmann R, Ruffert K, Schütte M, Ammon A, Kesztyüs T, Kaplan E, Nagel G. Evaluation of the importance and relevance of dose intensity using epirubicin and cyclophosphamide in metastatic breast cancer: interim analysis of a prospective randomized trial. Semin Oncol 1994; 21(suppl 1):10–16.
16. Meyer RM, Quirt IC, Skillings JR, Cripps MC, Bramwell VHC, Weinerman BH, Gospodarowicz MK, Burns BF, Sargeant AM, Shepherd LE, Zee B, Hryniuk WM. Escalated as compared with standard doses of doxorubicin in BACOP therapy for patients with non-Hodgkin's lymphoma. N Engl J Med 1993; 329:1770–1776.

17. Zuckerman KS. Efficacy of intensive, high-dose anthracycline-based therapy in intermediate- and high-grade non-Hodgkin's lymphomas. Semin Oncol 1994; 21(suppl 1):59–64.

18. Smith MA, Ungerleider RS, Horowitz ME, Simon R. Influence of doxorubicin dose intensity on response and outcome for patients with osteogenic sarcoma and Ewing's sarcoma. J Natl Cancer Inst 1991; 83:1460–1470.

19. Stone RM, Berg DT, George SL, Dodge RK, Paciucci PA, Schulman P, Lee EJ, Moore JO, Powell BL, Schiffer CA. Granulocyte-macrophage colony-stimulating factor after initial chemotherapy for elderly patients with primary acute myelogenous leukemia. N Engl J Med 1995; 332:1671–1677.

20. Dombret H, Chastang C, Fenaux P, Reiffers J, Bordessoule D, Bouabdallah R, Mandelli F, Ferrant A, Auzanneau G, Tilly H, Yver A, Degos L. A controlled study of recombinant human granulocyte colony-stimulating factor in elderly patients after treatment for acute myelogenous leukemia. N Engl J Med 1995; 332:1678–1683.

21. Chevallier B, Chollet P, Merrouche Y, Roche H, Fumoleau P, Kerbrat P, Genot JY, Fargeot P, Olivier JP, Fizames C, Clavel M, Yver A, Chabernaud VC. Lenograstim prevents morbidity from intensive induction chemotherapy in the treatment of inflammatory breast cancer. J Clin Oncol 1995; 13:1564–1571.

22. Dhingra K, Singletary E, Strom E, Sahin A, Esparza L, Valero V, Booser D, Walters R, Hortobagyi G. Randomized trial of g-csf (filgrastim)-supported dose-intensive neoadjuvant chemotherapy in locally advanced breast cancer (abstr). Proc Am Soc Clin Oncol 1995; 14:94(76).

23. O'Shaughnessy JA, Denicoff AM, Venzon DJ, Danforth D, Pierce LJ, Frame JN, Bastian A, Ghosh B, Goldspiel B, Miller L, Dorr FA, Keegan P, Ben-Baruch N, Mrose H, Noone M, Cowan KH. A dose intensity study of FLAC (5-fluorouracil, leucovorin, doxorubicin, cyclophosphamide) chemotherapy and Escherichia coli-derived granulocyte-macrophage colony-stimulating factor (GM-CSF) in advanced breast cancer patients. Ann Oncol 1994; 5:709–716.

24. Scinto AF, Ferraresi V, Campioni N, Tonachella R, Piarulli L, Sacchi I, Giannarelli D, Cognetti F. Accelerated chemotherapy with high-dose epirubicin and cyclophosphamide plus r-met-HUG-CSF in locally advanced and metastatic breast cancer. Ann Oncol 1995; 6:665–671.

25. Doroshow JH, Somlo G, Ahn C, Baker P, Rincon A, Forman S, Akman S, Chow W, Coluzzi P, Hamasaki V, Leong L, Margolin K, Molina A, Morgan R, Raschko J, Shibata S, Tetef M, Yen Y, Brent J. Prognostic factors predicting progression-free and overall survival in patients with responsive metastatic breast cancer treated with high-dose chemotherapy and bone marrow stem cell reinfusion (abstr). Proc Am Soc Clin Oncol 1995; 14:319(942).

26. Langleben A, Ahlgren P, Burdette-Radoux S, Donato M, Bahary J-P, Lisbona R, Kosiuk J, Shibata H, Milne C, Leyland-Jones B, DiPietro N. Ultra high dose anthracycline combination therapy, with peripheral blood stem cell, G-CSF, and ADR-529 support (abstr). Proc Am Soc Clin Oncol 1995; 14:321(948).

27. Eilber F, Eckardt J, Rosen G, Forscher C, Selch M, Fu Y-S. Preoperative therapy for soft tissue sarcoma. Hematol Oncol Clin North America 1995; 9:817–823.

28. Curley SA, Newman RA, Dougherty TB, Fuhrman GM, Stone DL, Milokajek JA, Guercio S, Guercio A, Carrasco CH, Kuo MT, Hohn DC. Complete hepatic venous isolation and extracorporeal v chemofiltration as treatment for human hepatocellular carcinoma: a phase I study. Ann Surg Oncol 1994; 1:389–399.

29. Perez-Soler R, Priebe W. Anthracycline antibiotics with high liposome entrapment: structural features and biological activity. Cancer Res 1990; 50:4260–4266.

30. Gill PS, Espina BM, Muggia F, Cabriales S, Tulpule A, Esplin JA, Liebman HA, Forssen E, Ross ME, Levine AM. Phase I/II clinical and pharmacokinetic evaluation of liposomal daunorubicin. J Clin Oncol 1995; 13:996–1003.

31. Harrison M, Tomlinson D, Stewart S. Liposomal-entrapped doxorubicin: an active agent in AIDS-related Kaposi's sarcoma. J Clin Oncol 1995; 13:914–920.

32. Uziely B, Jeffers S, Isacson R, Kutsch K, Wei-Tsao D, Yehushua Z, Libson E, Muggia FM, Gabizon A. Liposomal doxorubicin: antitumor activity and unique toxicities during two complementary phase I studies. J Clin Oncol 1995; 13:1777–1785.

33. Kleinerman ES, Snyder JS, Jaffe N. Influence of chemotherapy administration on monocyte activation by liposomal muramyl tripeptide phosphatidylethanolamine in children with osteosarcoma. J Clin Oncol 1991; 9:259–267.

34. Shi F, MacEwen G, Kurzman ID. In vitro and in vivo effect of doxorubicin combined with liposome-encapsulated muramyl tripeptide on canine monocyte activation. Cancer Res 1993; 53:3986–3991.

35. Vail DM, MacEwen EG, Kurzman ID, Dubielzig RR, Helfand SC, Kisseberth WC, London CA, Obradovich JE, Madewell BR, Rodriguez CO, Fidel J, Susaneck S, Rosenberg M. Liposome-encapsulated muramyl tripeptide phosphatidylethanolamine adjuvant immunotherapy for splenic hemangiosarcoma in the dog: a randomized multi-institutional clinical trial. Clin Cancer Res 1995; 1:1165–1170.

36. Higashi S, Shimizu M, Nakashima T, Iwata K, Ichiyama F, Tateno S, Tamura S, Setoguchi T. Arterial-injection chemotherapy for hepatocellular carcinoma using monodispersed poppy-seed oil microdroplets containing fine aqueous vesicles of epirubicin. Cancer 1995; 75:1245–1254.

37. Lee RJ, Low PS. Folate-mediated tumor cell targeting of liposome-entrapped doxorubicin in vitro. Biochim Biophys Acta 1995; 1233:134–144.

38. Trail PA, Willner D, Lasch SJ, Henderson AJ, Hofstead S, Casazza AM, Firestone RA, Hellström I, Hellström KE. Cure of xenografted human carcinomas by BR96-doxorubicin immunoconjugates. Science 1993; 261:212–215.

39. Sugarman S, Murray JL, Saleh M, LoBuglio AF, Jones D, Daniel C, LeBherz D, Brewer H, Healey D, Kelley S, Hellstrom KE, Onetto N. A phase I study of BR96-doxorubicin in patients with advanced carcinoma expressing the Lewis[Y] antigen (abstr). Proc Am Soc Clin Oncol 1995; 14:473(1532).

40. Stastny JJ, Das Gupta TK. The use of daunomycin-antibody immunoconjugates in managing soft tissue sarcomas: nude mouse xenograft model. Cancer Res 1993; 43:5740–5744.

41. Ahmad I, Longenecker M, Samuel J, Allen TM. Antibody-targeted delivery of doxorubicin entrapped in sterically stabilized liposomes can eradicate lung cancer in mice. Cancer Res 1993; 53:1484–1488.

42. Svensson HP, Vrudhula VM, Emswiler JE, MacMaster JF, Cosand WL, Senter PD, Wallace PM. In vitro and in vivo activities of a doxorubicin prodrug in combination with monoclonal antibody β-lactamase conjugates. Cancer Res 1995; 55:2357–2365.

43. Mukhopadhyay B, Mukhopadhyay A, Basu SK. Enhancement of tumouricidal activity of daunomycin by receptor-mediated delivery. Biochem Pharmacol 1993; 46:919–924.

44. Doughty JC, Anderson JH, Willmott N, McArdle CS. Intra-arterial administration of Adriamycin-loaded albumin microspheres for locally advanced breast cancer. Postgrad Med J 1995; 71:47–49.

45. Kartner N, Riordan JR, Ling V. Cell surface P-glycoprotein associated with multidrug resistance in mammalian cell lines. Science 1983; 221:1285–1288.

46. Bell DR, Gerlach JH, Kartner N, Buick RN, Ling V. Detection of P-glycoprotein in ovarian cancer: a molecular marker associated with multidrug resistance. J Clin Oncol 1985; 3:311–315.

47. Higgins CF. The ABC of channel regulation. Cell 1995; 82:693–696.

48. Fan D, Buccana CD, Beltran PJ, Gutman M, Yoon SS, Sanchez R, Campbell JE, Wang YF, Bielenberg D, Fidler IJ. High cell density and large tumor volume down-regulate the expression of the mdr1 gene in the CT-26 murine colon carcinoma and the KM12 human colon carcinoma (abstr). Proc Am Assoc Cancer Res 1994; 35:351(2089).

49. Muller C, Ling V. P-glycoprotein stability is affected by serum deprivation and high cell density in multidrug resistant cells (abstr). Proc Am Assoc Cancer Res 1992; 33:452(2701).

50. Schuurhuis GJ, van Heijningen THM, Cervantes A, Pinedo HM, de Lange JHM, Keizer HG, Broxterman HJ, Baak JPA, Lankelma J. Changes in subcellular doxorubicin distribution and cellular accumulation alone can largely account for doxorubicin resistance in SW-1573 lung cancer and MCF-7 breast cancer multidrug resistant tumour cells. Br J Cancer 1993; 68:898–908.

51. Molinari A, Cianfriglia M, Meschini S, Calcabrini A, Arancia G. P-glycoprotein expression in the Golgi apparatus of multidrug-resistant cells. Int J Cancer 1994; 59:789–795.

52. Schuurhuis GJ, Broxterman HJ, Cervantes A, van Heijningen THM, de Lange JHM, Baak JPA, Pinedo HM, Lankelma J. Quantitative determination of factors contributing to doxorubicin resistance in multidrug-resistant cells. J Natl Cancer Inst 1989; 81:1887–1892.

53. Muller C, Goubin F, Ferrandis E, Cornil-Scharwtz I, Bailly JD, Bordier C, Bénard J, Sikic BI, Laurent G. Evidence for transcriptional control of human mdr1 gene expression by verapamil in multidrug-resistant leukemic cells. Mol Pharmacol 1994; 47:51–56.

54. Safa AR. Photoaffinity labeling of P-glycoprotein in multidrug-resistance cells. Cancer Invest 1993; 11:46–56.

55. Safa AR, Agresti M, Bryk D, Tamai I. N-(p-Azido-3-[$^{125}$I]iodophenethyl)spiperone binds to specific regions of P-glycoprotein and another multidrug binding protein, spiperophilin, in human neuroblastoma cells. Biochemistry 1994; 33:256–265.

56. Ueda K, Okamura N, Hirai M, Tanigawara Y, Saeki T, Kioka N, Komano T, Hori R. Human P-glycoprotein transports cortisol, aldosterone, and dexamethasone, but not progesterone. J Biol Chem 1992; 267:24248–24252.

57. Lang A, de Giuli R, Lehnert M. Effects of prolonged drug exposure on P-glycoprotein resistance differ for various cytotoxic agents (abstr). Proc Am Soc Clin Oncol 1995; 14: 182(412).

58. Ferry DR, Russell MA, Kerr DJ. [$^3$H]-Taxol binds to a drug acceptor site which is allosterically coupled to the vinblastine-selective site of P-glycoprotein (abstr). Proc Am Assoc Cancer Res 1994; 35:349(2078).

59. Husain SR, Rahman A. Mechanism of interaction of taxol with P-glycoprotein in multidrug resistant cells (abstr). Proc Am Assoc Cancer Res 1994; 35:357(2129).

60. Holmes FA, Newman RA, Madden T, Valero V, Fraschini G, Walters RS, Booser DJ, Buzdar AU, Wiley J, Hortobagyi GN. Schedule dependent pharmacokinetics in a phase I trial of Taxol and doxorubicin as initial chemotherapy for metastatic breast cancer (abstr). Ann Oncol 1994; 5(suppl 5):197(489).

61. Kang Y, Perry RR. Effect of $\alpha$-interferon on P-glycoprotein expression and function and on verapamil modulation of doxorubicin resistance. Cancer Res 1994; 54:2952–2958.

62. Fogler WE, Pearson JW, Volker K, Ariyoshi K, Watabe H, Riggs CW, Wiltrout RH, Longo DL. Enhancement by recombinant human interferon alfa of the reversal of multidrug resistance by MRK-16 monoclonal antibody. J Natl Cancer Inst 1995; 87:94–104.

63. Dufour P, Feugeas O, Bergerat JP, Oberling F. Modulation of adriamycin cytotoxicity on K562 and K562 adri by interferon $\alpha$, all trans retinoic acid and their combination (abstr). Proc Am Assoc Cancer Res 1994; 35:282(1687).

64. Cardarelli CO, Aksentijevich I, Pastan I, Gottesman MM. Differential effects of P-glycoprotein inhibitors on NIIH3T3 cells transfected with wild-type (G185) or mutant (V185) multidrug transporters. Cancer Res 1995; 55:1086–1091.

65. Mogul MJ, Duran GE, Fleming WH, Jaffrezou JP, Chen G, Brophy NA, Sikic BI. Resistance to modulation in multidrug resistant cells co-selected with cyclosporine and doxorubicin (abstr). Proc Am Assoc Cancer Res 1994; 35:352(2096).

66. Chen G, Jaffrezou J-P, Flemming WH, Duran GE, Sikic BI. Prevalence of multidrug resistance related to activation of the mdr1 gene in human sarcoma mutants derived by single-step doxorubicin selection. Cancer Res 1994; 54:4980–4987.

67. Hill BT, Deuchars K, Hosking LK, Ling V, Whelan RDH. Overexpression of P-glycoprotein in mammalian tumor cell lines after fractionated x irradiation in vitro. J Natl Cancer Inst 1990; 82:607–612.

68. Chaudhary PM, Roninson IB. Induction of multidrug resistance in human cells by transient exposure to different chemotherapeutic drugs. J Natl Cancer Inst 1993; 84:632–639.

69. Schuetz JD, Schuetz EG, Furuya KN, Sun D. Estrogenic induction of human mdr in the human hepatoblastoma HepG2 (abstr). Proc Am Assoc Cancer Res 1994; 35:555(3305).

70. Kato S, Nishimura J, Yufu Y, Ideguchi H, Umemura T, Nawata H. Modulation of expression of multidrug resistance gene (mdr-1) by Adriamycin. FEBS Lett 1992; 308:175–178.

71. Thierry AR, Rahman A, Dritschilo A. A new procedure for the preparation of liposomal doxorubicin: biological activity in multidrug-resistant tumor cells. Cancer Chemother Pharmacol 1994; 35:84–88.

72. Mickisch GH, Rahman A, Pastan I, Gottesman MM. Increased effectiveness of liposome-encapsulated doxorubicin in multidrug-resistant-transgenic mice compared with free doxorubicin. J Natl Cancer Inst 1992; 84:804–805.

73. Kobayashi H, Dorai T, Holland JF, Ohnuma T. Reversal of drug sensitivity in multidrug-resistant tumor cells by an MDR1 (PGY1) ribozyme. Cancer Res 1994; 54:1271–1275.

74. Evans CH, Baker PD. Decreased P-glycoprotein expression in multidrug-sensitive and -resistant human myeloma cells induced by the cytokine leukoregulin. Cancer Res 1992; 52:5893–5899.

75. Quattrone A, Papucci L, Morganti M, Coronnello M, Mini E, Mazzei T, Colonna FP, Garbesi A, Capaccioli S. Inhibition of mdr1 gene expression by antimessenger oligonucleotides lowers muiltiple drug resistance. Oncol Res 1994; 6:311–320.

76. Beketic-Oreskovic L, Duran GE, Chen G, Dumontet C, Sikic BI. Decreased mutation rate for cellular resistance to doxorubicin and suppression of mdr1 gene activation by the cyclosporin PSC 833. J Natl Cancer Inst 1995; 87:1593–1602.

77. Morgan RJ, Margolin K, Raschko J, Akman S, Leong L, Somlo G, Scanlon K. Ahn C, Carroll M, Doroshow JH. Phase I trial of carboplatin and infusional cyclosporine in advanced malignancy. J Clin Oncol 1995; 13:2238–2246.

78. Sugimoto Y, Hrycyna CA, Aksentijevich I, Pastan I, Gottesman MM. Coexpression of a multidrug-resistance gene (mdr1) and herpes simplex virus thymidine kinase gene as part of a bicistronic messenger RNA in a retrovirus vector allows selective killing of mdr1-transduced cells. Clin Cancer Res 1995; 1:447–457.

79. Doroshow JH, Metz MZ, Matsumoto L, Winters KA, Sakai M, Muramatsu M, Kane SE. Transduction of NIH 3T3 cells with a retrovirus carrying both human mdr1 and glutathione s-transferase π produces broad-range multidrug resistance. Cancer Res 1995; 55:4073–4078.

80. Goldstein LJ, Galski H, Fojo A, Willingham M, Lai S-L, Gazdar A, Pirker R, Green A, Crist W, Brodeur GM, Lieber M, Cossman J, Gottesman MM, Pastan I. Expression of a multidrug resistance gene in human cancers. J Natl Cancer Inst 1989; 81:116–124.

81. Erlichman C, Moore M, Thiessen JJ, Kerr IG, Walker S, Goodman P, Bjarnason G, DeAngelis C, Bunting P. Phase I pharmacokinetic study of cyclosporin A combined with doxorubicin. Cancer Res 1993; 53:4837–4842.

82. Bartlett NL, Lum BL, Fisher GA, Brophy NA, Ehsan MN, Halsey J, Sikic BI. Phase I trial of doxorubicin with cyclosporine as a modulator of multidrug resistance. J Clin Oncol 1994; 12:835–842.

83. Rushing DA, Raber SR, Rodvold KA, Piscitelli SC, Plank GS, Tewksbury DA. The effects of cyclosporine on the pharmacokinetics of doxorubicin in patients with small cell lung cancer. Cancer 1994; 74:834–841.

84. Sonneveld P, Durie BGM, Lokhorst HM, Marie J-P, Solbu G, Suciu S, Zittoun R, Lowenberg B, Nooter K. Modulation of multidrug-resistant multiple myeloma by cyclosporin. Lancet 1992; 340:255–259.

85. Sparano JA, Wiernik PH, Leaf A, Dutcher JP. Infusional cyclophosphamide, doxorubicin, and etoposide in relapsed and resistant non-Hodgkin's lymphoma: evidence for a schedule-dependent effect favoring infusional administration of chemotherapy. J Clin Oncol 1993; 11:1071–1079.

86. Wilson WH, Bryant G, Bates S, Fojo A, Wittes RE, Steinberg SM, Kohler DR, Jaffe ES, Herdt J, Cheson BD, Chabner BA. EPOCH chemotherapy: Toxicity and efficacy in relapsed and refractory non-Hodgkin's lymphoma. J Clin Oncol 1993; 11:1573–1582.

87. Wilson WH, Bates SE, Fojo A, Bryant G, Zhan Z, Regis J, Wittes R, Jaffe ES, Steinberg SM, Herdt J, Chabner BA. Controlled trial of dexverapamil, a modulator of multidrug resistance, in lymphomas refractory to EPOCH chemotherapy. J Clin Oncol 1995; 13:1995–2004.

88. Pinedo HM, Giaccone G. P-glycoprotein—a marker of cancer-cell behavior. N Engl J Med 1995; 333:1417–1419.

89. Pilarski LM, Belch AR. Circulating monoclonal B cells expressing P-glycoprotein may be a reservoir of multidrug-resistant disease in multiple myeloma. Blood 1994; 83:724–736.

90. Grogan TM, Spier CM, Salmon SE, Matzner M, Rybski J, Weinstein RS, Scheper RJ, Dalton WS. P-glycoprotein expression in human plasma cell myeloma: correlation with prior chemotherapy. Blood 1993; 81:490–495.

91. Sonneveld P, Schoester M, de Leeuw K. Clinical modulation of multidrug resistance in multiple myeloma: effect of cyclosporine on resistant tumor cells. J Clin Oncol 1994; 12: 1584–1591.

92. Cornelissen JJ, Sonneveld P, Schoester M, Raaijmakers HGP, Nieuwenhuis HK, Dekker AW, Lokhorst HM. MDR-1 expression and response to vincristine, doxorubicin, and dexamethasone chemotherapy in multiple myeloma refractory to alkylating agents. J Clin Oncol 1994; 12:115–119.

93. Christen RD, McClay EF, Plaxe SC, Yen SSC, Kim S, Kirmani S, Wilgus LL, Heath DD, Shalinsky DR, Freddo JL, Braly PS, O'Quigley J, Howell SB. Phase I/pharmacokinetic study of high-dose progesterone and doxorubicin. J Clin Oncol 1993; 11:2417–2426.

94. Woods KE, Grant S, Yanovich S, Gewirtz DA. Variable effects of tamoxifen on human hematopoietic progenitor cell growth and sensitivity to doxorubicin. Cancer Chemother Pharmacol 1994; 33:509–514.

95. Panasci L, Damian S, Damian Z, Batist G, Leyland-Jones B. Synergistic reversal of adriamycin resistance in breast cancer cell lines by tamoxifen and Megace (abstr). Proc Am Soc Clin Oncol 1993; 12:59(37).

96. Leonessa F, Jacobson M, Boyle B, Lippman J, McGarvey M, Clarke R. Effect of tamoxifen on the multidrug-resistant phenotype in human breast cancer cells: Isobologram, drug accumulation, and $M_r$ 170,000 glycoprotein (gp170) binding studies. Cancer Res 1994; 54: 441–447.

97. Gruol DJ, Zee MC, Trotter J, Bourgeois S. Reversal of multidrug resistance by RU 486. Cancer Res 1994; 54:3088–3091.

98. Hyafil F, Vergely C, Du Vignaud P, Grand-Perret T. In vitro and in vivo reversal of multidrug resistance by GF120918, an acridonecarboxamide derivative. Cancer Res 1993; 53: 4595–4602.

99. de Valeriola D, Brassinne C, Lucas C, Tueni E, Awada A, Parmentier N, Bleiberg H, Piccart M. Lack of interference of S9788 with the pharmacokinetics of Adriamycin (abstr). Proc Am Assoc Cancer Res 1995; 36:234(1392).

100. Cole SPC, Bhardwaj G, Gerlach JH, Mackie JE, Grant CE, Almquist KC, Stewart AJ, Jurz EU, Duncan AMV, Deeley RG. Overexpression of a transporter gene in a multidrug-resistant human lung cancer cell line. Science 1992; 258:1650–1654.

101. Cole SPC, Sparks KE, Fraser K, Loe DW, Grant CE, Wilson GM, Deeley RG. Pharmacological characterization of multidrug resistant MRP-transfected human tumor cells. Cancer Res 1994; 54:5902–5910.

102. Zaman GJR, Flens MJ, van Leusden MR, de Haas M, Mulder HS, Lankelma J, Pinedo HM, Scheper RJ, Baas F, Broxterman HJ, Borst P. The human multidrug resistance-associated protein MRP is a plasma membrane drug-efflux pump. Proc Natl Acad Sci USA 1994; 91:8822–8826.

103. Nooter K, Westerman AM, Flens MJ, Zaman GJR, Scheper RJ, van Wingerden KE, Burger H, Oostrum R, Boersma T, Sonneveld P, Gratama JM, Kok T, Eggermont AMM, Bosman FT, Stoter G. Expression of the multidrug resistance-associated protein (MRP) gene in human cancers. Clin Cancer Res 1995; 1:1301–1310.

104. Zaman GJR, Versantvoort CHM, Smit JJM, Eijdems EWHM, de Haas M, Smith AJ, Broxterman HJ, Mulder NH, de Vries EGE, Baas F, Borst P. Analysis of the expression of MRP, the gene for a new putative transmembrane drug transporter, in human multidrug resistant lung cancer cell lines. Cancer Res 1993; 53:1747–1750.

105. Jedlitschky G, Leier I, Buchholz U, Center M, Keppler D. ATP-dependent transport of glutathione S-conjugates by the multidrug resistance-associated protein. Cancer Res 1994; 54:4833–4836.

106. Ishikawa T, Akimaru K, Kuo MT, Priebe W, Suzuki M. How does the MRP/GS-X pump export doxorubicin? J Natl Cancer Inst 1995; 87:1639–1640.

107. Scheper RJ, Broxterman HJ, Scheffer GL, Kaaijk P, Dalton WS, van Heijningen THM, van Kalken CK, Slovak ML, de Vries EGE, van der Valk P, Meijer CJLM, Pinedo HM. Overexpression of a $M_r$ 110,000 vesicular protein in non-P-glycoprotein-mediated multidrug resistance. Cancer Res 1993; 53:1475–1479.

108. Slovak ML, Ho JP, Cole SPC, Deeley RG, Greenberger L, de Vries EGE, Broxterman HJ, Scheffer GL, Scheper RJ. The LRP gene encoding a major vault protein associated with drug resistance maps proximal to MRP on chromosome 16: evidence that chromosome breakage plays a key role in MRP or LRP gene amplification. Cancer Res 1995; 55:4214–4219.

109. Izquierdo MA, van der Zee AGJ, Vermorken JB, van der Valk P, Belien JAM, Giaccone G, Scheffer GL, Flens MJ, Pinedo HM, Kenemans P, Meijer CJLM, de Vries EGE, Scheper RJ. Drug resistance-associated marker Lrp for prediction of response to chemotherapy and prognoses in advanced ovarian carcinoma. J Natl Cancer Inst 1995; 87:1230–1237.

110. Lothstein L, Savranskaya L. Overexpression of a novel 190 kDa protein associated with resistance against N-benzyladriamycin-14-valerate (AD 198) (abstr). Proc Am Assoc Cancer Res 1994; 35:342(2036).

111. Nakagawa M, Schneider E, Dixon KH, Horton J, Kelley K, Morrow C, Cowan KH. Reduced intracellular drug accumulation in the absence of P-glycoprotein (mdr1) overexpression in mitoxantrone-resistant human MCF-7 breast cancer cells. Cancer Res 1992; 52:6175–6181.

112. Hamaguchi K, Godwin AK, Yakushiji M, O'Dwyer PJ, Ozols RF, Hamilton TC. Cross-resistance to diverse drugs is associated with primary cisplatin resistance in ovarian cancer cell lines. Cancer Res 1993; 53:5225–5232.

113. Kwok TT. Characteristics of Adriamycin resistant sublines selected from human squamous carcinoma A431 cells (abstr). Proc Am Assoc Cancer Res 1994; 35:651(3880).

114. Brown GA, McPherson JP, Gu L, Hedley DW, Toso R, Deuchars KL, Freedman MH, Goldenberg GJ. Relationship to DNA topoisomerase II α and β expression to cytotoxicity of antineoplastic agents in human acute lymphoblastic leukemia cell lines. Cancer Res 1995; 55:78–82.

115. Riou J-F, Grondard L, Petitgenet O, Abitbol M, Lavelle F. Altered topoisomerase I activity and recombination activating gene expression in a human leukemia cell line resistant to doxorubicin. Biochem Pharmacol 1993; 46:851–861.

116. Smith PJ, Soues MS, Falk SJ, Hill BT. G1/S checkpoint evasion and resistance to a topoisomerase II poison (doxorubicin) in human breast tumor cell lines (abstr). Proc Am Assoc Cancer Res 1994; 35:25(147).

117. Zwelling LA, Bales E, Altschuler E, Mayes J. Circumvention of resistance by doxorubicin, but not by idarubicin, in a human leukemia cell line containing an intercalator-resistant form of topoisomerase II: evidence for a non-topoisomerase II-mediated mechanism of doxorubicin cytotoxicity. Biochem Pharmacol 1993; 45:516–520.

118. McPherson JP, Brown GA, Goldenberg GJ. Characterization of a DNA topoisomerase II gene rearrangement in Adriamycin-resistant P388 leukemia: expression of a fusion messenger RNA transcript encoding topoisomerase II and the retinoic acid receptor locus. Cancer Res 1993; 53:5885–5889.

119. Mirski SEL, Cole SPC. Cytoplasmic localization of a mutant $M_r$ 160,000 topoisomerase II is associated with the loss of putative bipartite nuclear localization signals in a drug-resistant human lung cancer cell line. Cancer Res 1995; 55:2129–2134.

120. Ganapathi R, Kamath N, Constantinou A, Grabowski D, Ford J, Anderson A. Effect of the calmodulin inhibitor trifluoperazine on phosphorylation of P-glycoprotein and topoisomerase II: relationship to modulation of subcellular distribution, DNA damage and cytotoxicity of doxorubicin in multidrug resistant L1210 mouse leukemia cells. Biochem Pharmacol 1991; 41:R21–R26.

121. Yalowich JC, Ritke MK, Allan WP, Murray NR, Fields AP. Bryostatin 1 upregulates topoisomerase II phosphorylation and potentiates VP-16 activity in VP-16 resistant K562 leukemia cells (abstr). Proc Am Assoc Cancer Res 1995; 36:342(2036).

122. Sehested M, Jensen PB. Uncoupling the DNA topoisomerase II catalytic cycle at 4 distinct steps by the drugs aclarubicin, VP-16, clerocidin and ICRF-187 (abstr). Proc Am Assoc Cancer Res 1995; 36:447(2669).

123. Jensen PB, Jensen PS, Demant EJF, Friche E, Sorensen BS, Sehested M, Wassermann K, Vindelov L, Westergaard O, Hansen HH. Antagonistic effect of aclarubicin on daunorubicin-induced cytotoxicity in human small cell lung cancer cells: relationship to DNA integrity and topoisomerase II. Cancer Res 1991; 51:5093–5099.

124. Kaufmann SH. Antagonism between camptothecin and topoisomerase II-directed chemotherapeutic agents in a human leukemia cell line. Cancer Res 1991; 51:1129–1136.

125. Capranico G, Butelli E, Zunino F. Change of the sequence specificity of daunorubicin-stimulated topoisomerase II DNA cleavage by epimerization of the amino group of the sugar moiety. Cancer Res 1995; 55:312–317.

126. Gudkov AV, Zelnick CR, Kazarov AR, Thimmapaya R, Suttle DP, Beck WT, Roninson IB. Isolation of genetic suppressor elements, inducing resistance to topoisomerase II-interactive cytotoxic drugs, from human topoisomerase II cDNA. Proc Natl Acad Sci USA 1993; 90:3231–3235.

127. Gudkov AV, Kazarov AR, Thimmapaya R, Axenovich SA, Mazo IA, Roninson IG. Cloning mammalian genes by expression selection of genetic suppressor elements: association of kinesin with drug resistance and cell immortalization. Proc Natl Acad Sci USA 1994; 91: 3744–3748.

128. Kaufmann SH, Karp JE, Jones RJ, Miller CB, Schneider E, Zwelling LA, Cowan K, Wendel K, Burke PJ. Topoisomerase II levels and drug sensitivity in adult acute myelogenous leukemia. Blood 1994; 83:517–530.

129. Kubo A, Nakagawa K, Fukuoka M, Yoshikawa A, Hirashima TK, Yana T, Masuda N, Matsui K, Kusunoki Y, Kawase I, Takada M. Identification of point mutations in the alpha-topoisomerase II cDNA from human small cell lung cancer treated previously with etoposide (abstr). Proc Am Assoc Cancer Res 1995; 36:447(2664).

130. van der Zee AGJ, de Vries EGE, Hollema H, Kaye SB, Brown R, Keith WN. Molecular analysis of the topoisomerase IIα gene and its expression in human ovarian cancer. Ann Oncol 1994; 5:75–81.

131. van der Zee AGJ, de Jong S, Keith WN, Hollema H, Boonstra H, de Vries EGE. Quantitative and qualitative aspects of topoisomerase I and IIα and β in untreated and platinum/cyclophosphamide treated malignant ovarian tumors. Cancer Res 1994; 54:749–755.

132. Brock I, Hipfner DR, Nielsen BS, Jensen PB, Deeley RG, Cole SPC, Sehested M. Sequential coexpression of the multidrug resistance genes MRP and mdr1 and their products in VP-16 (etoposide)-selected H69 small cell lung cancer cells. Cancer Res 1995; 55: 459–462.

133. Gekeler V, Beck J, Noller A, Wilisch A, Frese G, Neumann M, Handgretinger R, Ehninger G, Probst H, Niethammer D. Drug-induced changes in the expression of MDR-associated genes: investigations on cultured cell lines and chemotherapeutically treated leukemias. Ann Hematol 1994; 69:S19–S24.

134. Toffoli G, Simone F, Gigante M, Boiocchi M. Comparison of mechanisms responsible for resistance to idarubicin and daunorubicin in multidrug resistant LoVo cell lines. Biochem Pharmacol 1994; 48:1871–1881.

135. Kamath N, Grabowski D, Ford J, Kerrigan D, Pommier Y, Ganapathi R. Overexpression of P-glycoprotein and alterations in topoisomerase II in P388 mouse leukemia cells selected in vivo for resistance to mitoxantrone. Biochem Pharmacol 1992; 44:937–945.

136. Schneider E, Horton JK, Yang C-H, Nakagawa M, Cowan KH. Multidrug resistance-associated protein gene overexpression and reduced drug sensitivity of topoisomerase II in a human breast carcinoma MCF7 cell line selected for etoposide resistance. Cancer Res 1994; 54:152–158.

137. Evans CD, Mirski SE, Danks MK, Cole SPC. Reduced levels of topoisomerase IIα and IIβ in a multidrug-resistant lung-cancer cell line. Cancer Chemother Pharmacol 1994; 34:242–248.

138. Withoff S, Versantvoort CHM, Broxterman HJ, de Vries EGE, Mulder NH. Drug resistance associated factors in a small cell lung carcinoma cell line and its sublines with different Adriamycin resistance factors (abstr). Proc Am Assoc Cancer Res 1994; 35:364(2171).

139. Izquierdo MA, Neefjes JJ, El Matahari A, Scheffer GL, Flens MJ, Ploegh HL, Scheper RJ. Contribution to multidrug resistance of the transporter associated with antigen presentation TAP1 (abstr). Proc Am Assoc Cancer Res 1995; 36:323(1924).

140. Izquierdo MA, Shoemaker RH, Flens MJ, Scheffer GL, Wu L, Prater TR, Scheper RJ. Overlapping phenotypes of multidrug resistance among disease-oriented panels of human cancer cell lines (abstr). Proc Am Assoc Cancer Res 1995; 36:323(1923).

141. Zyad A, Benard J, Tursz T, Clarke R, Chouaib S. Resistance to TNF-α and Adriamycin in the human breast cancer MCF-7 cell line: relationship to MDR1, MnSOD, and TNF gene expression. Cancer Res 1994; 54:825–831.

142. Lenz JH, Danenberg KD, Uziely B, Muggia FM, Danenberg PV. Co-regulation of thymidylate synthase and MDR in patients with breast cancer (abstr). Proc Am Soc Clin Oncol 1994; 13:125(298).

143. Redmond A, Moran E, Clynes M. Multiple drug resistance in the human ovarian carcinoma cell line OAW42-A. Eur J Cancer 1993; 29A:1078–1081.

144. Volm M, Mattern J. Detection of multiple resistance mechanisms in untreated human lung cancer. Onkologie 1993; 16:189–194.

145. Kerr JFR, Winterford CM, Harmon BV. Apoptosis: its significance in cancer and cancer therapy. Cancer 1994; 73:2013–2026.

146. Thakkar NS, Potten CS. Abrogation of Adriamycin toxicity in vivo by cycloheximide. Biochem Pharmacol 1992; 43:1683–1691.

147. Thakkar NS, Potten CS. Inhibition of doxorubicin-induced apoptosis in vivo by 2-deoxy-D-glucose. Cancer Res 1993; 53:2057–2060.

148. Skladanowski A, Konopa J. Adriamycin and daunomycin induce programmed cell death (apoptosis) in tumor cells. Biochem Pharmacol 1993; 46:375–382.

149. Frankfurt OS, Seckinger D, Sugarbaker EV. Pleiotropic drug resistance and survival advantage in leukemic cells with diminished apoptotic response. Int J Cancer 1994; 59:217–224.

150. Holm B, Jensen PB, Sehested M, Hansen HH. In vivo inhibition of etoposide-mediated apoptosis, toxicity, and antitumor effect by the topoisomerase II-uncoupling anthracycline aclarubicin. Cancer Chemother Pharmacol 1994; 34:503–508.

151. Lotem J, Sachs L. Hematopoietic cytokines inhibit apoptosis induced by transforming growth factor β1 and cancer chemotherapy compounds in myeloid leukemic cells. Blood 1992; 80:1750–1757.

152. Zaleskis G, Berleth E, Verstovsek S, Ehrke MJ, Mihich E. Doxorubicin-induced DNA degradation in murine thymocytes. Mol Pharmacol 1994; 46:901–908.

153. Martin DS, Stolfi RL, Colofiore JR, Nord LD, Sternberg S. Biochemical modulation of tumor cell energy in vivo: II. A lower dose of Adriamycin is required and a greater antitumor activity is induced when cellular energy is depressed. Cancer Invest 1994; 12:296–307.

154. Miller T, Beausang LA, Meneghini M, Lidgard G. Death-induced changes in the nuclear matrix: the use of anti-nuclear matrix antibodies to study agents of apoptosis. Biotechniques 1993; 15:1042–1049.

155. Hockenbery D, Nunez G, Milliman C, Schreiber RD, Korsmeyer SJ. Bcl-2 is an inner mitochondrial membrane protein that blocks programmed cell death. Nature 1990; 348: 334–336.

156. Silvestrini R, Veneroni S, Daidone MG, Benini E, Boracchi P, Mezzetti M, Di Fronzo G, Rilke F, Veronesi U. The Bcl-2 protein: a prognostic indicator strongly related to p53 protein in lymph node-negative breast cancer patients. J Natl Cancer Inst 1994; 86:499–504.

157. Ohmori T, Podack ER, Nishio K, Takahashi M, Miyahara Y, Takeda Y, Kubota N, Funayama Y, Ogasawara H, Ohira T, Ohta S, Saijo N. Apoptosis of lung cancer cells caused by some anti-cancer agents (MMC, CPT-11, ADM) is inhibited by Bcl-2. Biochem Biophys Res Commun 1993; 192:30–36.

158. Reed JC, Kitada S, Takayama S, Miyashita T. Regulation of chemoresistance by the Bcl-2 oncoprotein in non-Hodgkin's lymphoma and lymphocytic leukemia cell lines. Ann Oncol 1994; 5(suppl 1):S61–S65.

159. Campos L, Rouault J-P, Sabido O, Oriol P, Roubi N, Vasselon C, Archimbaud E, Magaud J-P, Guyotat D. High expression of Bcl-2 protein in acute myeloid leukemia cells is associated with poor response to chemotherapy. Blood 1993; 81:3091–3096.

160. McLaughlin P, Hagemeister FB, Swan F, Cabanillas F, Romaguera J, Rodriguez MA, Lee MS, Pate O, Sarris A, Younes A. Intensive conventional-dose chemotherapy for stage IV low-grade lymphoma: high remission rates and reversion to negative of peripheral blood Bcl-2 rearrangement. Ann Oncol 1994; 5(suppl 2):S73–S77.

161. Krajewski S, Blomqvist C, Franssila K, Krajewska M, Wasenius V-M, Niskanen E, Nordling S, Reed JC. Reduced expression of proapoptotic gene Bax is associated with poor response rates to combination chemotherapy and shorter survival in women with metastatic breast adenocarcinoma. Cancer Res 1995; 55:4471–4478.

162. Froesch B, Stahel RA, Ludke G, Zangemeister-Wittke U. Combination of doxorubicine-immunoconjugates and molecular intervention in Bcl-2 oncogene expression to overcome drug resistance in small cell lung cancer (abstr). Proc Am Assoc Cancer Res 1995: 36:341 (2032).

163. Lasorella A, Iavarone A, Israel MA. Differentiation of neuroblastoma enhances Bcl-2 expression and induces alterations of apoptosis and drug resistance. Cancer Res 1995; 55: 4711–4716.

164. Lowe SW, Ruley HE, Jacks T, Housman DE. p53-dependent apoptosis modulates the cytotoxicity of anticancer agents. Cell 1993; 74:957–967.

165. Lane DP. A death in the life of p53. Nature 1993; 362:786–787.

166. Kuerbitz SJ, Plunkett BS, Walsh WV, Kastan MB. Wild-type p53 is a cell cycle checkpoint determinant following irradiation. Proc Natl Acad Sci USA 1992; 89:7491–7495.

167. Harris CC, Hollstein M. Clinical implications of the p53 tumor-suppressor gene. N Engl J Med 1993; 329:1318–1327.

168. Dittmer D, Pati S, Zambetti G, Chu S, Teresky AK, Moore M, Finlay C, Levine AJ. Gain of function mutations in p53. Nature Genet 1993; 4:42–46.

169. Lowe SW, Bodis S, McClatchey A, Remington L, Ruley HE, Fisher DE, Housman DE, Jacks T. p53 status and the efficacy of cancer therapy in vivo. Science 1994; 266:807–810.

170. Chin K-V, Ueda K, Pastan I, Gottesman MM. Modulation of activity of the promoter of the human MDR1 gene by Ras and p53. Science 1992; 255:459–462.

171. Zastawny RL, Salvino R, Chen J, Benchimol S, Ling V. The core promoter region of the P-glycoprotein gene is sufficient to confer differential responsiveness to wild-type and mutant p53. Oncogene 1993; 8:1529–1535.

172. Nguyen KT, Liu B, Ueda K, Gottesman MM, Pastan I, Chin K-V. Transactivation of the human multidrug resistance (MDR1) gene promoter by p53 mutants. Oncol Res 1994; 6:71–77.

173. Scanlon KJ, Ishida H, Kashani-Sabet M. Ribozyme-mediated reversal of the multidrug-resistant phenotype. Proc Natl Acad Sci USA 1994; 91:11123–11127.

174. Charpin C, Vielh P, Duffaud F, Devictor B, Andrac L, Lavaut MN, Allasia C, Horschowski N, Piana L. Quantitative immunocytochemical assays of P-glycoprotein in breast carcinomas: correlation to messenger RNA expression and to immunohistochemical prognostic indicators. J Natl Cancer Inst 1994; 86:1539–1545.

175. Toth K, Arredondo MA, Vaughn MM, Johnston PG, Freedman A, Fung V, Slocum HK, Allegra C, Rustum YM. Relationship between mdr1 P-glycoprotein, mutated p53 and thymidylate synthase expression on paraffin-sections of human primary breast carcinomas by immunohistochemical methods (abstr). Proc Am Assoc Cancer Res 1995; 36: 335(1993).

176. Krontiris T. Oncogenes. N Engl J Med 1995; 333:303–306.

177. Burt RK, Garfield S, Johnson K, Thorgeirsson SS. Transformation of rat liver epithelial cells with v-H-ras or v-raf causes expression of MDR-1, glutathione-S-transferase-P and increased resistance to cytotoxic chemicals. Carcinogenesis 1988; 9:2329–2332.

178. Peters GJ, Wets M, Keepers YPAM, Oskam R, Van Ark-Otte J, Noordhuis P, Smid K, Pinedo HM. Transformation of mouse fibroblasts with the oncogenes H-ras or trk is associated with pronounced changes in drug sensitivity and metabolism. Int J Cancer 1993; 54:450–455.

179. Nooter K, Boersma AWM, Oostrum RG, Burger H, Jochemsen AG, Stoter G. Constitutive expression of the c-H-ras oncogene inhibits doxorubicin-induced apoptosis and promotes cell survival in a rhabdomyosarcoma cell line. Br J Cancer 1995; 71:556–561.

180. Woessner RD, Chung TDY, Hofmann GA, Mattern MR, Mirabelli CK, Drake FH, Johnson RK. Differences between normal and ras-transformed NIH-3T3 cells in expression of the 170kD and 180kD forms of topoisomerase II. Cancer Res 1990; 50:2901–2908.

181. Tortora G, Ciardiello F, Damiano V, Pepe S, Bianco C, di Isernia G, Davies SL, North P, Harris AL, Hickson ID, Bianco AR. Cyclic AMP-dependent protein kinase type I is involved in hypersensitivity of human breast cells to topoisomerase II inhibitors. Clin Cancer Res 1995; 1:49–56.

182. Hollander MC, Fornace AJ. Induction of fos RNA by DNA-damaging agents. Cancer Res 1989; 49:1687–1692.

183. Muss HB, Thor AD, Berry DA, Kute T, Liu ET, Koerner F, Cirrincione CT, Budman DR, Wood WC, Barcos M, Henderson IC. c-erbB-2 expression and respnse to adjuvant therapy in women with node-positive early breast cancer. N Engl J Med 1994; 330:1260–1266.

184. Keith WN, Douglas F, Wishart GC, McCallum HM, George WD, Kaye SB, Brown R. Co-amplification of erbB2, topoisomerase IIα and retinoic acid receptor α genes in breast cancer and allelic loss at topoisomerase I on chromosome 20. Eur J Cancer 1993; 29A:1469–1475.

185. Harris L, Tang C, Yang D, Lupu R. Induction of chemotherapy sensitivity in MCF-7 breast cancer cells by heregulin (abstr). Proc Am Assoc Cancer Res 1995; 36:426(2539).

186. Matsumura K, Isola J, Chew K, Henderson C, Smith HS, Harris AL, Hickson ID, Waldman F. Topoisomerase IIα deletion as well as amplification associated with erbB2 amplification in breast cancer (abstr). Proc Am Assoc Cancer Res 1994; 35:454(2708).

187. Bhushan A, Kimberly PJ, Tritton T. Association of erbB-2 oncogene protein with response to Adriamycin in MCF-7 breast cancer cells (abstr). Proc Am Assoc Cancer Res 1995; 36:329(1960).

188. Schneider J, Rubio M-P, Barbazan M-J, Rodriguez-Escudero FJ, Seizinger BR, Castresana JS. P-glycoprotein, HER-2/neu, and mutant p53 expression in human gynecologic tumors. J Natl Cancer Inst 1994; 86:850–855.

189. Rasbridge SA, Gillett CE, Seymour A-M, Patel K, Richards MA, Rubens RD, Millis RR. The effects of chemotherapy on morphology, cellular proliferation, apoptosis and onco-protein expression in primary breast carcinoma. Br J Cancer 1994; 70:335–341.

190. Tsai C-M, Yu D, Chang K-T, Wu L-H, Perng R-P, Ibrahim NK, Hung M-C. Enhanced chemoresistance by elevation of p185$^{neu}$ levels in HER-2/neu-transfected human lung can-cer cells. J Natl Cancer Inst 1995; 87:682–684.

191. Tsai C-M, Chang K-T, Perng R-P, Mitsudomi T, Chen M-H, Kadoyama C, Gazdar AF. Correlation of intrinsic chemoresistance of non-small-cell lung cancer cell lines with HER-2/neu gene expression but not with ras gene mutations. J Natl Cancer Inst 1993; 85:897–901.

192. Dati C, Antoniotti S, Taverna D, Perroteau I, De Bortoli M. Inhibition of c-erbB-2 onco-gene expression by estrogens in human breast cancer cells. Oncogene 1990; 5:1001–1006.

193. Zhang L, Hung M-C. Sensitization of the Her-2/neu-overexpressing non-small-cell lung cancer cells to chemotherapeutic drugs by tyrosine kinase inhibitor, emodin. Oncogene 1996; 12:571–576.

194. Zhang Y, Yu D, Xia W, Hung M-C. Her-2/neu-targeting cancer therapy via adenovirus-mediated E1A delivery in an animal model. Oncogene 1995; 10:1947–1954.

195. Park JW, Hong K, Carter P, Asgari H, Guo LY, Keller GA, Wirth C, Shalaby R, Kotts C, Wood WI, Papahadjopoulos D, Benz CC. Development of anti-p185$^{HER2}$ immunolipo-somes for cancer therapy. Proc Natl Acad Sci USA 1995; 92:1327–1331.

196. Rodrigues ML, Presta LG, Kotts CE, Wirth C, Mordenti J, Osaka G, Wong WLT, Nuijens A, Blackburn B, Carter P. Development of a humanized disulfide-stabilized Anti-p185$^{HER2}$ Fv-β-lactamase fusion protein for activation of a cephalosporin doxorubicin prodrug. Can-cer Res 1995; 55:63–70.

197. Zuckier G, Tritton TR. Adriamycin causes up regulation of epidermal growth factor re-ceptors in actively growing cells. Exp Cell Res 1983; 148:155–161.

198. Kwok TT, Sutherland RM. Epidermal growth factor reduces resistance to doxorubicin. Int J Cancer 1991; 49:73–76.

199. Kwok TT, Mok CH, Menton-Brennan L. Up-regulation of a mutant form of p53 by dox-orubicin in human squamous carcinoma cells. Cancer Res 1994; 54:2834–2836.

200. Armstrong DK, Kaufmann SH, Ottaviano YL, Furuya Y, Buckley JA, Isaacs JT, Davidson NE. Epidermal growth factor-mediated apoptosis of MDA-MB-468 human breast cancer cells. Cancer Res 1994; 54:5280–5283.

201. Meyers MB, Merluzzi VJ, Spengler BA, Biedler JL. Epidermal growth factor receptor is increased in multidrug-resistant Chinese hamster and mouse tumor cells. Proc Natl Acad Sci USA 1986; 83:5521–5525.

202. Yang JM, Hait WM. Regulation of the function of P-glycoprotein by epidermal growth factor through phospholipase C (abstr). Proc Am Assoc Cancer Res 1995; 36:333(1985).

203. Aboud-Pirak E, Hurwitz E, Bellot F, Schlessinger J, Sela M. Inhibition of human tumor growth in nude mice by a conjugate of doxorubicin with monoclonal antibodies to epider-mal growth factor receptor. Proc Natl Acad Sci USA 1989; 86:3778–3781.

204. Baselga J, Norton L, Masui H, Pandiella A, Coplan K, Miller WH, Mendelsohn J. Antitu-mor effects of doxorubicin in combination with anti-epidermal growth factor receptor monoclonal antibodies. J Natl Cancer Inst 1993; 85:1327–1333.

205. Sivam GP, Martin PJ, Reisfeld RA, Mueller BM. Therapeutic efficacy of a doxorubicin immunoconjugate in a preclinical model of spontaneous metastatic human melanoma. Cancer Res 1995; 55:2352–2356.

206. Fanidi A, Harrington EA, Evan GI. Cooperative interaction between c-myc and Bcl-2 proto-oncogenes. Nature 1992; 359:554–556.

207. Fornari FA, Jarvis WD, Grant S, Orr MS, Randolph JK, White FKH, Gewirtz DA. Growth arrest and cell death associated with down-regulation of c-myc expression in MCF-7 breast tumor cells following acute exposure to doxorubicin (abstr). Proc Am Assoc Cancer Res 1995; 36:453(2700).

208. Randolph JK, Chawla J, Fornari F, Gewirtz DA. Biochemical and molecular perturbations associated with growth arrest and cell death in MCF-7 breast tumor cells treated with idarubicin (4-demethoxydaunorubicin) (abstr). Proc Am Assoc Cancer Res 1995; 36: 453(2701).

209. Lotem J, Sachs L. Regulation by Bcl-2, c-myc, and p53 of susceptibility to induction of apoptosis by heat shock and cancer chemotherapy compounds in differentiation-competent and -defective myeloid leukemic cells. Cell Growth Differ 1993; 4:41–47.

210. Bordow SB, Haber M, Madafiglio J, Cheung B, Marshall GM, Norris MD. Expression of the multidrug resistance-associated protein (MRP) gene correlates with amplification and overexpression of the N-myc oncogene in childhood neuroblastoma. Cancer Res 1994; 54:5036–5040.

211. Schwartz EL, Sartorelli AC. Structure-activity relationships for the induction of differentiation of HL-60 human acute promyelocytic leukemia cells by anthracyclines. Cancer Res 1982; 42:2651–2655.

212. Jeannesson P, Ginot L, Manfait M, Jardillier J-C. Induction of hemoglobin synthesis in human leukemic K 562 cells by Adriamycin. Anticancer Res 1984; 4:47–52.

213. Craig RW, Frankfurt OS, Sakagami H, Takeda K, Bloch A. Macromolecular and cell cycle effects of different classes of agents inducing the maturation of human myeloblastic leukemia (ML-1) cells. Cancer Res 1984; 44:2421–2429.

214. Fujii Y, Yuki N, Takeichi N, Kobayashi H, Miyazaki T. Differentiation therapy of a myelomonocytic leukemia (c-WRT-7) in rats by injection of lipopolysaccharide and daunomycin. Cancer Res 1987; 47:1668–1673.

215. Rocchi P, Ferreri AM, Simone G, Prodi G. Epirubicin-induced differentiation of human neuroblastoma cells in vitro. Anticancer Res 1987; 7:247–250.

216. Supino R, Mariani M, Colombo A, Prosperi E, Croce AC, Bottiroli G. Comparative studies on the effects of doxorubicin and differentiation inducing agents on B16 melanoma cells. Eur J Cancer 1992; 28A:778–783.

217. Tsuchiya KS, Kanbe T, Hori M, Uehara Y, Takahashi Y, Takeuchi T. Distinct effects of clinically used anthracycline antibiotics on ras oncogene-expressed cells. Biol Pharm Bull 1993; 16:908–911.

218. Fornari FA, Jarvis WD, Grant S, Orr MS, Randolph JK, White FKH, Mumaw VR, Lovings ET, Freeman RH, Gewirtz DA. Induction of differentiation and growth arrest associated with nascent (nonoligosomal) DNA fragmentation and reduced c-myc expression in MCF-7 human breast tumor cells after continuous exposure to a sublethal concentration of doxorubicin. Cell Growth Differ 1994; 5:723–733.

219. Schaefer A, Dressel A, Lingelbach K, Schmidt CA, Steinheider G, Marquardt H. Induction of differentiation in Friend-erythroleukemia cells by aclacinomycin A: early transient decrease in c-myc and c-myb mRNA levels. Leukemia 1992; 6:828–833.

220. Maragoudakis ME, Peristeris P, Missirlis E, Aletras A, Andriopoulou P, Haralabopoulos G. Inhibition of angiogenesis by anthracyclines and titanocene dichloride. Ann N Y Acad Sci 1994; 732:280–293.

221. Lau DHM, Duran GE, Lewis AD, Sikic BI. Metabolic conversion of methoxymorpholinyl doxorubicin: from a DNA strand breaker to a DNA cross-linker. Br J Cancer 1994; 70:79–84.

222. Geroni C, Pesenti E, Broggini M, Belvedere G, Tagliabue G, D'Incalci M, Pennella G, Grandi M. L1210 cells selected for resistance to methoxymorpholinyl doxorubicin appear specifically resistant to this class of morpholinyl derivatives. Br J Cancer 1994; 69:315–319.

223. Begleiter A, Leith MK, Johnston JB. Activity of 3'-(3-cyano-4-morpholinyl)-3'-deamino-adriamycin in sensitive and resistant L5178Y lymphoblasts in vitro. Cancer Res 1994; 54: 482–486.

224. van der Graff WTA, Mulder NH, Meijer C, de Vries EGE. The role of methoxymorpholino anthracycline and cyanomorpholino anthracycline in a sensitive small-cell lung-cancer cell line and its multidrug-resistant but P-glycoprotein-negative and cisplatin-resistant counterparts. Cancer Chemother Pharmacol 1995; 35:345–348.

225. Vasey PA, Bissett D, Strolin-Benedetti M, Poggesi I, Breda M, Adams L, Wilson P, Pacciarini MA, Kaye SB, Cassidy J. Phase I clinical and pharmacokinetic study of 3'-deamino-3'-(2-methoxy-4-morpholinyl)doxorubicin (FCE 23762). Cancer Res 1995; 55:2090–2096.

226. Priebe W, Perez-Soler R. Design and tumor targeting of anthracyclines able to overcome multidrug resistance: a double-advantage approach. Pharmacol Ther 1993; 60:215–234.

227. Zou Y, Ling YH, Van HT, Priebe W, Perez-Soler R. Antitumor activity of free and liposome-entrapped annamycin, a lipophilic anthracycline antibiotic with non-cross-resistance properties. Cancer Res 1994; 54:1479–1483.

228. Glaves D, Rustum Y, Bernacki RJ, Raghavan D, Israel M. Therapeutic activity of a nitrosourea: anthracycline hybrid (AD312) against human bladder, lung and ovarian carcinoma xenografts (abstr). Proc Am Assoc Cancer Res 1995; 36:392(2338).

229. Israel M, Krishan A, Wellham LL. Antitumor activity of 2-chlorethylnitrosoureidodaunorubicin (AD 312) in nude mice bearing xenografts of FCC-8 human lung adenocarcinoma (abstr). Proc Am Assoc Cancer Res 1995; 36:396(2359).

230. Arcamone F. Design and synthesis of anthracycline and distamycin derivatives as new, sequence-specific, DNA-binding pharmacological agents. Gene 1994; 149:57–61.

231. Farquhar D, Rosenblum MG, Cherif A, Nelson JA, Kenten JH. Melanoma-selective antitumor anthracyclines (abstr). Proc Am Assoc Cancer Res 1995; 36:396(2358).

# 14

## Cellular Mechanisms of Cisplatin Resistance

**Jeroen Oldenberg**
*The Netherlands Cancer Institute, Amsterdam, The Netherlands*

**Gerrit Los**
*University of California, San Diego, Cancer Center, La Jolla, California*

### INTRODUCTION

Since the discovery of cisplatin (*cis*-diamminedichloroplatinumII) or cDDP in 1965 (1) by its antibacterial action, the drug has become one of the most active and widely used anticancer drugs. Cisplatin has a proven efficacy against a variety of malignancies and is used in the treatment of solid tumors such as ovarian and testicular cancer, as well as head and neck, lung, and cervical carcinomas; breast cancer is also recognized as a potential target for cisplatin therapy. Furthermore, it is also used in combination chemotherapy for a variety of other malignancies. Extraordinarily good results are attained in the treatment of testicular cancer. Moreover, in ovarian cancer, remission rates of up to 50% have been documented (2).

Unfortunately, the clinical use of cisplatin is limited by its dose-dependent side effects such as severe nephrotoxicity, myelosuppression, and damage to the nervous system. Also the initial response of several tumor types is often followed by a relapse caused by either primary resistance or the development of secondary (acquired) drug resistance of the tumor. This acquired resistance to cisplatin occurs rapidly both in vitro and in vivo, and it is a major obstacle to effective chemotherapy.

Cisplatin is a neutral square-planar platinum(II) complex (3) (see Fig. 1a). After entry of cisplatin into the cytoplasm, the binding of the two chloride ligands will become unstable as a result of the lower intracellular chloride concentration. As a consequence, the ligand displacement reaction presumably will lead to activation of the molecule. One chloride ligand is displaced by a water molecule, so cisplatin becomes a (mono) aquated, charged electrophile that reacts with nucleophilic sites on cellular macromolecules. Because cisplatin contains two reactive sites, a second reaction takes place, resulting in the formation of bifunctional platinum-DNA adducts. Approximately 1% of the total cellular platinum will react with the DNA, the presumed critical target of cisplatin's cytotoxic action (4,5). Upon reaching the DNA, the binding between cisplatin and the DNA induces interstrand cross-links and intrastrand adducts (see Fig. 1b). The interstrand cross-links represent only 1–5% of the platinum-induced lesions

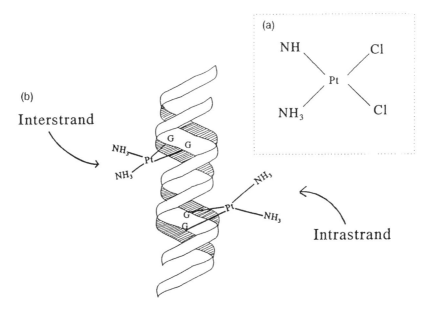

**Figure 1** (a) Cisplatinum is a neutral square-planar platinum (II) complex. (b) Binding between cisplatinum and DNA induces interstrand cross-links and intrastrand adducts.

(6). Therefore, the intrastrand adducts are recognized as the major lesions (>50%). These adducts consist of cisplatin cross-linked to two neighboring deoxyguanosines at their N(7) positions [cDDP(NH3)$_2$(dGpdG)] and approximately in 25% between adjacent adenines and guanines [cDDP(NH3)$_2$(dApdG)]. In less than 10%, two guanines are separated by one or more intervening bases. These cisplatin-GG and cisplatin-AG adducts cause a local unwinding of 13° of the DNA strand and a 35° kink in naked DNA (7). The causal relationship between adduct formation and cell death is obvious. However, how the adducts bring about cell death is not clear. The binding of cisplatin to DNA is not in itself sufficient to cause cell death. Cisplatin adducts inhibit DNA replication and transcription, but most cells are capable of repairing the damaged DNA. In addition, cellular damage produced by cisplatin provokes a programmed response that results in the activation of some genes, the inactivation of others, major shifts in cellular metabolism, and cell cycle progression, eventually triggering apoptosis. The latter is in agreement with other studies showing that proliferating cells are much more sensitive to the toxicity of the drug, indicating cell-cycle associated events involved in cisplatin cytotoxicity (8–11).

## PHARMACOKINETICS AND HYPOTHETICAL MECHANISMS OF RESISTANCE

In order to get a better understanding of the processes involved in the emergence of cisplatin resistance, we pictured a diagram representing the route of transport for cisplatin (see Fig. 2). The first barrier to be taken is the cell membrane. Any alterations

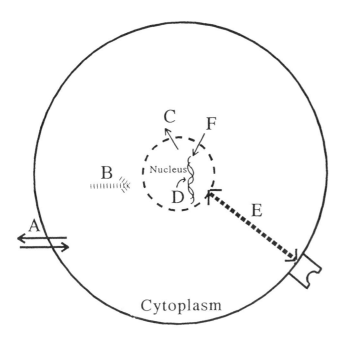

**Figure 2**   Route of transport for cisplatin.

in the cell membrane could lead to a change in drug transport over the cell membrane. Considering the latter, reduced platinum accumulation, which is often a hallmark for platinum resistance, could be the result of a decreased drug influx, an increased drug efflux, or a combination of both. After the drug has passed through the cell membrane, it encounters a milieu with a chloride concentration approximately five times lower than in the extracellular space. This leads to the above-mentioned exchange reaction in which a chloride ligand is substituted by an $H_2O$ molecule, producing an aquated charged electrophile platinum complex that can react with cellular proteins, small nucleophilic molecules such as glutathione and methionine, RNA, and DNA. Upon reaching the nucleus, the aquated monofunctional platinum complex will be rearranged to the critical bifunctional lesions. These bifunctional lesions may have possibly lethal consequences for the cell.

A second potential mechanism of resistance is the increased detoxification of cisplatin molecules by increased thiol-containing compounds such as glutathione (GSH), glutathione-S-transferase and/or metallothioneins. Despite the detoxification, a certain percentage of the drug entering the tumor cell will reach the nucleus, with potentially lethal consequences. But before entering the nucleus, drug molecules will encounter a second barrier, the nuclear membrane. The latter might be another cause of resistance.

The critical target for cisplatin is DNA. Therefore, the enhanced ability to remove the DNA lesions by excision repair enzymes such as DNA polymerase may have major consequences for the emergence of resistance. Further, one can speculate that resistant cells might be tolerant of unrepaired lesions in DNA. The latter was demonstrated by the fact that resistant cells had higher levels of DNA adducts than the parent cell at an equitoxic dose level (12). Little is known about the role oncogenes play in the emergence of cisplatin resistance. However, platinum resistance can be modulated by *c-Ha-ras* and *c-myc* (13). The involvement of these genes in cisplatin resistance is an interesting development and may give new insights into the mechanisms of drug resistance.

Treatment of tumor cells with clinically relevant exposure to cisplatin activates an injury response that eventually induces death via an apoptotic mechanism. Very little is known about the specifics of any of the signal-transduction pathways activated by the cisplatin injury and several of these pathways might be involved in cisplatin resistance. Since trans-DDP, the geometric isomer of cisplatin, binds to DNA and blocks replication but is ineffective as an antitumor agent (14,15), the biological activity of cisplatin cannot be explained only by its ability to damage DNA.

## Accumulation and Drug Transport of Cisplatin

Although the mechanism by which cisplatin enters the cell is still unelucidated (see Table 1), reduced accumulation of cisplatin is a consistent finding in many cisplatin-resistant cell lines from a variety of species (16). Decreased accumulation of cisplatin has been described in resistant murine L1210 cells (17,18), human head and neck squamous cell carcinomas (19), ovarian cancer cells (5,20–22), rat colon adenocarcinoma cells (23), human prostate tumor (24), Chinese hamster ovary cells (25), mouse NIH 3T3 cells (26), human lung cancer cells (27), and a human testicular nonseminomatous germ cell line (28). In other resistant cell lines, however, the cisplatin accumulation is comparable to that in the sensitive cells—for example, human small cell lung cancer cells (29,30) and human cervical carcinoma cells (31). A study performed at the Netherlands Cancer Institute indicated that decreased accumulation of cisplatin occurred at low levels of drug resistance and did not change when cells attained higher

**Table 1**  Factors Affecting the Accumulation of Cisplatin

| Accumulation affected by | Effect | Ref. |
|---|---|---|
| Aldehydes | Unable to permeate membrane and block 50% of the cisplatin uptake | 48, 49 |
| Amino acids | Interference of amino acids with cisplatin accumulation | 39, 40 |
| $Na^+$, $K^+$-ATPase | Reduced accumulation | 124 |
| c-Ha-ras | Increased accumulation | 26 |
| Composition of cell membrane | Regulates passive diffusion | 35 |
| Ouabain | Inhibition of accumulation | 41 |
| Increased PKC activity | Increased cisplatin accumulation | 44 |
| $Ca^{2+}$/calmodulin pathway | Decreased accumulation | 46 |
| Gated channel | Facilitated diffusion | 47 |
| GS-X pump | Export of GS-platinum complexes | 58–60, 65, 79 |
| MRP/LRP | Facilitates transport of GS-platinum complexes | 61, 66–69 |

levels of resistance (23). Most studies indicated a decrease in cellular platinum content varying from two- to fivefold despite resistance levels of 20-fold or even more. It turned out, however, that the accumulation of cisplatin is a primary determinant in the DNA platination and consequently cell kill (23,32).

*Reduced Uptake of Cisplatin into Cisplatin-Resistant Cells*

The way in which cisplatin enters the cell still remains uncertain. The agent could pass the cell membrane by passive diffusion through the lipid bilayer of the plasma membrane (33,34). Experiments with cisplatin-resistant ovarian carcinoma cells indicated changes in the lipid content of the membrane of resistant variants (35). Also, membrane proteins may interfere with the accumulation of cisplatin, for reduced drug accumulation in resistant squamous carcinoma cells was accompanied with a marked decrease in the SQM1 membrane protein (36).

Reduced drug accumulation could also be the result of increased efflux or a combination of both reduced influx and increased efflux. Resistant A2780-CP cells eliminate platinum more rapidly than sensitive cells (5). In contrast, resistance in human ovarian carcinoma cells incubated with a tritium-labeled cisplatin analogue [($^3$H)DEP] is accounted for primarily by lower initial uptake rather than changes in efflux. At steady state, the resistant cells eventually accumulated more free [($^3$H)DEP] than the sensitive cells (37). It has also been suggested that mitochondria may play an important role in the cellular pharmacology of cisplatin. Mitochondrial defects can be linked to an elevated plasma membrane potential decreasing cisplatin accumulation in ovarian carcinoma cells (21). Although transport of cisplatin across the cell membrane is still not fully elucidated, understanding of the involvement of the nuclear membrane in cisplatin resistance is scarcely to come by. Experiments in a resistant human squamous carcinoma cell line showed a decreased intranuclear-cytoplasmatic drug ratio in comparison with the sensitive cells (38).

*Factors Influencing Cisplatin Uptake*

A wide variety of pharmacological circumstances influence the entry of cisplatin into tumor cells. It has long been assumed that cisplatin enters the cell by passive diffusion (33); however, recent work indicated that mechanisms other than passive diffusion might be involved in the accumulation of cisplatin (16). The latter is supported by the findings that the accumulation of cisplatin: (1) can be inhibited by concomitant incubation with certain amino acids (39,40); (2) is energy dependent, $Na^+$ dependent, and ouabain inhibitable (16,41); (3) is not greatly affected by changes in pH (42); and (4) is inhibited by aldehydes (43). In addition, the accumulation of cisplatin is affected by a number of intracellular signaling pathways including protein kinase C (PKC) (44), epidermal growth factor (EGF) (45), and the $Ca^{2+}$/calmodulin pathway (46), suggesting their involvement in the regulation of cisplatin uptake.

A working model that accommodates most of the existing observations concerning cisplatin accumulation into cisplatin-sensitive and cisplatin-resistant cells has recently been published by Gately and Howell (47). This elegant model envisions that approximately one-half of the initial drug uptake rate is the result of passive diffusion and that the other half occurs by facilitated diffusion through a gated channel. The model would propose that the flux through the channel is regulated by phosphorylation cascades initiated by activation of protein kinase A, protein kinase C, or by the calmodulin-dependent kinase (47), which is similar to the regulation of a variety of gated channels.

This model is further strengthened by (1) the ability of aldehydes that are unable to permeate the membrane to block 50% of the uptake (48,49), suggesting that critical amino groups of the channel are exposed on the external surface of the cell; (2) the fact that ouabain inhibits 50% of the initial uptake (41,16) suggesting that ion gradients maintained by this ATPase are critical to the function of this channel; and (3) by the fact that the intracellular platinum content increases at higher temperatures due to increased membrane permeability (50). An important observation is that in no case has it been reported that accumulation can be inhibited by more than 50% (47). In view of the latter, and presuming that the gated channel is lost during the selection of drug-resistant variants, the accumulation of platinum compounds into resistant cells could be inhibited by as much as 50%, which is in agreement with the current literature. Furthermore, it has been shown that analogues of cisplatin that are more lipophilic do not exhibit decreased accumulation in resistant cells and show less cross-resistance (51–54). These findings are in agreement with this theoretical model because such analogues are less dependent on a gated channel for entry into the cell. In addition, the model allows for modulation of the flux through the channel and permits the design of specific experiments addressing the role of membrane transport in the accumulation of cisplatin into the cell.

### Active Transport Mechanisms Involved in the Accumulation of Platinum

Among the several potential mechanisms of acquired resistance to various chemotherapeutic agents, the P-glycoprotein pump is the most consistently described factor as an indicator of multidrug resistance. However, the P-glycoprotein (MDR1) pump that modulates chemotherapy resistance particularly by determining the drug efflux of the membrane appears to play no role in resistance to cisplatin compared to its function in, for example, doxorubicin resistance (55,56). Hydroxyurea is presumed to accelerate loss of amplified MDR1 genes and thus P-glycoprotein. As expected, cisplatin resistance in ovarian carcinoma cells could not be overcome by hydroxyurea (57).

Recently, in human epidermoid carcinoma cells (KCP-4 cells), an active efflux pump for cisplatin-conjugates has been discovered (58,59). In these tumor cells, it was shown that the ATP-dependent glutathione S-conjugate export pump (GS-X pump), which exports the bis-(glutathionato)platinum(II) (GS-platinum) complex, could contribute to cellular cisplatin resistance. In resistant human leukemia HL-60 cells, the GS-X pump is functionally overexpressed and related to cell proliferation. Further, its function is essentially linked to a variety of biological phenomena including oxidative stress and detoxification (60). In addition to the GS-X pump, Müller et al. demonstrated that overexpression of the MRP (multidrug resistance-associated protein) gene in human cancer cells increased the ATP-dependent glutathione S-conjugate carrier activity in plasma membrane vesicles isolated from the human tumor cells (61), suggesting MRP-mediated efflux of glutathione S-conjugates from cells. A possible link between MRP and the GS-X pump would hypothetically link MRP, a 180- to 190-kd glycoprotein mainly located in the plasma membrane and associated with multidrug resistance in human cells (62–64), to glutathione S-conjugate mediated resistance such as resistance to cisplatin. It is, however, clear that overexpression of the GS-X pump does not necessarily have to result in cisplatin resistance (65).

Another transport protein has recently been identified, the 110-kd lung resistance-related protein (LRP) (66). The overexpression of LRP is often, but not always, paralleled by overexpression of MRP (67,68). A study screening 61 unselected human tumor cell lines of a NIH panel demonstrated that expression of *LRP*, more than *MDR* or *MRP*, correlated with a broad pattern of cytostatic drug resistance, including the non-*MDR* drugs like cisplatin. Furthermore, *LRP* is an important prognostic factor for poor clinical performance in ovarian cancer, a cancer most commonly treated with platinum drug–based chemotherapy (69).

## Glutathione and/or Glutathione-S-Transferase

Glutathione (GSH) is a predominantly intracellular nonprotein sulfhydryl compound that plays a part in a variety of cellular functions including metabolism, transport, heat protection, detoxification, and repair of cellular injury (70,71) (see Table 2). Glutathione is found in a wide range of mammalian cells.

Under normal conditions, the majority of glutathione exists in the reduced form. Reactive oxygen or other harmful substances are removed in the glutathione oxidation-reduction cycle in which glutathione is oxidized to GSSG by the action of glutathione peroxidase. Glutathione reductase (GR) is a NADPH-dependent enzyme that helps to maintain cellular levels of reduced glutathione—and by that keeping cellular GSSG levels low. The conjugation of diverse electrophilic groups with the reduced sulfhydryl moiety of glutathione is catalyzed by the isoenzymes of glutathione-S-transferase (GST) resulting in the formation of thioethers (72). This reaction detoxifies compounds by covalent attachment of glutathione to potentially harmful electrophilic substances.

The role that glutathione and glutathione-S-transferase play in noncancer cells is well established. In fact, tumor cells may be able to mediate drug resistance through an increase of cellular glutathione and/or glutathione-S-transferase concentrations. Elevation in cellular glutathione content has been associated with drug-resistant phenotypes developed in several cases of resistance to alkylating agents. Increased levels of glutathione have been demonstrated in cisplatin-resistant murine leukemia cells (17), human ovarian carcinoma cells (73–75), rat colon adenocarcinoma cells (23), human small cell lung carcinoma (27), human melanoma cells (76), mouse mammary tumor cell line (77), and human bladder carcinoma (78). In other resistant tumor cell lines however, no elevated glutathione levels were detected (22,28).

The exact mechanism by which glutathione could diminish cisplatin's cytotoxic action has not been established. Several possibilities can be examined—for example, alterations of membrane transport. Recently, the role of glutathione in membrane transport has been established. The ATP-dependent glutathione S-conjugate export pump, named GS-X pump, has been shown to eliminate a potentially cytotoxic glutathione-

**Table 2** Glutathione and Cisplatin Resistance

| Role of glutathione | Effect | Ref. |
|---|---|---|
| Cytoplasmic thiols | Detoxification | 23, 77, 80, 82 |
| Nuclear GSH levels | Repair/adducts | 76, 82 |
| GSH-related enzymes | Detoxification | 55, 72, 91, 92 |
| GS-X pump | Efflux | 58–60, 65, 79 |
| Quenching mono-adducts | Decrease of bifunctional lesions | 80, 83 |
| DNA repair | Facilitates repair | 84, 85, 103, 104 |

platinum (GS-platinum) complex from tumor cells, thus modulating glutathione (GSH)-associated resistance to cisplatin (79).

A second possible mode of action is the direct inactivation of cisplatin in the cytosol by the binding of cisplatin to the sulfhydryl residue of glutathione, preventing it from reaching the DNA (80). Whether this mechanism actually plays a significant role is still circumstantial. In some studies, it was found that the elevated glutathione level was not intercepting intracellular cisplatin on its way to the nucleus (81). Correction of the reduced cisplatin accumulation was already sufficient to reach equal DNA platination in resistant rat colon adenocarcinoma cells, implying that glutathione had no effect on initial DNA platination (23). In contrast, depletion of the elevated glutathione levels resulted in an increase of platinum bound to the DNA in resistant human small cell lung cancer cells (82).

A third potential mechanism by which glutathione reduces cisplatin cytotoxicity involves the reaction of monofunctional adducts in DNA with glutathione to produce a glutathione-platinum-deoxyguanosine cross-link, thereby reducing toxicity through quenching monofunctional lesions before they can be rearranged to the more toxic bifunctional lesions (80,83). A fourth role glutathione might play is at the nuclear level, facilitating the repair of cisplatin-induced damage. The effect of glutathione on DNA repair, after treatment with cisplatin, was studied in resistant human ovarian and lung carcinoma cell lines. Experimentally lowering the glutathione concentration appeared to (partially) inhibit DNA repair (84,85).

Whether elevated glutathione levels play a significant role in resistant tumor cells or whether it is a general phenomenon in potential harmful chemotherapeutic treatments is still not clarified. If glutathione really is involved in cisplatin resistance, experimentally lowering the cellular glutathione content should reverse resistance. Intracellular glutathione levels can be reduced by incubation of the cells with dl-buthionine-S-R-sulfoximine (BSO). BSO is a specific inhibitor of the enzyme gamma-glutamyl cysteine synthetase, which is a crucial enzyme in the synthesis of glutathione. In several studies, resistant cells were sensitized to cisplatin after depletion of glutathione with BSO (82,86,87). In other studies, however, no significant effect of BSO treatment was observed (17). It might be that only simple depletion of glutathione is not sufficient to decrease resistance. In the absence of BSO, the glutathione synthesis is rapidly switched on, and the effect of glutathione depletion is set aside. It was shown that only after prolonged incubation with BSO did resistant cells become sensitized to cisplatin (88). If glutathione plays a major role at the nuclear rather than at the cytoplasmatic level, the cellular compartmentalization would be of importance. Besides, the effect of BSO on intracellular compartments (for example, nucleus or mitochondria) is unclear. In rat hepatocytes, the cytoplasmic compartment contains 85–90% of the total glutathione, whereas the mitochondria contain about 10–15%. Treatment with glutathione synthase inhibitor diethylmaleate (DEM) demonstrated that the two cytoplasmic compartments exhibit different rates of glutathione depletion. Exposure to DEM reduced cytoplasmic glutathione to 40% of control values without affecting mitochondrial glutathione (89). The same phenomenon could be valid for the nucleus. Elevated glutathione levels in the nucleus were shown in resistant human small cell lung cancer cells (82). In these cells, BSO pretreatment resulted in reduced nuclear glutathione levels. Another study, however, demonstrated the relative inefficiency of BSO pretreatment in reducing nuclear glutathione levels (90). Consequently, this could result in an underestimation of the resistance mechanism by glutathione.

The activity of glutathione transferases may also be a factor in determining drug response. Glutathione-S-transferases (GST) are a widely distributed glutathione-dependent group of enzymes that may participate in cisplatin resistance. In a human small cell lung cancer cell line (U-1906 L) resistant to cisplatin and doxorubicin, the total glutathione (GSH plus GSSG) level was 40% lower, whereas the activity of glutathione-S-transferase isoenzyme π was significantly higher (91). Another human small cell lung cancer cell line also showed increased glutathione-S-transferase activity and an over-expression of glutathione-S-transferase mRNA. The $IC_{50}$ concentrations (i.e., drug concentrations required for 50% growth inhibition) were decreased by treatment with ethacrynic acid, a potential modulator (inhibition) of glutathione-S-transferase activity. Transfection of a human alpha-glutathione-S-transferase ($\alpha$-GST) cDNA into murine NIH3T3 cells resulted in increased resistance to chemotherapeutic agents (92).

Whether glutathione can be qualified as a cisplatin-resistant phenotype or not, an increase in glutathione levels is demonstrated in many cisplatin-resistant cell lines. Moreover, the very broad cross-resistance to other chemotherapeutic agents (melphalan, etoposide, paclitaxel, and carboplatin) may, at least in part, be the direct result of glutathione-mediated drug resistance (73), indicating a major role of glutathione in the cisplatin-resistant phenotype.

## Metallothioneins

The involvement of metallothionein in acquired resistance to cisplatin is rather controversial. Metallothioneins are a family of inducible intracellular proteins rich in sulfhydryl groups, which are thought to play a role in the metabolism and storage of zinc, cadmium, copper, or other heavy metals. Metallothioneins are low-molecular-weight (6100–7000) proteins that contain 33% of their amino acids as cysteine and account for large percentages of the intracellular thiol content. Cells that have been selected for resistance to cadmium have elevated cellular amounts of metallothionein and exhibit some cross-resistance to cisplatin. Hence, metallothioneins are a potential candidate for involvement in the binding of cisplatin (93) (Table 3).

In case of exposure to electrophilic agents, the abundant nucleophilic sulfhydryl groups in metallothionein can interact with many toxins. Consequently, the binding of platinum(II) depends on the availability of sulfhydryl groups in metallothionein. The binding of platinum(II) to metallothionein is associated with the replacement of metals previously bound to metallothionein, particularly zinc; other metals such as cadmium or possibly copper are not as readily released by platinum(II). Furthermore, it has been demonstrated that selective blocking of sulfhydryl groups by performic acid oxidation almost completely prevents platinum binding by metallothionein (93). The

**Table 3** Metallothionein and Cisplatin Resistance

| Involvement of metallothionein | Effect | Ref. |
| --- | --- | --- |
| Increased cytoplasmic MT level | Detoxification | 28, 29, 93–95, 97, 98 |
| Genes (transfection with metallothionein-II$_A$) | Increased MT levels → Detoxification | 94 |

transcription of the metallothionein gene family is controlled by metals as well as other stimuli such as epinephrine, glucocorticoids, heat, or cytokines (94).

Cells may protect themselves against toxic metals through inducement of the synthesis of metallothioneins. In some cisplatin-resistant cell lines, increased levels of these cysteine-rich proteins can be detected (29). Induction of metallothionein synthesis through incubation with heavy metals (e.g., cadmium) has been demonstrated to increase resistance to cisplatin in human small cell lung cancer cells (29), human epithelial cells (95), and human ovarian carcinoma cells (96). A critical side note could be added to these studies: exposure to heavy metals may not only induce metallothionein synthesis but also induce other detoxification systems, such as glutathione, that may influence cisplatin resistance. Human ovarian carcinoma cells that were resistant to $CdCl_2$ were obtained by chronic culture in $CdCl_2$. The metallothionein-rich (23-fold elevated) variant was 3.2-fold resistant to $CdCl_2$ and 4.1-fold resistant to cisplatin; however, in vitro selection with cisplatin did not trigger metallothionein synthesis. Further, in other experiments it was shown that the strongly elevated metallothionein levels implicated only a low-level cisplatin resistance (97). In resistant L1210-PDD, the basis for the resistance is neither an increased level of metallothioneins nor an enhanced ability to increase the synthesis of metallothionein after drug exposure (98). The outcome of another study was that cisplatin appears to be unable to stimulate the biosynthesis of metallothionein, but cisplatin can be bound in vivo by already existing metallothionein in liver and kidney (93). Frequently, cisplatin-resistant cells do not exhibit any resistance to cadmium, suggesting that resistance is not modulated by metallothionein (99). However, cells transfected with bovine papilloma virus expression vectors containing DNA encoding human metallothionein-$II_A$ were resistant to cisplatin and several other chemotherapeutic agents (94). Furthermore, mouse C127 cells transfected with human metallothionein-II gene became resistant to cisplatin and alkylating agents (94).

Metallothionein elevations in cisplatin-resistant species have been demonstrated and may thus be involved in the cellular response to cisplatin. But this may be rather a secondary effect rather than an effective protection mechanism against cisplatin. Moreover, there is little proof of a detailed mechanism by which metallothioneins decrease cisplatin's cytotoxicity. Thus far, it has not been established that increased metallothioneins are capable of reducing the amount of DNA platination. Future analysis might elucidate more of the relationship between metallothionein and cisplatin resistance.

## DNA Repair

The possibility of increased repair as a mechanism of resistance has been studied extensively (see Table 4). The total amount of platinated DNA is the outcome of an equilibrium between platinum–DNA adduct formation and removal. Moreover, cisplatin resistance can be mediated by decreased initial platinum–DNA adduct formation, by a better DNA repair, or by a combination of the two. The level of DNA platination early after incubation (initial DNA platination) might be a gauge of the drug's facility to reach the nucleus and may be a reasonable predictor of sensitivity to the chemotherapeutic drug. In a study with six cell lines, a correlation was found between initial platination levels and the cells' sensitivity to cisplatin (100). Adduct half-lives, however, did not correlate with the sensitivities of the cells for the drug. We demonstrated that increased repair correlated with increasing resistance in resistant colon

**Table 4**  DNA Repair and Cisplatin Resistance

| Mechanism | Effect on | Ref. |
|---|---|---|
| Nucleotide excision repair enzymes | Repair of platinum DNA adducts | 105–107 |
| Increased DNA repair capacity | Level of resistance | 5, 17, 28, 101, 102 |
| Gene-specific repair | Interstrand cross-links | 108–110 |
| ERCC, XPAC, XPCC | Repair of interstrand cross-links | 112–115 |
| Tolerance | Removal of all platinum adducts | 22, 75, 102 |
| XPE binding factor | Recognition of DNA damage | 120 |

carcinoma cells and that the adduct ratios after 48 h were in closer agreement with resistance ratios than those for initial adducts, underlining the important of repair as one of the mechanisms involved in platinum resistance. As described in L1210 cells, the removal of the adducts occurred in a biphasic manner (101). This decrease in adduct formation was shown in sensitive as well as resistant cells; however, the resistant cells exhibited a more efficient repair (23). Although cells appear to remove more adducts as resistance increased, only a twofold increase in removal was detectable in cells 100-fold resistant compared with cells 20-fold resistant to cisplatin, indicating that additional mechanisms have to be involved in more resistant cells (101). This is also true for several other resistant cell lines such as human ovarian cancer cells (74,102), murine leukemia L1210 cells (which removed up to four times as many adducts during the rapid phase of repair) (101), and human testicular nonseminomatous germ cell lines (28).

*Role of Intracellular Thiols*

Because drug accumulation is one of the major determinants for initial adduct formation, intracellular thiols may be involved in removing cisplatin from the DNA. In addition, cellular thiols, such as glutathione, may facilitate DNA repair. Glutathione is necessary for the activity of various cellular enzymes, including some DNA polymerases. Glutathione is also essential for the synthesis of the DNA precursors deoxyribonucleotidetriphosphates (dNTP). The depletion of glutathione may inhibit repair through the reduction of the dNTP supply, although the requirement for repair synthesis would be very small when compared to what is needed for DNA replication (103). Experiments with BSO significantly inhibit the DNA repair processes in ovarian carcinoma cells (104).

*Enzymes Involved in DNA Repair*

Because platinum–DNA adducts are chemically stable, adducts can only be removed from DNA by the enzymatic process of repair. The importance of an adequate DNA repair system has been demonstrated in cell lines that show a lack of DNA repair. Defective removal of cisplatin-induced DNA damage in these cells resulted in a distinct hypersensitivity to the drug (105). Nucleotide excision repair is believed to be the main mechanism by which adducts are removed. The successive steps include recognition of the induced platinum-DNA lesion followed by incision of a damaged strand at or near the modified nucleotide together with several adjacent nucleotides, subsequently followed by filling in the resulting gap by DNA polymerases ($\alpha$ and $\beta$). Alterations of these enzymes involved in repair could mediate resistance. In fact, a cisplatin-resistant subline exhibited elevated polymerase $\beta$ activity (106). Human ovarian cancer cells, incubated once a week for 1 h with cisplatin, exhibited elevated DNA polymerase $\beta$ mRNA levels and activity (107).

Another nuclear enzyme potentially involved in cisplatin resistance is topoisomerase II. This is an important nuclear enzyme involved in DNA replication and possibly the DNA repair process. Resistance to cisplatin may be mediated by alterations in this enzyme. Elevated topoisomerase II activity has been shown in murine L1210 leukemia cells resistant to cisplatin. Opposite results were obtained in L1210 cells resistant to doxorubicin (a topoisomerase II inhibitor), which contained a lower amount of the enzyme (55).

Not only is the overall capacity to remove platinum-DNA lesions of importance, but repair of specific adducts may be more critical than others. In an experiment with human ovarian tumor cells, it was shown that the parental cells appeared proficient in removal of the intrastrand adduct platinum-AG but deficient in removal of the major adduct platinum-GG and the bifunctional platinum-$(GMP)_2$ lesion, whereas the resistant subline appeared proficient in removal of all four platinum-DNA adducts (22). In addition, repair of platinum damage in specific regions of the genome may be an important aspect of repair in resistant cells. It has been demonstrated that up to 20% more of the platinum-DNA lesions are repaired in critical genes compared with less important regions of the DNA (108,109). Quantitating the DNA damage for total genomic lesions and at the level of individual genes in two cisplatin-resistant human cancer cell lines demonstrated that the initial DNA platination was higher in the parental cell line but the total genomic repair of inter- as well as intrastrand lesions was not increased in the resistant cell lines. These differences in initial platination were not observed at the gene level. Also, no increase in the repair efficiency of intrastrand adducts in the DHFR gene were determined. However, a marked and consistent repair difference between parental and the resistant cells was seen for the gene-specific repair of cisplatin interstrand cross-links. For three genes, the DHFR, MDR1, and $\delta$-globin, these cross-links were removed much more efficiently in the resistant cells (110).

That not all tumor cells mediate their resistance by means of a better repair has been shown in two human ovarian cell lines. These cell lines, established from patients previously treated with alkylating agents but not with cisplatin, expressed a greater than 23-fold difference in cisplatin sensitivity in vitro. No significant modification of cisplatin accumulation was noted, and there was only marginally lower total platination of DNA in the resistant type. Also the overall ability to remove platinum-DNA lesions was less, with an apparent inability to remove either the major platinum-GG or platinum-GMP intrastrand adducts. And more important, significantly more of the interstrand cross-links were induced in the resistant cells. These data suggest the existence of increased tolerance of certain types of cisplatin-induced DNA damage (75). In accordance with this observation, some of the studies in ovarian cancer cells show higher DNA platination in resistant cells at equitoxic incubation concentrations (22,111). Tolerance as a mechanism of resistance might also be involved in other cell lines. Resistant human ovarian tumor cells, for example, tolerate significantly more adducts than do the parent cells (22).

*Excision Repair Genes*

In the past several years, there has been growing interest in the detection of genes that might be involved in cisplatin resistance—and vice versa, the elucidation of excision repair mechanisms has been advanced greatly by the cloning of human genes involved in the pathway of repair. The activation of oncogenes as well as loss of tumor suppressor gene product activity could be involved. Cell lines deficient in DNA repair have been DNA-corrected, resulting in the cloning of the designated group of excision repair cross-complementing (ERCC) genes and XPAC and XPCC genes (112). The ERCC and XP proteins may be involved in recognition of DNA damage of endonucleolytic incision at damaged sites, or they may play a role in the disassembly of chromatin structure to allow access for repair enzymes.

The role of the above-mentioned genes was investigated in excision-repair-deficient Chinese hamster ovary (CHO) cells. These cells were transfected with the human ERCC-1 gene and subsequently treated with cisplatin. These transfected CHO cells removed interstrand cross-links from the DHFR gene efficiently. In contrast, the transfected cells repaired the intrastrand adducts in the DHFR gene inefficiently. These data suggest that the ERCC-1 gene is more involved in repair of interstrand cross-links than in removal of intrastrand adducts (113). The most significant difference found in a study with ovarian and testicular teratoma cell lines was the inherent levels of expression of ERCC-1 between these two cell lines. The ovarian cells showed 30- or 50-fold higher ERCC-1 levels than the testicular teratoma cells. This difference could account, at least in part, for the high sensitivity of human teratomas for cisplatin (114). Tumor tissues from cancer patients who were clinically resistant to cisplatin showed a 2.6-fold higher expression of ERCC-1 (115). In addition, some proteins may also be regulatory products that control the expression of repair genes (113).

The role of other genes also has been studied. Transformation of a human mammary epithelial cell line by the *ras* oncogene resulted in an 2.7-fold increased resistance to cisplatin, a feature associated with a reduced proportion of induced interstrand cross-links and a higher efficiency in their removal (116).

## Genes and Signal-Transduction Pathways

The target of cisplatin therapy is binding of the agent to the DNA and thereby damaging the genome, probably leading to cell death (see Table 5). However, the biological activity of cisplatin cannot be explained only by its ability to damage the DNA.

*Gene Products*

According to this hypothesis, a mechanism that recognizes the cisplatin-DNA lesions, subsequently triggering a cellular response leading to cell death, may exist. In view of

**Table 5** Recognition of DNA Damage

| Mechanism | Effect | Ref. |
|---|---|---|
| HMG1, SSRP1 | Recognize specific cisplatin-DNA lesions | 117–119 |
| XPE-binding factor | Damage-recognition | 120 |
| Cisplatin inducible proteins ($b_{130}$ & $b_{95}$) | Damage-recognition | 121 |

the latter, it has been shown that several proteins—for example, the SSRP1 (structure specific recognition protein) and the HMG1 (high mobility group proteins)—are involved in recognizing specific cisplatin-DNA structures (117,118). Whether these proteins play a role in resistance is as yet unclear. Resistant human liver carcinoma cells (111-fold) and adenocarcinoma cells (1152-fold) were obtained by stepwise increases in cisplatin incubation. Gel electrophoresis revealed increases in 52-kd protein(s) in both the soluble cytosolic and crude membrane fractions in both cell lines. Moreover, the amount of this protein was proportional to the degree of resistance (119).

Effective DNA repair in cells depends on an efficient coupling of the repair enzymes to the target domain of the damaged chromosomal DNA. A potential factor that is capable of recognizing cisplatin-damaged DNA and is involved in repair is the XPE binding factor. Because this factor is deficient in complementation group E of xeroderma pigmentosum cells, which are characterized by defective DNA repair, as well as elevated in cisplatin-resistant cells, it has been proposed that increased expression of XPE binding factor mediates cisplatin drug resistance (120). In the same cell line, two other cisplatin-inducible proteins b130 and b95 were determined (121). Tumor necrosis factor (TNF) is a cytokine that exerts potent cytostatic and cytotoxic activity against a wide range of murine and human tumor cell lines. In order to augment the direct cytotoxic effects and prevent the development and emergence of resistant subclones, the combination of chemotherapeutic agents and TNF have been utilized (122). Alterations in cellular biochemistry that are associated with the development of resistance to tumor necrosis factor may also be involved in resistance to cisplatin. Human cervical carcinoma cells cultured in the presence of escalating amounts of TNF developed resistance to the substance. It was shown that tyrosine kinase activity associated with EGF receptor was threefold higher than that expressed in the parental line. In addition, these cervical carcinoma cells showed a three- to fivefold increased sensitivity to the antiproliferative effects of cisplatin. Selection for resistance to TNF appears to correlate with both altered EGF receptor expression and less resistance to cisplatin, which may be mediated through lesions in DNA repair processes (31).

*Oncogenes*

The relationship between oncogenes and drug resistance has been demonstrated by transfection studies (Table 6). The role of *c-myc* in cisplatin resistance has been studied in NIH3T3 cells (123). Cells transfected with *c-myc* acquired resistance to anticancer agents (123). The $IC_{50}$ values for all the drugs (cDDP, hCPA, melphalan, ADR, and CPT-11) except VP-16 were significantly higher than those in the parental cells. Cells transformed with *H-ras*—in contrast to *K-ras* transfected cells—showed an increase in resistance to cisplatin compared with the parental cells. It was concluded that induction of cisplatin resistance by *H-ras* is mainly the result of a reduction of accumulation and an impairment of $Na^+$ $K^+$-ATPase activity in the membrane fraction (124). Moreover, resistance to cisplatin can be avoided by suppression of the *H-ras* function (124). The oncogenes of the ras family encode a homologous 21-kd protein, p21, which plays a role in signal-transduction processes.

*Bcl-2* is an oncogene and one of the genes involved in the pathway leading to apoptosis. The ability of this proto-oncogene to contribute to chemotherapy resistance by inhibiting drug-induced programmed cell death has been studied in a neuroblastoma cell line (125). It was found that these cells, when transfected with *Bcl-2*, showed increased (dose-dependent) tolerance to DNA damage. Further, the *Bcl-2* gene might

**Table 6**  Genes/Proteins Involved in Cisplatin Resistance

| Gene | Effect on | Ref. |
|---|---|---|
| *H-ras* | Na+, K+-ATPase, accumulation | 124,127 |
| *Bcl-2* | Inhibition of apoptosis | 125, 127 |
| *c-Ha-ras* | Impairment of drug accumulation | 26 |
|  | Increased MT content |  |
| *c-myc* | Accumulation of cisplatin | 123, 127 |
| *c-fos, c-jun* | Early response genes | 127, 129, 130 |
| *p53* (mutant) | Transfection of p53 (mutant) resulted in resistance | 128 |
| Protein |  |  |
|   HSPs | Protection against toxic stimuli | 132–134 |

HSPs = heat shock proteins.

delay, or in some instances prevent, the activation of the death program, allowing time for DNA repair, which by itself could allow the cell to develop resistance. Treatment of murine leukemia (L1210) cells and a resistant subline with cisplatin led only in the parental cells to the typical morphological changes such as fragmentation of DNA into oligonucleosome-size fragments typical for apoptosis. Treatment with protein kinase C inhibitor staurosporine induced features of apoptosis in both cell lines. Another explanation for the involvement of *Bcl-2* in platinum resistance could be the fact that the apoptotic cell death operates through different, endonuclease-mediated, signal-transduction pathways—among them, one possibly defective in the cisplatin-resistant cells (126). In addition, cisplatin-resistant human prostate (PC3) cells overexpressing *Bcl-2* (two to threefold) also overexpressed *c-myc, c-jun*, and *H-ras* mRNA. The latter suggest that other oncogenes besides *Bcl-2* are involved in the emergence of platinum resistance (127). This was confirmed in a murine keratinocyte cell line (PAM 212) transformed with different oncogenes (*v-H-ras, v-myc* and a mutant *p53* suppressor gene [*mp53*]). It was demonstrated that the oncogenes *v-H-ras* and *mp53* induced resistance to cisplatin (128).

Several cytotoxic drugs, including cisplatin, enhance the mRNA expression of *c-fos* and *c-jun*, immediate early response genes (129). Also, protein kinase C (PKC) activity, which is involved in growth factor signal-transduction, is affected by cisplatin (130) and therefore potentially involved in platinum resistance. Agents such as quercetin, TPA, tamoxifen, and staurosporine may, as a result of inhibition of protein kinase C, enhance the antiproliferative effect of cisplatin (131).

*Genes of the Heat Shock Family*

Heat shock proteins (HSPs) are highly conserved throughout evolution. Therefore, it is not entirely surprising that they play crucial roles in a wide variety of cellular processes. By binding to other proteins, the molecular chaperonins such as hsp60 and 70 may regulate their activity, help them to fold, and inhibit incorrect interactions between highly adhesive hydrophobic protein surfaces. It is for these reasons that HSPs and in particular molecular chaperoning may play a role in the development of drug resistance by protecting the cell from toxic stimuli (132). Recently, a cDNA was isolated that was associated with clinically relevant levels of platinum resistance and was identified as the terminal portion of the mitochondrial hsp60 chaperonin (133). Nakata et al.

demonstrated that the expression of hsp60 was closely related to the emergence of cisplatin resistance (134). Based on their findings, they concluded that the increase of hsp60 level in cisplatin-resistant cells was not caused by a general induction of molecular chaperonins as an overall defense mechanism but was much more a unique event, associated with the early development of cisplatin resistance. In view of the latter, hsp60 might be involved in molecular pathways dealing with cellular injury; e.g., there are indications that hsp60 is induced by DNA relaxation, which itself can be induced by specific chemicals (135), suggesting a role in the DNA repair pathway.

## THERAPEUTIC IMPLICATIONS

In an effort to overcome cisplatin resistance, six major strategies have been developed dealing with drug exposure, transport, synergistic interaction with nonplatinum drugs, and the development of new analogues (see Table 7).

### Increase of Drug Exposure

Because cell lines obtained from patients with clinically refractory tumors often show less than a fivefold level of resistance, at least some of these patients might be expected to respond to increased chemotherapeutic doses. Unfortunately, toxic side effects currently limit the magnitude of dose escalations that can be achieved.

**Table 7**  Major Strategies for Overcoming Cisplatin Resistance

| Strategy | Successful attempts | Ref. |
|---|---|---|
| Increase in drug exposure | Reduction in toxicity | 136–139, 140–142 |
| | Change in route of administration | 2, 143, 172 |
| | Combination with heat | 145, 146 |
| Modulation of resistance mechanisms | Nifedipine | 157, 158 |
| | Aphidicolin | 153, 155, 159 |
| | Shock waves/hyperbaric $O_2$ | 147, 148 |
| | Nicotinamide | 156 |
| | Propargylglycine | 149, 150 |
| | Quercetin | 131 |
| | BSO/Ethacrynic acid | 23, 82, 86, 88, 152 |
| Synergistic interactions | Tamoxifen, Taxol (paclitaxel), temozolomide, amphotericin B, topotecan, cyclosporin A | 73, 159, 160, 162, 164–169, 171 |
| New analogues | - Carbo-, ipro-, tetraplatin and dicarboxylate compounds | 27, 74, 171, 173, 174 |
| Detection | GST-π expression | 180 |
| | Neuroendocrine markers | 179 |
| | Damage in leukocyte DNA | 181 |
| Tests in models | Animals | 176, 177 |
| | Clinical | 176 |
| | Prediction | 175 |

*Reduced Toxicity*

Improvements in supportive care, such as extensive hydration, chemoprotective agents such as sodium thiosulfate, stem cell progenitor rescue, and cytokines may permit evaluation of more dose-intensive regimens. Sodium thiosulfate was the first drug to be introduced into clinical study and convincingly showed that the intraperitoneal cisplatin therapy could be intensified without incurring nephrotoxicity. Further, anemia and neurotoxicity were also reduced. However, nausea and vomiting have been considerable, and the gain in therapeutic effect beyond the peritoneum is unclear (136–138). The nervous system could be protected by treatment with an ACTH (4-9) analogue (139). Better antiemetics may enhance the therapeutic index of cisplatin. The effect of pretreatment, using thiols such as glutathione, on the pharmacokinetics of total and free platinum was investigated in 12 patients suffering from non–small cell lung cancer or pleural mesothelioma. Patients who had been pretreated with glutathione showed both an increased rate of platinum elimination and extent of platinum tissue distribution and, as a consequence of the latter, might prolong the residence time of the drug in the body. Glutathione pretreatment might diminish cisplatin's nephrotoxicity without reducing its antitumor action (140). Nephrotoxicity might also be prevented by the induction of metallothionein synthesis. A study has shown that administration of bismuth subnitrate, which led to the induction of metallothionein synthesis, resulted in a substantial reduction of cisplatin-induced renal toxicity without compromising its antitumor activity (141).

Recently high-dose chemotherapy of solid tumors combined with autologous bone marrow transplantation has been suggested. Advention of hematopoietic growth factors and the rescue by the peripheral stem cells to reduce the duration of myeloid aplasia. For the treatment of primary resistant gonadal germ cell tumors, the effectiveness of this therapy has been demonstrated. However, for the treatment of chemoresistant extragonadal germ cell tumors, particularly for primary mediastinal tumors, the degree of resistance may be too high to be overcome by intensive therapies. The exact place of high-dose chemotherapy in the field of intraperitoneal and breast cancer treatment has to be established (142).

*Change Route of Administration*

Dose intensification can be achieved by locoregional administration of the drug. In an animal model, collagen chemoembolization of the liver resulted in up to 200-fold elevated platinum concentrations (143). In ovarian cancer, regional application of chemotherapy has considerable potential. The large pharmacological advantage of intraperitoneal administration can be translated into improved survival. In a clinical study, the therapeutic index was improved by changing the route of administration of the drug from intravenous to intraperitoneal in patients with residual small volume ovarian cancer who had failed to respond to intravenous cisplatin (144). In the treatment of solid tumors, diminished access of chemotherapeutic agents to cells in (peritoneal) tumors will result in lack of total eradication of that tumor, especially in resistant types. Improvement in locoregional chemotherapy will therefore be based on the penetration of drugs into peritoneal tumors. One way is to increase the temperature in the region of the tumor (2).

*Combining Heat with Cisplatin*

A possible method of overcoming resistance is the combination of cisplatin therapy and (locoregional) heat. Hyperthermia facilitated the uptake of cisplatin into tumor cells and increased cytotoxicity. Intraperitoneal cisplatin combined with heat resulted in 4.1 times higher platinum concentrations in tumors in an animal model. However, the combination therapy also enhances the toxic side effects of cisplatin, although renal toxicity was less than in whole-body hyperthermia (145). In Chinese hamster ovary cells resistant to cisplatin, a combined treatment of hyperthermia and cisplatin resulted in increased accumulation at elevated temperatures and consequently increased cytotoxicity (146).

## Modulation of Resistance Mechanisms

Hypothetically, modulation of resistance mechanisms can be achieved by interference with each particular mechanism of resistance.

### Transport

Because decreased accumulation of cisplatin is a frequently recognized feature of resistance, attempts have been made to manipulate platinum transport. One method is use of shock waves and cisplatin. Extracorporeal shock-wave lithotripsy is one of the clinical procedures in the treatment of renal stones. Side effects of shock waves indicated that exposure of parenchymatous organs induces hemorrhage and vessel-wall damage. These unwanted side effects might be used positively to overcome chemotherapy resistance. The reduced growth of subcutaneously implanted rodent tumors was significantly more effective after combined treatment than either monotherapy. A transient increase in cisplatin uptake upon exposure to shock waves was suggested as a major cause (147).

Resistance to chemotherapy is common in bulky hypoxic tumors such as epithelial ovarian cancer. Promotion of neovascularization by hyperbaric oxygen (HBO) may help overcome cisplatin resistance. Neovascularization may result in increased tumor perfusion. Experiments in an animal (mouse) model with subcutaneously inoculated human epithelial ovarian cancer cells showed enhanced response to cisplatin after hyperbaric oxygen therapy. This response appeared to be related to increased vascularity (148).

### Detoxification Systems

Attempts have been made to manipulate the activity of the detoxification systems that exist in resistant tumor cells. One possible method considers the inhibition of metallothionein synthesis. Propargylglycine (PPG), a specific inhibitor of the cystathionein pathway, was injected into mice bearing a murine bladder tumor. That resulted in a decrease of the intracellular free cysteine pool, thereby lowering the metallothionein synthesis. Metallothionein concentrations in tumor and kidneys were significantly increased after induction with $ZnSO_4$, with subsequently reduced renal toxicity and increased cisplatin resistance. Treatment with PPG, however, could clearly overcome the metallothionein-mediated resistance without compromising the protective effect exerted by renal metallothionein on nephrotoxicity (149,150). In vitro depletion of glutathione by BSO results in decreasing intracellular thiol contents and, often, decreasing resistance. Clinically, however, this combination does not appear to be of use because of the danger of aggravating its nephrotoxicity (151). Another method of modifying intracellular thiols may be the use of ethacrynic acid, which (in vitro) inhibits glutathione-S-transferase and lowers glutathione levels (152). The combination of cisplatin and this agent might produce less toxicity; however, its clinical efficacy remains to be established.

### DNA Repair

In attempts to overcome cisplatin resistance, agents that inhibit DNA repair have been tested. Experiments with two recently established human ovarian carcinoma cell lines have been used to study the effect of aphidicolin glycinate (APG). The effect of this specific competitive inhibitor of DNA polymerase α on the formation and repair of four platinum-DNA adducts was studied. Aphidicolin adheres to nucleotide-binding sites on DNA polymerase α, thereby causing an incomplete repair process and accumulation of DNA lesions. Unfortunately, there were no significant differences observed in both the total DNA platination and repair of DNA lesions (153). Aphidicolin reversibly inhibits DNA polymerase α and δ and has antiproliferative effects in vitro. In resistant A2780-CP cells, aphidicolin glycinate increased the cytotoxicity about twofold and caused a significant delay in the time required for repair of the cisplatin-DNA lesions (154). In both a sensitive and resistant reticular cell sarcoma, a moderate potentiation of activity of cisplatin by aphidicolin glycinate was observed (155). The activity of poly(ADP-ribose) polymerase (PARP), a nuclear enzyme, is stimulated when DNA breaks are induced after treatment with DNA-damaging agents. This enzyme has been postulated to play a role in cisplatin resistance by modulation of DNA excision repair. Therefore, inhibition of this enzyme might overcome cisplatin resistance. Nicotinamide, an inhibitor of PARP, has been shown to be able to reverse cisplatin resistance in a rat ovarian tumor cell line both in vitro and in vivo (156).

### Signal Transduction Pathways

Nifedipine, which is a dihydropyridine calcium channel blocker and a modulator of P-glycoprotein–mediated *MDR*, has been tested in human testicular tumor cell lines with different chemosensitivities. The combination of cisplatin and nifedipine was tested in nude mice that underwent heterotransplantation with these human testicular tumor cells. An increased antitumor effect was observed—remarkable because cisplatin resistance is thought not to be related to the *MDR* phenotype, whereas nifedipine is thought to interfere with this particular mechanism of drug resistance (157). On that account, the effect may be mediated through interference of the agent in calcium-mediated drug resistance. Further, the increased antitumor activity was, in vivo, associated with a considerable increase in overall toxicity.

In multidrug-resistant human glioblastoma GB-1 cells, significantly more resistant to cisplatin than the parental cells, it was determined that calcium channel blockers enhance the antitumor activity of cisplatin. Not only was cytotoxicity significantly increased but also the DNA fragmentation assay demonstrated that synergism between cisplatin and nifedipine led to apoptosis (158).

## Synergistic Interaction with Other Drugs

In order to overcome cisplatin resistance, the combination of cisplatin and other (chemotherapeutic) agents has been used. Amphotericin B is a macrolide polyene antibiotic that is used in the therapy of fungal diseases. It is believed to potentiate the activity of several chemotherapeutics, possibly by increasing membrane permeability.

In human larynx carcinoma cells, amphotericin B was able to potentiate cisplatin toxicity selectively in the resistant cells, without having any such effects in the parental cells (159). In another study, it was also demonstrated that amphotericin B was capable of significantly increasing cisplatin cytotoxicity in resistant human ovarian carcinoma cells but not in the parental cells.

Cyclosporin A is an immunosuppressive agent used extensively in organ transplantation. It inhibits the initial activation of lymphocytes and other critical pathways of the immune system. It has been demonstrated that cyclosporin A is able to reverse cisplatin resistance (160). Possibly, cyclosporin A can modulate the expression of oncogenes (161,162). In a phase I study of patients suffering from ovarian carcinoma, the combination of cyclosporin and cisplatin resulted in a 25% response rate. Renal toxicity appeared to be the dose-limiting factor (163).

Efforts to identify new drugs with activity against resistant cells may lead to therapeutic success. One such drug, paclitaxel, has shown great promise in the treatment of ovarian and metastatic breast cancers and malignant melanoma. It appears to promote and stabilize microtubule assembly, leading to mitotic arrest and eventual cell death. Particularly encouraging are the response rates for paclitaxel in patients with ovarian cancer that is refractory to cisplatin. In these patients, response rates have ranged from 20–38% (164).

Clinical studies have shown that tamoxifen is an important component of combination drug therapy for several different tumor types. In a recent clinical study, it was demonstrated that in patients with malignant melanoma documented to be resistant to single-agent cisplatin, the addition of tamoxifen to the next cycle resulted in a response rate of 32% (165). Further, it has been demonstrated that tamoxifen is able to delay the emergence of resistance to cisplatin in vitro for cell lines representative of two important types of human malignancy, melanoma and ovarian carcinoma. In addition to decreasing the rate of development of cisplatin resistance, tamoxifen also decreases the absolute magnitude of resistance to cisplatin that develops over a given period of time (166). Furthermore, although the interaction between tamoxifen and cisplatin is synergistic in cisplatin-resistant human malignant melanoma cells, it is not clear by which mechanism the cytotoxicity is modulated. It was shown that this synergistic effect was not dependent upon PKC activity (166).

Paclitaxel is a highly active single agent as therapy for previously untreated as well as doxorubicin-refractory metastatic breast cancer, with associated response rates of 62% and 20–48%, respectively. Early data suggest that administering biweekly paclitaxel and cisplatin to previously untreated metastatic breast cancer patients is associated with high response rates (167).

Cisplatin-based chemotherapy cures approximately 85% of patients suffering from metastatic testicular germ cell cancer. Cisplatin-resistant sublines of human nonseminomatous testicular germ cell cancer have been shown to be sensitive to temozolomide, a new imidazotetrazine that also can cross the blood-brain barrier in mice (168).

Intraperitoneal cisplatin-refractory ovarian cancer may be treated with topotecan, a water-soluble camptothecin analogue. Cisplatin-resistant human ovarian carcinoma cells (A2780) inoculated intraperitoneally into mice were treated with topotecan. Twelve of the 15 animals were found to be tumor free. It was suggested that the high responsiveness to the drug might be related to the elevated expression of the target enzyme topoisomerase I (169).

## New Analogues

A possible approach to improving the therapeutic index and successful therapy can be the use of newly developed platinum analogues. Nowadays, the research into platinum analogues has several aims: (1) activity by the oral route; (2) less toxicity; and (3) activity against cisplatin-resistant cancer (170). Nine platinum analogues are currently in clinical development, of which carboplatin [cis-diamminecyclobutane1,1-dicarboxylato-platinum(II)] has been investigated extensively in both the experimental and clinical setting (171). Carboplatin was developed primarily to circumvent the side effects of cisplatin. It is less nephrotoxic, neurotoxic, and emetogenic than cisplatin. Because a high drug concentration in the peritoneal cavity contributes to a large extent to the penetration of the drug from the peritoneal cavity directly into the tumor, carboplatin with its favorable toxicity profile is a good candidate for intraperitoneal chemotherapy. However, despite increased doses, the capacity of carboplatin to penetrate into peritoneal tumor cells is lower than that of cisplatin (172).

New platinum analogues may be able to circumvent cisplatin resistance. In two pairs of human ovarian carcinoma cells, acquired resistance has been established. A novel class of platinum(IV) complex, ammine/amine platinum(IV) dicarboxylates—completely circumventing resistance in the cell line that is resistant predominantly because of reduced uptake—showed cross-resistance to the other cell line (where resistance appears likely to have occurred at the DNA level). This suggests that this new platinum analogue is capable of circumventing acquired cisplatin resistance due to decreased intracellular accumulation but is not able to overcome resistance at the level of DNA platination and removal (173). However, in two resistant human lung cancer cell lines, the efficacy of the compound was determined, but reduced accumulation played a role in only one of the two lines. The ability of the compound to circumvent such an accumulation barrier, therefore, cannot alone explain the effect (27). In human ovarian carcinoma cells, cisplatin resistance was attributable to the inhibition of formation of bifunctional DNA lesions. This resistance could be circumvented by the non-cross-resistant properties of JM221 (ammine bis butyrato cyclohexylamine dichloro-platinum [IV]), which were attributable to both improved transport properties and the circumvention of DNA repair mechanisms (174).

## Tests in Models

One possibility is to mimic strategies for reversal of drug resistance using a model. In one study, experimental data were compared with model predictions (175). In resistant cells with high levels of glutathione, short-term cell survival was dose dependent, and even high doses of cisplatin did not eliminate all of these cells. Addition of an inhibitor of glutathione synthesis (BSO) did, however, augment elimination of the resistant cells. Resistant cells with low levels of glutathione could be eliminated with high cisplatin doses or coadministration of the drug and BSO. The results were comparable in qualitative accuracy and predictability to results with the model.

In another (clinical) model, three human ovarian carcinoma lines derived from the same patient before and after cisplatin therapy were established intraperitoneally in nude mice. The availability of tumor variants derived from the same patient, similar in several phenotypes but with different sensitivities to cisplatin, makes such a model suitable for investigating acquired resistance (176). Another in vivo model in which treatment for cisplatin-resistant tumor types can be studied involves the use of Scid mice. These mice may have a higher transplantability rate than do nude mice (177).

Because it is not known whether the resistance mechanisms could change as a consequence of chemotherapy, this was characterized in a clinical study. In 37 patients, a comparison was made of the changes in chemosensitivity between the original tumors and recurrent tumors after responses. The results suggest that locally recurred tumors may become resistant to the agents previously administered. Remarkably, the distantly recurred tumors did not necessarily become resistant to the agents administered (178).

## Detection

Because several tumor types (for example, lung cancer cells) respond only in a few cases, there have been attempts to determine whether some subset of patients might have an increased likelihood of benefiting from chemotherapy. Neuroendocrine markers might be prospectively indicative of a more responsive tumor type in non–small cell lung cancer cells. When patients whose neuroendocrine markers were identified retrospectively were included, 44% responded to cisplatin-based chemotherapy, compared to 13% with no markers present (179). In a clinical study, the expression of glutathione-S-transferase-π was examined immunohistochemically in relation to the response to chemotherapy with cisplatin. Among the ovarian tumors showing positive glutathione-S-transferase-π staining, 90.9% were drug resistant, whereas negative staining signified drug resistance in 35.3% of the cases. Moreover, survival of patients with glutathione-S-transferase-π positive tumors was also significantly shorter than that of those with glutathione-S-transferase-π negative tumors. Glutathione-S-transferase-π expression in tumor cells in patients with epithelial ovarian cancer may be a potential marker of poor prognosis (180).

Research into drug resistance in cancer has led to the observation that peripheral blood cells may provide a way to assess an individual's susceptibility to chemotherapy. Analysis of platinum-DNA adduct formation in peripheral leukocyte DNA of patients receiving carboplatin and cisplatin chemotherapy showed consistently higher platinum-adduct levels in the group of responders. This suggests that an individual's innate (genetic or acquired) ability to protect cellular DNA has a substantive impact on disease response to platinum-based therapy, and that this innate ability may be common to both normal and malignant cells (181).

The above-mentioned clinically useful approaches for modulation of cisplatin resistance emphasize the need for continued research on potential strategies.

## CONCLUSION

Resistance to chemotherapy is a major therapeutic problem in medical oncology and continues to be a challenge. Nearly half of all patients with cancer have malignancies that are intrinsically resistant to chemotherapy. The remainder of the patients may acquire resistance during the clinical course despite being initially sensitive to chemotherapy. It has been estimated that drug resistance is involved in more than 90% of cancer mortality (164). Therefore, understanding the detailed biochemical mechanisms of cisplatin resistance and devising strategies to circumvent this resistance is important for research and clinical aims.

None of the above-mentioned mechanisms is predominant: usually, resistance is modulated through two or three separate mechanisms. Further, each individual tumor type may be unique in the resistance mechanisms used. A better understanding of the underlying molecular basis of these mechanisms may result in reliable methods for routine detection and classification of cisplatin resistance. This better screening, combined with new developments in the field of experimental therapies, will permit improvements in the therapeutic approach to cisplatin-resistant cancers. Although cisplatin will ultimately be replaced by compounds that have a greater cytotoxic spectrum, over the short term, cisplatin will continue to play an important role in both clinical practice and oncological research.

## REFERENCES

1.  Rosenberg B, Von Camp L, Krigas T. Inhibition of cell division in Escherichia coli by electrolysis products from a platinum electrode. Nature 1965; 205N698–699.
2.  Los G, McVie JG. Experimental and clinical status of intraperitoneal chemotherapy. Eur J Cancer 1990; 26(6):755–762.
3.  Eastman A. Mechanisms of resistance to cisplatin. In: Ozols RF, ed. Molecular and Clinical Advances in Anticancer Drug Resistance. Boston: Kluwer Academic Publishers, 1991:233–249.
4.  Andrews PA. Anticancer drug resistance. In: Goldstein LJ, Ozols RF, eds. Advances in Molecular and Clinical Research. Boston: Kluwer Academic Publishers, 1994.
5.  Parker RJ, Eastman A, Bostick-Bruton F, Reed E. Acquired cisplatin resistance in human ovarian cancer cells is associated with enhanced repair of cisplatin-DNA lesions and reduced drug accumulation. J Clin Invest 1991; 87:772–777.
6.  Eastman A. The formation, isolation and characterization of DNA adducts produced by anticancer platinum complexes. Pharmacol Ther 1987; 34:155–166.
7.  Bellon SF, Coleman JH, Lippard SJ. DNA unwinding produced by site-specific intrastrand cross-links of the antitumor drug cis-diamminedichloroplatinum(II). Biochemistry 1991; 30: 8026–8035.
8.  Kerr JFR, Winterford CM, Harmon BV. Apoptosis: its significance in cancer and cancer therapy. Cancer 1994; 73:2013–2026.
9.  Sorenson CM, Eastman A. The mechanism of cis-diamminedichloroplatinum(II) induced cytotoxicity: the role of G2 arrest and DNA double strand breaks. Cancer Res 1988; 48:4484–4488.
10.  Eastman A. Activation of a programmed cell death by anticancer agents: cisplatin as a model system. Cancer Cells 1990; 2:275–280.
11.  Donaldson KL, Goolsby GL, Wahl AF. Cytotoxicity of the anticancer agents cisplatin and Taxol during cell proliferation and the cell cycle. Int J Cancer 1994; 57:847–855.
12.  Sklar M. Increased resistance to cis-diamminedichloroplatinum(II) in NIH 3T3 cells transformed by ras oncogenes. Cancer Res 1988; 48:793–797.
13.  Strandberg MC, Bresnick E, Eastman A. The significance of DNA cross-linking to cis-diamminedichloroplatinum(II)-induced cytotoxicity in sensitive and resistant lines of murine leukemia L1210 cells. Chem Biol Interact 1982; 39:169–180.
14.  Pinto AL, Lippard SJ. Sequence-dependent termination of in vitro DNA synthesis by cis- and trans-diamminedichloroplatinum(II). Proc Natl Acad Sci USA 1985; 82:4616–4619.
15.  Ciccarelli RB, Solomon MJ, Varshavsky A, Lippard SJ. In vivo effects of cis- and trans-diamminedichloroplatinum (II) on SV 40 chromosomes: differential repair, DNA protein cross-linking and inhibition of replication. Biochemistry 1985; 24:7533–7540.
16.  Andrews PA, Howell SB. Cellular pharmacology of cisplatin: perspective on mechanisms of acquired resistance. Cancer Cells 1990; 2:35–43.

17. Richon VM, Schulte N, Eastman A. Multiple mechanisms of resistance to cis-diamminedichloroplatinum(II) in murine leukemia L1210 cells. Cancer Res 1987; 47:2056–2061.

18. Waud WR. Differential uptake of cis-diamminedichloroplatinum(II) by sensitive and resistant murine L1210 leukemia cells. Cancer Res 1987; 46:6242–6245.

19. Teicher BA, Holden SA, Herman TS, Alvarez Sotomayor E, Khandekar V, Rosbe KW, Brann TW, Korbut TT, Frei E. Characteristics of five human tumor cell lines and sublines resistant to cis-diamminedichloroplatinum(II). Int J Cancer 1991; 47:252–260.

20. Mellish KJ, Kelland LR. Mechanisms of acquired resistance to the orally active platinum-based anticancer drug bis-acetato-ammine-dichloro-cyclohexylamine platinum(IV) (JM216) in two human ovarian carcinoma cell lines. Cancer Res 1994; 54:6194–6200.

21. Andrews PA, Albright KD. Mitochondrial defects in cis-diamminedichloroplatinum(II)-resistant human ovarian carcinoma cells. Cancer Res 1992; 52:1895–1901.

22. Dempke WCM, Shellard SA, Hosking LK, Fichtinger-Schepman AMJ, Hill B. Mechanisms associated with the expression of cisplatin resistance in a human ovarian tumor cell line following exposure to fractionated x-irradiation in vitro. Carcinogenesis 1992; 13(7):1209–1215.

23. Oldenburg J, Begg AC, van Vught MJH, Ruevekamp M, Schornagel JH, Pinedo HM, Los G. Characterization of resistance to cis-diamminedichloroplatinum(II) in three sublines of CC531 colonadenocarcinoma cell line in vitro. Cancer Res 1994; 54:487–493.

24. Metcalfe SA, Cain K, Hill BT. Possible mechanism for differences in sensitivity to cisplatinum in human prostate tumor cell lines. Cancer Lett 1986; 31:163–169.

25. Wallner KE, DeGregorio MW, Li GC. Hyperthermic potentiation of cis-diamminedichloroplatinum(II) cytotoxicity in chinese hamster ovary cells resistant to the drug. Cancer Res 1986; 46:6242–6245.

26. Isonichi S, Hom DK, Thiebaut FB, Mann SC, Andrews PA, Basu A, Lazo JS, Eastman A, Howell SB. Expression of the c-Ha-ras oncogene in mouse NIH3T3 cells induces resistance to cisplatin. Cancer Res 1991; 51:5903–5909.

27. Twentyman PR, Wright KA, Mistry P, Kelland LR, Murrer BA. Sensitivity to novel platinum compounds of panels of human lung cancer cell lines with acquired and inherent resistance to cisplatin. Cancer Res 1992; 52:5674–5680.

28. Kelland LR, Mistry P, Abel G, Freidlos F, Loh SY, Roberts JJ, Harrap KR. Establishment and characterization of an in vitro model of acquired resistance to cisplatin in a human testicular nonseminomatous germ cell line. Cancer Res 1992; 52:1710–1716.

29. Kasahara K, Fujiwara Y, Nishio K, Ohmori T, Sugimoto Y, Komiya K, Matsuda T, Saijo N. Metallothionein content correlates with the sensitivity of human small cell lung cancer cell lines to cisplatin. Cancer Res 1991; 51:3237–3242.

30. Hospers GAP, Mulder NH, de Jong B, de Ley L, Uges DRA, Fichtinger-Schepman AMJ, Schepter RJ, de Vries EGE. Characterization of a human small cell lung carcinoma with acquired resistance to cis-diamminedichloroplatinum in vitro. Cancer Res 1988; 48:6803–6807.

31. Nishikawa K, Rosenblum MG, Newman RA, Pandita TK, Hittelman WN, Donato NJ. Resistance of human cervical carcinoma cells to tumor necrosis factor correlates with their increased sensitivity to cisplatin: evidence of a role for DNA repair and epidermal growth factor receptor. Cancer Res 1992; 52:4758–4765.

32. Bungo M, Fujiwara Y, Kasahara K, Nakagawa K, Ohe Y, Sasaki Y, Irino S, Saijo N. Decreased accumulation as a mechanism of resistance to cis-diamminedichloroplatinum(II) in human non-small cell lung cancer cell lines: relation to DNA damage and repair. Cancer Res 1990; 50:2549–2553.

33. Gale GR, Morris CR, Atkins LM, Smith AB. Binding of an antitumor platinum compound to cells as influenced by physical factors and pharmacologically active agents. Cancer Res 1973; 33:813–818.

34. Binks SP, Dobrota M. Kinetics and mechanism of uptake of platinum based pharmaceuticals by the rat small intestine. Biochem Pharmacol 1990; 40:1329–1336.

35. Mann SC, Andrews PA, Howell SB. Comparison of lipid content, surface membrane fluidity, and temperature dependence of cis-diamminedichloroplatinum(II) accumulation in sensitive and resistant human ovarian carcinoma cells. Anticancer Res 1988; 8:1211–1216.

36. Bernal SD, Speak JA, Boeheim K, Dreyfuss AI, Wright JE, Teicher BA, Rosowsky A, Tsao SW, Wong YC. Reduced membrane protein associated with resistance of human squamous carcinoma cells to methotrexate and cis-platinum. Mol Cell Biochem 1990; 95:61–70.

37. Jekunen AP, Hom DK, Alcaraz JE, Eastman A, Howell SB. Cellular pharmacology of dichloro(ethylenediamine) platinum(II) in cisplatin sensitive and resistant human ovarian carcinoma cells. Cancer Res 1994; 2680–2687.

38. Teicher BA, Holden SA, Kelley MJ, Shea TC, Cucchi CA, Rosowsky A, Henner WD, Frei III E. Characterization of a human squamous carcinoma cell line resistant to cis-diamminedichloroplatinum(II). Cancer Res 1987; 47:388–393.

39. Byfield JE, Calabro-Jones PM. Further evidence for carrier mediated uptake of cis-dichlorodiammine platinum. Proc Am Assoc Cancer Res 1982; 23:167.

40. Scanlon KJ, Safirstein RL, Thies H, Gross RB, Waxman S, Guttenplan JB. Gross inhibition of amino acid transport by cis-diamminedichloroplatinum(II) derivatives in L1210 murine leukemia cells. Cancer Res 1983; 43:4211–4215.

41. Andrews PA, Velury S, Mann SC, Howell SB. Cis-diamminedichloroplatinum(II) accumulation in sensitive and resistant human ovarian cells. Cancer Res 1988; 48:68–73.

42. Atema A, Buurman KJH, Noteboom E, Smets LA. Potentiation of DNA-adduct formation and cytotoxicity of platinum-containing drugs by low pH. Int J Cancer 1993; 54:1–7.

43. Dornish JM, Peterson EO. Modulation of cis-dichlorodiammineplatinum by benzaldehyde derivatives. Cancer Lett 1989; 46:63–68.

44. Basu A, Lazo JS. Sensitization of human cervical carcinoma cells to cis-diamminedichloroplatinum(II) by byrostatin. Cancer Res 1992; 52:3119–3124.

45. Christen RD, Hom DK, Porter DC, Andrews PA, Macleod CL, Halfstrom L, Howell SB. Epidermal growth factor regulates the in vitro sensitivity of human ovarian carcinoma cells to cisplatin. J Clin Invest 1990; 86:1632–1640.

46. Kikuchi Y, Iwano I, Miyauchi M, Sasa H, Nagata I, Kuki E. Restorative effects of calmodulin antagonists on reduced cisplatin uptake by cisplatin-resistant human ovarian carcinoma cells. Gynecol Oncol 1990; 39:199–203.

47. Gately DP, Howell SB. Cellular accumulation of the anticancer agent cisplatin: a review. Br J Cancer 1993; 67:1171–1176.

48. Dornish JM, Melvik JE, Pettersen EO. Reduced cellular uptake of cis-diamminedichloroplatinum(II) by benzaldehyde. Anticancer Res 1986; 6:583–588.

49. Dornish JM, Pettersen EO, Oftebro R. Modifying effect of cinnamaldehyde and cinnamaldehydes derivatives on cell inactivation and cellular uptake of cis-diamminedichloroplatinum(II) in human NHIK 3025 cells. Cancer Res 1989; 49:3917–3921.

50. Los G, Vugt van M, Vlist van der M, den Engels L, Pinedo HM. The effect of heat on the interaction of cisplatin and carboplatin with cellular DNA. Biochem Pharmacol 1993; 46:1229–1237.

51. Kraker AJ, Moore CW. Accumulation of cis-diamminedichloroplatinum(II0 and platinum analogs by platinum resistant murine leukemia cells in vitro. Cancer Res 1988; 48:9–13.

52. Kelland LR, Mistry P, Abel G, Loh SY, O'Neill CF, Murrer BA, Harrap KR. Mechanism-related circumvention of acquired cis-diamminedichloroplatinum(II) resistance using two pairs of human ovarian carcinoma cell lines by ammine/amine platinum(IV) dicarboxylates. Cancer Res 1992; 53:3857–3864.

53. Los G, Mutsaers PHA, Ruevekamp M, McVie JG. The use of oxaliplatin versus cisplatin in intraperitoneal chemotherapy in cancers restricted to the peritoneal cavity. Cancer Lett 1990; 51:109–117.

54. Sharp SY, Mistry P, Valenti MR, Bryant AP, Kelland LR. Selective potentiation of platinum drug cytotoxicity in cisplatin-sensitive and -resistant ovarian carcinoma cell lines by amphotericin B. Cancer Chemother Pharmacol 1994; 35:137–143.

55. Mestdagh N, Pommery N, Saucier J-M, Hecquet B, Fournier C, Slomianny C, Teisier E, Henichart J-P. Chemoresistance to doxorubicin and cisplatin in a murine cell line, analysis of P-glycoprotein, topoisomerase II activity, glutathione and related enzymes. Anticancer Res 1994; 14:869–874.

56. Veneroni S, Zaffaroni N, Daidone MG, Benini E, Villa R, Silvestrini. Expression of P-glycoprotein and in vitro or in vivo resistance to doxorubicin and cisplatin in breast and ovarian cancers. Eur J Cancer 1994; 30A(7):1002–1007.

57. Christen RD, Shalinsky DR, Howell SB. Enhancement of the loss of multiple drug resistance by hydroxyurea. Semin Oncol 1992; 19(3 suppl 9):94–100.

58. Fujii R, Mutoh M, Niwa K, Yamada K, Aikou T, Nakayawa M, Kuwano M, Akiyama S-I. An active efflux system for cisplatin in cisplatin-resistant human KB cells. Jpn J Cancer Res 1994; 85:426–433.

59. Fujii R, Mutoh M, Sumizawa T, Chen Z, Yoshimura A, Akiyama S. Adenosine triphosphate-dependent transport of leukotriene C4 by membrane vesicles prepared from cisplatin-resistant human epidermoid carcinoma tumor cells. J Natl Cancer Inst 1994; 86:1781–1784.

60. Ishikawa T, Wright CD, Ishizuka H. GS-X pump is functionally overexpressed in cis-diamminedichloroplatinum (II)-resistant human leukemia HL-60 cells and down-regulated by cell differentiation. J Biochem 1994; 269(46):29085–29093.

61. Muller M, Meijer C, Zaman GJR, Borst P, Scheper RJ, Mulder NH, de Vries EGE, Jansen PLM. Overexpression of the gene encoding the multidrug resistance-associated protein results in increased ATP-dependent glutathione S-conjugate transport. Proc Natl Acad Sci USA 1994; 91:13033–13037.

62. Cole SP, Bhardwaj G, Gerlach JH, Mackie JE, Grant CE, Almquist KC, Stewart AJ, Kurz EU, Duncun AMV, Deeley RG. Overexpression of a transporter gene in multidrug resistant human lung cancer cell line. Science 1992; 258:1650–1654.

63. Zaman GJR, Flens MJ, van Leusden MR, de Haas M, Mulder HS, Lankema J, Pinedo HM, Scheper RJ, Baas F, Broxterman HJ, Borst P. The human multidrug resistance-associated protein MRP is a plasma drug efflux pump. Proc Natl Acad Sci USA 1994; 91:8822–8826.

64. Flens MJ, Izquierdo MA, Scheffer GL, Fritz JM, Meijer CJLM, Scheper RJ, Zaman GJR. Immunochemical detection of multidrug resistance-associated protein MRP in human multidrug resistance tumor cells by monoclonal antibodies. Cancer Res 1994; 54:4557–4563.

65. De Vries EGE, Müller M, Meijer C, Jansen PLM, Mulder NH. Role of the glutathione S-conjugate pump in cisplatin resistance. J Natl Cancer Inst 1995; 87:537–538.

66. Scheper RJ, Broxterman HJ, Scheffer GL, Kaaijk P, Dalton WS, van Heijningen THM, van Kalken CK, Slovak ML, de Vries EGE, van der Valk P, Meijer CJLM, Pinedo HM. Overexpression of $M_r$ 110,000 vesicular protein in non P-glycoprotein-mediated multidrug resistance. Cancer Res 1993; 53:1475–1479.

67. Scheffer GL, Wijngaard PLJ, Flens MJ, Izquierdo MA, Slovak ML, Pinedo HM, Meijer CJLM, Clevers HC, Scheper RJ. The drug resistance related protein LRP is a major vault protein. Proc Am Assoc Cancer Res 1995; 36:1921.

68. Izquierdo MA, Schoemaker RH, Flens MJ, Scheffer GL, Wu L, Prater TL, Scheper RJ. Overlapping phenotype of multidrug resistance among disease-oriented panels of human cancer cell lines. Proc Am Assoc Cancer Res 1995; 36:1923.

69. Scheper RJ, Scheffer GL, Flens M, Izquierdo MA, van der Valk P, Broxterman HJ, Pinedo HM, Meijer CJLM, Clevers HC. Molecular and clinical characterization of the LRP protein associated with non-P-glycoprotein multidrug resistance. Proc Am Assoc Cancer Res 1994; 35:2050.

70. Ozols RF, O'Dwyer PJ, Hamilton TC, Young RC. The role of glutathione in drug resistance. Cancer Treat Rev 1990; 17(suppl A):45–50.

71. Arrick BA, Nathan CF. Glutathione metabolism as determinant of therapeutic efficacy: a review. Cancer Res 1984; 44:4224–4232.

72. Cazenave LA, Moscow JA, Meyers CE, Cowan KH. Glutathione S-transferase and drug resistance. In: Ozols RF, ed. Drug Resistance in Cancer Therapy. Boston: Kluwer Academic Publishers, 1989:171–188.

73. Hamaguchi K, Godwin AK, Yakushiji M, O'Dwyer PJ, Ozols RF, Hamilton TC. Cross-resistance to diverse drugs is associated with primary cisplatin resistance in ovarian cancer cell lines. Cancer Res 1993; 53:5225–5232.

74. Behrens BC, Hamilton TC, Masuda H, Grotzinger KR, Whang-Peng J, Louie KG, Knutsen T, McKoy WM, Young RC, Ozols RF. Characterization of a cis-diamminedichloroplatinum(II)-resistant human ovarian cancer cell line and its use in evaluation of platinum analogues. Cancer Res 1987; 47:414–418.

75. Shellard SA, Hosking LK, Hill BT. Anomalous relationship between cisplatin sensitivity and the formation and removal of platinum-DNA adducts in two human ovarian carcinoma cell lines in vitro. Cancer Res 1991; 51:4557–4564.

76. Hansson J, Fichtinger-Schepman AMJ, Edgren M, Ringborg U. Comparative study of two human melanoma cell lines with different sensitivities to mustine and cisplatin. Eur J Cancer 1991; 27)8):1039–1045.

77. Muller MR, Wright KA, Twentyman PR. Differential properties of cisplatin and tetraplatin with respect to cytotoxicity and perturbation of cellular glutathione levels. Cancer Chemother Pharmacol 1991; 28:273–276.

78. Bedford P, Walker MC, Sharma HL, Perera A, Mcauliffe CA, Masters JRW, Hill BT. Factors influencing the sensitivity of two human bladder carcinoma cell lines to cis-diamminedichloroplatinum(II). Chem Biol Interact 1987; 61:1–15.

79. Ishikawa T, Ali-Osman F. Glutathione-associated cis-diamminedichloroplatinum metabolism and ATP-dependent efflux from leukemia cells. J Biol Chem 1993; 268:20116–20125.

80. Eastman A. Cross-linking of glutathione to DNA by cancer chemotherapeutic platinum coordination complexes. Chem Biol Interact 1987; 61:241–248.

81. Sekiya S, Oosaki T, Andoh S, Suzuki N, Akaboshi M, Takamizawa H. Mechanisms of resistance to cis-diamminedichloroplatinum(II) in a rat ovarian carcinoma. Eur J Cancer Clin Oncol 1989; 25:429–437.

82. Meijer C, Mulder NH, Hospers GAP, Uges DRA, de Vries EGE. The role of glutathione in resistance to cisplatin in a human small cell lung cancer cell line. Br J Cancer 1990; 62:72–77.

83. Micetich K, Zwelling LA, Kohn KW. Quenching of DNA platinum(II) monoadducts as a possible mechanism of resistance to cis-diamminedichloroplatinum(II) in L1210 cells. Cancer Res 1983; 43:3609–3613.

84. Lai GM, Ozols RF, Young RC, Hamilton TC. Effect of glutathione on DNA repair in cisplatin-resistant human ovarian cancer cell lines. J Natl Cancer Inst 1989; 81:535–539.

85. Meijer C, Mulder NH, Hospers GAP, Uges DRA, de Vries EGE. The role of glutathione in resistance to cisplatin in a human small cell lung cancer cell line. Br J Cancer 1990; 62:72–77.

86. Hromas RA, Andrews PA, Murphy MP, Burns CP. Glutathione depletion reverses cisplatin resistance in murine L1210 leukemia cells. Cancer Lett 1987; 34:9–13.

87. Hromas RA, Barlogie B, Meyn RE, Andrews PA, Burns CP. Diverse mechanisms and methods of overcoming cis-platinum resistance in L1210 leukemia cells. Proc Am Assoc Cancer Res 1985; 26:1030.

88. Andrews PA, Schiefer MA, Murphy MP, Howell SB. Enhanced potentiation of cisplatin cytotoxicity in human ovarian carcinoma cells by prolonged glutathione depletion. Chem Biol Interact 1988; 65:51–58.

89. Meredith MJ, Reed DJ. Status of the mitochondrial pool of glutathione in the isolated hepatocyte. J Biol Chem 1982; 257:3747–3753.

90. Edgren M, Revesz L. Compartmentalised depletion of glutathione in cells treated with buthionine sulfoximine. Br J Radiol 1987; 670:723–724.

91. Hao X, Bergh J, Brodin O, Hellman U, Mannervik B. Acquired resistance to cisplatin and doxorubicine in a small cell lung cancer cell line is correlated to elevated expression of glutathione-linked detoxification enzymes. Carcinogenesis 1994; 15(6):1167–1173.

92. Lewis AD, Duran GE, Sikic BI. Transfection of a full length alpha class glutathione-s-transferase cDNA confers resistance to chemotherapeutic agents. Proc Am Assoc Cancer Res 1992; 33:497.

93. Zelazowski AJ, Garvey JS, Hoeschele JD. In vivo and in vitro binding of platinum to metallothionein. Arch Biochem Biophys 1984; 229(1):246–252.

94. Kelly SL, Basu A, Teicher BA, Hacker MP, Hamer DH, Lazo JS. Overexpression of metallothionein confers resistance to anticancer drugs. Science 1988; 241:1813–1815.

95. Bakka A, Endresen L, Johnsen ABS, Edminson PD, Rugstad HE. Resistance against cis-diamminedichloroplatinum(II) in cultured cells with high content of metallothioneins. Toxicol Appl Pharmacol 1981; 61:215–226.

96. Murphy MP, Andrews PA, Howell SB. Metallothionein mediated cisplatin and melphalan resistance in human ovarian carcinoma. Proc Am Assoc Cancer Res 1985; 26:344.

97. Koropatnik J, Pearson J. Zinc treatment, metallothionein expression, and resistance to cisplatin in mouse melanoma cells. Somat Cell Mol Genet 1990; 16:529–537.

98. Farnworth P, Hillcoat B, Roos I. Metallothionein-like protein and cell resistance to cis-diammineplatinum(II) in L1210 cells. Cancer Chemother Pharmacol 1990; 25:411–417.

99. Eastman A, Schulte N, Sheibani N, Sorenson CM. Mechanisms of resistance to platinum drugs. In: Nicolini M, ed. Platinum and Other Metal Coordination Compounds in Cancer Chemotherapy. Boston: Martinus Nijhoff, 1988:178–196.

100. Terheggen PMAB, Emondt JY, Floot BGJ, Dijkman R, Schrier PI, Den Engelse L, Begg AC. Correlation between cell killing by cis-diamminedichloroplatinum(II) in six mammalian cell lines and the binding of a cis-diamminedichloroplatinum(II)-DNA antiserum. Cancer Res 1990; 50:3556–3561.

101. Eastman A, Schulte N. Enhanced DNA repair as a mechanism of resistance to cis-diamminedichloroplatinum(II). Biochemistry 1988; 27:4730–4734.

102. Johnson SW, Swiggard LM, Handel JM, Brennan JM, Godwin AK, Ozols RF, Hamilton TC. Relationship between platinum-DNA adduct formation and removal and cisplatin cytotoxicity in cisplatin-sensitive and -resistant human ovarian cancer cells. Cancer Res 1994; 54:5911–5916.

103. Meijer C, Mulder NH, de Vries EGE. The role of role of detoxifying systems in resistance of tumor cells to cisplatin and Adriamycin. Cancer Treat Rev 1990; 17(suppl A):45–50.

104. Masuda H, Ozols RF, Lai GM, Fojo A, Rothenberg M, Hamilton TC. Increased DNA repair as a mechanism of acquired resistance to cis-diamminedichloroplatinum(II) in human ovarian cancer cell lines. Cancer Res 1988; 48:5713–5716.

105. Plooy ACM, van Dijk M, Berends F, Lohman PHM. Formation and repair of DNA interstrand cross-links in relation to cytotoxicity and unscheduled DNA synthesis induced in control and mutant human cells, treated with cis-diamminedichloroplatinum(II). Cancer Res 1985; 45:4178–4184.

106. Kraker AJ, Moore CW. Elevated DNA polymerase beta activity in cis-diamminedichloroplatinum(II) resistant P388 murine leukemia cell line. Cancer Lett 1988; 38:307–314.

107. Scanlon KJ, Kashani-Sabet M, Miyachi M, Sowers LC, Rossi J. Molecular basis of cisplatin resistance in human carcinomas: model systems and patients. Anticancer Res 1989; 9:1301–1312.

108. Bohr VA. Gene specific repair. Carcinogenesis 1991; 12:1983–1992.

109. Jones JC, Zhen W, Reed E, Parker RJ, Sancar A, Bohr VA. Gene-specific formation and repair of cisplatin instrastrand adducts and interstrand cross-links in chinese hamster ovary cells. J Biol Chem 1991; 266:7101–7107.

110. Zhen W, Link CJ, O'Connor PM, Reed E, Parker R, Howell SB, Bohr VA. Increased gene-specific repair of cisplatin interstrand cross-links in cisplatin resistant human ovarian cancer cell lines. Mol Cell Biol 1992; 3689–3698.

111. Johnson SW, Swiggard LM, Handel JM, Brennan JM, Godwin AK, Ozols RF, Hamilton TC. Relationship between platinum-DNA adduct formation and removal and cisplatin cytotoxicity in cisplatin-sensitive and -resistant human ovarian cancer cells. Cancer Res 1994; 54:5911–5916.
112. Weeda G, Hoeijmakers JHJ, Bootsma D. Bioessays 1993; 15:249–258.
113. Larminat F, Bohr VA. Role of human ERCC-1 gene in gene-specific repair of cisplatin-induced DNA damage. Nucleic Acids Res 1994; 22(15):3005–3010.
114. Taverna P, Hansson J, Scanlon KJ, Hill BT. Gene expression in X-irradiated human tumour cell lines expressing cisplatin resistance and altered DNA repair capacity. Carcinogenesis 1994; 15(9):2053–2056.
115. Dabholkar M, Bostick-Bruton F, Weber C, Bohr VA, Egwuagu C, Reed E. ERCC-1 and ERCC-2 expression in malignant tissues from ovarian cancer patients. J Natl Cancer Inst 1992; 84:1512–1517.
116. Levy E, Baroche C, Barret JM, Alapetite C, Salles B, Averbeck D, Moustacchi E. Activated *ras* oncogene and specifically acquired resistance to cisplatin in human mammary epithelial cells: induction of DNA cross-links and their repair. Carcinogenesis 1994; 15(5):845–850.
117. Pil PM, Lippard SJ. Specific binding of chromosomal protein HMG1 to DNA damaged by the anticancer drug cisplatin. Science 1992; 256:234–237.
118. Bruhn SL, Pil PM, Essigman JM, Housman DE, Lippard SJ. Isolation and characterization of human cDNA clones encoding a high mobility group box that recognize structural distortions to DNA caused by binding of the antitumor agent cisplatin. Proc Natl Acad Sci USA 1992; 89:2307–2311.
119. Shen DW, Akiyama S, Schoenlein P, Pastan I, Gottesman MM. Characterization of high-level cisplatin-resistant cell lines established from a human hepatoma cell line and human KB adenocarcinoma cells: cross-resistance and protein changes. Br J Cancer 1995; 71(4): 676–683.
120. Chu G, Chang E. Cisplatin-resistant cells express increased levels of a factor that recognizes damaged DNA. Proc Natl Acad Sci USA 1990; 87:3324–3327.
121. Chao CCK, Huang S-L, Lee L-Y, Chao SL. Identification of inducible damage-recognition proteins that are overexpressed in HeLa cells resistant to cis-diamminedichloroplatinum(II). Biochem J 1991; 277:875–878.
122. Regenass U, Muller M, Curschellas E, Matter A. Anti-tumor effects of human tumor necrosis factor in combination with chemotherapeutic agents. Int J Cancer 1987; 39: 266–273.
123. Niimi S, Nakagawa K, Yokota J, Tsunokawa Y, Nishio K, Terashima Y, Shibuya M, Terada M, Saijo N. Resistance to anticancer drugs in NIH3T3 cells transfected with c-myc and/or c-H-ras genes. Br J Cancer 1991; 63:237–241.
124. Shinohara N, Ogiso Y, Arai T, Takami S, Nonomura K, Koyanagi T, Kuzumaki N. Differential Na$^+$, K$^+$-ATPase activity and cisplatin sensitivity between transformants induced by H-ras and those induced by K-ras. Int J Cancer 1994; 58:672–677.
125. Dole M, Nunez G, Merchant AK, Maybaum J, Rode CK, Bloch CA. Bcl-2 inhibits chemotherapy-induced apoptosis in neuroblastoma. Cancer Res 1994; 54:3253–3259.
126. Segal-Bendirdjian E, Jacquemin-Sablon A. Cisplatin resistance in a murine leukemia cell line is associated with a defective apoptotic process. Exp Cell Res 1995; 218(1):201–212.
127. Sihna BK, Yamazaki H, Eliot HM, Schneider E, Borner MM, O'Connor PM. Relationships between proto-oncogene expression and apoptosis induced by anticancer drugs in human prostate tumor cells. Biochem Biophys Acta 1995; 1270(1):12–18.
128. Sanchez-Prieto R, Vargas JA, Carnero A, Marchetti E, Romero J, Durantez A, Lacal JC, Ramon y Cajal S. Modulation of cellular chemoresistance in keratinocytes by activation of different oncogenes. Int J Cancer 1995; 60(2):235–243.
129. Kashani-Sabet M, Wang W, Scanlon KJ. Cyclosporin A suppresses cisplatin-induced c-fos gene expression in ovarian carcinoma cells. J Biol Chem 1991; 265:11285–11288.

130. Rubin E, Kharbanda S, Gunji H, Weichselbaum R, Kufe D. Cis-diamminedichloroplatinum (II) induces c-jun expression in human myeloid leukemia cells: potential involvement of a protein kianse C-dependent signaling pathway. Cancer Res 1992; 52:878–882.

131. Hofmann J, Doppler W, Jakob A, Maly K, Posch L, Uberall F, Grunicke HH. Enhancement of the antiproliferative effect of cis-diamminedichloroplatinum(II) and nitrogen mustard by inhibitors of protein kinase C. Int J Cancer 1988; 42:382–388.

132. Oesterreich S, Weng C-N, Qui M, Hilsenbeck SG, Osborne CK, Fuqua AW. The small heat shock protein hsp27 is correlated with the growth and drug resistance in human breast cancer cell lines. Cancer Res 1993; 53:4443–4448.

133. Enns RE, Howell SB. Isolation of a gene associated with resistance to cisplatin. New York: Plenum Press, 1991:213–220.

134. Nakata B, Barton RM, Robbins TK, Howell SB, Los G. Association between $hsp60$ mRNA levels and cisplatin resistance in human head and neck cancer cell lines. Int J Oncol 1994; 6:1425–1432.

135. Mizushima T, Natori S, Sekimizu K. Relaxation of supercoiled DNA associated with induction of heat shock proteins in Escherichia coli. Mol Gen Genet 1993; 238:1–5.

136. Muggia FM. Introduction: cisplatin update. Semin Oncol 1991; 18(suppl 3):1.

137. Howell SB, Pfeifle CE, Wung WE, Olshen RA, Lucas WE, Yon JL, Green M. Intraperitoneal cisplatin with cystemic thiosulfate protection. Ann Intern Med 1982; 97:845–851.

138. Markman M, Cleary S, Pfeifle CE, Howell SB. High dose intracavitary cisplatin with intravenous thiosulfate: low incidence of serious neurotoxicity. Cancer 1987; 56:2364–2368.

139. vanderHoop RG, Vecht CJ, van der Burg MEL, Elderson A, Boogerd W, Heimans JJ, Vries EP, van Houwelingen JC, Jennekens FGI, Gispen WH, Neyt JP. Prevention of cisplatin neurotoxicity with an ACTH (4-9) analog in patients with ovarian cancer. N Engl J Med 1990; 322:89–94.

140. Leone R, Fracasso ME, Soresi E, Cimino G, Tedeschi M, Castoldi D, Monzani V, Colombi L, Usari T, Bernareggi A. Influence of glutathione administration on the disposition of free and total platinum in patients after administration of cisplatin. Cancer Chemother Pharmacol 1992; 29:385–390.

141. Naganuma A, Satoh M, Imura N. Prevention of lethal and renal toxicity of cis-diamminedichloroplatinum(II) by induction of metallothionein synthesis without compromising its antitumor activity in mice. Cancer Res 1987; 47:983–987.

142. Lotz JP, Pene F, Bouleuc C, Andre T, Gisselbrecht C, Bonnak H, Merad Z, Esteso A, Miccio-Bellaiche A, Avenin D, et al. Therapeutic intensification and hematopoietic stem cell autotransplantation in the treatment of solid tumors in adults: principles, realization and application to the treatment of germ cell, trophoblastic, breast, ovarian and small-cell bronchial tumors. Rev Med Intern 1995; 16(1):43–54.

143. Daniels JR, Sternlicht M, Daniels A. Collagen chemoembolization: pharmacokinetics and tissue tolerance of cis-diamminedichloroplatinum(II) in porcine liver and rabbit kidney. Cancer Res 1988; 108:340–344.

144. Brenner DE. Intraperitoneal chemotherapy: a review. J Clin Oncol 1986; 4:1135–1147.

145. Los G, Sminia P, Wondergem J, Mutsaers PHA, Havemen J, ten Bokkel Huinink D, Smals O, Gonzalez-Gonzalez D, McVie GJ. Optimisation of intraperitoneal cisplatin therapy with regional hyperthermia in rats. Eur J Cancer 1991; 27(4):472–477.

146. Wallner KE, DeGregorio MW, Li GC. Hyperthermic potentiation of cis-diamminedichloroplatinum(II) cytotoxicity in chinese hamster ovary cells resistant to the drug. Cancer Res 1986; 46:6242–6245.

147. Weiss N, Delius M, Gambihler S, Eichholtz-Wirth H, Dirschedl P, Brendel W. Effect of shock waves and cisplatin on cisplatin-sensitive and resistant rodent tumors in vivo. Int J Cancer 1994; 58:693–699.

148. Alagoz T, Buller RE, Anderson B, Terrell KL, Squatrito RC, Neimann TH, Tatman DJ, Jebson P. Evaluation of hyperbaric oxygen as a chemosensitizer in the treatment of epithelial ovarian cancer in xenografts in mice. Cancer 1995; 75(9):2313–2322.

149. Satoh M, Kloth DM, Kadhim SA, Chin JL, Naganuma A, Imura N, Cherian MG. Modulation of both cisplatin nephrotoxicity and drug resistance in murine bladder tumor by controlling metallothionein synthesis. Cancer Res 1993; 53:1829–1832.

150. Satoh M, Cherian GM, Imura N, Shimizu H. Modulation of resistance to anticancer drugs by inhibition of metallothionein synthesis. Cancer Res 1994; 54:5255–5257.

151. Ishikawa M, Takayanagi Y, Sasaki K. The deleterious effect of buthionine sulfoximine, a glutathione depleting agent, on the cisplatin toxicity in mice. Jpn J Pharmacol 1990; 52:652–655.

152. O'Dwyer P, LaCreta F, Nash S, Tinsley P, Schilder R, Clapper R. Phase I study of thiotepa in combination with the glutathione transferase inhibitor ethacrynic acid. Cancer Res 1991; 51:6059–6065.

153. Dempke WCM, Shellard SA, Fichtinger-Schepman AMJ, Hill BT. Lack of significant modulation of the formation and removal of platinum-DNA adducts by aphidicolin glycinate in two logarithmically-growing ovarian tumour cell lines in vitro. Carcinogenesis 1991; 12(3):525–528.

154. Masuda H, Tanaka T, Matsuda H, Kusaba I. Increased removal of DNA bound platinum in a human ovarian cancer cell line resistant to cis-diamminedichloroplatinum(II). Cancer Res 1990; 50:1863–1866.

155. Damia G, Tagliabue G, Zucchetti M, Davoli E, Sessa C, Cavalli F, D'Incalci M. Activity of aphidicolin glycinate alone or in combination with cisplatin in a murine ovarian tumor resistant to cisplatin. Cancer Chemother Pharmacol 1992; 30:459–464.

156. Chen G, Zeller WJ. Reversal of acquired cisplatin resistance by nicotinamide in vitro and in vivo. Cancer Chemother Pharmacol 1993; 33:157–162.

157. Bokemeyer C, Dunn T, Harstrick A, Lerch T, Poliwoda H, Schmoll H-J. Modulation of cytostatic drugs by nifedipine in two heterotransplanted human testicular-cancer cell lines differing in their sensitivity to standard agents. Int J Cancer 1994; 56:452–456.

158. Kondo S, Yin D, Morimura T, Takeuchi J. Combination therapy with cisplatin and nifedipine inducing apoptosis in multi-drug resistant human glioblastoma cells. J Neurosurg 1995; 82(3):469–474.

159. Beketic-Oreskovic L, Osmak M. Modulation of resistance to cisplatin by amphotericin B and aphidicolin in human larynx carcinoma cells. Cancer Chemother Pharmacol 1995; 35:327–333.

160. Stratton JA, DiSaia PJ. Reversal of cisplatinum (CDDP) resistance by cyclosporine A (CsA) in xenografts of fresh human ovarian carcinoma. Proc Am Assoc Cancer Res 1988; 29:479.

161. Flanagan WM, Corthesy B, Bram RJ, Crabtree GR. Nuclear association of a T-cell transcription factor blocked by KF-506 and cyclosporin A. Nature 1991; 352:803–806.

162. Foxwell BM, Mackie A, Ling V, Ryffel B. Identification of the multidrug resistance-related P-glycoprotein as a cyclosporine binding protein. Mol Pharmacol 1989; 36:543.

163. Manetta A, Boyle J, Berman ML, Disaia PJ, Lentz S, Liao SL, Mutch D, Slater L. Cyclosporin enhancement of cisplatin chemotherapy in patients with refractory gynecologic cancer. Cancer 1994; 73(1):196–199.

164. Perez RP, Hamilton TC, Ozols RF, Young RC. Mechanisms and modulation of resistance to chemotherapy in ovarian cancer. In: Resistance to chemotherapy in ovarian cancer. Cancer 1993; 71(suppl):4.

165. McClay EF, McClay ME, Albright KA, Jones JA, Christen R, Alcaraz J, Howell SB. Tamoxifen modulation of cisplatin resistance in patients with metastatic melanoma. Cancer 1993; 72:1914–1918.

166. McClay EF, Albright KD, Jones JA, Christen RD, Howell SB. Tamoxifen delays the development of resistance to cisplatin in human melanoma and ovarian cancer cell lines. Br J Cancer 1994; 70:449–452.

167. O'Shaughnessy JA, Cowan KH. Current status of paclitaxel in the treatment of breast cancer. Breast Cancer Res Treat 1995; 33(1):27–37.

168. Pera MF, Koberle B, Masters JR. Exceptional sensitivity of testicular germ cell tumour cell lines to the new anti-cancer agent, temozolomide. Br J Cancer 1995; 71(5):904–906.

169. Pratesi G, Tortoreto M, Corti C, Giardini R, Zunino F. Successful local regional therapy with topotecan of intraperitoneally growing human ovarian carcinoma xenografts. Br J Cancer 1995; 71(3):525–528.

170. Muggia FM, Los G. Platinum resistance: laboratory findings and clinical implications. Stem Cells 1993; 11:182–193.

171. Christian MC. The current status of new platinum analogs. Semin Oncol 1992; 19(6):720–733.

172. Los G, Verdegaal EME, Mutsaers PHA, McVie JG. Penetration of carboplatin and cisplatin into rat peritoneal tumor nodules after intraperitoneal chemotherapy. Cancer Chemother Pharmacol 1991; 28:159–165.

173. Kelland LR, Mistry P, Abel G, Loh SY, O'Neill CF, Murrer BA, Harrap KR. Mechanism-related circumvention of acquired cis-diamminedichloroplatinum(II) resistance using two pairs of human ovarian carcinoma cell lines by ammine/amine platinum(IV) dicarboxylates. Cancer Res 1993; 52:3857–3864.

174. McKeage MJ, Abel G, Kelland LR, Harrap KR. Mechanisms of action of an orally administered platinum complex [ammine bis butyro cyclohexylamine dichloroplatinum (IV) (JM221)] in intrinsically cisplatin-resistant human ovarian carcinoma in vitro. Br J Cancer 1994; 69:1–7.

175. Slate D, Michelson S. Drug resistance-reversal strategies: comparison of experimental data with model predictions. J Natl Cancer Inst 1991; 83:1574–1580.

176. Masazza G, Lucchini V, Tomasoni A, Peccatori F, Lampasona V, Giudici G, Mangioni C, Biondi A, Giavazzi R. Malignant behaviour and resistance to cisplatin of human ovarian carcinoma xenografts established from the same patient at different stages of the disease. Cancer Res 1991; 51:6358–6362.

177. Heike Y, Takahashi M, Ohira T, Arioka H, Funayama Y, Nishio K, Ogasawara H, Saijo N. In vivo screening models of cisplatin-resistant human lung cancer cell lines using SCID mice. Cancer Chemother Pharmacol 1995; 35:200–204.

178. Nio Y, Tamura K, Kawabata K, Masai Y, Hayashi H, Ishigami S, Araya S, Inamura M. Anticancer chemosensitivity changes between the original and recurrent tumors after successful chemotherapy selected according to the sensitivity assay. Ann Surg 1995; 221(1):89–99.

179. Shaw GL, Gazdag AF, Phelps R, Linnoila RI, Ihde DC, Johnson BE, Oie HK, Pass HI, Steinberg SM, Ghosh BC, Walsh TE, Nesbitt JC, Cotelingham JD, Minna JD, Mulshine JL. Individualized chemotherapy for patients with non-small cell lung cancer determined by prospective identification of neuroendocrine markers and in vitro drug sensitivity testing. Cancer Res 1993; 53:5181–5187.

180. Hamada S, Kamada M, Furumoto H, Hirao T, Aono T. Expression of glutathione S-transferase-$\pi$ in human ovarian cancer as an indicator of resistance to chemotherapy. Gynecol Oncol 1994; 52:313–319.

181. Parker RJ, Gill I, Tarone R, Vionnet JA, Grunberg S, Muggia FM, Reed E. Platinum-DNA damage in leukocyte DNA of patients receiving carboplatin and cisplatin chemotherapy, measured by atomic absorption spectrometry. Carcinogenesis 1991; 12(7):1253–1258.

# 15

## Radiation Response in Chemotherapy-Resistant Tumors

**Patrick Miller, Michael Nejad, and David S. Shimm**
*University of Arizona Health Sciences Center,*
*Tucson, Arizona*

### INTRODUCTION

Clinical reports of the treatment of many types of malignancies (including head and neck, ovarian, cervical, and non–small cell lung cancer) suggest that tumors initially resistant to chemotherapy, or that become resistant after treatment with chemotherapy, are more likely to be resistant to radiation (1–9). With the frequent and increasing use of combined-modality therapy in clinical practice, an understanding of possible cross-resistance between chemotherapy and radiation is essential. This chapter will focus on (1) identifying the clinical problem of radiation resistance in chemotherapy-resistant tumors; (2) reviewing the proposed mechanisms of radiation resistance; and (3) analyzing current research that may provide further insight into how cells respond and possibly become resistant to radiation.

### CLINICAL RADIATION RESISTANCE

The treatment of head and neck cancer demonstrates the phenomenon of chemotherapy resistance associated with radiation resistance. Tumors that demonstrate a complete response to induction chemotherapy have improved local control and survival compared with tumors that have less than a complete response. Tumors with less than complete responses are frequently not sensitive to subsequent radiation. In fact, tumors that respond poorly to induction chemotherapy have a lower response to subsequent radiation and do worse in terms of local control and survival than do tumors treated with radiation alone. However, a complete response to chemotherapy followed by radiation therapy does not translate into improved survival over radiation alone. This is an important point for several reasons. First, it suggests that chemotherapy and radiation act on the same populations of cells. If they acted on separate populations, one would expect an additive effect from the combined treatment. Second, it suggests that chemotherapy can have effects on cells other than lethality. Death of sensitive cells may select a more resistant remaining population. Some have suggested that response to chemotherapy predicts the response to radiation (10) but does not cause lethality in a separate group of cells. In head and neck cancer, chemotherapy—at worst—may alter a population of cells to be radioresistant.

This phenomenon is demonstrated in a recent randomized study reported by Jaulerry and colleagues (11). They randomized 208 patients with locally advanced squamous cell carcinomas of the head and neck to receive local therapy with or without induction chemotherapy. The chemotherapy regimen used in the first trial included two cycles of a combination of cisplatin, bleomycin, vindesine, and mitomycin C. The subsequent trial changed to three cycles of cisplatin, continuous-infusion 5-fluorouracil, and vindesine. The radiation therapy was given using standard techniques to a dose of 55 Gy. If the response was greater than 50%, the treatment was continued to 70 Gy. If the response was less, a surgical resection was attempted. Figures 1A and 1B

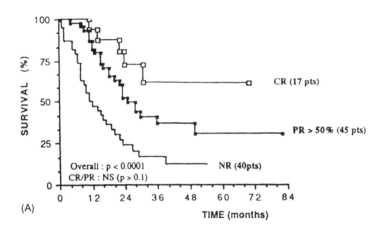

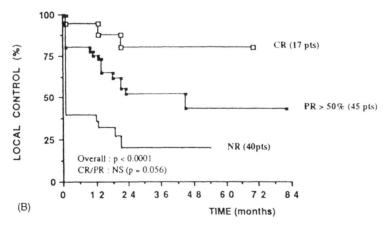

**Figure 1**   (A) Local control and (B) survival according to the initial response to chemotherapy. Tumors that demonstrate a complete response to chemotherapy appear to have an improvement in local control and survival. (From Ref. 11.)

show that tumors that respond well to chemotherapy have improved survival and local control, respectively. However, Figures 2A and 2B show that combined treatment does not lead to improved survival or local control over the entire population. Figure 3 reveals the answer to this apparent paradox. Here we see that patients treated with radiation alone do not do statistically poorer than patients treated with chemotherapy and radiation, regardless of their response to chemotherapy. Note that even if a complete radiation response is obtained after a chemotherapy failure, the patients have a significantly worse rate of local failure than those who have no chemotherapy and a complete radiation response. This suggests that the chemotherapy may be altering the tumor, and that even a subsequent complete radiation response leaves behind resistant cells. Similar results can be abstracted from many other studies in head and neck cancer (1,2,6,8).

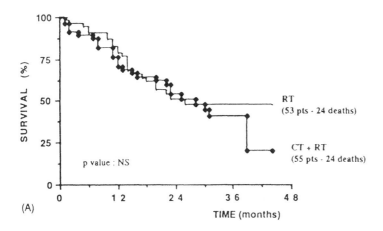

(A)

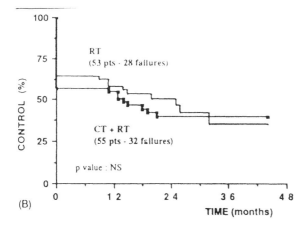

(B)

**Figure 2** (A) Overall local control and (B) survival for patients treated with radiation alone or combined modality therapy. When compared with radiation therapy alone, no improvement in local control or survival is seen in the combined therapy group. (From Ref. 11.)

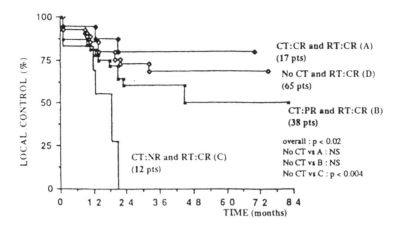

**Figure 3** Local control according to response to initial chemotherapy and/or radiotherapy. Failure to obtain a complete response to chemotherapy predicts for an ultimate failure to radiotherapy, even if a temporary complete response to radiation is obtained. Tumors that develop resistance to chemotherapy appear to be developing a cross-resistance to radiotherapy. (From Ref. 11.)

A similar phenomenon has been observed in ovarian cancer, cervical cancer, and non–small cell lung cancer. Hacker et al. at UCLA (3) reported on the use of whole abdominal irradiation as salvage therapy in patients with residual ovarian cancer at second-look surgery following chemotherapy. Of 22 patients with minimal residual disease (less than or equal to 5 mm), 15 responded to primary chemotherapy. Forty percent of those were clinically disease-free at 19 to 41 months of follow-up. Conversely, all patients with the same amount of residual disease, but who failed to respond to chemotherapy, went on to progress despite radiation therapy and die of their disease. At least two other reports confirm this finding in ovarian cancer (4,5).

In cervical cancer, a recent report of 260 patients with advanced disease (9) treated by epirubicin and cisplatin followed by pelvic radiation indicated that although tumor response to chemotherapy was common, subsequent radiotherapy was less effective at controlling disease than was primary radiotherapy. Alternative hypotheses were proposed, but it is likely that some effect was due to a change in the tumor cell biology.

Finally, in a randomized trial of radiation therapy with and without induction chemotherapy for non–small cell lung cancer (12), a similar correlation between chemotherapy and radiation was found. In that study, 155 patients were evaluated, 78 in the combined-modality arm and 77 in the radiation-alone arm. In the combined-modality arm, 17 patients had a partial response to chemotherapy, and six went on to have a complete response to radiation. Of the eight patients who had less than a partial response, only one had a complete response to radiation. Of the 50 patients judged to have stable disease after induction chemotherapy, only three had a complete response after radiotherapy.

Tumors in other sites show similar phenomena, with chemotherapy either predicting but not enhancing radiation response, or in some cases leading to a worse radiation response, regardless of chemotherapy response. Though there may be some alternate explanations for the altered radiation response, such as a time delay in commencing radiation required by induction chemotherapy, there is mounting clinical evidence, and emerging experimental evidence, to suggest that prior exposure to chemotherapy may lead to the development of cross-resistance to radiation in some types of human cancer.

## CELLULAR AND BIOCHEMICAL CHANGES IN RADIATION RESISTANCE

Initial investigations into the relationship between chemotherapy and radiation resistance focused primarily on characterizing the radiation response in cell lines generated from clinically drug-resistant tumors. Drug resistance has also been generated in cell lines by continuous incubation or stepwise selection in particular chemotherapeutic agents. In either case, subsequent studies involved examining survival curve parameters of these in vitro cell lines. Using Dq, Do, and N values from these cell survival curves, or the alpha/beta values (see Fig. 4) along with assays to detect sublethal and potentially lethal damage repair (Fig. 5A and B), it is possible to detect cell lines that have altered sensitivity to radiation (13–17). Subsequent studies have attempted to determine the mechanisms for this observed phenomenon.

One mechanism that has been proposed by several authors is the alteration of the level of intracellular glutathione. Batist et al. (18) isolated a doxorubicin-resistant human breast cancer cell line, which was shown to have the multidrug-resistant phenotype. Because the magnitude of the decrease in drug accumulation was not sufficient to account for the overall resistance, they sought other mechanisms, and found overexpression of a novel anionic glutathione transferase. Subsequent experiments

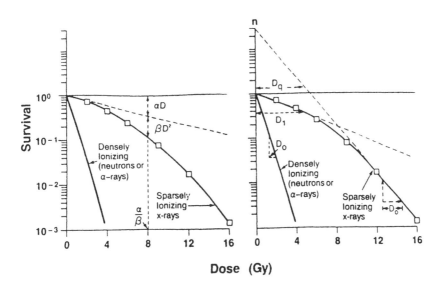

**Figure 4**  Survival curves for mammalian cells exposed to radiation. They are described by the alpha/beta ratio, or by the Do or D1, and N or Dq, which describe the slope of the curve and the shoulder region. By examining these parameters it is possible to determine if one cell line is more or less sensitive to a given dose of radiation. (From Hall EJ. Radiobiology for the Radiologist. 4th ed. Philadelphia: Lippincott, 1994:33.)

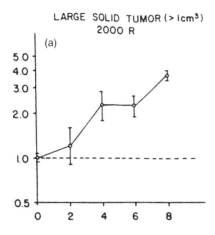

LARGE SOLID TUMOR (> 1 cm³)
2000 R

TIME (hours) BETWEEN IRRADIATION AND EXPLANT

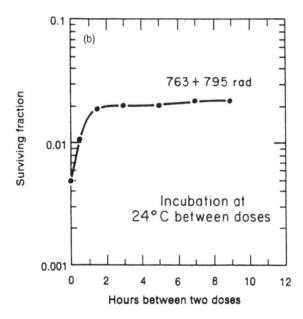

**Figure 5** Demonstration of (a) potentially lethal damage (PLD) repair and (b) sublethal damage repair, two additional methods commonly used to assay for response and sensitivity to radiation. (a, from Elkind MM, Sutton-Gilbert H, Moses WB, Alescio T, Swain RW. Radiat Res 25:359, 1965. b, from Little JB, Hahn GM, Frindel E, Tubiana M. Radiology 106:689–694, 1973.)

confirmed that this cell line was radiation-resistant, and the alteration of glutathione metabolism was of a magnitude sufficient to account for the level of radiation resistance (19).

At least four other investigators have shown that glutathione levels correlate with radiation resistance. Ozols and colleagues established cell lines from patients at a time when their tumors were resistant to chemotherapy and also developed drug-resistant lines in vitro. Glutathione levels correlated well with in vitro radiation sensitivity, and depletion of glutathione levels with L-buthionine sulfoximine (BSO) restored radiation sensitivity. Godwin et al. (20), Oshita et al. (21), and Prezioso et al. (22) all have developed drug-resistant cell lines with alterations in cellular glutathione pathways. Each of these lines also exhibits some degree of radiation resistance. Unfortunately, clinical attempts to reverse resistance by depleting glutathione (with the use of BSO) have not proved fruitful. Still, it is likely that the cellular level of glutathione or other free-radical scavenging counterparts plays a role in the cells' response to radiation. And clearly, the levels of glutathione are altered in drug-resistant cells.

Other biochemical changes not clearly linked to drug resistance have been found to result in radiation resistance. Differing levels of expression of thymidine kinase and basic fibroblast growth factor (bFGF) have both recently been found to lead to radiation resistance in different cell lines. Using a rodent glioma cell line, Al-Nabulsi and colleagues (23) found that the lack of expression of thymidine kinase made cells significantly more sensitive to clinically relevant doses of radiation. The sensitivity was further isolated to an inability of these cells to repair sublethal DNA damage. All other radiobiological responses, including other aspects of DNA repair, and differences in cell cycle kinetics, were unchanged. Thus, it may be possible to target the thymidine kinase gene to enhance radiation response clinically.

Another proposed mechanism of radiation resistance is the alteration of radiation-induced programmed cell death (apoptosis). Studying alterations of this pathway (24), Fuks et al. have found that an endothelial cell line given clinically relevant radiation doses and then exposed to basic fibroblast growth factor will be protected from undergoing apoptosis. These findings were extended to the point of protecting mice from the effects of lethal radiation pneumonitis with doses of bFGF.

A second area of research in radiation resistance involves oncogenes associated with an altered radiation response. Kasid et al. (25) were the first to report an association between altered radiosensitivity in a human tumor cell line and overexpression of a specific oncogene. They had established a tumor cell line from a patient with a laryngeal cancer, which had progressed during radiation therapy, and noted that the cell line was radiation-resistant in culture. In an attempt to uncover genes that might be responsible for the observed radiation resistance, they transfected NIH/3T3 cells with DNA from this cell line. The transfectants were then probed for various human oncogenic sequences, including v-*myv*, N-*myc*, v-*myc*, v-K-*ras*, N-*ras*, v-H-*ras*, c-*myc*, and c-*raf*; and for human papilloma viral DNA. The only oncogene to hybridize was *raf*. It was then possible to show that an antisense strand of RNA was able to bind the *raf* gene and to reverse the radiation resistance. This finding clearly implicated *raf* in the radiation-resistant phenotype. These findings were supported by studies conducted at the National Cancer Institute (NCI) and Walter Reed Hospital involving an analysis of the noncancerous skin fibroblasts from a cancer-prone family (26). The fibroblasts were not transformed or malignant, but they were found to be radiation resistant. On analysis the researchers detected a three- to eightfold elevation in the expression of c-*myc*, and activation of the c-*raf*-1 oncogene.

The *ras* oncogene has been reported to be involved in both resistance and sensitivity to radiation. Sklar transfected *ras* genes from a bladder cancer line, a Hodgkin's disease line, and a leukemia line into NIH 3T3 cells, and analyzed their response to radiation. He found the transformed cells resistant to radiation (27). Others have been unable to confirm this (28). Both *ras* and *raf* oncogene products are associated with membranes, the *ras* gene product being a G protein located in the plasma membrane, whereas *raf* produces a membrane-associated protein kinase. Shimm et al. (29) studied the effect of the *src* oncogene activation on radiation sensitivity. They found that *src* activation made no difference in the radiation response of drug-sensitive cell lines. However, in a multidrug-resistant cell line, *src* activation led to a significant increase in radiation resistance. In a review, Pirollo and colleagues (30) recently proposed a mechanism for the interaction of the various oncogenes. They postulated that growth factors or other extracellular factors interact with membrane-associated receptors. These factors in turn can function via *ras* activation to stimulate intracellular kinases such as *raf*. These activated intracellular proteins work at the nuclear level to alter the biological response to radiation. Certainly, there are gaps in our understanding of this pathway, but it does give some form to a previously unconnected series of observations.

Two other genes, *Bcl-2* and p53, have been found to have some effect on radiation sensitivity. *Bcl-2* is a protein of molecular weight 25 kd that is associated with the inner mitochondrial membrane (31). Its normal cellular function appears to be to inhibit apoptosis. The mechanism of this inhibition is not fully understood, but involves a number of factors, including oncogene expression and growth factor and cytokine levels. In addition, *Bcl-2* may exert its effect by altering levels of oxygen free radicals. Askew et al. have shown that expression of c-myc can increase the apoptotic pathway in a myeloid cell line dependent on interleukin-3 (IL-3) (32). *Bcl-2* expression suppresses this increase. Transforming growth factor (TGF) beta-1 has also been shown to be involved in the apoptotic pathway (33), and *Bcl-2* likewise is able to suppress this stimulatory effect. Other studies have implicated superoxide dismutase and decreased oxygen free-radicals with *Bcl-2* protection from undergoing apoptosis. The exact effect that *Bcl-2* has on irradiated cells is not clear, though certainly *Bcl-2* acts on pathways that have been shown to influence radiation sensitivity. Clearly, for radiation to exert its maximal effect on cells, *Bcl-2* inhibition of apoptosis must be overcome (34).

The p53 tumor suppressor gene encodes for a 53-kd nuclear protein that has undergone mutation in about half of all human cancers (35). It has been implicated in regulation of the cell cycle, DNA transcription and repair, and apoptosis (36). Importantly, several reports have found that alterations of the p53 protein can lead to radiation resistance. Studies in transgenic mice expressing mutant p53 alleles have shown radiation resistance in a variety of hematopoietic tumors (37). In addition, rat embryos transfected with mutant p53 alleles (38), as well as some human squamous cell carcinoma cell lines with altered p53 (39), have shown radiation resistance. The role of p53 in DNA repair has been demonstrated for UV-damaged cells (40), and it is possible that altered DNA repair may be responsible for the resistance to x-irradiation. Another possibility is that p53 functions as a checkpoint, and that a malfunction of this process leads to altered radiation sensitivity.

## CHECKPOINTS AND THEIR ROLE IN RADIATION RESPONSE

Dividing eukaryotic cells traverse the stages of the cell cycle from $G_1$ to S, to $G_2$, to M. To ensure successful and proper division, cells must faithfully complete DNA replication, DNA repair, and chromosome segregation. Cells guarantee the success of these events by using checkpoint controls. In the presence of incomplete replication, damaged DNA, or improper spindle assembly, checkpoints arrest the cell cycle at one of four points: the $G_1$/S transition, S phase, late S or $G_2$ phase, or M phase (41,42). Checkpoint controls are universally conserved and observed in all eukaryotic organisms studied from budding yeast to humans (43–45). Similar systems appear to govern the cell division of prokaryotic organisms, such as *Escherichia coli*, where DNA damage blocks cell division via a checkpoint pathway that is part of the SOS response (46). Defects in checkpoint controls can lead to aberrant cell division, genomic instability, and cell death.

The budding yeast, *Saccharomyces cerevisiae*, provides a model system for studying the genes and mechanistic pathways of checkpoint control. To ensure that chromosomes are intact prior to segregation, entry into mitosis should be blocked until both replication and repair can be completed. Studies of budding yeast mutants led to the discovery of six genes that, in the presence of incompletely replicated chromosomes, damaged DNA, or both are required to arrest cell cycle progression during late S phase or $G_2$ phase (late S/$G_2$): *MEC1*, *MEC2*, *MEC3*, *RAD9*, *RAD17*, and *RAD24* (47). The arrest phenotype of each of these genes has been well characterized using a variety of DNA damage–inducing sources including UV and x-ray irradiation, DNA replication mutants (*cdc9*/DNA ligase, *cdc2*/Pol II, *cdc13*/telomere replication), and chemical mutagens. The late S/$G_2$ arrest requires all six of the checkpoint proteins. Cells mutant for any one of the checkpoint genes continue to divide in the presence of DNA damage, resulting in dramatic (>90%) declines in cell viability.

In addition to being required for arresting cells in late S/$G_2$ in the presence of DNA damage, *MEC1* and *MEC2* are essential for growth, and they appear to have functional roles in a distinct S phase specific–arrest. In contrast to other checkpoint mutants, *mec1-1* and *mec2-1* mutants both fail to arrest in the presence of hydroxyurea (HU), a DNA synthesis inhibitor (47). Strains wild-type for *MEC1* and *MEC2*, with mutations in any or all of the other four checkpoints, are still HU resistant. These observations indicate that there may be many mechanisms by which cells arrest division during various stages of the cell cycle.

Although the checkpoint phenotype of these genes has been properly characterized using genetic deletions (nulls) and loss-of-function mutations, the mechanism of cell cycle arrest, as well as interacting and target proteins, remains elusive. However, analysis of checkpoint protein sequences has yielded clues about how checkpoints may function. *RAD24* has limited homology to an important replication protein (RF-C, encoded by *CDC44* in yeast) (48). *RAD17* shows homology to the *Rec1* exonuclease of *Ustilago maydis* (49). *MEC2* contains a protein kinase domain that is essential for checkpoint control and normal cell growth. *MEC1* contains a domain that encodes a lipid kinase that is essential for checkpoint function. Mutants in both *MEC1* and *MEC2* are defective for the transcriptional induction of several genes, including DNA damage–inducible (*DIN*) genes (50). All of the evidence considered together strongly suggests that, at least in budding yeast, checkpoints are intricately involved in DNA metabolism processes, such as repair and replication, in addition to being required for cell cycle arrest.

Checkpoint controls are evident in humans when irradiated cells arrest at cell cycle stages corresponding to checkpoint control points in budding and fission yeast. However, few checkpoint genes in humans have been identified. One human checkpoint gene that has been identified is the tumor suppressor gene *p53*. Mutations in the *p53* tumor suppressor gene result in the loss of a $G_1$/S checkpoint and appear to be intricately linked to tumorigenesis (51). Mutations or loss of the *p53* gene are the most common genetic alteration found in sporadic nonfamilial cancers, lending support to the theory that checkpoints are important in the prevention of cancer (52).

Checkpoint defects appear to be tightly correlated with cancer. There are two main types of mutations that lead to the development of cancer: those mutations that directly lead to neoplastic behavior, and those that indirectly result in neoplastic behavior by increasing the rate at which mutations arise (47). Checkpoints appear to be intricately involved in the latter. Budding yeast strains carrying a mutation in the RAD9 gene are viable but lose chromosomes at a rate 20 times higher than RAD9+ strains (53). It has been hypothesized that this high rate of chromosome loss is the ultimate result of an accumulation of uncorrected errors, due to the checkpoint defect. Similar genomic instability appears to play a role in the transformation of human cells.

Cancer cells typically display aneuploid genomes with many amplified genes and chromosomal rearrangements (42,51,54). In humans, failure of checkpoint controls can contribute to the generation of cancer by increasing genomic instability. Mutations in the *p53* tumor suppressor gene not only lead to loss of a $G_1/S$ checkpoint, but also increase the incidence of gene amplification, aneuploidy, immortalization, and ability to be transformed by *ras* (51,52).

An understanding of the mechanism by which checkpoints arrest cell division, and the status of checkpoints in malignant cells, may help in the understanding of radiation and chemotherapy response, and of cancer treatment in general (47). Most chemotherapeutic drugs act by blocking DNA replication, damaging DNA, or inhibiting spindles. Other changes found in chemotherapy-treated cells include overexpression of P-glycoprotein (55,56) and other membrane proteins (57), as well as alterations in topoisomerases (58). Cytogenetic alterations have also been found in drug-resistant cells (59). Some of these changes undoubtedly alter the cell's ability to detoxify oxygen-mediated damage, and others may affect the cell's checkpoint control system. Neoplastic cells that escape the hoped-for result of chemotherapy, that is, death, may end up with enhanced ability to perform these functions. Certainly not all changes will lead to radiation resistance, but many are candidates for further investigation.

## SUMMARY

Clinical experience suggests that tumors that are resistant to chemotherapy may be resistant to radiation. Whether the radiation resistance is due to a cellular change caused by chemotherapy is not known with certainty, but some experimental evidence suggests this is the case. Designers of clinical trials must continue to search for ways to more effectively integrate chemotherapy and radiation, and the sequencing of the two modalities is crucial. Approaches with concurrent therapy might avoid the generation of cross-resistant tumor populations, but result in added normal tissue toxicity.

## REFERENCES

1. Al-Kourainy K, Kish J, Ensley J, Tapazoglou E, Jacobs J, Weaver A, Crissman J, Cummings G, Al-Sarraf M. Achievement of superior survival for histologically negative versus histologically positive clinically complete responders to cisplatin combination in patients with locally advanced head and neck cancer. Cancer 1987; 59:223–238.

2.  Ervin T, Clark J, Weichselbaum R, Fallon B, Miller D, Fabian R, Posner M, Norris C, Tuttle S, Schoenfeld D, Price K, Frei E. An analysis of induction and adjuvant chemotherapy in the multidisciplinary treatment of squamous cell carcinoma of the head and neck. J Clin Oncol 1987; 5:10–20.

3.  Hacker N, Berek J, Burnison C, Heintz P, Juillard G, Lagasse L. Whole abdominal radiation as salvage therapy for epithelial ovarian cancer. Obstet Gynecol 1985; 65:60–66.

4.  Hainsworth J, Malcolm A, Johnson D, Burnett L, Jones H, Greco F. Advanced minimal residual ovarian carcinoma: abdominopelvic irradiation following combination chemotherapy. Obstet Gynecol 1983; 61:619–623.

5.  Hoskins W, Lichter A, Whittington R, Artman L, Bibro M, Park R. Whole abdominal and pelvic irradiation in patients with minimal disease at second-look reassessment for ovarian carcinoma. Gynecol Oncol 1985; 20:271–280.

6.  Jacobs J, Pajak T, Kinzie J, Al-Sarraf M, Davis L, Hanks G, Weigensberg I, Leibel S. Induction chemotherapy in advanced head and neck cancer—a Radiation Therapy Oncology Group study. Arch Otolaryngol Head Neck Surg 1987; 113:193–197.

7.  Jeremic B, Shibamoto Y, Acimovic L, Djuric L. Randomized trial of hyperfractionated radiation therapy with or without concurrent chemotherapy for stage III non-small-cell lung cancer. J Clin Oncol 1995; 13:452–458.

8.  Pfister D, Harrison L, Strong E, Shah J, Spiro R, Kraus D, Armstrong J, Zelefsky M, Fass D, Weiss M, Wang R, Schantz S, Bosl G. Organ-function preservation in advanced oropharynx cancer: results with induction chemotherapy and radiation. J Clin Oncol 1995; 13: 671–680.

9.  Tattersall M, Lorvidhaya V, Vootiprux V, Cheirsilpa A, Wong F, Azhar T, Lee H, Kang S, Manalo A, Yen S, Kampono N, Aziz F. Randomized trial of epirubicin and cisplatin chemotherapy followed by pelvic radiation in locally advanced cervical cancer. J Clin Oncol 1995; 13:444–451.

10. Stell PM. Adjuvant chemotherapy in head and neck cancer. Semin Radiat Oncol 1992; 2: 195–205.

11. Jaulerry C, Rodriguez J, Brunin F, Jouve M, Mosseri V, Point D, Pontvert D, Validire P, Zafrani B, Blaszka B, Asselain B, Pouillart P, Brugere J. Induction chemotherapy in advanced head and neck tumors: results of two randomized trials. Int J Radiat Oncol Biol Phys 1992; 23:483–489.

12. Dillman R, Seagren S, Propert K, Guerra J, Eaton W, Perry M, Carey R, Frei E, Green M. A randomized trial of induction chemotherapy plus high-dose radiation versus radiation alone in stage III non-small-cell lung cancer. N Engl J Med 1990; 323:940–945.

13. Louie K, Behrens B, Kinsella T, Hamilton T, Grotzinger K, McKoy W, Winker M, Ozols R. Radiation survival parameters of antineoplastic drug-sensitive and -resistant human ovarian cancer cell lines and their modulation by buthionine sulfoximine. Cancer Res 1985; 45:2110–2115.

14. Zuckerman J, Raffin T, Brown J, Newman R, Etiz B, Sikic B. In vitro selection and characterization of a bleomycin-resistant subline of B16 melanoma. Cancer Res 1986; 46:1748–1753.

15. Lehnert S, Greene D, Batist G. Radiation response of drug-resistant variants of a human breast cancer cell line. Radiat Res 1989; 118:568–580.

16. Miller PR, Hill AB, Slovak M, Shimm D. Radiation response in a doxorubicin resistant human fibrosarcoma cell line. Am J Clin Oncol 1992; 15:216–221.

17. Shimm D, Olson S, Hill A. Radiation resistance in a multidrug resistant human T-cell leukemia line. Int J Radiat Oncol Biol Phys 1988; 15:931–936.

18. Batist G, Tulpule A, Sinha B, Katki A, Myers C, Cowans K. Overexpression of a novel anionic glutathione transferase in multidrug resistant human breast cancer. J Biol Chem 1986; 261: 15544–15549.

19. Lehnert S, Greene D, Batist G. Radiation response of drug-resistant variants of a human breast cancer cell line. Radiat Res 1989; 118:568–580.

20. Godwin A, Meister A, O'Dwyer P, Huang C, Hamilton T, Anderson M. High resistance to cisplatin in human ovarian cancer cell lines is associated with a marked increase of glutathione synthesis. Proc Natl Acad Sci USA 1992; 89:3070–3074.

21. Oshita F, Fujiwara Y, Saijo N. Radiation sensitivities in various anticancer-drug-resistant human lung cancer cell lines and mechanisms of radiation cross-resistance in a cisplatin-resistant cell line. J Cancer Res Clin Oncol 1992; 119:28–34.

22. Prezioso J, Shields D, Wang N, Rosenstein M. Role of gamma-glutamyltranspeptidase-mediated glutathione transport on the radiosensitivity of B16 melanoma variant cell lines. Int J Radiat Oncol Biol Phys 1994; 30:373–381.

23. Al-Nabulsi I, Takamiya Y, Voloshin Y, Dritschilo A, Martuza R, Jorgensen T. Expression of thymidine kinase is essential to low dose radiation resistance of rat glioma cells. Cancer Res 1994; 54:5614–5617.

24. Fuks Z, Persaud R, Alfieri A, McLoughlin M, Ehleiter D, Schwartz J, Seddon A, Cordon-Cardo C, Haimovitz-Freidman A. Basic fibroblast growth factor protects endothelial cells against radiation-induced programmed cell death in vitro and in vivo. Cancer Res 1994; 54:2582–2590.

25. Kasid U, Pfeifer A, Weichselbaum RR, Dritschilo A, Mark GE. Effect of antisense c-raf-1 on tumorigenicity and radiation sensitivity of a human squamous carcinoma. Science 1989; 243:1354–1356.

26. Chang EH, Pirollo KF, Zou ZQ, Cheung HY, Lawler EL, Garner R, White E, Bernstein WB, Fraumeni JW Jr, Blattner WA. Oncogenes in radioresistant, noncancerous skin fibroblasts from a cancer-prone family. Science 1987; 237:1036–1038.

27. Sklar MD. The ras oncogenes increase the intrinsic resistance of NIH 3T3 cells to ionizing radiation. Science 1988; 239:645–647.

28. Harris JF, Chambers AF, Tam AS. Some ras-transformed cells have increased radiosensitivity and decreased repair of sublethal radiation damage. Radiat Res 1990; 16:39–48.

29. Shimm DS, Miller PR, Lin T, Moulinier P, Hill AB. Effects of v-src oncogene activation on radiation sensitivity in drug-sensitive and in multidrug-resistant rat fibroblasts. Radiat Res 1992; 129:149–156.

30. Pirollo KF, Tong YA, Villegas Z, Chen Y, Chang EH. Oncogene-transformed NIH 3T3 cells display radiation resistance levels indicative of a signal transduction pathway leading to the radiation-resistance phenotype. Radiat Res 1993; 135:234–243.

31. Hockenberry D, Nunez G, Milliman C, Schreiber R, Korsmeyer S. Bcl-2 is an inner mitochondrial membrane protein that blocks programmed cell death. Nature 1990; 348:334–336.

32. Askew D, Ashmun R, Simmons B, Cleveland J. Constitutive c-myc expression in an IL-3-dependent myeloid cell line suppresses cell cycle arrest and accelerates apoptosis. Oncogene 1991; 6:1915–1922.

33. Selvakumaran M, Lin H-K, Sjin R, Reed JC, Liebermann DA, Hoffman B. The novel primary response gene MyD118 and the proto-oncogenes myb, myc, and bcl-2 modulate transforming growth factor beta 1-induced apoptosis of myeloid leukemia cells. Mol Cell Biol 1994; 14:2352–2360.

34. Chen M, Quintans J, Fuks Z, Thompson C, Kufe DW, Weichselbaum RR. Suppression of Bcl-2 messenger RNA production may mediate apoptosis after ionizing radiation, tumor necrosis factor alpha, and ceramide. Cancer Res 1995; 55(5):991–994.

35. Harris CA, Hollstein M. Clinical implications of the p53 tumor-suppressor gene. N Engl J Med 1993; 329:1318–1327.

36. Prives C, Manfredi J. The p53 tumor suppressor protein: meeting review. Genes Dev 1993; 7:529–534.

37. Lee JM, Bernstein A. p53 mutations increase resistance to ionizing radiation. Proc Natl Acad Sci USA 1993; 90:5742–5746.

38. Pardo F, Su M, Borek C, Preffer F, Dombkowski D, Gerweck L, Schmidt E. Transfection of rat embryo cells with mutant p53 increases the intrinsic radiation resistance. Radiat Res 1994; 140:180–185.
39. Jung M, Notario V, Dristschilo A. Mutations in the p53 gene in radiation-sensitive and -resistant human squamous carcinoma cells. Cancer Res 1992; 52:6390–6393.
40. Smith ML, Chen IT, Zhang Q, O'Connor PM, Fornace AJ Jr. Involvement of the p53 tumor suppressor in repair of u.v.-type DNA damage. Oncogene 1995; 10:1053–1059.
41. Murray AW. Creative blocks: cell-cycle checkpoints and feedback controls. Nature 1992; 359:599–604.
42. Hartwell LH, Weinert TA. Checkpoints: controls that ensure the order of cell cycle events. Science 1989; 246:629–634.
43. Weinert TA, Hartwell LH. The RAD9 gene controls the cell cycle response to DNA damage in Saccharomyces cerevisiae. Science 1988; 241:317–322.
44. Hartwell LH. Defects in a cell cycle checkpoint may be responsible for the genomic instability of cancer cells. Cell 1992; 71:543–546.
45. Enoch T, Carr AM, Nurse P. Fission yeast genes involved in coupling mitosis to completion of DNA replication. Genes Dev 1992; 6:2035–2046.
46. Walker GC. E. coli and S. typhimurium: cellular and molecular biology. Reidhart FC, ed. Washington, DC: American Society of Microbiology, 1987.
47. Weinert TA, Kiser GL, Hartwell LH. Mitotic checkpoint genes in budding yeast and the dependence of mitosis on DNA replication and repair. Genes Dev 1994; 8:652–665.
48. Howell EA, McAlear MA, Rose D, Holm C. CDC44: a putative nucleotide-binding protein required for cell cycle progression that has homology to subunits of replication factor C. Mol Cell Biol 1994; 14:255–267.
49. Thelen MP, Onel K, Holloman WK. The REC1 gene of Ustilago maydis involved in the cellular response to DNA damage encodes an exonuclease. J Biol Chem 1994; 269:747–754.
50. Kiser GL, Weinert TA. A transcriptional regulation role for the MEC and RAD checkpoint genes in yeast and an hierarchy of gene function. Cell [submitted].
51. Livingstone LR, White A, Sprouse J, Livanos E, Jacks T, Tlsty TD. Altered cell cycle arrest and gene amplification potential accompany loss of wild-type p53. Cell 1992; 70:923–935.
52. Donehower LA, Harvey M, Slagle BL, McArthur MJ, Montgomery CA Jr, Butel JS, Bradley A. Mice deficient for p53 are developmentally normal but susceptible to spontaneous tumours. Nature 1992; 356:215–221.
53. Weinert TA, Hartwell LH. Characterization of RAD9 of Saccharomyces cerevisiae and evidence that its function acts posttranslationally in cell cycle arrest after DNA damage. Mol Cell Biol 1990; 10:6554–6564.
54. Hollstein M, Sidransky D, Vogelstein B, Harris CC. p53 mutations in human cancers. Science 1991; 253:49–53.
55. Kartner N, Riordan J, Ling V. Cell surface P-glycoprotein associated with multidrug resistance in mammalian cell lines. Science 1983; 221:1285–1288.
56. Riordan J, Deuchars K, Kartner K, Alon N, Trent J, Ling V. Amplification of P-glycoprotein genes in multidrug-resistant mammalian cell lines. Nature 1985; 316:817–819.
57. Norris M, Haber M, King M, Davey R. Atypical multidrug-resistance in CCRF-CEM cells selected for high level methotrexate resistance: reactivity to monoclonal antibody C219 in the absence of P-glycoprotein expression. Biochem Biophys Res Commun 1989; 165:1435–1441.
58. Danks M, Schmidt C, Cirtain M, Suttle P, Beck W. Altered catalytic activity of and DNA cleavage by DNA topoisomerase II from human leukemic cells selected for resistance to VM-26. Biochemistry 1988; 27:8861–8869.
59. Slovak M, Hoeltge G, Trent J. Cytogenetic alterations associated with the acquisition of doxorubicin resistance: possible significance of chromosome 7 alterations. Cancer Res 1987; 47:6646–6652.

# 16

## Preclinical In Vivo Models of Drug Resistance

**Beverly A. Teicher**
*Dana Farber Cancer Institute, Harvard Medical School, Boston, Massachusetts*

Relative resistance to cytotoxic therapies, existing prior to therapy or acquired over the course of therapy, is a major clinical problem (1–3). Preclinical models of various types have been applied to the elucidation of the mechanisms of resistance to therapy and have been used to develop clinically relevant approaches to overcoming such resistance (4–6). Breast cancer, among the major solid tumors, is an example of a malignancy where resistance to cytotoxic therapies such as the antitumor alkylating agents can develop (7,8).

### IN VIVO MODELS AND END POINTS

The earliest in vivo preclinical tumor models were leukemias grown as ascites tumors. The end point of experiments with these tumors was most often an increase in life span. As solid tumor models were developed, the appropriate end points devised were tumor growth delay or tumor control of a primary implanted tumor. These assays require that drugs be administered at doses producing toxicity tolerable to normal tissue so that the response of the tumor to the treatment can be observed for a relatively long period of time. These end points cannot be applied to the high-dose setting in which normally lethal doses of anticancer therapies can be administered with normal tissue support such as bone marrow transplantation. Response to high-dose therapies can be assessed by use of excision assays (9).

One important difference between excision assays and the in situ assays of increase in life span, tumor growth delay, or local tumor control is that excision assays require removal of the tumor from the environment in which it was treated. This difference and the nature of the assay procedure leads to a number of advantages and disadvantages in using excision assays rather than in situ assays. The ability to measure cell survival directly is important because it gives basic information about what is perhaps the ultimate definitive cellular effect. Tumor excision assays also allow greater accuracy and finer resolution between various therapeutic regimens than do the in situ assays. Supralethal treatments can be tested. Perhaps the greatest disadvantage of excision assays is that extended treatment regimens cannot be used because of tumor cell loss and tumor cell proliferation over the treatment time; thus, an excision assay provides a static picture of tumor response at a short time after treatment.

The survival of tumor cells from tumors treated in vivo and then excised is often determined by in vitro colony formation. This requires use of tumor models that grow well in vivo and also have a high plating efficiency in vitro (ideally on the order of 20%). However, in vivo colony formation such as spleen colony formation for leukemias is also often used as an excision assay end point. The use of excision assays to determine survival of tumor cells after treatment in vivo with a range of drug doses can provide insights concerning both treatment efficacy and tumor biology.

## TUMOR EXCISION ASSAY

Historically the use of clonogenicity—that is, the ability of single cells to proliferate to form a colony of at least 50 cells—has been to determine the effectiveness of different types of antitumor therapies since the seminal publication of the method by Hewitt and Wilson (10). As the focus of preclinical research evolved from the leukemias and lymphomas to solid tumors, several tumor systems were developed that grew well in vivo and had plating efficiencies (10–20%) from in vivo implants into cell culture suitable for colony-forming assays (11–18). The tumor excision/colony-forming assay has been a highly effective tool for understanding dose response of chemotherapeutic agents as well as radiation therapy, hyperthermia, and so forth in vivo. Until now, the tumor cell survival assay has been applied most exclusively to the response of the primary tumor to therapy. Recently, however, tumor cell survival assay has been applied to the detection of metastatic disease as well as to the therapeutic response of tumor in several organs.

## IN VIVO RESISTANT EMT-6 TUMOR LINES

These studies were performed in the EMT-6/Parent murine mammary carcinoma tumor line that was originally developed as an in vivo/in vitro line by Rockwell et al. (11) and the EMT-6 in vivo alkylating agent–resistant sublines of the original tumor developed by Teicher et al. (19). The in vivo alkylating agent–resistant EMT-6 murine mammary tumors were made resistant to cis-diamminedichloroplatinum (II) (CDDP), carboplatin, cyclophosphamide, or thiotepa in vivo by treatment of tumor-bearing animals with the drug during a 6-month period (19). In spite of high levels of in vivo resistance, no significant resistance was observed when the cells from these tumors were exposed to the drugs in vitro in monolayer culture. The pharmacokinetics of CDDP and cyclophosphamide were altered in animals bearing the respective resistant tumors. The resistance of all tumor lines except for the EMT-6/thiotepa decreased during 3 to 6 months' in vivo passage in the absence of drug treatment. These studies indicated that very high levels of resistance to anticancer drugs can develop through mechanisms that are expressed in vivo but not in monolayer culture (19). The survival of bone marrow colony-forming units–granulocyte-macrophage (CFU-GM), an alkylating agent–sensitive normal tissue, was assessed in mice bearing the EMT-6/Parent tumor or the in vivo resistant EMT-6/CDDP, EMT-6/CTX, EMT-6/Thio, and EMT-6/carboplatin tumors (20). The survival pattern of the bone marrow CFU-GM recapitulated the survival of the tumor cells, mimicking the development of resistance and reversion to sensitivity upon removal of the selection pressure for each of the four alkylating agents. When the EMT-6/Parent tumor was implanted in the opposite hind limb of animals bearing the EMT-6/CDDP or EMT-6/CTX tumor, the survival of the parental tumor cells after treatment of the animals with the appropriate antitumor alkylating agent was enhanced. The EMT-6/CDDP tumor was cross-resistant to cyclophosphamide and high-dose melphalan, whereas the EMT-6/CTX tumor was somewhat resistant to CDDP and markedly sensitive to etoposide (VP-16). In each case, the survival pattern of the bone marrow CFU-GM reflected the survival of the tumor cells. These results indicated that the presence of an alkylating agent–resistant tumor in an animal can affect the drug response of tissues distal to that tumor (20). The expression of several early-response genes and genes associated with malignant disease was assessed in the EMT-6/Parent tumor and the EMT-6/CTX and EMT-6/CDDP in vivo resistant tumor lines growing as tumors or as monolayers in culture (21). In the absence of treatment the levels of mRNA for the genes c-jun, c-fos, c-myc, Ha-ras and p53 were increased in the EMT-6/CTX and EMT-6/CDDP compared with the EMT-6/Parent tumor while the expression of erb-2 was similar in all three tumors. Although the cells from each of the three tumors showed increased expression of early-response genes after exposure to CDDP (100 $\mu$mol/L, 2 h) or 4-hydroperoxycyclophosphamide (100 $\mu$mol/L, 2 h) in culture, these changes were absent or very small in mRNA extracted from tumor tissue. C-jun and erb-2 were detectable in liver. There was increased expression of both of these genes in the livers of tumor-bearing animals compared with non-tumor-bearing animals. The highest expression of both c-jun and erb-2 occurred in the livers of animals bearing the EMT-6/CDDP tumor. Treatment of the animals with CDDP or cyclophosphamide, in general, resulted in increased expression of both genes 6 h after treatment. The increased expression of these genes may impart metabolic changes in the tumors or hosts that contribute to the resistance of these tumors to specific antitumor alkylating agents (21). Although the EMT-6/Parent tumor is estrogen receptor positive, the EMT-6/CTX and EMT-6/CDDP tumors are estrogen receptor negative. The resistant tumor lines are also much more aggressively metastatic than the EMT-6/Parent tumor line.

Several observations, including the fibrous nature of the resistant tumors, the increased metastatic potential of the resistant tumors, and the altered pharmacokinetics of the drugs in the resistant-tumor-bearing hosts, led to the hypothesis that transforming growth factor-$\beta$ (TGF-$\beta$) might be integrally involved in in vivo antitumor akylating agent resistance in the EMT-6 tumor lines. Because it is difficult to maintain increased systemic levels of TGF-$\beta$ by administering the protein to mimic the resistance phenotype, administration of TGF-$\beta$–neutralizing antibodies or the naturally occurring TGF-$\beta$ inhibitor, decorin, to animals bearing the resistant tumors in an attempt to reverse the resistance was chosen as the experimental design to address the hypothesis.

Transforming growth factor-$\beta$ is a widely occurring cytokine (22). TGF-$\beta_1$ along with other cytokines such as basic fibroblast growth factor, platelet-derived growth factor, tumor necrosis factor, and interleukin-1 are involved in tissue remodeling, such as wound healing after injury. Excessive or sustained production of TGF-$\beta_1$ is a key factor in tissue fibrosis (23,24). In breast cancer patients, high plasma concentrations of TGF-$\beta_1$ measured after induction chemotherapy but prior to high-dose combination alkylating agent therapy with autologous bone marrow transplantation have been shown to strongly correlate with the risk of hepatic venoclusive disease and idiopathic inter-

**Table 1**  Number of Intratumoral Vessels in the EMT-6/Parent,
EMT-6/CTX, and EMT-6/CDDP Tumors as Determined by CD31 and
Factor VIII Immunohistochemical Staining

| Tumor | Intratumoral vessels[a] | |
|---|---|---|
|  | Factor VIII | CD31 |
| EMT-6/Parent | 4.2 ± 2.4 | 28.7 ± 10.0 |
| EMT-6/CTX | 8.0 ± 2.9 | 51.2 ± 27.4 |
| EMT-6/CDDP | 9.1 ± 6.2 | 47.1 ± 10.5 |

[a]Mean numbers of intratumoral vessels in 10 high-power (200×) fields.

stitial pneumonitis (25). In another clinical study, persistently elevated plasma TGF-$\beta_1$ levels were a strong predictor for developing symptomatic pneumonitis after thoracic radiotherapy (26). Muir et al. (27) found that high levels of TGF-$\beta$ expression in prostate carcinoma biopsies from patients correlated sith failure of the tumors to respond to hormonal withdrawal. In a cell culture study using human MCF-7 breast carcinoma, it was found that marked alterations in the levels of TGF-$\beta$ (and TGF-$\alpha$) may play a role in the molecular events that are involved in the progression of these cells from

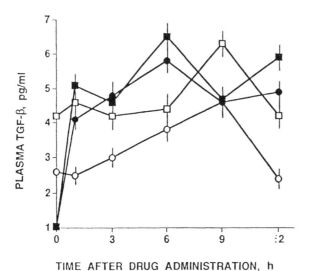

**Figure 1**  Time course of plasma levels of transforming growth factor-$\beta$ in animals bearing the EMT-6/Parent tumor after a single dose of cyclophosphamide (250 mg/kg) (●) or a single dose of CDDP (20 mg/kg) (■), in animals bearing the EMT-6/CTX tumor after a single dose of cyclophosphamide (250 mg/kg) (○) or in animals bearing the EMT-6/CDDP tumor after a single dose of CDDP (□). Points are the means of three independent determinations; bars are the SEM.

estrogen-responsive to estrogen-autonomous growth (28). Welch et al. (29) found that TGF-$\beta_1$ may modulate metastatic potential of mammary tumor cells by controlling their ability to break down and penetrate basement membrane barriers. TGF-$\beta_1$ was found to strongly stimulate the ability of human glioma cells to migrate and invade in cell culture (30). In the clinic, expression of TGF-$\beta_1$ correlates with decreased survival, presumably due to its invasion-promoting action (30).

Both the EMT-6/CTX and EMT-6/CDDP tumors have a higher number of intratumoral vessels than the EMT-6/Parent tumor (Table 1). Animals bearing the resistant tumors have higher plasma levels of TGF-$\beta$ than animals bearing the parent tumors; however, upon treatment with cytotoxic therapies, there is a greater rise in plasma TGF-$\beta$ levels in animals bearing the parent tumor than in animals bearing the resistant tumors (Fig. 1). In situ hybridization for the TGF-$\beta$ mRNA and immunohistochemical staining for TGF-$\beta$ protein showed that the resistant tumor levels of this growth factor are higher than those of the parent tumor prior to treatment; after cytotoxic therapy, however, the increase in TGF-$\beta$ is greater in the parent tumor than in the resistant tumors (Figs. 2 and 3).

The potential role of transforming growth factor-$\beta$ in in vivo resistance was examined by administration of transforming growth factor-$\beta$ neutralizing antibodies to animals bearing the EMT-6/Parent tumor or the antitumor alkylating agent–resistant tumors, EMT-6/CTX or EMT-6/CDDP (19–21,31). Treatment of tumor-bearing animals with anti–TGF-$\beta$ antibodies by intraperitoneal injection daily on days 0 through

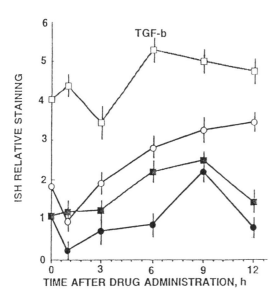

**Figure 2**  Time course of relative transforming growth factor-$\beta$ mRNA staining by in situ hybridization (ISH) in tumor sections of EMT-6/Parent tumor (●) and EMT-6/CTX tumor (○) after treatment of the tumor-bearing animal with cyclophosphamide (250 mg/kg) and of EMT-6/Parent tumor (■) and EMT-6/CDDP tumor (□) after treatment of the tumor-bearing animal with CDDP (20 mg/kg). Points are the means of three independent determinations; bars are the SEM.

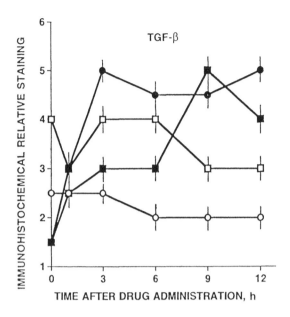

**Figure 3** Time course of relative transforming growth factor-$\beta$ protein by immunohistochemical staining of tumor sections of EMT-6/Parent tumor (●) and EMT-6/CTX tumor (○) after treatment of the tumor-bearing animal with cyclophosphamide (250 mg/kg) and of EMT-6/Parent tumor (■) and EMT-6/CDDP tumor (□) after treatment of the tumor-bearing animal with CDDP (20 mg/kg). Points are the means of three independent determinations; bars are the SEM.

8 after tumor cell implantation increased the sensitivity of the EMT-6/Parent tumor to cyclophosphamide CDDP and markedly increased the sensitivity of the EMT-6/CTX tumor to cyclophosphamide and the EMT-6/CDDP tumor to CDDP as determined by tumor cell survival assay (Figs. 4 and 5). Bone marrow CFU-GM survival was determined from these same animals. The increase in the sensitivity in the tumors upon treatment with the anti–TGF-$\beta$ antibodies was also observed in increased sensitivity of the bone marrow CFU-GM to cyclophosphamide and CDDP (Figs. 6 and 7) (19–21, 31).

Treatment of nontumor-bearing animals with the anti–TGF-$\beta$ regimen did not alter blood ATP or serum glucose level but did decrease serum lactate levels. This treatment also decreased hepatic glutathione, glutathione-S-transferase, glutathione reductase, and glutathione peroxidase in nontumor-bearing animals by 40–60% but increased hepatic cytochrome $P_{450}$ reductase in these normal animals. Animals bearing the EMT-6/CTX and EMT-6/CDDP tumors had higher serum lactate levels than normal or EMT-6/Parent tumor–bearing animals; these were decreased by the anti–TGF-$\beta$ regimen. Treatment of animals bearing any of the three tumors with the anti–TGF-$\beta$ regimen decreased by 30–50% the activity of hepatic glutathione-S-transferase and glutathione peroxidase and increased by 35–80% the activity of hepatic cytochrome $P_{450}$ reductase (19–21,31).

The generation stroma in tumors is markedly influenced by the malignant cells (32). Altered expression of chondroitin sulfate proteoglycan has been associated with

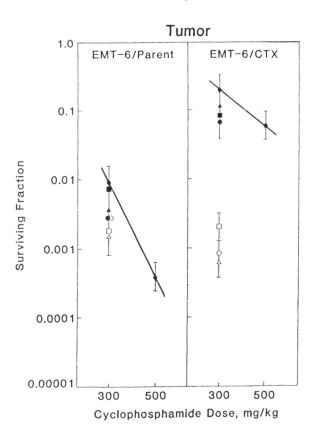

**Figure 4** Survival of EMT-6/Parent tumor cells and EMT-6/CTX tumor cells from tumors treated in vivo with cyclophosphamide alone on day 8 (◆); anti–TGF-β 2G7 (1 mg/kg, I.P.) days 4–8, then cyclophosphamide on day 8 (■); anti–TGF-β 4A11 (1 mg/kg, I.P.) days 4–8, then cyclophosphamide on day 8 (▲); anti–TGF-β 2G7 (1 mg/kg, I.P.) + anti–TGF-β 4A11 (1 mg/kg, I.P.) days 4–8, then cyclophosphamide on day 8 (●); anti–TGF-β 2G7 (1 mg/kg, I.P.) days 0–8, then cyclophosphamide on day 8 (□); anti–TGF-β 4A11 (1 mg/kg, I.P.) days 0–8, then cyclophosphamide on day 8 (△); anti–TGF-β 2G7 (1 mg/kg, I.P.) + anti–TGF-β 4A11 (1 mg/kg, I.P.) days 0–8, then cyclophosphamide on day 8 (○). Points are the means of three independent experiments; bars are the SEM.

tumor development and progression (32). The levels of decorin, a leucine-rich proteoglycan involved in the regulation of matrix assembly and cell proliferation, have been found to be elevated in colon carcinoma. The structure of the decorin gene has been elucidated (32). A transforming growth factor-β (TGF-β)–negative element was present in the promoter region of the decorin gene. Decorin is a naturally occurring inhibitor of TGF-β. By binding to TGF-β, decorin neutralizes the growth factor, essentially removing it from the cellular microenvironment (33). TNF-α may be involved in the regulation of decorin gene expression. Decorin binds to collagen type I or fibrillar collagen, but that binding does not necessarily correlate with inhibition of fibrillogenesis (34,35). Administration of human recombinant decorin to glomerulonephritic rats inhibited the production of extracellular matrix, a hallmark of the disease (36).

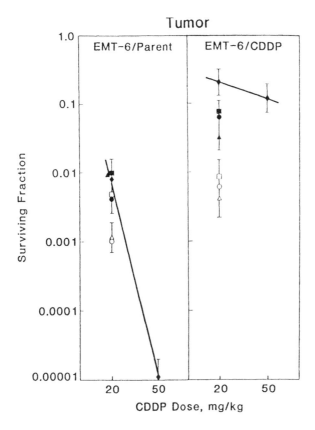

**Figure 5** Survival of EMT-6/Parent tumor cells and EMT-6/CTX tumor cells from tumors treated in vivo with CDDP alone on day 8 (♦); anti–TGF-β 2G7 (1 mg/kg, I.P.) days 4–8, then CDDP on day 8 (■); anti–TGF-β 4A11 (1 mg/kg, I.P.) days 4–8, then CDDP on day 8 (▲); anti–TGF-β 2G7 (1 mg/kg, I.P.) + anti–TGF-β 4A11 (1 mg/kg, I.P.) days 4–8, then CDDP on day 8 (●); anti–TGF-β 2G7 (1 mg/kg, I.P.) days 0–8, then CDDP on day 8 (□); anti–TGF-β 4A11 (1 mg/kg, I.P.) days 0–8, then CDDP on day 8 (△); anti–TGF-β 2G7 (1 mg/kg, I.P.) + anti–TGF-β 4A11 (1 mg/kg, I.P.) days 0–8, then CDDP on day 8 (○). Points are the means of three independent experiments; bars are the SEM.

Transfection of the decorin gene into the skeletal muscle of glomerulonephritic rats resulted in reduced glomerular TGF-β and decreased extracellular matrix accumulation (37).

Treatment of tumor-bearing animals with the naturally occurring TGF-β inhibitor, decorin, did not alter the sensitivity of the parent tumor to cyclophosphamide or to CDDP as determined by tumor cell survival assay (Fig. 8) (38). However, administration of decorin increased the sensitivity of the EMT-6/CTX tumor to cyclophosphamide and of the EMT-6/CDDP tumor to CDDP so that the drug resistance of these tumors was nearly ablated. A similar pattern was observed in the drug response of the

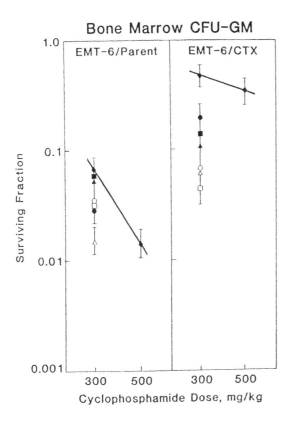

**Figure 6**  Survival of bone marrow colony-forming units–granulocyte-macrophage (CFU-GM) from the same animals shown in Figure 4. Bone marrow was taken from the femurs of the animals at the time of tumor excision. Points are the means of three independent experiments; bars are the SEM.

bone marrow CFU-GM of animals bearing each of the three tumors (38). Further investigation of decorin as an agent to prevent or reverse therapeutic resistance is warranted.

## METASTATIC DISEASE

The initial study of the response of metastatic tumor to high-dose alkylating agent therapy was carried out in mice bearing the EMT-6/Parent tumor implanted subcutaneously in the hind leg, using cyclophosphamide as the treatment agent. The tumor-bearing animals were treated with cyclophosphamide (300 mg/kg or 500 mg/kg) by intraperitoneal injection on day 8 after tumor cell implantation, when the primary tumors were about 200 mm$^3$ in volume. On day 9, the animals were sacrificed; tumor, liver, lungs, blood, bone marrow, brain, and spleen were removed from the animals. The tissues were minced with crossed scalpels, then treated with DNase and collagenase

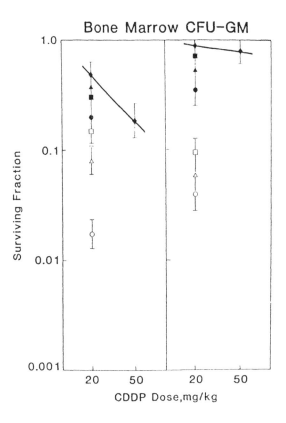

**Figure 7** Survival of bone marrow CFU-GM from the same animals shown in Figure 5. Bone marrow was taken from the femurs of the animals at the time of tumor excision. Points are the means of three independent experiments; bars are the SEM.

to disaggregate the tissues into single cells. The enzyme exposure time was varied, depending on the tisue, to optimize cell yield from each tissue. Known numbers of nucleated cells from each tissue were then plated in monolayer culture under conditions suitable for tumor cell proliferation (39). After 10 days, colonies were stained and counted. In Figure 9, the resulting data are expressed as colonies per $10^6$ cells plated from each tissue. In the absence of treatment, the primary tumor produced $2 \times 10^4$ colonies per $10^6$ cells; about 6,000, 1,000, and 500 colonies grew from the liver, lungs, and blood per $10^6$ cells, respectively. Many fewer colonies about 25, 2, and 1.5— grew from the bone marrow, brain, and spleen per $10^6$ cells, respectively. These data, then, indicate the relative abundance of viable malignant cells in the respective normal tissues of the host. Next, the response to therapy of tumor depending on the organ in which the tumor was located was determined. Figure 10 presents these data traditionally as surviving fraction versus dose of cyclophosphamide. The blood and spleen are shown on the lower axis because no colonies grew from these tissues at either dose of cyclophosphamide. On the other hand, although the number of tumor cells in the brain were relatively few, most of them survived treatment of the host with cyclophosphamide.

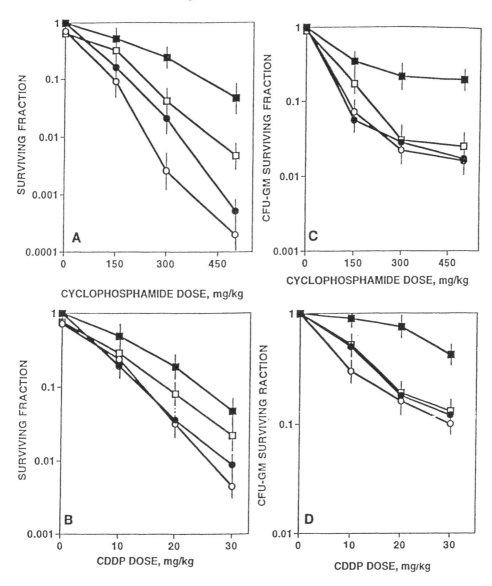

**Figure 8** Panel A. Survival of tumor cells from animals bearing the EMT-6/Parent tumor (●,○) or bearing the EMT-6/CTX tumor (■,□) after treatment with various doses of cyclophosphamide alone (●,■) or along with administration of decorin (4.5 mg/kg, I.V.) on days 0–8 (○.□). Points are the means of three independent experiments; bars are the SEM. Panel B. Survival of tumor cells from animals bearing the EMT-6/Parent tumor (●,○) or bearing the EMT-6/CDDP tumor (■,□) after treatment with various doses of CDDP alone (●,■) or along with administration of decorin (4.5 mg/kg, I.V.) on days 0–8 (○,□). Points are the means of three independent experiments; bars are the SEM. Panel C. Survival of bone marrow CFU-GM from animals bearing the EMT-6/Parent tumor (●,○) or bearing the EMT-6/CTX tumor (■,□) after treatment with various doses of cyclophosphamide alone (●,■) or along with administration of decorin (4.5 mg/kg, I.V.) on days 0–8 (○,□). Points are the means of three independent experiments; bars are the SEM. Panel D. Survival of bone marrow CFU-GM from animals bearing the EMT-6/Parent tumor (●,○) or bearing the EMT-6/CDDP tumor (■,□) after treatment with various doses of CDDP alone (●,■) or along with administration of decorin (4.5 mg/kg, I.V.) on days 0–8 (○,□). Points are the means of three independent experiments; bars are the SEM.

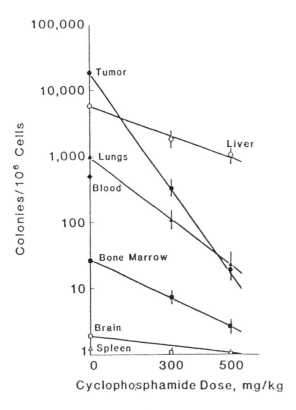

**Figure 9**   Colonies per $10^6$ cells from tissues of animals bearing EMT-6/Parent tumors either without treatment or after cyclophosphamide (300 or 500 mg/kg). The animals were treated on day 7 after tumor implant, and tissues were excised on day 8.

Tumor metastatic to the liver, bone marrow, and lungs was also less responsive to treatment with cyclophosphamide than the primary tumor (39).

The reason(s) for the differential responsiveness of the EMT-6/Parent tumor depending on location of the tumor in the host are manifold. The first is the great heterogeneity of drug distribution throughout the host. The second may be the capacity of the surrounding normal tissue to detoxify the drug. The third may be differences in the expression of genes involved in drug detoxification in the tumor cells depending on the molecular environment (organ or tissue) in which they are located. Figure 2 also shows the response of the primary tumor and metastatic disease in animals bearing the EMT-6/CTX tumor after treatment with cyclophosphamide. As was seen with animals bearing the EMT-6/Parent tumor, tumor cells in the blood and spleen were eradicated by the drug treatment. Response of tumor in the other organ sites followed a pattern similar to that of the EMT-6/Parent tumor; however, relative treatment resistance was clear in both primary and metastatic disease. Understanding the mechanisms involved in the sensitivity/resistance of tumors to chemotherapy, coupled with the development of a clinically relevant means of ensuring tumor sensitivity to treatment, is an important continuing endeavor (39).

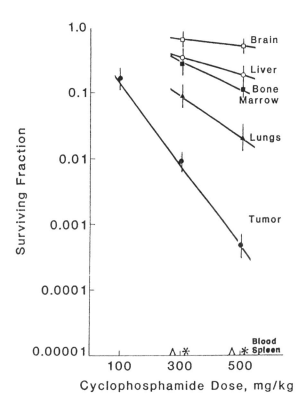

**Figure 10**   Survival of EMT-6/Parent or EMT-6/CTX cells from various tissues of animals treated with various doses of cyclophosphamide.

## CONCLUSIONS

Achieving a therapeutically meaningful impact on the resistance of the EMT-6/CTX and EMT-6/CDDP tumors has been very difficult. Traditional approaches to antitumor alkylating agent resistance, such as administration of thiol-depleting agents or administration of the "chemosensitizer" etanidazole, were not effective in restoring drug sensitivity to these tumors. The fibrous nature of the resistant tumors and the increased metastatic potential of the resistant tumors compared to the EMT-6/Parent tumor led to the hypothesis that transforming growth factor-β might be important in the genesis and maintenance of the in vivo resistant phenotype (19–21,31).

The key to understanding mechanisms of therapeutic resistance in vivo lies in understanding the response of the tumor and host to exposure to cytotoxic therapy and how specific factors of that response after repeated fractions or courses of therapy result in a tumor that is no longer responsive to cytotoxic therapy. The initiation of a cytokine cascade or storm by repeated exposure to cytotoxic therapy has been recognized for several years in radiation therapy (40–44). The connection between this early burst of cytokine production and a perpetual production of transforming factor-β leading to post-irradiation pulmonary fibrosis has also been established (40). In the EMT-6 in vivo alkylating agent–resistant tumor lines, a connection has been established between increased levels of transforming growth factor-β and drug resistance (31,45). The repeated induction of a cytokine cascade by sequential fractions of radiation or courses of chemotherapy may result in a metastable increase in transforming growth factor-β levels and to therapeutic resistance. Animals bearing EMT-6/CDDP tumors have higher circulating levels of TGF-β than do animals bearing the EMT-6/Parent tumor; however, when exposed to a cytotoxic insult (cyclophosphamide or CDDP), a rapid and sustained induction of TGF-β occurred in animals bearing the EMT-6/Parent tumor—whereas in animals bearing the resistant tumors, a lesser and more short-lived induction of TGF-β occurred. Focusing on the tumor tissue, transcription of TGF-β was induced by the cytotoxic therapies. A marked increase in TGF-β protein occurred in the EMT-6/Parent tumors that paralleled the changes seen in the circulating blood.

Decorin is a well-known, ubiquitous proteoglycan of the chondroitin sulfate/dermatansulfate proteoglycan family (32–37). Altered expression of chondroitin sulfate proteoglycan in the stroma of solid tumors, especially of human colon carcinoma, has been well established (32). Proteoglycans are polyanionic and interact with a variety of growth factors and cytokines. Yamaguchi et al. (33) reported that decorin binds to TGF-β via its core protein and sequesters the TGF-β, thus neutralizing the effects of that growth factor. Since then, potential medical applications for decorin in disease states involving overexpression of TGF-β have been explored either by administration of decorin (36) or by gene therapy expressing increased levels of decorin in vivo (37,47).

Administration of TGF-β neutralizing antibodies to animals over the growth period of the EMT-6/CTX and EMT-6/CDDP tumors reversed the resistance of these tumors to cyclophosphamide and CDDP, respectively (31). Although administration of multiple doses of TGF-β neutralizing antibodies was efficacious in restoring the sensitivity of the in vivo resistant tumors, it is unlikely that administration of multiple doses of TGF-β neutralizing antibodies will be feasible clinically. Recombinant human decorin has been shown to bind to and neutralize TGF-β (36). In the current study, administration of decorin restored drug sensitivity to the EMT-6/CTX and EMT-6/CDDP tumors.

The reason most patients with cancer are not cured by cytotoxic anticancer therapies is that their disease becomes less responsive to the therapy and/or their normal tissues reach a limit of tolerance to the therapy. It appears that malignant cells can become tolerant to the cytotoxic therapies. Many mechanisms for the development of this "drug tolerance" or "drug resistance" have been elucidated in cell culture; however, the translation of these observations in isolated malignant cells to drug resistance in tumors has been problematic (19,45). In vivo survival advantage to repeated cytotoxic insults may be achieved by the induction of factors that are operative in complex tissues and require normal cells. Therapeutically relevant methods for interfering with or blocking these processes may prevent the development of therapeutic resistance and allow many more patients to be cured.

## REFERENCES

1. Teicher BA, Cucchi CA, Lee JB, Flatow JL, Rosowsky A, Frei E III. Alkylating agents: in vitro studies of cross-resistance patterns. Cancer Res 1986; 46:4379–4383.

2. Teicher BA, Hilden SA, Cucchi CA, Cathcart KNS, Korbut TT, Flatow JL, Frei E III. Combination of N,N',N''-triethylenethiophosphoramide and cyclophosphamide in vitro and in vivo. Cancer Res 1988; 48:94–100.

3. Teicher BA, Holden SA, Kelley MJ, Shea TC, Cucchi CA, Rosowsky A, Henner WD, Frei E III. Characterization of a human squamous carcinoma cell line resistant to cis-diammine-dichloroplatinum(II). Cancer Res 1987; 47:388–393.

4. Teicher BA. Mechanisms of resistance in oncology. In: Teicher BA, ed. New York: Marcel Dekker, 1993.

5. Teicher BA, Frei E III. Development of alkylating agent-resistant human tumor cell lines. Cancer Chemother Pharmacol 1988; 21:292–298.

6. Teicher BA, Holden SA, Herman TS, Alvarez Sotomayor E, Khandekar V, Rosbe KW, Brann TW, Korbut TT, Frei E III. Characteristics of five human tumor cell lines and sublines resistant to cis-diamminedichloroplatinum(II). Int J Cancer 1991; 47:252–260.

7. Frei E III, Teicher BA, Holden SA, Cathcart KNS, Wang Y. Preclinical studies and clinical correlation of the effect of alkylating dose. Cancer Res 1988; 48:6417–6423.

8. Frei E III, Teicher BA, Cucchi CA, Rosowsky A, Flatow JL, Kelley MJ, Genereux P. Resistance to alkylating agents: basic studies and therapeutic implications. In: Woolley PVI, Tew KD, eds. Mechanisms of Drug Resistance in Neoplastic Cells. New York: Academic Press, 1988:69–87.

9. Hill RP. Excision assays. IN: Kallman RF, ed. Rodent Tumor Models in Experimental Cancer Therapy. New York: Pergamon Press, 1987:67–75.

10. Hewitt HB, Wilson CW. A survival curve for mammalian leukemia cells irradiated in vivo. Br J Cancer 1959; 13:69–75.

11. Rockwell SC, Kallman RF, Fajardo LF. Characteristics of serially transplanted mouse mammary tumor and its tissue-culture-adapted derivative. J Natl Cancer Inst 1972; 49:735–747.

12. Courtenay VD. A soft agar colony assay for Lewis lung tumour and B16 melanoma taken directly from the mouse. Br J Cancer 1976; 34:39–45.

13. Hill RP. An appraisal of in vivo assays of excised tumours. Br J Cancer 1980; 41(Suppl 4):230–239.

14. Courtenay VD, Smith IE, Peckham MJ, Steel GG. In vitro and in vivo radiosensitivity of human tumour cells obtained from a pancreatic xenograft. Nature 1976; 263:771–772.

15. Jung H. Radiation effects on tumours. In: Broerse JJ, Barendsen GW, Kal HB, van der Kogel AJ, eds. Radiation Research. Amsterdam: M. Nijhoff, 1983:427–434.

16. Kelley SD, Kallman RF, Rapacchietta D, Franko AJ. The effect of X-irradiation on cell loss in five solid murine tumors, as determined by the 125IUdR method. Cell Tissue Kinetics 1981; 14:611–624.

17. Twentyman PR, Brown JM, Gray JW, Franko AJ, Scoles MA, Kallman RF. A new mouse tumor model (RIF-1) for a comparison of endpoint studies. J Natl Cancer Inst 1980; 64:595–604.

18. Teicher BA, Rose CM. Perfluorochemical emulsions can increase tumor radiosensitivity. Science 1984; 223:934–936.

19. Teicher BA, Herman TS, Holden SA, Wang Y, Pfeffer MR, Crawford JM, Frei E III. Tumor resistance to alkylating agents conferred by mechanisms operative only in vivo. Science 1990; 247:1457–1461.

20. Teicher BA, Chatterjee D, Liu J-T, Holden SA, Ara G. Protection of bone-marrow granulocyte-macrophage colony-forming units in mice bearing in vivo alkylating-agent-resistant EMT-6 tumors. Cancer Chemother Pharmacol 1993; 32:315–319.

21. Chatterjee D, Liu JT, Northey D, Teicher BA. Molecular characterization of the in vivo alkylating agent resistant murine EMT-6 mammary carcinoma tumors. Cancer Chemother Pharmacol 1995; 35:423–431.

22. Border WA, Noble NA. Transforming growth factor β in tissue fibrosis. N Engl J Med 1994; 331:1286–1292.

23. Beck LS, DeGuzman L, Lee WP, Xu Y, Siegel MW, Amento EP. One systemic administration of transforming growth factor-β1 reverses age- or glucocorticoid-impaired wound healing. J Clin Invest 1993; 92:2841–2849.

24. Sporn MB, Roberts AB. A major advance in the use of growth factors to enhance wound healing. J Clin Invest 1993; 92:2565–2566.

25. Anscher MS, Peters WP, Reisenbichler H, Petros WP, Jirtle RL. Transforming growth factor β as a predictor of liver and lung fibrosis after autologous bone marrow transplantation for advanced breast cancer. N Engl J Med 1993; 328:1592–1598.

26. Anscher MS, Murase T, Prescott DM, Marks LB, Reisenbichler H, Bentel GC, Spencer D, Sherouse G, Jirtle RL. Changes in plasma TGFβ levels during pulmonary radiotherapy as a predictor of the risk of developing radiation pneumonitis. Int J Radiat Oncol Biol Phys 1994; 30:671–676.

27. Muir GH, Butta A, Shearer RJ, Fisher C, Dearnaley DP, Flanders KC, Sporn MB, Colletta AA. Induction of transforming growth factor beta in hormonally treated human prostate cancer. Br J Cancer 1994; 69:130–134.

28. Herman ME, Katzenellenbogen BS. Alterations in transforming growth factor-α and -β production and cell responsiveness during the progression of MCF-7 human breast cancer cells to estrogen-autonomous growth. Cancer Res 1994; 54:5867–5874.

29. Welch DR, Fabra A, Motowo N. Transforming growth factor β stimulates mammary adenocarcinoma cell invasion and metastatic potential. Proc Natl Acad Sci USA 1990; 87:7678–7682.

30. Merzak A, McCrea S, Koocheckpour S, Pilkington GJ. Control of human glioma cell growth, migration and invasion in vitro by transforming growth factor β1. Br J Cancer 1994; 70:199–203.

31. Teicher BA, Holden SA, Ara G, Chen G. Transforming growth factor-β in in vivo resistance. Cancer Chemother Pharmacol 1996; 37:601–609.

32. Iozza R, Cohen I. Altered proteoglycan gene expression and the tumor stroma. Experientia 1993; 49:447–455.

33. Yamaguchi Y, Mann DM, Ruoslahti E. Negative regulation of transforming growth factor-β by the proteoglycan decorin. Nature 1990; 346:281–284.

34. Schonherr E, Hausser H, Beavan L, Kresse H. Decorin type I collagen interaction. J Biol Chem 1995; 270:8877–8883.

35. Bittner K, Liszio C, Blumberg P, Schonherr E, Kresse H. Modulation of collagen gel contraction by decorin. Biochem J 1996; 314:159–166.

36. Border WA, Noble NA, Yamamoto K, Harper JR, Yamaguchi Y, Pierschbacher MD, Ruoslahti E. Natural inhibitor of transforming growth factor-β protects against scarring in experimental kidney disease. Nature 1992; 360:361–364.

37. Isaka Y, Brees D, Ikegaya K, Kaneda Y, Imai E, Noble N, Border W. Gene therapy by skeletal muscle expression of decorin prevents fibrotic disease in rat kidney. Nature 1996; 2:418–423.

38. Teicher B, Maehara Y, Kakeji Y, Ara G, Keyes S, Wong J, Herbst R. Reversal of in vivo drug resistance by the transforming growth factor-β inhibitor decorin. Int J Cancer, in press.

39. Holden S, Emi Y, Kakeji Y, Northey D. Host distribution and response to antitumor alkylating agents of EMT-6 tumor cells from subcutaneous tumor implants. Cancer Chemother Pharmacol, in press.

40. Rubin P, Johnston CJ, Williams JP, McDonald S, Finkelstein JN. A perpetual cascade of cytokines postirradiation leads to pulmonary fibrosis. Int J Radiat Oncol Biol Phys 1995; 33:99–109.

41. McBride WH. Cytokine cascades in late normal tissue radiation responses. Int J Radiat Oncol Biol Phys 1995; 33:233–234.

42. Anscher MS, Jirtle RL. Role of transforming growth factor-β and hepatocyte growth factor in late normal tissue effects of radiation. Radiat Oncol Invest 1994; 1:305–313.

43. Rodemann HP, Bamberg M. Cellular basis of radiation-induced fibrosis. Radiother Oncol 1995; 35:83–90.
44. Randall K, Coggle JE. Expression of transforming growth factor-β1 in mouse skin during the acute phase of radiation damage. Int J Radiat Biol 1995; 68:301–309.
45. Teicher BA. In vivo resistance to antitumor alkylating agents. In: Teicher BA, ed. Drug Resistance in Oncology. New York: Marcel Dekker, 1993:263–290.
46. Takeuchi Y, Kodama Y, Matsumoto T. Bone matrix decorin binds TGF-β and enhances its bioactivity. J Biol Chem 1994; 269:32634–32638.
47. Santra M, Skorski T, Calabretta B, Lattime E, Iozzo R. De novo decorin gene expression suppresses the malignant phenotype in human colon cancer cells. Proc Natl Acad Sci USA 1995; 92:7016–7020.

# Index

*About the Editor*

SAMUEL D. BERNAL is Professor of Medicine at the University of California, Los Angeles, UCLA School of Medicine, and Chief of Hematology and Oncology at the UCLA/San Fernando Valley Program, Sepulveda Veterans Administration Medical Center, California. The coeditor of *Lung Cancer Differentiation* (Marcel Dekker, Inc.) and the author or coauthor of over 75 papers, book chapters, and abstracts, he is a member of the International Association for the Study of Lung Cancer, the Developmental Therapeutics Review Board of the National Cancer Institute, the American Association for Cancer Research, and the American Society of Clinical Oncology. Dr. Bernal received the B.S. degree (1969) in chemistry from the University of Illinois, Chicago, and the Ph.D. degree (1974) in biochemical pathology and the M.D. degree (1975) from the University of Chicago, Illinois. He was trained in internal medicine at Johns Hopkins Hospital, Baltimore, Maryland, and in medical oncology at the Dana-Farber Cancer Institute and Harvard Medical School, Boston, Massachusetts.

Printed and bound by CPI Group (UK) Ltd, Croydon, CR0 4YY

17/10/2024

01775700-0013